COLOR PLATE I

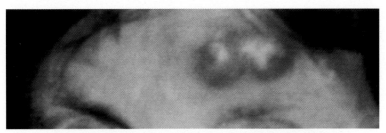

Sadick, **Fig 3**

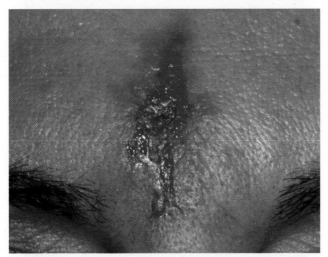

Sadick, **Fig 4**

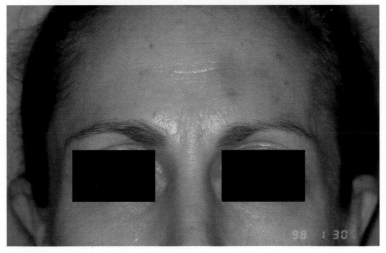

Sadick, **Fig 9**

COLOR PLATE II

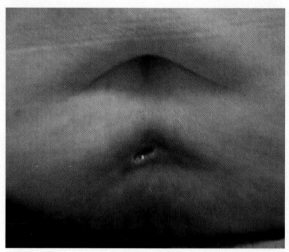

Sadick, Fig 14

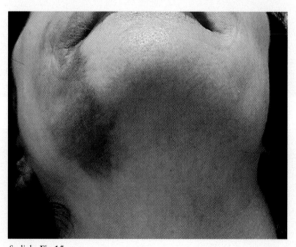

Sadick, Fig 15

COLOR PLATE III

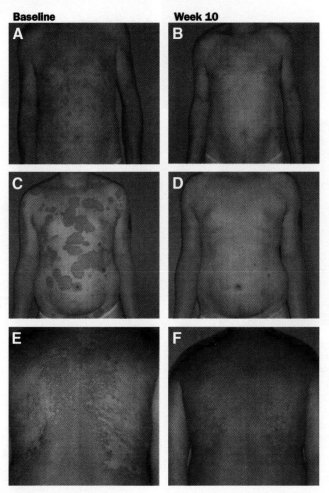

Abstract 3–9, **Fig 5**

COLOR PLATE IV

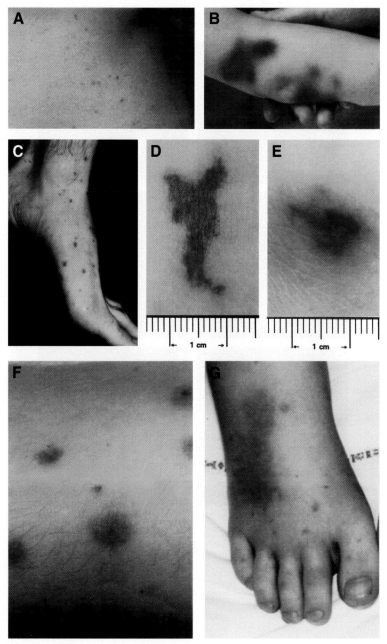

Abstract 4–6, **Fig 1**

COLOR PLATE V

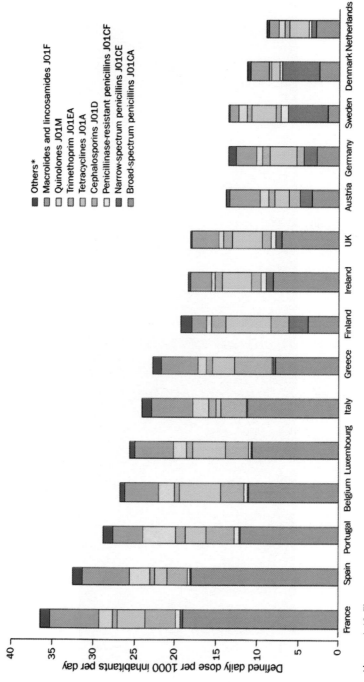

Abstract 4–19, Figure

COLOR PLATE VI

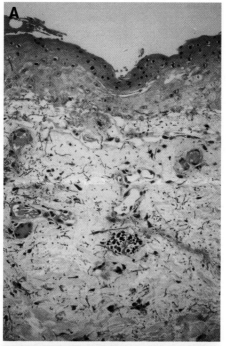

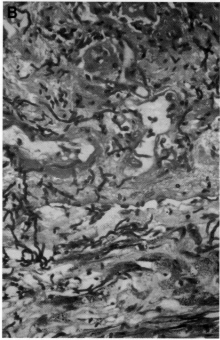

Abstract 5–1, **Fig 1**

COLOR PLATE VII

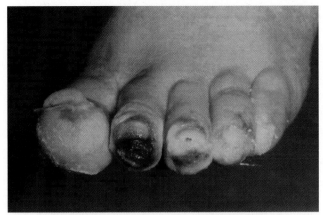

Abstract 5–2, **Fig 1**

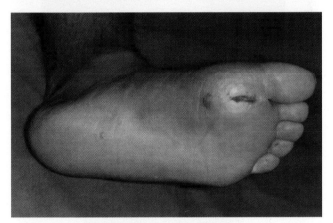

Abstract 5–2, **Fig 2**

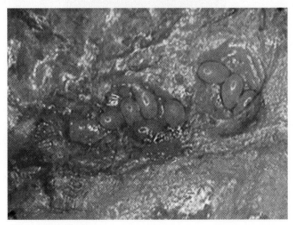

Abstract 8–1, **Fig 4**

COLOR PLATE VIII

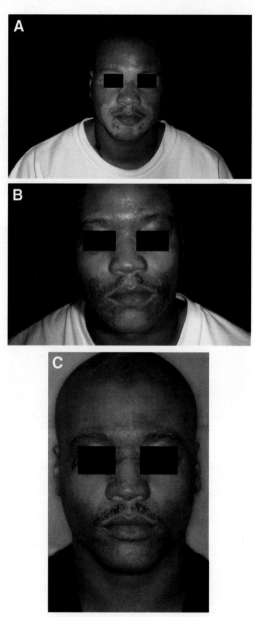

Abstract 11–1, Fig 1

COLOR PLATE IX

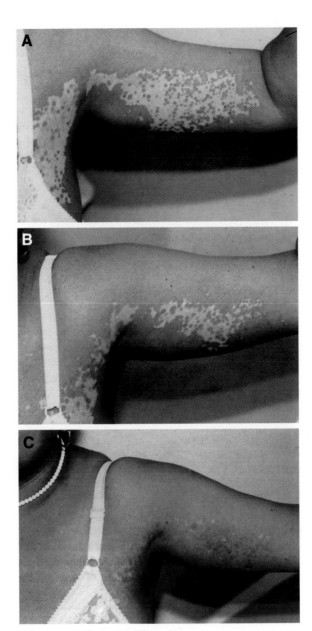

Abstract 11–2, **Fig 1**

COLOR PLATE X

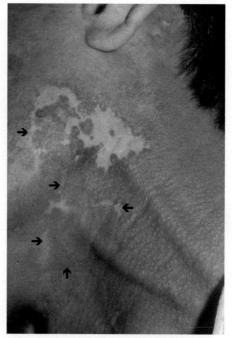

Abstract 12–3, **Fig 2**

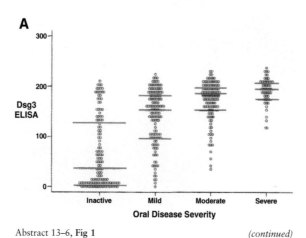

Abstract 13–6, **Fig 1**

(continued)

Fig 1 (continued)

B

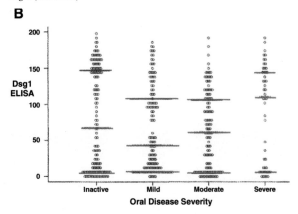

C

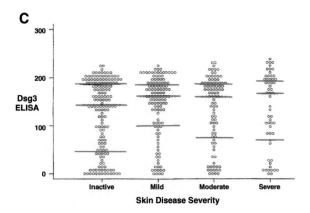

D

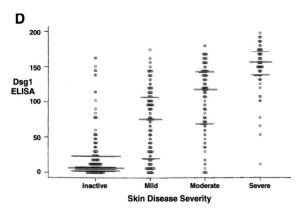

COLOR PLATE XII

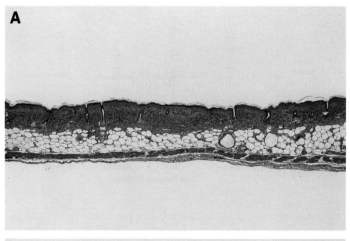

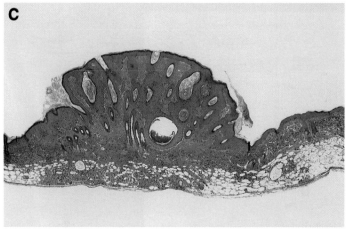

Abstract 14–2, **Fig 1**   *(continued)*

COLOR PLATE XIII

Fig 1 (continued)

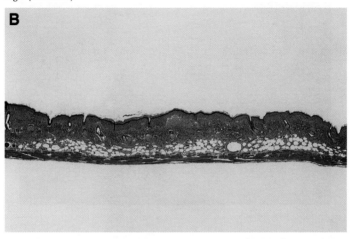

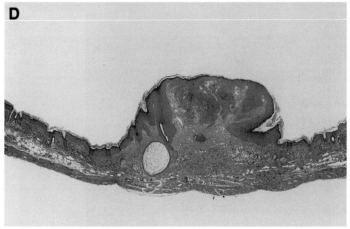

COLOR PLATE XIV

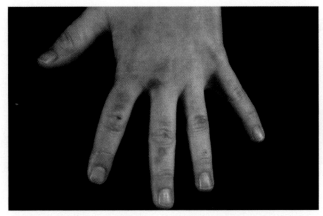

Abstract 14–5, **Fig 1**

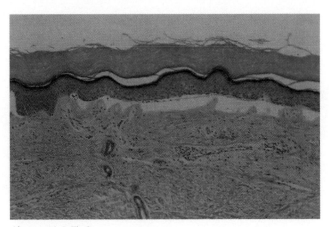

Abstract 14–5, **Fig 2**

COLOR PLATE XV

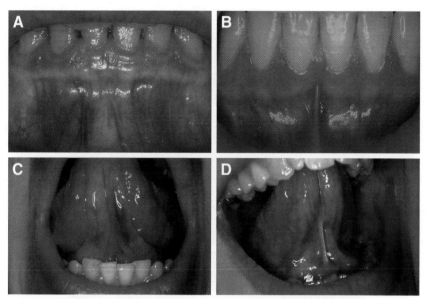

Abstract 15–1, **Figure**

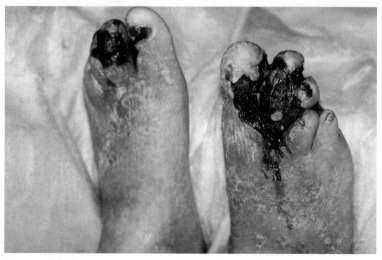

Abstract 18–4, **Figure**

COLOR PLATE XVI

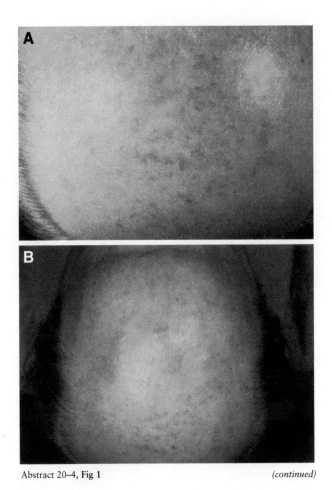

Abstract 20–4, **Fig 1** *(continued)*

COLOR PLATE XVII

Fig 1 (continued)

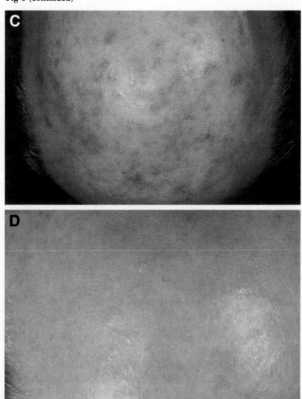

COLOR PLATE XVIII

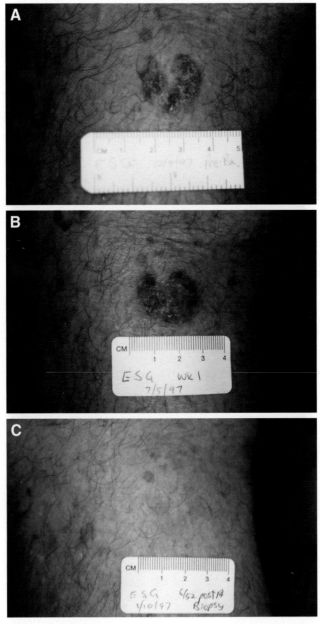

Abstract 20–5, **Fig 1**

COLOR PLATE XIX

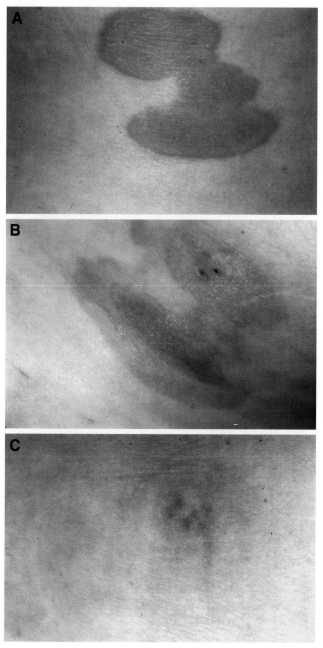

Abstract 22–5, **Fig 1**

COLOR PLATE XX

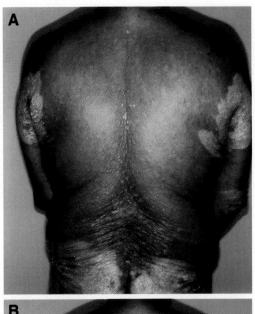

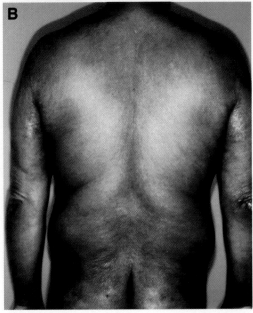

Abstract 22–8, Fig 1

Complications of Excisional and Reconstructive Surgery

STUART J. SALASCHE, MD

Clinical Professor, University of Arizona Health Sciences Center; Research Scientist, University of Arizona Cancer Center, Tucson

Complications and untoward events are the "dark side" of cutaneous surgery. Despite mastering anatomy and wound healing, learning sterile technique and good surgical technique, taking an appropriate history, and supplying the patient with clear postoperative instructions, the surgeon sees that bad things still happen. When they do occur, negative emotions of guilt and blame are generated and medical-legal issues may rear their ugly heads. But at the core of the matter, there is a patient who needs help. Supplying this aid to resolve the problem in a timely, competent, professional, and enthusiastic manner usually supercedes these other issues and often makes them disappear. Most patients recognize that their doctors are human and that everything does not always go as planned. What they expect is that the doctors care and want to help resolve the problem.

Hopefully, this compilation of complications and the attendant discussions will help circumvent them from being repeated unnecessarily.

Acute Complications

Every surgical procedure, if not properly attended to in relation to sterile technique and good surgical technique, becomes prone to one or more of the acute complications of bleeding, infection, necrosis, and dehiscence. The initiating events that are consistently associated with these adverse events are drug-related interference with coagulation, inadequate intraoperative hemostasis, excessive tension on the wound edges, and intraoperative contamination of the wound with pathogenic organisms.[1-3] To compound matters, one of these complications may eventuate into one or more of the others. For example, blood in the wound bed, in the form of a hematoma, may serve as a favorable environment for bacterial proliferation and wound infection that terminates in complete disruption of the wound and dehiscence (Fig 1).

Bleeding problems are the most common of the acute complications. They can take the form of persistent intraoperative bleeding or delayed bleeding in the postoperative period. In the latter situation, if the blood cannot egress from the sutured wound, it collects within the wound bed as a hematoma.[4]

Being prepared to deal with bleeding problems begins with a review of the patient's medical history and medication list.[5-7] A significant proportion of patients will be on one or more pharmaceutical agents that are either anticoagulant or antiplatelet. The anticoagulants (warfarin) block thrombin generation and fibrin clot formation, while antiplatelet agents (aspirin, ticlodipine, clopidogrel, abciximab, tirofiban, epitifibatide) inhibit thromboxane A2 and platelet aggregation. For years, there has been a perception that intraoperative and postoperative hemostasis would be

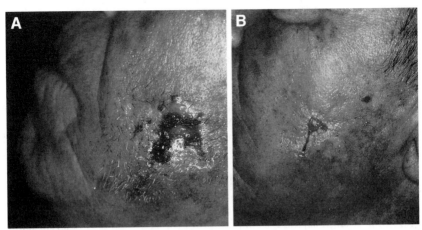

FIGURE 1.—**A,** Wound infection with crust and exudates. **B,** Dehiscence apparent as infection resolves.

deleteriously affected by such medications; consequently, they have often been discontinued, in consultation with the patient's medical doctor, for the perioperative period. However, current recommendations have come full circle on this issue as recent literature has indicated that there are only few adverse outcomes from continuing antithrombotic therapy (more intraoperative time for hemostasis), but a significant number of systemic disasters actually do occur, including cerebrovascular accidents, myocardial infarctions, deep vein thrombosis, emboli, and vascular occlusion.[8-15] The risks of stopping antithrombotic agents in patients with legitimate risk factors seems to outweigh the relative inconvenience of minor wound site bleeding, which can be managed by meticulous intraoperative hemostasis and appropriate immobilizing dressings. Caution should be exercised to keep repairs and reconstructions as simple as possible; the surgeon should not attempt high-risk tissue rearrangements and full-thickness skin grafts (FTSGs).

The main postoperative bleeding problem is hematoma formation (Fig 2). When discovered within a day or two of the procedure, it is usually in the setting of the patient calling in to report blood from the surgical site is leaking through the suture line and soaking through the dressing.[1] Identifying hematomas within 48 hours of surgery allows the clot to be easily evacuated after sterile cleansing of the area, injecting anesthesia, and taking down the stitches to expose the wound bed. Once this is done, the wound can be resutured. Beyond this time, the clot becomes organized and adherent to the walls of the wound. At this stage, the hematoma has to be manually debrided and the wound left open to heal by second intention. Many small hematomas do not become evident until the time of suture removal. It is often best to let the clot liquefy (fibrinolysis) and reabsorb naturally. If loculation of the fluid occurs, it can be drained by inserting a large bore needle (#18 or larger) and aspirating the serum-like fluid. Flaps

seem to be particularly vulnerable to hematoma formation as free radicals are released that compromise blood flow and may result in necrosis.[16,17]

Wound infections are surprisingly infrequent in dermatologic surgery. This is despite the fact that most surgery takes place in an outpatient setting with many of the procedures being "clean" rather than adhering to strict antiseptic routine.[18-24] Wound infections are usually due to a combination wound contamination during surgery combined with reduced local host defenses (tension on wound edges).

They become apparent 4 to 8 days after surgery, usually by signs and symptoms that are exaggerations of the normal wound healing process that include erythema, edema, and warmth. Pain and tenderness are not normal and should prompt suspicion while exudation is pathognomonic with a wound infection (Fig 1). It is most appropriate to obtain a Gram stain along with a culture and sensitivity before initiating antibiotic therapy. The latter should consist of the regional anti-staphylococcus drug of choice until the culture results are known. Also, as the sutures may retard drainage and healing, they should be removed. Drainage may be improved in situations with copious purulent discharge by placing a wick of thin gauze strips into the wound bed. The wick is changed on a daily basis or every other day until the discharge remits and clean granulation tissue appears. In instances such as this, the wound must heal by second intention and be revised some time in the future if necessary. Most of the time, steri strips can be placed after suture removal to maintain wound orientation and more directed healing. Most surgeons do not rely on prophylactic

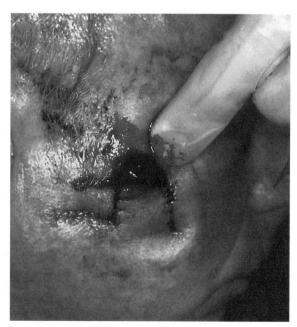

FIGURE 2.—Hematoma under transposition flap.

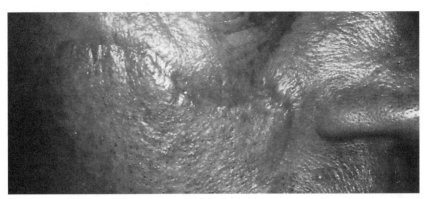

FIGURE 3.—Wide, depressed scar secondary to wound edge necrosis.

antibiotics unless the patient is immunosuppressed or the wound is in an intertriginous area such as the groin or axilla.[25,26]

As wound infections disrupt normal wound healing events, frequent sequelae are poor cosmetic result, wound dehiscence, and partial necrosis of the wound edges (Fig 1B).

Necrosis of the wound edges of a side-to-side closure is invariably due to poor surgical technique that in one way or another compromises the blood flow. Tension is the usual initiating event and is caused by either insufficient undermining or securing the suture knots too tightly. Conversely, excessive undermining may create flap-like conditions wherein the blood must flow too great a distance through the subdermal plexus to the wound edge. The result of poor perfusion is cell death and formation of an eschar. As will be discussed later with flap necrosis, it is best to await spontaneous demarcation of the slough rather than debride it to avoid causing more damage.[1,27,28] The end result is often a widened depressed scar line that may require revision (Fig 3).

Wound dehiscence is most frequently the sequela of a wound infection or necrosis, but it may be due to faulty suturing technique or early suture removal. Most surgical wounds require the support of buried subcuticular stitches to sustain closure during the first several postoperative weeks when there is very little innate tensile strength in the wound. Even minor trauma or physical activity may result in dehiscence in wounds lacking subcuticular sutures (Fig 4). Posttraumatic dehiscence may be resutured within the first 24 hours as all the requisite wound healing cells and cytokines have already been recruited, but those due to other causes should probably be allowed to heal by second intention.

Flap Design Complications

Flaps are at once the most rewarding and the most difficult of surgical repair options. At the same time, the surgeon must be cognizant of where extra skin can be recruited, how it is best rearranged to fill the defect, what the arrangement of the often complicated scar lines will look like, and what tension-stress relationships will develop. Flap design planning also must take into consideration whether or not the free margins will be affected by the tension vector of closure and if the natural concavities of the face will be effaced as the newly recruited tissue is draped into place.[27,28]

One of the most common errors in flap design is to have an excessively long flap in relation to the pedicle width. In random flaps, the blood supply to all portions of the flap (especially to its most distal edge) must traverse through the subdermal plexus. Two possible errors in design have dire consequences. The first is not creating the flap pedicle wide enough to sustain blood flow to its most distal portion (or conversely, designing the body of the flap too long in relation to the width of the pedicle). The other is excessively undermining the pedicle, which, in effect, lengthens the body of the flap. Both may result in insufficient perfusion to the distal flap margin with ischemia and, consequently, necrosis. All these problems are compounded in random pattern advancement and rotation flaps because, with these flaps, the most distant portion of the flap is also the point of highest tension (Fig 5). Accordingly, the already tenuous point furthest from the pedicle has the potential added stress of closure under tension.[27-33] Cigarette smoking potentiates this precarious nature of flaps and adds considerably to the risk of necrosis.[34-36]

Another flap planning mishap involves the distance the flap must travel and be sewn into place under no tension. In some flap designs, such as the axial pattern midline forehead flap, the pedicle is twisted at its base at the glabella before being interpolated into place at a distant point, usually on the lower portion of the nose. This problem is obviated by measuring the exact distance to the defect with a piece of gauze that acts as a flap surrogate. This template can be used to draw out the flap on the forehead

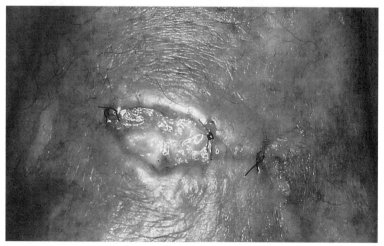

FIGURE 4.—Traumatic dehiscence.

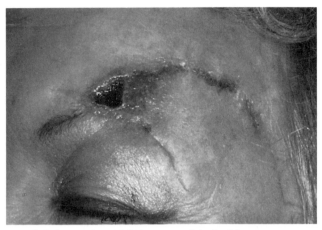

FIGURE 5.—Full-thickness and partial-thickness necrosis in distal flap.

and will help avoid this problem. The same lesson obviously applies to all cutaneous flaps, even those with apparently predictable excursions.

Many principles of modern reconstruction are based on a detailed understanding of the cosmetic units of the face and the boundary or junction lines that separate one cosmetic unit from the other.[37-39] Defects are best closed within a single cosmetic unit or from skin from an adjacent unit that shares similar skin color and texture. The scar lines camouflage best if placed within the junction lines such as the melolabial fold, nasofacial sulcus, or eyebrow hairline, as these are places where shadows and lines are expected by the inspecting eye. If this is not feasible, tissue should be borrowed from an adjacent cosmetic unit and designed to fill the defect and fit into the boundary lines and relaxed skin tension lines. When a flap or

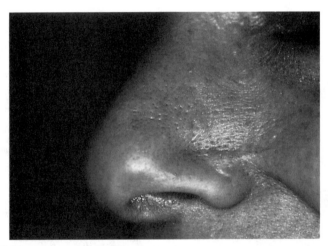

FIGURE 6.—Scar crosses junction line.

excision lines cross perpendicular to these lines, the deformity is readily apparent and distracting (Fig 6). Defects that involve more than one cosmetic unit often do best when they are repaired as separate defects.

Finally, flap design should take the hills and valleys of the face into account. Convexities of the face include the tip of the nose, the malar eminence, and the chin. There are concavities such as the nasofacial sulcus, the medial canthus, the alar crease, the labial-mental crease, and the philtrum that must be maintained to give the face a pleasing and symmetric appearance. Obliteration of the nasofacial sulcus can give the nose a broadened and disproportionate look. There are several reasonable approaches to avoid these problems. One might be to reconstruct defects that involve multiple cosmetic units as separate repairs. In this way, junction lines are maintained in their normal position. Another method is to use suspension stitches that tack the deep dermis into periosteum and maintain the concavity.[40]

Pincushion Deformity

Some flaps, particularly those with a curved or rounded design, tend to develop a bulky, humped appearance. The central portion of the flap domes upward while the scar lines appear depressed or inverted. The prototype situation for this complication is the melolabial (formerly nasolabial) transposition flap that utilizes fatty cheek skin to repair defects of the ala nasi and lower nasal sidewall (Fig 7). It is believed that the deformity results from inward (centripedal) contraction of the sheet of scar that forms beneath the undersurface of the flap and vertical contraction of the flap wound edge scars. The compressed tissue of the flap confined within this space buckles upward to give the characteristic pincushion or trapdoor appearance.[41-43]

Prevention consists of thinning (defatting) the flap to just below the subdermal plexus, widely undermining the recipient bed to create a wider base scar, and suturing techniques that evert the wound edges. Postoperative intralesional corticosteroids and massage complete the program. If a trapdoor deformity does form, surgical revision several months after surgery is optimal, as the wound has had a chance to mature by then. The technique involves incising into one of the suture lines and with sharp dissection, wedge out the offending excess fat and scar tissue. The wound edges are then redraped and excess skin is trimmed before resuturing.

Free Margins

The free margins are the discontinuities of the skin around the orifices of the face that include the eyelids, lips, nostril rim, eyebrows, and helix of the ears. Their importance lies in that they offer no opposing force to tension placed against them during surgical closure of defects in the anatomic vicinity.[28] Distortion of a free margin may be readily noticeable during the surgical procedure, or it may become apparent some weeks into the postoperative period. This delayed type of problem is due to the fact that as they mature, scars contract in all directions. Since there is no contravailing force, scar contraction may continue to the point that the

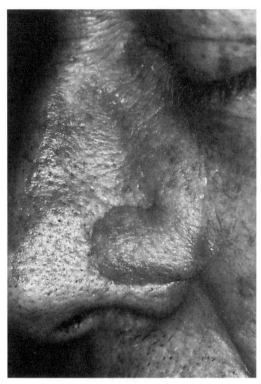

FIGURE 7.—Pincushion deformity of transposition flap.

free margin is pulled into a functional or cosmetic asymmetry in relation to its contralateral side (Fig 8). All types of surgical repairs, including side-to-side closures, tissue rearrangements (flaps), split-thickness skin grafts, and second intention healing can result in untoward pull on a free margin.

While elevation of an eyebrow may give the person a startled or quizzical appearance and uneven helical healing may result in a noticeable asymmetry, neither of these problems is of a functional nature. In contrast, ectropion of the lower eyelid may pull the puncta away from the globe, resulting in tearing (epiphora) and ultimately, the sequela of the dry eye syndrome. Upward pull of the nostril rim can impinge on the function of the internal nasal valve and interfere with the inspiration phase of breathing. Similarly, eclabion of either the upper or lower lip can result in loss of the oral seal required for phonation, eating, and drinking.

The key to avoiding free margin distortion is to be cognizant of the tension vector (TV) of closure. The TV is the summation of all the forces of closure expressed at a single point; usually designated as a single arrow. Each type of closure has a TV, except a FTSG for which inhibition of wound contraction is inherent in the design. Locating the TV is relatively easy to envision with side-to-side closures, but it becomes more complicated when planning the various tissue rearrangements or allowing the wound to heal by second intention. By understanding the TV, the surgeon can predict which closure may work best and choose the best option for that specific sized defect and patient. Patient variables include skin laxity, elasticity, redundancy, and degree of solar damage. A general rule is that the TV should lie parallel to the free margin, not perpendicular to it.

In the preoperative period, the surgeon can assess the strength of the lower eyelid by doing a "snap" test.[44] Pulling the skin of the lower lid away from the eyeball and then letting it go should result in the lid snapping quickly back into place. If the lid tone is poor, it only retracts very slowly and the surgeon is forewarned that it will tolerate very little tension (or weight) and should adjust the closure accordingly. Similarly, when working on the lower nose, document that the nostrils are symmetrical before the procedure. Asymmetry due to preexisting septal deviation may not take too much further displacement to cause a functional nostril rim problem.

Equally important is to assess and continually monitor the impact of closure tension during the procedure. This can be achieved by pulling the wound edges together with toothed forceps, skin hooks, or a "test" stitch. For wounds impinging on the lower eyelid, the patient is asked to sit up in a semi-reclining position, open their mouth, and gaze upward while performing one of the above impact tests. If the lid is pulled away from the globe during this "stress test," it can be assumed the same will occur with routine suturing and an alternative option should be sought.

The key to avoiding free margin problems is to know how to redirect the TV in a manner that will not put undo pull on it. Several techniques can be utilized to this end. They include off-set bias suturing, suspension (pexing or tacking) sutures, tissue rearrangements, and FTSGs. Off-set

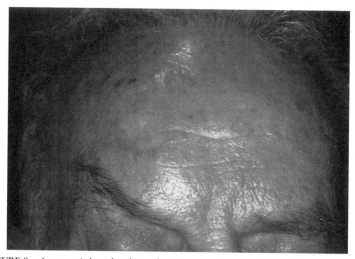

FIGURE 8.—Asymmetric lateral eyebrow elevation secondary to surgical repair.

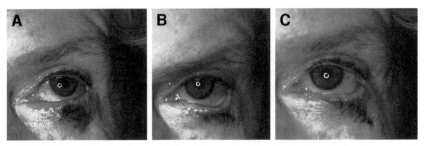

FIGURE 9.—**A,** Post-tumor removal defect. **B,** Ectropion when closed with vertical tension vector. **C,** Resutured with horizontal tension vector.

bias suturing is a method of skewed stitching that favorably alters the TV (usually 45°-60°) (Fig 9). It is usually accomplished with the buried subcuticular stitches. The downside to this technique is that it lengthens the wound and either creates or magnifies dogears at one or both ends of the wound.

Tacking sutures redirect the tension vector by anchoring them to the deep and sturdy periosteum.[40] This technique utilizes either absorbable or nonabsorbable suture material that is buried into the dermis 4 to 5 mm from the wound edge that is to be moved. It is then secured into an appropriate place in the periosteum at a point that, when tied off, will move the wound edge close to the free margin, but with all the tension directed to the periosteum. This has been most helpful for defects just above the eyebrow or involving the lower eyelid and/or cheek.

FTSGs have the ability to inhibit wound contraction if they are placed into position within a day or two of when the wound was created.[45,46] Full-thickness grafts are very helpful for defects of the lower lid that can utilize the redundant upper lid skin as a donor site.

Finally, flaps, especially transposition flaps are used to reorient the TV. Rhombic or bilobed transposition flaps are of great value for defects of the lower nose. With these flaps, all the tension is redirected to the single point where the secondary defect is closed. This allows for predictable and favorable disposition of the TV.

Full-Thickness Skin Grafts

An FTSG is often an excellent reconstruction choice for some defects on the nose and selected other sites on the face.[47-49] Complications for the most part are of 2 varieties: graft necrosis within the healing period and color, contour, and texture mismatches that occur within the early postoperative period.

Successful "take" of a FTSG depends on a series of events that reestablishes vascularization. Over the first several days, the graft is sustained by imbibing serum-like fluid from the surrounding tissue. Next, vessels in the wound bed connect with those in the undersurface of the graft (inosculation) and finally neoangiogenesis takes place. Necrosis is invariably due to poor vascularization of the tenuous graft that has been cut off completely from all sources of nourishment.

There are many things that can interfere with these physiological processes. The most critical non-technical insult is cigarette smoking.[35,36] Nicotine causes vasoconstriction and lowers perfusion as well as tissue oxygenation. Carbon monoxide in smoke competes with oxygen for hemoglobin binding sites resulting in hypoxia. All these mechanisms conspire to endanger graft survival. It has been recommended that potential graft patients stop smoking 2 days before surgery and maintain a smokeless state for 7 days after surgery. A word of caution: this type of behavior modification during stressful periods (such as excision and repair of a skin cancer) is often more wishful thinking than realistic.

More often, a technical surgical error is the cause of necrosis. The recipient site may not be capable of sustaining the graft (denuded cartilage or bone) and another option should have been chosen. Sometimes the graft is not defatted sufficiently, or a hematoma or seroma develops that prevents apposition of wound bed to the FTSG, or the graft is not adequately immobilized to prevent shearing movement between it and the bed. The use of basting sutures or a tie-over dressing may avoid the latter 2 situations.

Treatment of FTSG necrosis is usually disappointing (Fig 10). By the time the situation is discovered (often when the tie-over dressing is taken down), events are irreversible and the graft is doomed to either partial or full-thickness slough. The graft appears black or bluish-black and is usually dry. The best course of action is usually expectant as there are presently no therapeutic agents capable of reversing events if the scale has been tipped toward cell death. Over the next several days, it will become apparent how severe the damage will be. Obviously, the best outcome is when there is only partial thickness necrosis. If only the superficial dermis or even better, only the epidermis (autolysis) is involved, the dead cells shear off within a few days, leaving a moist but healthy surface. Continued daily dressing changes with an antibiotic ointment and a nonadherent dressing will eventuate in an outcome that is either close to perfect, if only

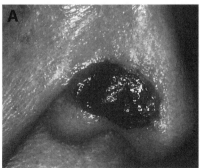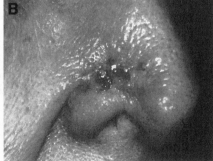

FIGURE 10.—A, Necrosis of full-thickness skin graft. B, Healing with contraction and elevation of nostril rim.

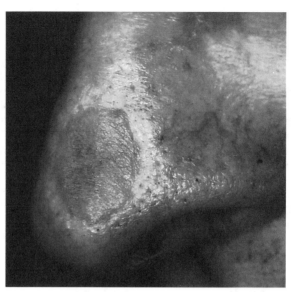

FIGURE 11.—Poor color and texture match of full-thickness graft.

the epidermis was involved, or depressed and shiny, if portions of the dermis were lost. If the damage is full-thickness, an adherent eschar will form and the wound will heal by second intention from the undersurface. It is probably best to allow the eschar to act as a biological dressing and allow it to separate spontaneously, as surgical debridement will only result in excess tissue damage. In most cases, a surgical revision will be required after the wound heals and matures.

Less serious but more frequent adverse sequelae of FTSG involve contour, color, and texture differences. Not uncommonly, FTSG covering deep defects of the nose appear depressed the first month after placement. This type of contour defect tends to correct itself over the ensuing several weeks as the dermal scar remodels. However, there are more permanent contour mismatches. Even though FTSG, for the most part, inhibits wound contraction, a certain amount will occur anyhow. This may result in a slight buckling and elevation of the graft as it becomes relatively larger than the wound bed it occupies (Figs 11 and 12). Contour differences also result from less than optimal suturing technique that dictates absolute matching of the graft edge to the surrounding skin around the entire perimeter. Despite attempts to choose donor skin that closely matches the color, texture, thickness, sebaceous quality, and pore size of the recipient skin, regional skin quality differences become apparent as the graft settles down.

Hydroquinone and tretinoin have been used topically with some success to address these problems. However, the mainstay modality to treat post-grafting color and contour discrepancies is spot dermabrasion carried out 6 weeks to a few months after surgery.[50,51] After local anesthesia, the entire

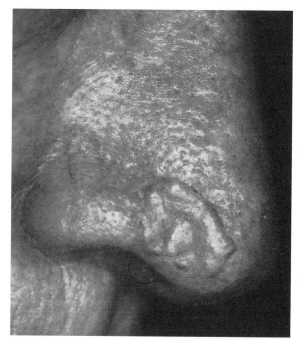

FIGURE 12.—Full-thickness skin graft; poor contour match.

graft and a few millimeters of surrounding skin is lightly dermabraded with a diamond frieze. It there are contour differences, these are sanded down until they match. Care should be taken not to accentuate the scar line separating the FTSG from the neighboring skin. Postoperative care consists of a topical antibiotic and nonadherent dressing until reepithelialization occurs. Recently, the resurfacing CO_2 laser has proven equally successful in correcting color and contour problems.

The Facial Nerve: Danger Zones of the Face

Knowledge of the surgical anatomy of the face is essential if the surgeon is to avoid damaging or cutting vital structures. The most important of these are the various branches of the seventh cranial or facial nerve.[44,52-54] Sometimes sacrificing one of these branches is an unavoidable sequela of removing a deeply invasive tumor. However, a true surgical complication exists when this occurs in the setting of electively removing a benign lipoma, an acne scar, an epidermal inclusion cyst, or an incorrectly diagnosed inflamed lymph node.

Being cognizant of the "danger zones" of the face will help avoid these mishaps. The main trunk of the facial nerve enters the substance of parotid gland after emerging from the stylomastoid foramen. Within the parotid gland, the nerve divides into its typical 5 branches (temporal, zygomatic, buccal, marginal mandibular, and cervical nerves). These branches then exit from the protection of the gland to run medially to innervate their designated muscles of facial expression on their lateral undersurface. For most of this distance, the nerves are protected by overlying dermis, subcutaneous fat, and fascia and only relatively deep incisions cause damage.

However, 2 areas on the face are particularly at risk because the nerves are relatively superficial and unprotected and are single rami in 85% of humans when they cross these "danger zones." One is a 2-cm wide strip of the temple ranging from the mid zygomatic arch upward across the temple toward the lateral forehead to an area about 1 to 3 cm above the lateral eyebrow. Within this zone, the temporal branch of the facial nerve traverses in the deep portion of the superficial temporalis fascia. With all but very invasive tumors, the nerve is protected by this well-defined fascial plane that is contiguous with the galea aponeurotica of the scalp. Severing this nerve usually results in permanent paresis of the frontalis muscle. The patient is unable to wrinkle the ipsilateral forehead, raise the eyebrow, or open the eye widely. This constitutes a real functional upper visual field gaze problem in elderly patients who often have dermatoclasia of the upper lid (Fig 13). Surgical repair of a motor nerve is rarely successful, and the best expedient measure is a brow-lift. Traction on the nerve during surgery may just cause temporary neuropraxis with similar symptoms lasting up to 6 months. An even more frequent occurrence is to cause a motor nerve block due to repeat injections of anesthesia during a multistage Mohs' micrographic surgery procedure. Many a sleepless night is spent awaiting return of function that usually does not occur until the following day.

The second danger zone on the face is along the jawline at the anterior border of the masseter muscle. This important landmark identifies where the facial artery and vein curve around the jaw from the neck and enter

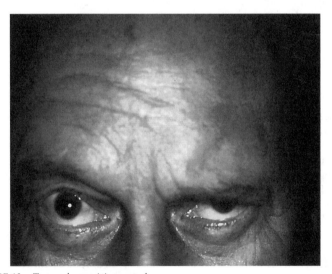

FIGURE 13.—Temporal nerve injury sequela.

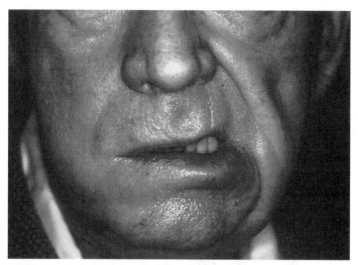

FIGURE 14.—Marginal mandibular nerve injury sequela.

onto the face. Just superficial to these vessels, the marginal mandibular courses transversely after leaving the parotid to innervate the lip depressors and the mentalis muscles. As there is no platysma muscle in this area, the nerve is relatively superficial and vulnerable. A particularly treacherous situation arises when attempting to excise old acne scars that arise secondary to inflamed acne cysts in this area. Adhesions often exist from the multitrack scars to the soft tissue below, and the surgeon finds himself deeper than he had anticipated. With the resultant paresis, the patient is unable to retract the corner of the mouth or depress the lower lip when

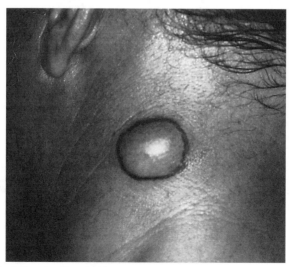

FIGURE 15.—Inflamed epidermal inclusion cyst in posterior triangle.

smiling (Fig 14). Even more functionally disabling are the results of cutting the Spinal Accessory or eleventh cranial nerve in the neck as it emerges from behind the sternocleidomastoid (SCM) muscle to innervate the trapezius and supraspinatous muscles. The nerve runs obliquely downward in the fascia virtually unprotected by any overlying muscle. This portion of the posterior triangle of neck is a frequent site for inflamed epidermal inclusion cysts and lymph nodes (Fig 15). To the unwary surgeon, transecting the nerve is a real threat. If this occurs, there is an inability to shrug the ipsilateral shoulder or easily abduct the arm from a rest position.

References

1. Salasche SJ: Acute surgical complications: Cause, prevention, and treatment. *J Am Acad Dermatol* 15:1163-1185, 1986.
2. Maloney ME: Management of surgical complications and suboptimal results, in Wheeland RG (ed): *Cutaneous Surgery*. Philadelphia, W.B. Saunders Co, 1994, pp 921-934.
3. Stasko T: Complications of cutaneous procedures, in Roenigk RKK, Roenigk HH Jr (eds): *Roenigk and Roenigk's Dermatologic Surgery: Principles and Practice.* New York, Marcel Dekker, 1996, pp 149-175.
4. Robinson JK: Management of hematomas, in Robinson JK, Arndt KA, Leboit PE, et al (eds): *Atlas of Cutaneous Surgery*. Philadelphia, W.B. Saunders Co, 1996, pp 73-77.
5. Selva-Nayagam PA, Hill DC: Preoperative assessment of the elderly patient. *J Geriatr Dermatol* 4:169-178, 1996.
6. Leshin B, Whitaker DC, Swanson NA: An approach to patient assessment and preparation in cutaneous oncology. *J Am Acad* 19:1081, 1981.
7. Petry JJ: Surgically significant nutritional supplements. *Plast Reconstr Surg* 97:233-240, 1996.
8. Otley CC, Fewkes JL, Frank SM, et al: Complications of cutaneous surgery in patients who are taking warfarin, aspirin, or nonsteroidal anti-inflammatory drugs. *Arch Dermatol* 132:161-166, 1996.
9. Billingsley EM, Maloney ME: Intraoperative and postoperative bleeding problems in patients taking warfarin, aspirin, and nonsteroidal anti-inflammatory agents: A prospective study. *Dermatol Surg* 23:381-385, 1997.
10. Schanbacher CF, Bennett RG: Postoperative stroke after stopping warfarin for cutaneous surgery. *Dermatol Surg* 26:785-789, 2000.
11. Schanbacher CF, Bennett RG: Regarding postoperative stroke after warfarin for cutaneous surgery [letter]. *Dermatol Surg* 27:91-92, 2001.
12. Goldman G: Regarding postoperative stroke after warfarin for cutaneous surgery [letter]. *Dermatol Surg* 27:90-91, 2001.
13. Bornstein NM: Antiplatelet drugs: How to select them and possibilities of combined treatment. *Cerebrovasc Dis* 11(Suppl 1):96-99, 2001.
14. Van De Graaff E, Steinhubl SR: Complications of oral antiplatelet medications. *Curr Cardiol Rep* 3:371-379, 2001.
15. Caliendo FJ, Halpern VJ, Marini CP, et al: Warfarin anticoagulation in the perioperative period: Is it safe? *Ann Vasc Surg* 13(1):11-16, 1999.
16. Mulliken J, Im M: The etiologic role of free radicals in hematoma-induced flap necrosis [discussion]. *Plast Reconstr Surg* 77:802, 1986.
17. Angel MF, Ramasastry SS, Swartz WM, et al: The critical relationship between free radicals and degree of ischemia: Evidence for tissue intolerance of marginal perfusion. *Plast Reconstr Surg* 81:233, 1988.
18. Futoryan T, Grande D: Postoperative wound infection rates in dermatologic surgery. *Dermatol Surg* 21:509-514, 1995.

19. Whitaker DC, Grande DJ, Johnson SS: Wound infection rate in dermatologic surgery. *J Dermatol Surg Oncol* 14:525-528, 1988.
20. Takegami KT, Siegle RJ, Ayers LW: Microbiologic counts during outpatient office-based cutaneous surgery. *J Am Acad Dermatol* 23:1149, 1990.
21. Sebben JE: Surgical preparation, facilities, and monitoring, in Roenigk RKK and Roenigk HH Jr (eds): *Roenigk and Roenigk's Dermatologic Surgery: Principles and Practice*. New York, Marcel Dekker, 1996, pp 1-24.
22. Haas AF: Antisepsis, in Robinson JK, Arndt KA, Leboit PE, et al (eds): *Atlas of Cutaneous Surgery*. Philadelphia, W.B. Saunders Co, 1996, pp 27-31.
23. Sebben JE: Sterile technique and the prevention of wound infection in office surgery: Part I. *J Dermatol Surg Oncol* 14:1364, 1988.
24. Sebben JE: Sterile technique and the prevention of wound infection in office surgery: Part II. *J Dermatol Surg Oncol* 15:38, 1989.
25. Haas AF, Grekin RC: Practical thoughts on antibiotic prophylaxis [letter]. *Arch Dermatol* 134:872-873, 1998.
26. Haas AF, Grekin RC: Antibiotic prophylaxis in dermatologic surgery. *J Am Acad Dermatol* 32:155-176, 1995.
27. Salasche SJ, Grabski WJ: Complications of flaps. *J Dermatol Surg Oncol* 17:132-140, 1991.
28. Salasche SJ: Complications of flaps, in Baker SR, Swanson NA (eds): *Local Flaps in Facial Reconstruction*. St Louis, Mosby, 545-585, 1995.
29. Myers B: Understanding flap necrosis [editorial]. *Plast Reconstr Surg* 78:813, 1986.
30. Kerrigan CL: Skin flap failure: Pathophysiology. *Plast Reconst Surg* 72:766-774, 1985.
31. Angel MF, Narayanan K, Swartz WM, et al: The etiologic role of free radicals in hematoma-induced flap necrosis. *Plast Reconstr Surg* 77:795-801, 1986.
32. Larrabee WF Jr, Holloway GA Jr, Sutton D: Wound tension and blood flow in flaps. *Ann Otol Rhino Laryngol* 93:112-115, 1984.
33. Myers B: Understanding flap necrosis [editorial]. *Plast Reconstr Surg* 78:813, 1986.
34. Nolan J, Jenkins RA, Kurihara K, et al: The acute effects of cigarette exposure on experimental skin flaps. *Plast Reconstr Surg* 75:544, 1985.
35. Goldminz D, Bennett R: Cigarette smoking and flap and full-thickness graft necrosis. *Arch Dermatol* 127:1012-1015, 1991.
36. Jensen JA, Goodson WH, Hopf HW, et al: Cigarette smoking decreases tissue oxygen. *Arch Surg* 126:1331, 1991.
37. Burget GC: Aesthetic reconstruction of the nose. *Clin Plast Surg* 12:463, 1985.
38. Burget GC, Menick FJ: The subunit principle in nasal reconstruction. *Plast Reconstr Surg* 76:239, 1985.
39. Dzubow LM, Zack L: The principle of cosmetic junctions as applied to reconstruction of defects following Mohs surgery. *J Dermatol Surg Oncol* 16:353, 1990.
40. Salasche SJ, Jarchow R, Feldman BD, et al: The suspension suture. *J Dermatol Surg Oncol* 13:973-978, 1987.
41. Hosokawa K, Susuki T, Kikui T, et al: Sheet of scar deformity: A hypothesis. *Ann Plast Surg* 25:134, 1990.
42. Koranda FC, Webster RC: Trapdoor effect in nasolabial flaps. *Arch Otolaryngol* 111:421, 1985.
43. Zielli JA: The bilobed flap for nasal reconstruction. *Arch Dermatol* 125:957-959, 1989.
44. Salasche SJ, Bernstein G, Senkarik M: *Surgical Anatomy of the Skin*. Norwalk, Conn, Appelton and Lange, 1988.
45. Walden J, Garcia H, Hawkins H, et al: Both dermal matrix and epidermis contribute to an inhibition of wound contraction. *Ann Plast Surg* 45:162-166, 2000.
46. Stephenson A, Griffiths R, La H-BT: Patterns of contraction in human full thickness skin grafts. *Br J Plast Surg* 53:397-402, 2000.
47. Johnson TM, Ratner D: *Skin grafts*, in Ratz JL (ed): *Textbook of Dermatologic Surgery*. Philadelphia, Lippincott-Raven, 1988, pp 201-221.
48. Gloster HM Jr: The use of full-thickness skin grafts to repair non-perforating nasal defects. *J Am Acad Dermatol* 42:1041-1050, 2000.

49. Salasche SJ, Feldman BD: Skin grafting: Perioperative technique and management. *J Dermatol Surg Oncol* 13:863-869, 1987.
50. Robinson JK: Improvement of the appearance of full-thickness skin grafts with dermabrasion. *Arch Dermatol* 123:1340-1345, 1987.
51. Nehal K, Levine V, Ross B, et al: Comparison of high-energy pulsed carbon dioxide laser resurfacing and dermabrasion in the revision of surgical scars. *Dermatol Surg* 24:647-650, 1998.
52. Flynn TC, Emmanouil P, Limmer B: Unilateral transient forehead paralysis following injury to the temporal branch of the facial nerve. *Int J Dermatol* 38:474-477, 1999.
53. Delmar H: Anatomy of the superficial parts of the face and neck. *Ann Chir Plast Esthet* 39:527-555, 1994.
54. Otani A, Otani L, Carlson KC: The superficial neurovasculature of the head and neck. *Semin Dermatol* 13:43-47, 1994.

Complications of Cosmetic Surgery

Neil S. Sadick, MD

Clinical Professor of Dermatology, Weill Medical College, Cornell University, New York

Complications may arise during cosmetic procedures, even at the hands of the skilled dermatologic surgeon. As in all surgical settings, fastidious technique is the most important factor in minimizing such events. However, even in the best circumstances, such adverse events do occasionally arise. Recognition, avoidance, and appropriate management of these untoward events can help to minimize the morbidity associated with such reactions.

Filler Substances: Bovine Collagen

Various bovine and cadaver-based collagen derivatives are used for the correction of rhytides and lipodystrophy. Adverse reactions associated with these fillers are listed in Table 1.

Localized Hypersensitivity Reactions

Localized hypersensitivity reactions may occur in 3% to 35% of treated individuals.[1] One percent to 3% of patients with a single negative skin test have a reaction at a treatment site. Between 0.5% and 1% of patients with 2 negative skin tests may have a similar hypersensitivity response. The large majority (more than 70%) of these positive skin test reactions occur within 72 hours. In rare cases, adverse reactions at test sites may occur 4 to 5 weeks after test dose placement. Hence long-term (up to 8 weeks) examination for potential positive test implant reactions should be carried out[2] (Fig 1).

Symptoms are characterized by erythema, induration, discoloration, or pruritus of the treatment site (Fig 2). Eighty percent of the reactions occur within 4 weeks after the sensitizing dose has been administered. Occasionally, a first occurrence may occur after years of repeated filler treatments. The mean duration of such hypersensitivity responses is 4 months, with a range of 1 to 9 months. Long-term sequelae are extremely unusual, although rare cases of residual firmness or discoloration have been reported.[3] The incidence of these localized hypersensitivity reactions increases when topical rejuvenation agents, such as retinoids or α-hydroxy acids, are used at the same time. Thus, it is recommended that these agents be

TABLE 1.—Adverse Events Associated With Collagen

Local hypersensitivity reactions
Systemic hypersensitivity reactions
Granulomatous reactions
Sterile abscesses
Local tissue necrosis
Activation of herpetic infection
Unilateral vision loss
Ectopal collagen deposition

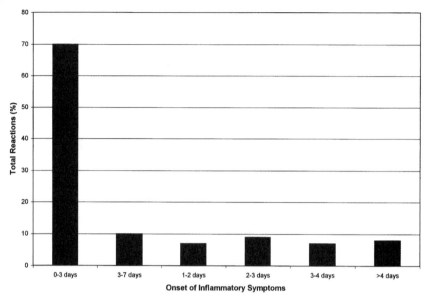

FIGURE 1.—Inflammatory symptoms at test site of Zyderm collagen (McGhan Medical, Santa Barbara, Calif). More than 70% of positive tests occur within 72 hours; however, hypersensitivity may be noted 4 to 5 weeks after test implant placement.

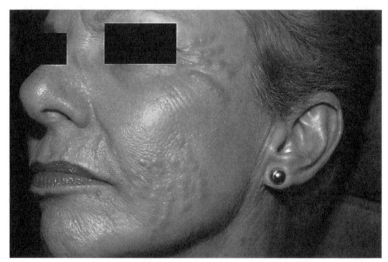

FIGURE 2.—Induration and erythema noted 24 hours after Zyderm I (McGhan Medical, Santa Barbara, Calif) implant at all injection sites. Patient had 2 negative skin tests.

TABLE 2.—Agents Used to Manage Collagen
Hypersensitivity Reactions

Antihistamines
Nonsteroidal anti-inflammatory drugs (NSAIDs)
Topical steroids
Intralesional steroids
System steroids
Tacrolimus

discontinued 2 weeks before and after collagen implantation to minimize the potential synergistic inflammatory potential.

Various therapeutic interventions have been used in the literature to minimize or shelter the course of this process; however, no controlled studies have been performed substantiating their efficacy[1-3] (Table 2).

Systemic Hypersensitivity Reactions

Significant systemic hypersensitivity reactions have rarely been reported and when they do occur, they usually occur within 48 to 72 hours after collagen implantation. Fever, malaise, and urticaria are common initial symptoms. Systemic steroids (prednisone, 60 mg/d) are often helpful in controlling symptoms associated with this reaction. Of note, it is usually necessary to continue treatment of such patients for 3 to 6 weeks after institution of therapy. Rapid taper of these relatively high dosages may lead to reactivation of symptoms.

Granulomatous Reactions

Rare granulomatous reactions consisting of palpable nodules have been described. These foreign body-type reactions have been reported despite negative skin tests.[4]

Sterile Abscesses

Sterile abscess-like reactions may occur in approximately 4 in 10,000 treated individuals. These reactions are believed to be secondary to type IV delayed hypersensitivity. The onset is usually 8 to 12 weeks after implantation (range, 7 days to 22 months) (Fig 3; see color plate I). This reaction usually occurs as painful small draining papules to large erythematous

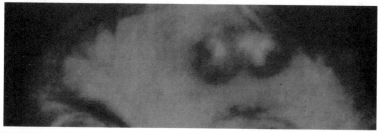

FIGURE 3.—Sterile abscess formation after Zyplast instillation, resolved spontaneously in a period of 60 days.

TABLE 3.—Management of Collagen-Induced Sterile
Abscess Formation

Needle aspiration or incision and drainage
Intralesional steroids (triamcinolone acetinide, 3-5 mg/mL)
Oral antibiotics (macrolide or tetracycline derivative)

nodules with induration. If these nodules are left untreated, they may be continuous or intermittent and last from several days to several weeks. These reactions, although usually resolving completely, have been associated with cases of scarring. Clinical approaches used for the treatment of collagen-induced abscesses are outlined in Table 3. Observational support is the treatment of choice, as other approaches have no supporting scientific validity.

Local Tissue Necrosis

This is perhaps the most serious consequence of collagen implantation. This vascular-occlusive phenomenon has been reported most often in the glabellar region, and has an incidence of 9 in 10,000 treated individuals. The onset of immediate blanching or cyanosis after instillation of the more concentrated Zyplast collagen should be a warning sign to the dermatologic surgeon. This is subsequently followed by progression to a white or blackened appearance within 72 hours. The presentation is that of a moist,

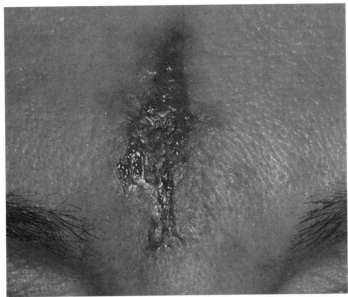

FIGURE 4.—Ulceration of the glabellar area after Zyderm II (McGhan Medical, Santa Barbara, Calif) implantation. The cause is believed to be related to vaso-occlusive phenomena.

TABLE 4.—Management of Suspected Post-Collagen Tissue Necrosis

Discontinue injection and massage gently
Immediate application of warm compresses
Nitroglycerin paste application every hour
Fastidious wound care
Laser resurfacing, dermabrasion, or surgical revision should be considered if a scar
   develops

pustular dry eschar that may be significant. Lesions frequently heal without difficulty; however, ensuing scar formation is not unusual[5] (Fig 4; see color plate I).

Technique modification that may help to minimize the occurrence of necrosis in the glabellar region is fastidious avoidance of vessels. This may be accomplished by limiting implantation to the more superficial portion of the dermis by using Zyderm I (McGhan Medical, Santa Barbara, Calif) collagen implants in danger zones (eg, glabellar furrows), as vaso-occlusion is thought to be the major mechanism by which necrosis occurs in this precarious location. Table 4 outlines steps to be instituted should an interruption of the local vasculopathy be suspected.[6]

Reactivation of Herpes Simplex

A careful history of recent herpetic outbreaks should be obtained during the initial patient consultation. If recent or frequent outbreaks are noted, antiviral prophylaxis should be considered. Lesions may mimic those of vaso-occlusive interglabellar necrosis (Fig 5). Appropriate Tzanck smear monoclonal antibody tests and cultures should be undertaken to differentiate these clinically similar ulceronecrotic patterns. Suggested prophylac-

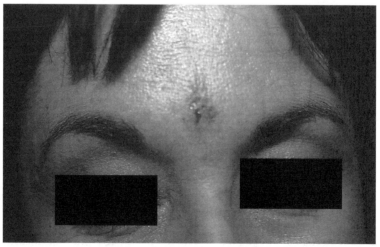

FIGURE 5.—Ulceration secondary to herpes simplex I reactivation. Clinical appearance may mimic interglabellar vaso-occlusive necrosis and must be differentiated by appropriate laboratory testing.

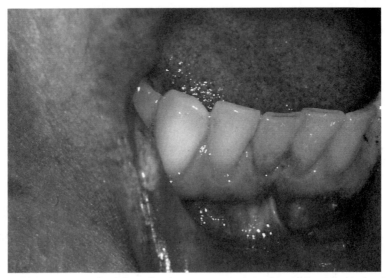

FIGURE 6.—Ectopic collagen formation may appear as papules or thin nodules with white hue. This phenomenon is most commonly noted in distensible epithelial anatomical areas such as the mucous membranes.

tic therapeutic regimens include valacyclovir (Valtrex) 500 mg twice daily for 3 days or famciclovir (Famvir) 250 mg twice daily for 3 days.

Unilateral Vision Loss

Occlusion of the retinal artery is believed to be associated with unilateral vision loss. Occlusion may be avoided by limiting the practitioner's injection technique to the outer margin of the orbital rim and aspirating air before injection to confirm localization of extravascular location.[3,6]

Ectopic Collagen Implantation

One of the most annoying problems for patients is persistent papular nodule formation caused by ectopic collagen implantation. These palpable nodules, although temporary, are often distressing to the patient. This occurs most often after lip augmentation (Fig 6). Fastidious technique, minimal overcorrection in the dermal anatomical locations, and postimplantation massage may help to minimize this phenomenon. If the patient is disturbed, ectopic deposition may be evacuated by incision and drainage through a Bard-Parker (BD Surgical Products, Franklin Lakes, NJ) number 11 blade.

Silicone

Silicone has re-emerged as a viable filler. It is currently FDA approved for ophthalmologic indications, but it has an off-label use as permanent filler (Silkone 1000, Alcon Laboratories, Fort Worth, Tex). The dermatologic surgeon may again begin to see adverse sequelae after administration of this substance.

The most common adverse reaction associated with silicone is nodular granuloma formation, which may appear as a painless nodule at the injection site (Fig 7). Implantation of excessive material that increases with time or ectopic migration of this inert material are the major causes of this adverse sequela.[7]

Intralesional injection of triamcinolone acetonide (3-5 mg/mL) has been attempted but is associated with disappointing results. Only incision and draining of this inert filler consistently has been shown to remove these disturbing palpable lesions.

Botox

Both botulinum toxin A (Botox Callergen Inc, Irvine, Calif) and botulinum toxin B (Elan Pharmaceuticals, San Diego, Calif) have gained increasing popularity and shown remarkable safety. However, these toxins are antigenic and have been associated with a pattern of similar adverse reactions (Table 5).

Blocking Antibody Formation

There is evidence that patients with neurologic conditions requiring larger amounts of A toxin (1000 IU or more) and selected patients undergoing cosmetic treatment may produce circulating neutralizing immunoglobin G antibotulinum toxin A[8] antibodies. This may result in therapeutic failure. The factors that cause antibodies to the toxin to develop in susceptible individuals are unknown. A cross-reactivity between A and B toxins has been seen. In addition, there is no definite correlation between antibody levels, number of injections, dilution practice, length of treatment, and total cumulative toxin dose.

Immunologic and treatment resistance have not been a significant problem in the aesthetic population yet. Keeping injection volumes low, avoid-

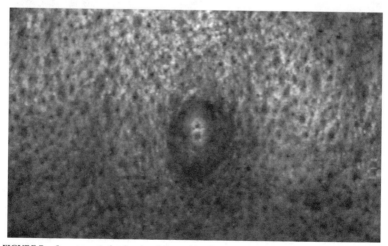

FIGURE 7.—Symptomatic forehead nodule resulting from excess implantation of silicone. Incision and drainage of this inert material is the only method to remove these unsightly lesions.

TABLE 5.—Adverse Reactions Associated With Botulinum Toxins
A and B

Antibody resistance
Idiosyncratic reactions (eg, nausea, fatigue, malaise, flulike symptoms, distant
  eruptions)
Distant electromyographic changes
Dry mouth
Ptosis
Pain
Localized reactions (eg, urticaria, erythema, edema)
Ecchymosis
Headache
Short-term hypesthesia

ing injections into the systemic circulation, and, when treating large muscles or multiple sites, spacing injections at 1-month intervals may help minimize the complications.

Idiosyncratic Reactions

Generalized reactions, including nausea, fatigue, malaise, flulike symptoms, and eruption at distant sites have been reported.

Ptosis

Transient ptosis is the most significant complication, and its onset is usually within 1 to 2 days. It is usually minimal (1-2 mm) and short lived (approximately 2 weeks) (Fig 8).

Ptosis may be minimized by following guidelines presented in Table 6. If significant ptosis does eventuate the application of iopidine (Apidomidine,

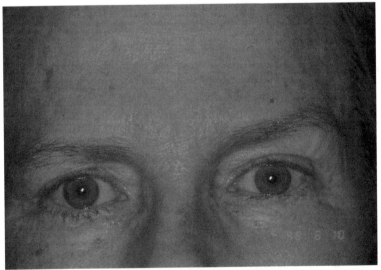

FIGURE 8.—Right lid ptosis secondary to Botox (Allergan, Inc, Irvine, Calif) injection. This laxity is usually less than 2 mm and often resolves within 1 to 2 weeks.

TABLE 6.—Methods of Minimizing Ptosis With Botulinum
Toxin Injections

Keep the dose low (8 to 15 U Botox A; 1000 to 1875 U Botox B)
  per corrugator
Inject the toxin adequately into the belly of the muscle
Avoid manipulating the area
Avoid injecting below level of cerebrum

Alan Laboratories, Fort Worth, Tex) 1 to 2 drops, 3 times per day until improvement occurs is indicated and may shorten the course of this problem. Similar effects have been noted with botulinum toxin B (Myobloc) as well.

Pain

Discomfort can be decreased with the use of preinjection topical anesthesia (Emla, Lastra Pharmaceuticals, West Borough, Ga) and small gauge needles, such as insulin and tuberculin needles and syringes. Myobloc (Botox B) has a more acid pH and is associated with slightly more pain than Botox (Botox A). However, discomfort may be minimized by diluting Myobloc with bacteriostatic 0.9 NaCl (Abbot Laboratories, North Chicago, Ill) to desired concentration.[9]

Technique modifications include pinching the skin and other underlying muscle, slowly inserting the needle bevel up through the opening of a pilosebaceous unit, and slowly injecting the solution to help diminish discomfort. Ice packs applied immediately before or after injection may ameliorate pain further.

Localized Reactions

Urticaria, edema, and erythema are localized reactions reported with Botox A and Botox B administration.[10] Localized hypersensitivity reactions may occur at treatment sites. This hypersensitivity is nonsystemic and may be treated by topical corticosteroids, H1 antihistamines, and posttreatment ice packs. Such reactions are not contraindications to further treatments. These lesions probably are related to local histamine and cytokine release.

Ecchymosis

Postinjection bruising (Fig 9; see color plate I) can be minimized by avoiding aspirin-containing products and antiplatelet agents (eg, NSAIDs), as well as oral vitamin E, and gingko biloba for 7 to 10 days before injection. Limiting the number of injections and postinjection digital pressure without manipulation may help reduce bruising. Other helpful reagents include topical vitamin K preparations and arnica montana.[11]

Headache

There have been sporadic reports of the onset of headaches after botulinum toxin injections, but more commonly, chronic tension and migraine

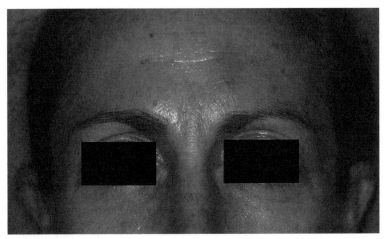

FIGURE 9.—Ecchymosis after Botox (Allergan, Inc, Irvine, Calif) injection may be minimized by fastidious injection technique and avoidance of aspirin and nonsteroidal anti-inflammatory drugs for 7 to 10 days before injection.

headaches are improved after the injection of botulinum toxin.[12] Standard analgesic agents may be used if temporary headaches ensue.[12]

Dry Mouth

Dry mouth was reported after the initial utilization of Myobloc (Botox B1) for neurologic indications, but further usage studies in the aesthetic venue have not shown this to be a problem.[13]

Short-term Hyperesthesia

In most cases, this rare postinjection sequela responds spontaneously within 48 to 72 hours. The exact mechanism of this reported complication is not known. Table 7 lists a summary of adverse reactions when performing Botox injections.

TABLE 7.—Technique Modifications for Limiting Adverse Reactions When Performing Botulinum Toxin Injections

Use of small-gauge needles and syringes (eg, insulin, tuberculin)
Two-hand placement using upward injection technique
Post-injection ice pack application
Avoidance of antiplatelet agents (eg, aspirin, nonsteroidal anti-inflammatory drugs [NSAIDs])
Use of products to minimize bruising (ie, vitamin K, Arnica montana)
Avoidance of supine position for 4 hours after injection
Frequent contraction of injected muscle groups for 4 hours after injection
Localization of muscle before treatment
Proper reconstitution, preoperation, and injection of toxin

TABLE 8.—Complications Related to Chemical Peeling
True Complication
Prolonged erythema (> 3 months)
Pigmentary change
Hypertrophic scarring
Atrophy
Systemic effects (eg, hepatic, renal, cardiac abnormalities)
Adverse Procedural Sequelae
Prolonged erythema (< 3 months)
Pigmentary changes
Colloid milia
Reactivation of Herpes simplex
Superficial bacterial or yeast infections
Demarcation problems

Chemical Peels

Reactions related to chemical peeling are divided into 3 complications and adverse procedural sequelae (Table 8).

Pigmentary Changes

Hyperpigmentation and hypopigmentation are noted most often with strong concentration medium and deep chemical peeling agents (Fig 10). These are also more common in darker phenotypic (Fitzpatrick IV-VI) individuals. UV light protection prepeel and postpeel is a major factor in preventing these sequelae. In high-risk individuals, spot peels and the use of lower potency peeling agents may help minimize this disturbing complication.

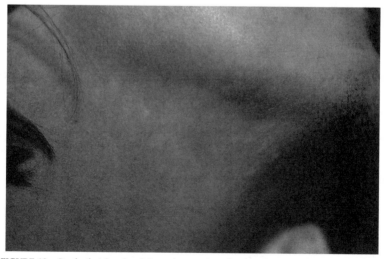

FIGURE 10.—Patchy facial and neck hypopigmentation after a combination Jessner and 35% trichloroacetic acid (TCA) peel.

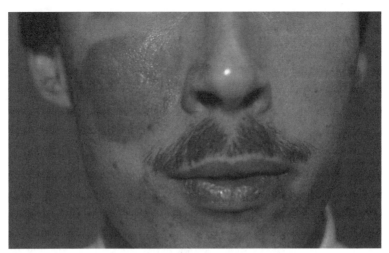

FIGURE 11.—Persistent erythema lasting more than 3 months followed by incipient scarring; a combined Jessner and 35% trichloroacetic acid (TCA) peel. Severe scarring was avoided by aggressive topical application of class I corticosteroid ointment (clobetasol propionate [Temovate] ointment, .05%, Glaxo, Greenville, NC).

Prolonged Erythema

Overaggressive technique (eg, multilayered applications, high concentrations of agents applied to high-risk areas such as the mandible, eyelid, and neck), and an intrinsic genetic scarring predisposition may lead to prolonged erythema (more than 3 months) as a form fruste of incipient scar formation (Fig 11).[14]

Early intervention with potent class I topical corticosteroids may help to minimize progression to scarring.

Scarring

Scarring resulting from chemical peeling usually is related to overaggressive application of the peeling agent or use of an inappropriate concentration match for a given anatomical site. It may be hypertrophic, atrophic, or combined in nature.[15]

High-potency topical or intralesional corticosteroids (intralesional triamcinolone acetonide, 3-5 mg/mL), Silastic gel, and the pulsed dye laser all have been used for treatment of the hypertrophic variant. Atrophic scars may be treated with the 1320 nm holmium yttrium aluminum garnet (YAG) laser (ICN/Cool Touch, Auburn, Calif). Scarring, although more common with deeper peeling agents (eg, phenol), may also be associated with superficial agents (eg, glycolic acid). The time of application and pH may play roles in this setting.

Systemic Effects

Hepatic, renal, and cardiac abnormalities are noted almost exclusively with phenol peeling.[12,16] Appropriate EKG and pulse oximetry monitoring and adequate hydration are the major factors necessary to avoid such complications.

Procedural Adverse Reactions: Pigmentary Changes and Prolonged Erythema

Transient pigmentary dyschromia and erythema lasting less than 3 months commonly are noted, particularly after medium and deep-depth chemical peeling. Observation and broad spectrum sunscreens such as Ti-Screen (Fisher, Irvine, Calif) or Shade UVA (Sherring Plough, Memphis, Tenn) are often all that are needed.[17]

Colloid Milia

Occlusive retention cysts are frequent and temporary minor sequelae of all facial ablative resurfacing procedures. Spontaneous resolution, the use of topical retinoids, or incision and drainage are typical interventions.

Reactivation of Latent Herpes Simplex

All forms of ablative facial rejuvenation may be associated with reactivation of herpes type I and II infection.[18] Prophylaxis has been previously discussed. Therapeutic intervention with valacyclovir 500 mg twice daily for 5 days or famciclovir 250 mg 3 times daily for 5 days should be instituted at an early suspected stage. UV avoidance is important.

Superficial Bacterial or Yeast Infections

Superficial bacterial infections with *Staphylococcus aureus*, *Pseudomonas aeruginosa*, or yeast infection from *Candida* species have been reported.[18] Manifestations include persistent crusting, erythema, and superficial erosions.[18] The role of prophylactic antibiotics has been debated; however, rapid intervention with fluoroquinolones (eg, twice-daily profloxacin 250 mg), if bacterial infection is suspected, or fluconazole 150 mg 4 times per day if yeast infection is documented by appropriate KOH stains and cultures, is indicated.

Demarcation Problems

Demarcation problems usually are caused by a lack of feathering in segmental cosmetic units. Creation of a tapering zone by use of a lighter concentration of a given peeling agent, or combined peeling with feathering in discreet areas with a different, less aggressive agent may help minimize this disturbing nonaesthetic sequela.[19,20] Anatomical areas where this problem commonly occurs are the neck, scalp, and periauricular and periorbital regions. Table 9 outlines measures reported to be helpful in minimizing chemical peel complications.

Microdermabrasion

One of the more popular noninvasive modalities in modern aesthetic practice, microdermabrasion has been associated with minimal complications. Only pigment streaking, noted more frequently in Fitzpatrick skin types IV-VI, and persistent erythema lasting more than 48 hours have been reported.[21,22] Hypersensitivity pulmonary disease resulting from aluminum

---

TABLE 9.—Measures Reported to Be Helpful in Minimizing Dermal Peel Complications

---

Sunscreens
Lower concentrations or blending of agents in danger zones (eg, upper lip, jawline, neck, eyelids)
Early treatment of pigment dyschromia (eg, hydroquinones, azelaic acid, kojic acid, retinoids)
Early treatment of incipient hypertrophic scars (eg, Silastic gel sheeting, topical and intralesional corticosteroids, imiquimod [Aldara])
Herpes prophylaxis: Valcyclovir (Valtrex) 50 mg twice daily for 5 days and famciclovir (Famvir) 250 mg twice daily for 5 days
Pretreatment and maintenance programs (eg, α-hydroxides, retinoids, vitamin C derivatives, micropeels)

---

oxide inhalation has not been a reported problem. The use of beginning treatments with conservative settings is advocated in those with dark skin and sensitive skin phenotypes.

Laser Resurfacing

The role of ablative laser resurfacing has diminished over the past several years. Newer hybrid and extended pulse duration technologies have minimized some of the complications, well recognized by physicians and patients, that have contributed to the lack of popularity of this useful modality. Table 10 divides these adverse sequelae into mild, moderate, and severe complications.

Postoperative Swelling

This universal reaction is often disturbing to patients. The use of postoperative semiocclusive dressings for the first 3 to 5 days after resurfacing may minimize this reaction, because this keeps the skin free of exudate and permits faster re-epithelialization.[23,24] These dressings also are helpful in diminishing crust formation, postoperative erythema, pain, and pruritus. Hydrogels, silicone polymer films, and foam-composite dressings are available. Alternatively, a short course of prednisone 40 to 50 mg/d for 3 days is helpful in this regard.

Erythema

More prolonged with CO_2 than Er-YAG modalities, erythema may last up to 3 to 6 months after resurfacing. One factor that may help to alleviate such prolonged erythema is the avoidance of topical corticosteroids that may exacerbate this phenomena and induce a state of tachyphylaxis.[25]

TABLE 10.—Side Effects and Complications of Laser Resurfacing

Mild	Moderate	Severe
Persistent erythema	Transient hyperpigmentation	Hypertrophic scarring
Transient edema	Local herpes simplex virus	Disseminated infection
Milia formation	reactivation	Ectropion
Acne flare	Superficial bacterial or fungal	Permanent hypopigmentation
Contact dermatitis	infection	
	Delayed hyperpigmentation	

Gentle skin care regimens incorporating hypogenic moisturizers, appropriate broad-spectrum sunscreen, or ascorbic acid derivatives (Celex C Skin Ceutricals, Dallas, Tex) are useful modalities minimizing this sequela. Such programs may be instituted 10 to 14 days after re-epithelialization of the resurfaced skin.

Infections with *P aeruginosa*, *S aureus*, and *Candida* species, as described in the section on chemical peeling, must also be considered in case of postresurfacing persistent erythema.[10,26] Herpes prophylaxis is unquestioned in the ablative resurfacing protocol. However, the role of antibacterial and antifungal prophylaxis is more in question and is used on an individual personal experience basis by laser surgeons.[27,28]

Acne and Milia

Occlusive cyst and pustule formation is common after facial resurfacing procedures and may be managed by incision and drainage. If acne flares, begin a short course of a tetracycline derivative (eg, Minocycline). Dynacin 100 to 200 mg/d is often helpful.

Hyperpigmentation

This common sequela may occur in up to 20% to 30% of resurfaced patients.[29] It usually appears 1 month after laser therapy.[29] Usually, it is transient; however, it is often bothersome to patients.[30] Treatment options include hydroquinones, glycolic acid, ascorbic acid, azelaic acid, and retinoid derivatives. The efficacy of pretreatment regimens in preventing this dyschromia is controversial.

Hypopigmentation

Post-laser hypopigmentation has been reported after both CO_2 and Er:YAG resurfacing, although more frequently with the former. It is rare

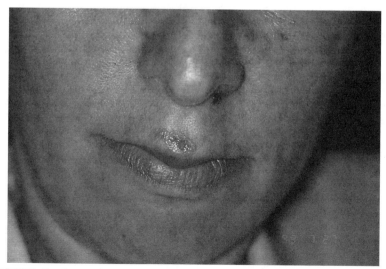

FIGURE 12.—Hypotrophic scarring of the upper lip after 3 passes with the CO_2 laser at 300 J/cm^2.

TABLE 11.—Treatment Options for Impending and Established Post-Laser Resurfacing Scarring

---

Steriods (topical class I superpotent or intralesional triamcinolone acetonide 3 to 10 mg/mL)
Silicone gel sheeting/ointment
Pressure and massage
Imiquimod (Aldara) (3M Pharmaceuticals, St Paul, MN) 585 to 600-nm pulsed-dye laser
Intralesional 5-fluorouracil (50 mg/mL) (2-50 mg) combined with 1% lidocaine (Xylocaine)

---

and onset may be delayed from 6 to 12 months. Predisposed areas include the perioral region and previously or aggressively treated facial zones.

Recently, the 308-nm excimer laser has been effective in inducing repigmentation in this setting.

Petechiae

This vascular fragility phenomenon is usually temporary. It is noted most often in patients who have or are simultaneously undergoing rhytidectomy procedures and are using topical retinoids or steroids.[31]

Scarring

This rare complication is the most dreaded after laser resurfacing. Danger zones are the mandible, neck, forehead, and preauricular zones (Fig 12). Prolonged erythema is a warning of impending cicatrization. Fibrosis may appear as soon as 1 month after surgery. The most common cause is overaggressive laser technique. Treatment options are listed in Table 11.[32]

Ectropion

This rare complication occurs most often in patients who have undergone previous blepharoplasty procedures or who have lid laxity. All patients should be evaluated before treatment. Overaggressive lid resurfacing is the major cause[33] and feathering techniques are most helpful. The Ten Commandments for minimizing adverse outcomes when performing laser resurfacing procedures are listed in Table 12.

Hair Transplantation

Advanced follicular unit and micro/minigraft hair transplantation techniques have significantly diminished the number of side effects once noted after hair replacement surgery. A list of reported common and rare complications are listed in Table 13.

Common complications such as perifollicular scarring, poor growth of grafts, inclusion cysts (Fig 13) and acquired posttransplanted hair kinking have diminished with the advent of the current micro/minigraft techniques.

The most common side effects, which are bothersome to patients, are excessive swelling and telogen effluvium.[34]

TABLE 12.—Measures Helpful in Reducing Complications When
Performing Laser Resurfacing

Preconditioning (eg, retinoids, α-hydroxy acids, hydroquinones, azelaic acid, kojic acid, vitamin C)
Test laser spot sessions in susceptible individuals (eg, history of scarring, dark phenotypic skin type V-VI individuals)
Minimize overlap of laser pulses (ie, stacking)
When using combined modalities, peel first, then use laser
Keep in cosmetic units
Treat danger zones (eg, neck, chin, lower lids) with extra caution
Minimize crust development by using appropriate postoperative lubricants and wound dressing
Appropriate use of prophylactic antiviral agents
Early and aggressive treatment of persistent red streaks (silicone dressings, topical and intralesional corticosteroids)
Institute early usage of bleaching creams (days 15-20) in dark-skinned individuals

Excessive swelling of the forehead, particularly when the frontal scalp is transplanted, may be minimized by instituting a 3-day postoperative course of prednisone 20 mg twice a day without tapering.

Shedding of hairs surrounding transplanted regions is common, particularly between fill-in sessions. Hair regrowth may be delayed several anagen cycles and may take from 6 to 12 months to regrow fully. This disturbing event should be discussed with the patient in the preoperative consultation.[35]

Of the listed rare complications, numbness and scar formation in the donor area are often disturbing to the patient. A long single-donor area strip, compared with wide, multistrip excisions, may enhance patient

TABLE 13.—Complications After Hair Transplantation Surgery

Common
Telogen effluvium
Nausea and vomiting from analgesics
Bleeding (< 5%)
Infection (< 1%)
Excessive swelling
Temporary headache
Temporary numbness of scalp
Scarring around grafts
Poor growth of grafts
Reactions to medications (< 1%)
Syncope (< 1%)
Occasional small ingrown hair causing a cyst (< 10%)
Acquired posttransplant hair kinking
Rare
Keloid formation
Complete failure of growth of transplanted hair
Persistent scalp pain
Total loss of donor hair
Permanent numbness of scalp
Notable scarring of donor area
Unnatural growth of transplanted hair
Allergic reactions or other non-medication-related problems

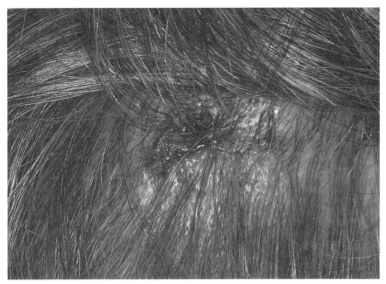

FIGURE 13.—Persistent posttransplant abscess formation caused by poor inward placement of recipient hair.

comfort and produce less scarring and postoperative paresthesias. This factor is more important than whether the donor area is closed by a staple or suturing technique.

Liposuction

True complications of tumescent liposuction are infrequently encountered and can be divided into uncommon, rare, and very rare (Table 14).

Uncommon Complications

The possibility of lidocaine toxicity must always be kept in mind, but this problem is infrequent, as long as the maximum ASDS/AAD*-recommended dose (55 mg/kg) is not exceeded.[36] Signs and symptoms of lidocaine toxicity include nausea and vomiting, altered consciousness, dysarthria, dizziness, paresthesias, muscle twitching, and seizures, and may culminate in respiratory failure.[37,38] A similar clinical picture and more likely scenario may occur as an allergic reaction to medications used in the perioperative period, such as analgesics or antibiotics.[39]

The large majority of complications related to tumescent liposuction are minor aesthetic concerns. Skin dimpling, irregular contours, nodularity, and mild asymmetry may ensue. It is generally advisable to wait at least 3 to 6 months before attempting to touch up a suboptimal result, as spontaneous improvement often occurs.

---

*American Society for Dermatologic Surgery/American Academy of Dermatology

TABLE 14.—Complications of Tumescent Liposuction

Uncommon
    Drug allergy versus toxicity
    Skin-surface irregularities
    Irregular contours
    Asymmetry
    Inadequate skin contraction
    Entry site scars
    Seromas
Rare
    Excessive bleeding or hematomas
    Wound infection
    Erythema ab igne
    Skin necrosis
    Syncope episodes
Very Rare
    Pulmonary embolism
    Deep vein thrombosis
    Pulmonary edema
    Massive generalized edema
    Intraperitoneal/intrathoracic penetration
    Necrotizing vasculitis
    Death versus cardiopulmonary arrest

Seromas may also appear in the early postoperative period. They represent a form of noninfectious panniculitis and usually appear as tender, indurated, warm subcutaneous masses with overlying erythema. They usually resolve spontaneously, but improvement may be accelerated with a short course of low-dose prednisone or a nonsteroidal anti-inflammatory agent. When doubt concerning an infectious etiology cannot be ruled out, appropriate cultures and antibiotics should be instituted.[40]

Rare Complications

Of the rare complications of tumescent liposuction, infection is the most serious concern. Bacterial infection may be superficial or, in its most severe form, may present as fulminant necrotizing fasciitis. More recently, cases of atypical mycobacterial infections secondary to *Mycobacterium avium-intracellulare* have been reported (Fig 14; see color plate II). This difficult to diagnose entity appears with areas of induration and purulence that progress to ulcerative necrotic lesions.[40]

Such considerations should be in the liposuction surgeon's mind when fever, persistent erythema, pain, and induration are manifested during the postoperative course.

Incision and drainage, cultures, surgical debridement, and appropriate antibiotic coverage are the cornerstones of therapy.

Very Rare Complications

Liposuction deaths have been reported, but they are rare in the hands of the dermatologic surgeon. The use of tumescent anesthesia with adherence to appropriate lidocaine toxicity guidelines is prudent. Conservative removal of fat at a given surgical session (5000 cc or less) and fastidious

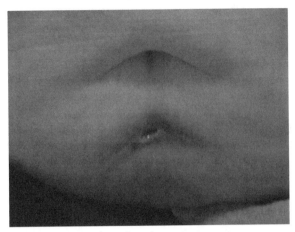

FIGURE 14.—Liposuction—atypical mycobacterium.

surgical septic technique with careful monitoring of fluids and medications will avoid this most dreaded complication.[41-44]

Lipotransfer

Complications from lipotransfer are rare and follow those associated with other fillers and the less serious and common complications of liposuction (Table 15).

The most consistent sequela of lipotransfer is prolonged edema. It may last from 2 weeks to 2 months and will resolve spontaneously.[45]

Bruising (Fig 15; see color plate II) and hematomas may occur because of sharp injection of local anesthesia, multiple passes with tunneling, or patients taking antiplatelet aggregating agents during the procedure.

Necrosis of grafted tissue has been reported. Forcing too much fat into a limited recipient site may kill grafted adipocytes or cause vaso-occlusion, which leads to subsequent necrosis.[46] Migration may occur by forcing too much fat into a recipient area during infiltration or by postoperative manipulation of the corrected area by strong digital pressure.[47]

The most common source for infection in facial recontouring has been the oral muscle. Unnoticed perforation of the oral mucosa during infiltra-

TABLE 15.—Complications of Lipotransfer

Bruising
Prolonged edema
Irregularities
Nodularity
Infection
Migration
Necrosis of grafted tissue

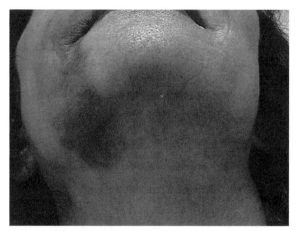

FIGURE 15.—After lipotransfer—bruising.

tion of the lip or buccal cheek can lead to contamination of the transplanted fatty tissue.[46-51]

Conclusion

An in-depth understanding of potential adverse sequelae related to aesthetic facial rejuvenation and available management approaches, should such a complication occur, will enable the dermatologic surgeon to reduce his or her complication profile and minimize the consequence of untoward events, resulting in improved patient care and satisfaction.

References

1. Stegman SJ, Chu S, Armstrong RC: Adverse reactions to bovine collagen implant: Clinical and histologic features. *J Dermatol Surg Oncol* 14(Suppl):39-48, 1988.
2. Charriere G, Bejot M, Schnitzler L, et al: Reactions to a bovine collagen implant. Clinical and immunologic study in 705 patients. *J Am Acad Dermatol* 21:1203-1208, 1989.
3. Labow TA, Silvers DN: Late reactions at Zyderm skin test sites. *Cutis* 35:154-158, 1985.
4. Overhold MA, Tschen JA, Font RL: Granulomatous reaction to collagen implant, light and electron microscopic observations. *Cutis* 51:95-98, 1993.
5. Parish LC, Witkowski JA: Collagen implants for soft tissue augmentation. *Int J Dermatol* 24:499-504, 1998.
6. Elson ML: Correction of dermal contour defects with the injectable collagen: Choosing and using these materials. *Semin Dermatol* 5:77-82, 1987.
7. Klein AW, Rish DC: Substances for soft-tissue augmentation: Collagen and silicone. *J Dermatol Surg Oncol* 11:337-339, 1985.
8. Matarasso SL: Complications of botulinum A exotoxin for hyperfunctional lines. *Dermatol Surg* 24:1249-1254, 1998.
9. Benedetto A: The cosmetic uses of botulinum toxin type A. *Int J Dermatol* 38:641-655, 1999.
10. Carruthers A, Kiene K, Carruthers J: Botulinum A exotoxin use in clinical dermatology. *J Am Acad Dermatol* 34:788-797, 1996.
11. Sadick NS: Overview of complications of nonspecific facial rejuvenation procedures. *Clin Plast Surg* 28:163-176, 2001.

12. Asken S: Unoccluded Baker-Gordon phenol peels: Review and update. *J Dermatol Surg Oncol* 15:998-1008, 1989.
13. Sadick NS: An initial study of the treatment of hyperkinetic facial wrinkles utilizing botulinum toxin B evaluation of a low dose 1800 unit injection region. *Derm Surg* 2002 (in publication).
14. Coleman WP III, Brody HJ: Advances in chemical peeling. *Dermatol Clin* 15:19-26, 1997.
15. Resnik SS, Resnik BI: Complications of chemical peeling. *Dermatol Clin* 13:309-312, 1995.
16. Alt TH: Occluded Baker-Gorden chemical peel: Review and update. *J Dermatol Surg Oncol* 15:980-993, 1989.
17. David L, Glassberg E, Lask G: Combined carbon dioxide laser resurfacing and trichloroacetic acid chemical peel. *Am J Cosmetic Surg* 9:153-158, 1992.
18. Resnik SS: Chemical peeling with trichloroacetic acid. *J Dermatol Surg Oncol* 10:549-550, 1984.
19. Moy LS, Myad H, Moy RL: Glycolic acid peels for the treatment of wrinkles and photoaging. *J Dermatol Surg Oncol* 19:203-246, 1993.
20. Stagnone JJ: Superficial peeling. *J Dermatol Surg Oncol* 15:924-930, 1989.
21. Ess SM, Steinegger AF, Ess HG, et al: Experimental study on the fibrogenic properties of different types of alumina. *Am Ind Hyg Assoc J* 54:360-391, 1993.
22. Rollin HB, Theodorou P, Kilroe-Smith TA: Deposition of aluminum in tissues of rabbits exposed to inhalation of low concentrations of Al_2O_2 dust. *Br J Ind Med* 48:389-391, 1991.
23. Ruiz-Esparza J, Gomez JMB, Gomez de la Torre OL: Wound care after laser resurfacing. A combination of open and closed methods using a new polyethylene mask. *Dermatol Surg* 24:79-81, 1998.
24. Suarez M, Fulton JE: A novel occlusive dressing for skin resurfacing. *Dermatol Surg* 24:567-570, 1998.
25. Rapaport MJ, Rapaport V: Prolonged erythema after facial laser resurfacing or phenol peel secondary to corticosteroid addiction. *Dermatol Surg* 25:781-785, 1999.
26. Ross EV, Amesbury EC, Basile A, et al: Incidence of postoperative infection or positive culture after facial laser resurfacing. A pilot study, a case report, and a proposal for a rational approach to antibiotic prophylaxis. *J Am Acad Dermatol* 39:975-981, 1998.
27. Alster TA, Nanis CA: Famciclovir prophylaxis of Herpes simplex virus reactivation after laser skin resurfacing. *Dermatol Surg* 25:242-246, 1999.
28. Fulton JE: Herpes simplex flare-ups following CO_2 laser resurfacing. *Am J Cosmetic Surg* 15:155-159, 1998.
29. Fulton JE: Complications of laser resurfacing: Methods of prevention and management. *Dermatol Surg* 24:91-99, 1997.
30. West TB, Alster TA: Effect of pretreatment on the incidence of hyperpigmentation following cutaneous CO_2 laser resurfacing. *Dermatol Surg* 25:90-99, 1999.
31. Ratner A, Tse Y, Marchell N, et al: Cutaneous laser resurfacing. *J Am Acad Dermatol* 41:365-389, 1999.
32. Fitzpatrick RE: Treatment of inflamed hypertrophic scars using intralesion 5-FU. *Dermatol Surg* 2:224-231, 1999.
33. Dover JS: Round-table discussion on laser skin resurfacing. *Dermatol Surg* 35:639-653, 1999.
34. Swinehart JM: Hair repair surgery: Corrective measures for improvement of older large-graft procedures and scalp scars. *Dermatol Surg* 25:523-529, 1998.
35. Bruno TG, Grecvo JF: Toxicity of local anesthetics in hair transplantation and facial plastic surgery. *Am J Cosmetic Surg* 14:453-456, 1997.
36. Coleman WB III: Noncosmetic application of liposuction. *J Dermatol Surg Oncol* 14:1085-1096, 1998.
37. Lillis PJ: Liposuction of the arms, calves and ankles. *Dermatol Surg* 23:1161-1168, 1997.

38. Lillis PJ: Liposuction of the knees, calves and ankles. *Dermatol Clin* 17:865-879, 1999.
39. Flynn TC, Narrins RS: Pre-operative evaluation of the liposuction patient. *Dermatol Clin* 17:729-734, 1999.
40. Chastain MA: A review of current concepts in tumescent liposuction. Part 2. *Cosmetic Dermatol* 15:25-34, 2002.
41. Grazier FM, deJong RN: Fatal outcomes from liposuction. *Census Group Cosmetic Surg Plast Reconstruct Surg* 105:436-446, 2000.
42. Rao RB, Ely ST, Hoffman RS: Deaths related to liposuction. *N Engl J Med* 340:1471-1475, 1999.
43. Laurence N, Clark RE, Flynn TC, et al: American Academy for Dermatologic Surgery guidelines of care for liposuction. *Dermatol Surg* 26:265-269, 2000.
44. Coleman WP III, Glogau RG, Klein JR, et al: Guidelines of care for liposuction. *J Am Acad Dermatol* 45:438-447, 2001.
45. Coleman SR: The technique of periorbital lipo-infiltration. *Operative Techniques Plast Reconstr Surg* 1:120-126, 1994.
46. Coleman SR: Facial recontouring with liposculpture. *Clin Plast Surg* 24:347-367, 1997.
47. Lewis CM: The current states of autologous fat grafting. *Aesthet Plast Surg* 17:109-112, 1993.
48. Gurney CE: Studies on the fate of free transplants of fat. *Proc Staff Meet Mayo Clin* 12:317, 1937.
49. Pinski KS: Fat transplantation autologous collagen. A decade of experience. *Am J Cosmetic Surg* 16:217-223, 1999.
50. Pinski KS: Fat transplantation and autologous collagen: A decade of experience. *Am J Cosmetic Surg* 16:217-224, 1996.
51. Drake LA, Dinehart SM, Former ER, et al: Guidelines of care for soft tissue augmentation: Fat transplantation. *J Am Acad Dermatol* 34:690-694, 1996.

Statistics of Interest to the Dermatologist

MARTIN A. WEINSTOCK, MD, PHD, AND MARGARET M. BOYLE, BS
Brown University Dermatoepidemiology Unit, Providence, RI

Morbidity and Mortality

Table   1 Reportable Infectious Diseases, United States
Table   2 AIDS/HIV: Geographic Distribution Worldwide
Table   3 AIDS: Cumulative Cases, United States
Table   4 Deaths from Selected Causes, United States
Figure 1 AIDS: Incidence Rates, United States
Table   5 Cancer Incidence, United States
Table   6 Melanoma: Incidence and Mortality, Whites, United States
Table   7 Melanoma: Five-Year Relative Survival
Table   8 Contact Dermatitis, Belgium

Health Care Delivery in the United States

Table   9 Dermatologists by Age, Sex, and Training
Table 10 Dermatologists by State
Table 11 Dermatology Trainees
Table 12 Diplomates of the American Board of Dermatology
Table 13 Physicians Certified in Dermatologic Subspecialties
Table 14 Dermatologic Outpatient Care
Table 15 Health Insurance Coverage
Table 16 Health Insurance Coverage by Family Income
Table 17 Health Maintenance Organization Market Penetration
Table 18 National Health Expenditures
Table 19 Expenditure for Consumer Advertising of Prescription Products, United States

Miscellaneous

Table 20 American Academy of Dermatology Skin Cancer Screening Program
Table 21 Leading Dermatology Journals

TABLE 1.—New Cases of Selected Reportable Infectious Diseases in the United States

	1940	1950	1960	1970	1980	1990	2000	2001*
AIDS	—	—	—	—	—	41,595	40,758	42,008†
Anthrax	76	49	23	—	1	0	1	16
Congenital Rubella	—	—	—	2	50	11	9	2
Congenital Syphilis	—	—	—	77	—	3,865	529	240
Diphtheria	15,536	5,796	918	435	3	4	1	2
Gonorrhea	175,841	286,746	258,933	600,072	1,004,029	690,169	358,995	326,346
Hansen's Disease	—	44	54	129	223	198	91	90
Lyme Disease	—	—	—	—	—	—	17,730	13,452
Measles	291,162	319,124	441,703	47,351	13,506	27,786	86	108
Plague	1	3	2	13	18	2	6	2
Rocky Mountain Spotted Fever	457	464	204	380	1,163	651	495	614
Syphilis (primary and secondary)	—	23,939	16,145	21,982	27,204	50,223	5,979	5,790
Toxic Shock Syndrome	—	—	—	—	—	322	135	128
Tuberculosis‡	102,984§	121,742§	55,494	37,137	27,749	25,701	16,377	12,294
U.S. population (millions)	132	151	179	203	227	249	281	285

Note: *Dash* indicates that data were not available.
*For 52 weeks ending December 29, 2001.
†Last update December 25, 2001.
‡Reporting criteria changed in 1975.
§Data include newly reported active and inactive cases.
(Data from Centers for Disease Control and Prevention: Summary of Notifiable Diseases, United States, 2001. *Morb Mortal Wkly Rep* 50 [51&52]:1169-1175, 2002; Centers for Disease Control and Prevention: Summary of Notifiable Diseases, United States, 2000. *Morb Mortal Wkly Rep* 49 [51&52]:1167-1174, 2001; Centers for Disease Control and Prevention: Annual summary 1984: Reported morbidity and mortality. *Morb Mortal Wkly Rep* 49 [53] [in press]; Centers for Disease Control and Prevention: Annual summary 1984: Reported morbidity and mortality. *Morb Mortal Wkly Rep* 45:1137-1141, 1996; Centers for Disease Control and Prevention: Annual summary 1984: Reported morbidity and mortality. *Morb Mortal Wkly Rep* 33:124-129, 1986; Centers for Disease Control and Prevention: Annual summary 1984: Reported morbidity and mortality. *Morb Mortal Wkly Rep* 43 [53]: 70-71, 1994.)

TABLE 2.—Acquired Immunodeficiency Syndrome and Human Immunodeficiency Virus Infection Worldwide

Estimated number of adults and children living with HIV/AIDS as of end of 2001 by region

Sub-Saharan Africa	28,100,000
South and South East Asia	6,100,000
Latin America	1,400,000
North America	940,000
East Asia and Pacific	1,000,000
Western Europe	560,000
Caribbean	420,000
Eastern Europe and Central Asia	1,000,000
North Africa and Middle East	440,000
Australia/New Zealand	15,000
TOTAL	36,260,000

Reported AIDS cases as of November 25, 2001

Africa	1,093,522
Americas	1,199,850
Eastern Mediterranean	10,007
South-Asia	193,657
Europe	251,021
Western Pacific	36,260
TOTAL	2,784,317

AFRICA

Algeria	501
Angola	6637
Benin	4957
Botswana	10,178
Burkina Faso	17,081
Burundi	25,361
Cameroon	18,986
Cape Verde	408
Central African Republic	7016
Chad	13,385
Comoros	27
Congo	40,643
Democratic Republic of the Congo	85,058
Ivory Coast	55,957
Equatorial Guinea	875
Eritrea	6873
Ethiopia	100,353
Gabon	5423
Gambia	637
Ghana	47,444
Guinea	8448
Guinea-Bissau	1160
Kenya	81,492
Lesotha	14,640
Liberia	532
Madagascar	42
Malawi	60,564
Mali	5263
Mauritania	532
Mauritius	70
Mozambique	25,024
Namibia	26,096
Niger	5598
Nigeria	54,280
Reunion	166
Rwanda	22,594
Sao Tome and Principe	89
Senegal	2912
Seychelles	41
Sierra Leone	317
South Africa	12,825
Swaziland	4787
United Republic of Tanzania	130,386
Togo	12,047
Uganda	55,861
Zambia	44,942
Zimbabwe	74,782

AMERICAS

Anguilla	5
Antigua and Barbuda	113
Netherlands Antilles	235
Aruba	37
Argentina	17,615
Bahamas	3498
Barbados	1199
Belize	393
Bermuda	424
Bolivia	217
Brazil	215,799
British Virgin Islands	20
Canada	19,153
Cayman Islands	26
Chile	3740

(Continued)

TABLE 2 (cont.)

Colombia	8433
Costa Rica	2102
Cuba	1135
Dominica	134
Dominican Republic	5440
Ecuador	1559
El Salvador	2985
French Guiana	641
Grenada	118
Guadeloupe	809
Guatemala	4233
Guyana	1615
Haiti	8902
Honduras	11,789
Jamaica	5544
Martinique	436
Mexico	47,870
Montserrat	8
Nicaragua	272
Panama	3526
Paraguay	469
Peru	9882
Saint Kitts and Nevis	68
Saint Lucia	136
Saint Vincent and the Grenadines	229
Suriname	550
Trinidad and Tobago	3384
Turks and Caicos Islands	39
United States	806,157
Uruguay	1365
Venezuela	7546

EASTERN MEDITERRANEAN

Afghanistan	—
Bahrain	82
Cyprus	137
Djibouti	1783
Egypt	314
Iran	215
Iraq	108
Jordan	95
Kuwait	66
Lebanon	147
Libyan Arab Jamahiriya	74
Morocco	913
Oman	484
Pakistan	210
Qatar	125
Saudi Arabia	414
Somalia	13
Sudan	4004
Syrian Arab Republic	71
Tunisia	541
United Arab Emirates	22
West Bank and Gaza Strip	33
Yemen	156

EUROPE

Albania	15
Austria	2127

Armenia	28
Azerbaijan	42
Belarus	28
Belgium	2846
Bulgaria	83
Bosnia and Harzagovina	35
Croatia	172
Czech Republic	151
Denmark	2325
Estonia	27
Finland	324
France	53,879
Georgia	49
Germany	20,460
Greece	2207
Hungary	389
Iceland	52
Ireland	711
Israel	707
Italy	48,488
Kazakhstan	47
Kyrgyzstan	27
Latvia	89
Lithuania	43
Luxembourg	155
Malta	51
Monaco	40
Netherlands	5423
Norway	710
Poland	1004
Portugal	8232
Republic of Moldova	33
Romania	7770
Russian Federation	451
San Marino	15
Slovakia	28
Slovenia	94
Spain	61,028
Sweden	1771
Switzerland	7207
Tajikstan	0
The Former Yugoslav Republic of Macedonia	43
Ukraine	2297
United Kingdom	17,993
Uzbekistan	11
Yugoslavia	922

SOUTHEAST ASIA

Bangladesh	10
Bhutan	3
Democratic Republic of Korea	0
India	8438
Indonesia	635
Maldives	11
Myanmar	2568
Nepal	415
Sri Lanka	93
Thailand	181,484

(Continued)

TABLE 2 (cont.)

WESTERN PACIFIC

American Samoa	1	Marshall Islands	2
Australia	8570	Micronesia (Federated States of)	4
Brunei Darussalam	18	Mongolia	2
Cambodia	9318	Nauru	0
China	1111	New Caledonia and	
Cook Islands	0	Dependencies	80
Fiji	15	New Zealand	746
French Polynesia	74	Niue	0
Guam	73	Northern Mariana Islands	5
Hong Kong Special		Palau	2
Administrative Region		Papua New Guinea	867
Of China	524	Philippines	508
Japan	2548	Samoa	8
Republic of Korea	186	Singapore	826
Kiribati	18	Solomon Islands	0
Lao People's Democratic		Tokelau	0
Republic	177	Tonga	9
Macao	21	Tuvalu	0
Malaysia	5204	Vanuatu	0
		Viet Nam	5332
		Wallis and Futuna Islands	1

(Data from World Health Organization, *Wkly Epidemiol Rec* 76:49:381-388, 2001.)

TABLE 3.—Patients With AIDS by Age Group and Exposure Category, July 2000 Through June 2001, and Cumulative Totals Through June 2001, United States

	July 2000- June 2001		Cumulative Total*	
	No.	(%)	No.	(%)
Adult/adolescent exposure category				
Men who have sex with men	13,293	(33%)	361,867	(46%)
Injecting drug use	7675	(19%)	197,091	(25%)
Men who have sex with men and inject drugs	1477	(4%)	50,066	(6%)
Hemophilia/coagulation disorder	103	(0%)	5234	(1%)
Heterosexual contact	6472	(16%)	85,738	(11%)
Receipt of blood transfusion, blood components, or tissue†	249	(1%)	8894	(1%)
Other/risk not reported or identified	11,431	(28%)	75,142	(10%)
Adult/adolescent SUBTOTAL	40,700	(100%)	784,032	(100%)
Pediatric (<13 years old) exposure category				
Hemophilia/coagulation disorder	0	(0%)	237	(3%)
Mother with/at risk for HIV infection	166	(86%)	8207	(91%)
Receipt of blood transfusion blood components, or tissue†	2	(1%)	382	(4%)
Other/risk not reported or identified	26	(13%)	168	(2%)
Pediatric SUBTOTAL	194	(100%)	8994	(100%)
TOTAL	40,894		793,026	

Note: Total includes 1 person whose sex is unknown.

*Includes persons known to be infected with human immunodeficiency virus type 2 (HIV-2). See *MMWR* 44:603-606, 1995.

†Forty-one adults/adolescents and 2 children developed AIDS after receiving blood screened negative for HIV antibody. Thirteen additional adults developed AIDS after receiving tissue, organs, or artificial insemination from HIV-infected donors. Four of the 13 received tissue, organs, or artificial insemination from a donor who was negative for HIV antibody at the time of donation. See *N Engl J Med* 326:726-732, 1992.

(Data from Centers for Disease Control and Prevention: *HIV/AIDS Surveillance Rep* 13[1]:12, 2001.)

TABLE 4.—Selected Causes of Death, United States, 1989 and 1999

Cause of Death	Number of Deaths	
	1989	1999
Malignant melanoma	6161	7215
Infections of the skin	812	983
Motor vehicle traffic accidents	46,586	40,965
Accident involving animal being ridden	106	110
Accidental drowning and submersion	4015	3529
Lightning	75	64
Homicide and legal intervention	22,909	17,287
All cancer	496,152	549,838
All causes	2,150,466	2,391,399

(Data from National Center for Health Statistics, Division of Vital Statistics. Personal communication, February 2002.)

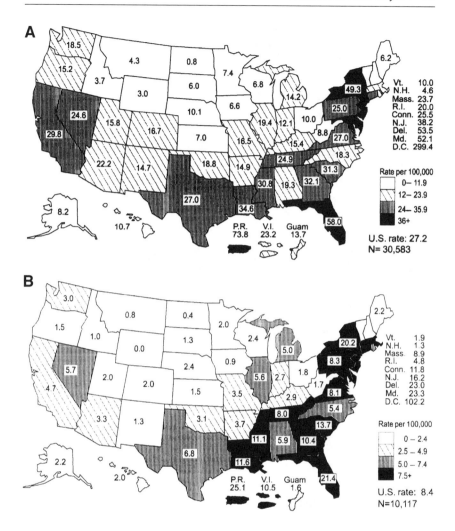

FIGURE 1.—Incidence rates of AIDS in the United States for cases reported July 2000 through June 2001, annual rates per 100,000 population. **A**, Male Adult/Adolescents; **B**, Female Adult/Adolescents. (Reprinted from Centers for Disease Control and Prevention. *HIV/AIDS Surveillance Rep*, 13[1]:10, 2001.)

TABLE 5.—Cancer Incidence in the United States: Ten Leading Sites, Both Sexes, All Ages, All Races

	Average Annual Percent Change	
	1992-1998	1973-1990
Melanomas of the skin	+2.8	+4.3
Non-Hodgkin's lymphoma	+0.1	+3.5
Breast (women only)	+1.2	+1.8
Corpus and uterus	+0.4	−2.5
Lung and bronchus	−1.6	+1.9
Leukemia	−1.4	+0.1
Urinary bladder	−0.9	+0.8
Colon/rectum	−0.7	+0.3
Oral cavity and pharynx	−1.9	−0.2
Prostate	−5.1	+3.4
All sites	−1.1	+1.2

(Data from Howe HL, Wingo PA, Thun MJ, et al: The annual report to the nation on the status of cancer, 1973-1998, featuring cancers with recent increasing trends. *J Natl Cancer Inst* 93 [11]:824-842, 2001; Ries LAG, Wingo PA, Miller DS, et al: Annual report to the nation on the status of cancer, 1973-1997, with a special section on colorectal cancer. *Cancer* 88 [10] :2398-2424, 2000; Wingo PA, Ries LAG, Rosenberg HM, et al: Cancer incidence and mortality, 1973-1985: A report card for the US. *Cancer* 82:1199, 1998.)

TABLE 6.—Melanoma Incidence and Mortality Rates Among US Whites

Year	Incidence	Mortality
1970	4.5	—
1973	6.2	1.7
1974	6.5	1.9
1975	7.2	1.9
1976	7.5	2.0
1977	8.3	2.1
1978	8.4	2.1
1979	8.9	2.2
1980	9.9	2.1
1981	10.4	2.2
1982	10.4	2.2
1983	10.2	2.3
1984	10.5	2.3
1985	11.7	2.3
1986	12.1	2.4
1987	12.3	2.4
1988	11.8	2.4
1989	12.5	2.5
1990	12.3	2.5
1991	13.2	2.5
1992	13.6	2.5
1993	13.3	2.5
1994	14.2	2.5
1995	15.2	2.5
1996	15.9	2.6
1997	16.2	2.5
1998	16.0	2.6

2002 estimate: 53,600 newly diagnosed cases and 7400 deaths

Note: Rates per 100,000 per year, and age-adjusted to the 1970 US standard population.
(Data from American Cancer Society, Inc, Surveillance Research. *Cancer Facts & Figures 2002* 4:2002; Ries LAG, Eisner MP, Kosary CL, et al [eds]: *SEER Cancer Statistics Review: 1973-1998.* National Cancer Institute, Bethesda, Md, 2001; Cutler SJ, Young JL: *Third National Cancer Survey: Incidence Data.* NCI Monogr, 41:22, 1975; National Cancer Institute. Personal communication.)

TABLE 7.—Melanoma Five-Year Relative Survival

Year	Whites	Blacks
	Year at Diagnosis	
1960-1963	60	—
1970-1973	68	—
1974-1976	80	66
1977-1979	82	51
1980-1982	83	60
1983-1985	85	76
1986-1988	88	65
1989-1996	89	70
1992-1997	89	61
	Stage at Diagnosis (1992-1997)	
Local	96	77
Regional	61	—
Distant	12	—

Notes: *Dash* indicates Insufficient data. Relative survival is the observed survival divided by the survival expected in a demographically similar subgroup of the general population. Survival estimates among blacks are imprecise because of the small numbers of cases observed.

(Data from Ries LAG, Eisner MP, Kosary CL, et al [eds]: *SEER Cancer Statistics Review: 1973-1998.* National Cancer Institute, Bethesda, Md, 2001; American Cancer Society, Inc, Surveillance Research. *Cancer Facts & Figures 2002.* 4:2002.)

TABLE 8.—Contact Dermatitis in Belgium: Proportion of Positive Patch Tests to Standard Chemicals in 363 Patients With at Least 1 Positive Reaction (Among 639 Patients Tested in 2001)

Nickel sulphate	35.5
Fragrance mix	15.7
Paraphenylenediamine	12.9
Balsam of Peru	10.7
Cobalt Chloride	8.3
Colophony	8.3
Potassium dichromate	8.3
Wool alcohols	6.3
Thiuram mix	5.2
Cl+ Me-isothiazolinone	3.3
Formaldehyde	2.7
Neomycin sulphate	2.7
Epoxy Resin	2.5
Mercapto mix	2.5
Paratertiarybutyl phenol-formaldehyde resin	2.5
Budesonide	2.2
Tixocortol pivalate	2.2
Isopropyl-phenylparaphenylenediamine	1.6
Mercaptobenzothiazole	1.6
Benzocaine	1.4
Sesquiterpene lactone mix	1.4
Paraben mix	0.8
Primin	0.5
Quaternium-15	0.5
Clioquinol	0.3

(Data from Goossens A, Universitaire Ziekenhuizen Leuven, Belgium. Personal communication, January 2002.)

TABLE 9.—Non-Federal Dermatologists by Age and Sex, 1991 and 2000

1991

Age Group	Men	Women	Total
under 35	745	716	1461
35-44	1838	805	2643
45-54	1777	265	2042
55-64	1020	88	1108
65 and older	626	32	658
TOTAL	6006	1906	7912

Country of Graduation	Men	Women
United States	7221	(91%)
Canada	119	(2%)
Other	572	(7%)
TOTAL	7912	(100%)

Board Certification	Men	Women
Certified	6376	(81%)
Not certified	1536	(19%)
TOTAL	7912	(100%)

2000

Age Group	Men	Women	Total
under 35	624	812	1436
35-44	1293	1233	2526
45-54	1892	785	2677
55-64	1582	224	1806
65 and older	956	74	1030
TOTAL	6347	3128	9475

Country of Graduation	Men	Women
United States	8905	(92%)
Canada	132	(1%)
Other	638	(7%)
TOTAL	9675	(100%)

Board Certification	Men	Women
Certified	7680	(79%)
Not certified	1995	(21%)
TOTAL	9675	(100%)

(Data from *Physician Characteristics and Distribution in the US, 2002* ed. Department of Physician Practice and Communication Information, Division of Survey and Data Resources, American Medical Association, 2002; and special tabulations. *Physician Characteristics and Distribution in the US, 1990.* Chicago, American Medical Association, 1990; and special tabulations.)

TABLE 10.—Number of Dermatologists per Million Population

State	1970		1980		1990		2000	
Alabama	13	(44)	17	(68)	18	(75)	22	(99)
Alaska	3	(1)	0	(0)	9	(5)	11	(7)
Arizona	15	(26)	27	(75)	26	(98)	31	(160)
Arkansas	9	(17)	16	(36)	20	(48)	23	(62)
California	27	(542)	34	(819)	40	(1157)	40	(1353)
Colorado	17	(38)	21	(61)	26	(91)	27	(116)
Connecticut	21	(65)	28	(87)	41	(136)	48	(162)
Delaware	11	(6)	17	(10)	15	(10)	18	(14)
District of Columbia	49	(37)	58	(37)	60	(37)	72	(63)
Florida	17	(116)	26	(55)	34	(431)	39	(628)
Georgia	13	(58)	21	(116)	24	(162)	30	(249)
Hawaii	23	(18)	26	(25)	30	(34)	33	(40)
Idaho	7	(5)	13	(12)	15	(15)	22	(29)
Illinois	16	(179)	21	(238)	24	(283)	30	(378)
Indiana	10	(54)	13	(73)	19	(104)	23	(140)
Iowa	12	(34)	18	(52)	24	(66)	27	(80)
Kansas	6	(13)	13	(30)	16	(39)	18	(53)
Kentucky	7	(23)	14	(52)	21	(79)	27	(110)
Louisiana	17	(61)	23	(97)	29	(129)	37	(164)
Maine	8	(8)	10	(11)	13	(16)	15	(19)
Maryland	14	(54)	29	(121)	39	(185)	44	(232)
Massachusetts	24	(137)	30	(173)	41	(243)	53	(335)
Michigan	16	(139)	21	(193)	27	(250)	29	(291)
Minnesota	20	(76)	24	(100)	29	(124)	36	(175)
Mississippi	7	(16)	9	(23)	11	(31)	17	(47)
Missouri	15	(70)	19	(94)	23	(120)	29	(160)
Montana	13	(9)	19	(15)	22	(18)	31	(28)
Nebraska	9	(13)	16	(25)	15	(24)	18	(30)
Nevada	12	(6)	19	(15)	20	(21)	25	(49)
New Hampshire	15	(11)	27	(25)	25	(28)	32	(39)
New Jersey	19	(134)	23	(168)	31	(245)	36	(305)
New Mexico	11	(11)	18	(23)	25	(41)	30	(55)
New York	27	(485)	31	(548)	42	(740)	50	(941)
North Carolina	13	(68)	21	(123)	26	(173)	33	(263)
North Dakota	13	(8)	12	(8)	27	(18)	26	(17)
Ohio	16	(166)	18	(196)	25	(265)	29	(327)
Oklahoma	14	(36)	16	(48)	17	(55)	21	(71)
Oregon	22	(47)	27	(71)	34	(95)	34	(118)
Pennsylvania	17	(198)	21	(247)	29	(340)	34	(421)
Puerto Rico	12	(33)	16	(51)	20	(72)	21	(81)
Rhode Island	17	(16)	28	(27)	43	(43)	61	(64)
South Carolina	7	(17)	12	(38)	21	(73)	26	(106)
South Dakota	9	(6)	0	(6)	17	(12)	25	(19)
Tennessee	11	(42)	15	(67)	22	(108)	28	(161)
Texas	15	(173)	20	(284)	23	(400)	26	(536)
Utah	13	(14)	19	(28)	25	(45)	14	(69)
Vermont	9	(4)	12	(6)	27	(15)	30	(18)
Virginia	14	(64)	22	(117)	26	(159)	28	(200)
Washington	14	(47)	22	(91)	29	(133)	28	(192)
West Virginia	8	(14)	13	(25)	13	(24)	15	(28)
Wisconsin	15	(66)	20	(93)	24	(115)	30	(162)
Wyoming	3	(1)	8	(4)	6	(3)	14	(7)
TOTAL	17	(3526)	23	(5207)	29	(7233)	34	(9473)

Note: Actual number in parenthesis.

(Data from *Physician Characteristics and Distribution in the US*, 2002 ed. Department of Physician Practice and Communication Information, Division of Survey and Data Resources, Chicago, American Medical Association, 2002, and special tabulations.)

TABLE 11.—Dermatology Trainees in the United States

Year Residency to Be Completed	Male Residents	Female Residents	Total
2002	139	175	314
2003	136	185	321
2004	153	183	336
2005	7	8	15
2006	5	2	7

(Data from American Academy of Dermatology. Personal communication, April 2002.)

TABLE 12.—Diplomates Certified by the American Board of Dermatology from 1933 to 2001

Decade Totals (Inclusive Dates)	Average Number Certified
1933-1940	69
1941-1950	74
1951-1960	76
1961-1970	112
1971-1980	247
1981-1990	271
1991-2000	295
2001	305

Year Totals	Actual Number Certified
1991	284
1992	297
1993	284
1994	308
1995	302
1996	295
1997	321
1998	294
1999	286
2000	283
2001	305
TOTAL 1933 through 2001	11,612

(Data from The American Board of Dermatology, Inc. Personal communication, February 2002.)

TABLE 13.—Physicians Certified in Dermatologic Subspecialties

Physicians Certified for Special Qualification in Dermatopathology, 1974-2001

Year	Dermatologists	Average Number Certified Pathologists	Total
1974-1975	108	44	302
1976-1980	54	49	515
1981-1985	37	34	351
1986-1990	11	14	125
		Actual Number Certified	
1991	21	18	39
1993	38	31	69
1995	39	49	88
1997	35	60	95
1998	12	27	39
1999	11	35	46
2000	11	36	47
2001	10	34	44
TOTAL 1974-2001	903	860	1763

Dermatologists Certified for Special Qualification in
Clinical and Laboratory Dermatologic Immunology, 1985-2001

Year	Number Certified
1985	52
1987	16
1989	22
1991	15
1993	5
1997	5
2001	6
TOTAL 1985-2001	121

Note: No special qualification examination for Dermatopathology was administered in 1992, 1994, and 1996. No special qualification examination in Clinical and Laboratory Dermatologic Immunology was administered in 1986, 1988, 1990, 1992, 1994, 1995, 1996, 1998, 1999, or 2000.

(Data from the American Board of Dermatology and the American Board of Pathology. Personal communication, February 2002.)

TABLE 14.—Visits to Non-Federal Office-Based Physicians in the United States, 1999
(Estimates in Thousands)

Diagnosis	Dermatologist		Type of Physician Other		All Physicians	
Acne vulgaris	5051	(15.4%)	*	*	6125	(0.8%)
Eczematous dermatitis	3432	(10.5%)	5007	(0.7%)	8439	(1.1%)
Warts	2016	(6.2%)	1959	(0.3%)	3975	(0.5%)
Skin cancer	1818	(5.6%)	1246	(0.2%)	3064	(0.4%)
Psoriasis	989	(3.0%)	*	*	1033	(0.1%)
Fungal infections	848	(2.6%)	1794	(0.2%)	2642	(0.3%)
Hair disorders	903	(2.8%)	*	*	1711	(0.2%)
Actinic keratosis	3733	(11.4%)	*	*	3746	(0.5%)
Benign neoplasm of the skin	1822	(5.6%)	1672	(0.2%)	3496	(0.5%)
All disorders	32,704	(100%)	724,029	(100%)	756,734	(100%)

Note: Percentage of visits for all disorders is in parentheses.
*Figure does not meet standard of reliability or precision.

(Data from the National Ambulatory Medical Care Survey 1999, National Center for Health Statistics, Centers for Disease Control and Prevention. Personal communication, February 2002.)

TABLE 15.—Health Insurance Coverage of the United States Population, 2000

	1-17 Years (%)	Adults Aged 18-64 Years (%)	Adults Aged 65 Years and Over (%)
Individually purchased insurance	8	6	28
Employer-provided private insurance	63	69	34
Public insurance, any type	23	10	97
Medicaid	20	6	10
No health insurance	12	18	1

Note: Some individuals have both public and private insurance, so the numbers will not add to 100%.
(Data from the Employee Benefit Research Institute, Washington, DC. Personal communication, January 2002.)

TABLE 16.—Nonelderly Population With Selected Sources of Health Insurance, by Family Income, 2000

Yearly Family Income Level	Employment-Based Coverage %	Individually Purchased %	Public %	Uninsured %	Total %
under $5000	15	12	37	40	100
$5000-$9999	15	11	52	27	100
$10,000-$14,999	24	11	36	34	100
$15,000-$19,999	38	10	28	30	100
$20,000-$29,999	53	8	19	25	100
$30,000-$39,999	67	7	13	17	100
$40,000-$49,999	74	6	10	14	100
$50,000 and over	86	5	5	8	100
TOTAL	67	7	14	16	100

Note: Details may not add to totals because individuals may receive coverage from more than one source.
(Data from Fronstin P, Employee Benefit Research Institute, Washington, DC. March 2002.)

TABLE 17.—Health Maintenance Organization (HMO) Market Penetration in the United States, January 1, 2001

HMO Penetration in Region	
Northeast	41%
Mid-Atlantic	35%
South Atlantic	26%
East South Central	24%
West South Central	20%
East North Central	25%
West North Central	30%
Mountain	34%
Pacific	49%
National	32%

HMO Penetration Top Ten Most Highly Penetrated Metropolitan Statistical Areas	
Jackson, Tenn	72%
Sacramento, Calif	72%
San Francisco, Calif	70%
Oakland, Calif	68%
Rochester, NY	68%
Vallejo-Fairfield-Napa, Calif	66%
Buffalo-Niagara Falls, NY	64%
New Haven-Meriden, Conn	64%
Madison, Wis	63%
Stockton-Lodi, Calif	61%

(Data from The InterStudy Competitive Edge: *Regional Market Analysis* 11.2 [January 1, 2001:15,19], InterStudy Publications, St Paul, Minn. Personal communication, February 2002.)

TABLE 18.—National Health Expenditures 1970 Compared With 2000

Spending Category	Billions of Dollars (%)			
	1970		2000*	
Total national expenditures	73	(100)	1316	(100)
Health services and supplies	68	(93)	1276	(97)
Personal health care	64	(87)	1151	(88)
Hospital care	28	(39)	424	(33)
Physician services	14	(19)	259	(20)
Dental services	28	(6)	60	(5)
Other professional services	1	(2)	78	(6)
Home health care	0	(<1)	36	(3)
Drugs and other medical nondurables	9	(12)	146	(11)
Prescription drugs	6	(8)	112	(8)
Other nondurable medical products	3	(5)	33	(3)
Vision products and other medical durables	2	(2)	15	(1)
Nursing home care	4	(6)	94	(7)
Other personal health care	1	(2)	40	(3)
Program administration and net cost of private health insurance	3	(4)	75	(5)
Government public health activities	1	(2)	50	(4)
Research and construction	5	(8)	41	(3)
Research†	2	(3)	21	(2)
Construction	3	(5)	20	(2)

*Figures for 2000 are projections. Numbers may not add to totals because of rounding. The health spending projections were based on the 1997 version of the National Health Expenditures (NHE) released in November 1998. Subsequent release of the NHE may not be consistent with these projections and should not be substituted for the 1997 historical estimates.
†Research and development expenditures of drug companies and other manufacturers and providers of medical equipment and supplies are excluded from research expenditures but are included in the expenditure class in which the product falls.
(Data from National Health Expenditures and Selected Economic Indicators, Levels and Average Percent Change: Selected Years, Office of the Actuary, Health Care Financing Administration, 1998.)

TABLE 19.—Spending on Consumer Advertising of Prescription Products, United States

Year	Dollars (in Millions)
2001	2479
2000	2150*
1999	1590
1998	1173
1997	844
1996	595
1995	313
1994	242
1993	165
1992	156
1991	56
1990	48
1989	12

*Estimated.
(Data from CMR, A Taylor Nelson Sofres Co. Personal communication, March 2002.)

TABLE 20.—Results of the American Academy of Dermatology Skin Cancer Screening Program, 1985-2001

Year	Number Screened	Suspected Diagnosis		
		Basal Cell Carcinoma	Squamous Cell Carcinoma	Malignant Melanoma
1985	32,000	1056	163	97
1986	41,486	3049	398	262
1987	41,649	2798	302	257
1988	67,124	4457	474	435
1989	78,486	6266	761	593
1990	98,060	7959	1069	872
1991	102,485	8110	1193	1062
1992	98,440	8403	1280	1054
1993	97,553	7067	1068	2465*
1994	86,895	6908	1235	1010
1995	88,934	7503	1317	1353
1996	94,363	8713	1656	1399
1997	99,554	8730	1685	1469
1998	89,536	6687	1308	1078
1999	89,916	5790	1136	635
2000	65,854	5074	1053	653
2001	70,562	5192	1102	642
TOTAL	1,342,897	103,762	17,200	15,336

*Number of cases included melanoma, "rule-out melanoma," and lentigo maligna.
(Data from American Academy of Dermatology: *2001 Skin Cancer Screening Program Statistical Summary Report*, March 2002.)

TABLE 21.—Leading Dermatology Journals

Journal	Total Citations in 2000	Number of Articles Published in 2000
Acta Dermato-Venereologica	3001	79
American Journal of Dermatopathology	1527	89
Annales de Dermatologie et de Venereologie	1136	206
Archives of Dermatology	10,589	206
Archives of Dermatological Research	1893	86
British Journal of Dermatology	9918	371
Clinics in Dermatology	728	65
Clinical and Experimental Dermatology	1476	137
Contact Dermatitis	3232	296
Current Problems in Dermatology	6	62
Cutis	1257	148
Dermatologic Clinics	1228	72
Dermatologic Surgery	1537	228
Dermatology	3041	210
European Journal of Dermatology	550	139
Experimental Dermatology	654	53
Hautarzt	1077	141
International Journal of Dermatology	2400	159
Journal of the American Academy of Dermatology	12,190	410
Journal of Cosmetic Science	9	9
Journal of Cutaneous Pathology	1371	90
Journal of Dermatological Science	562	92
Journal of Dermatological Treatment	155	50
Journal of the European Academy of Dermatology	224	55
Journal of Investigative Dermatology	15,329	304
Leprosy Review	482	34
Melanoma Research	986	71
Mycoses	1011	77
Pediatric Dermatology	1072	107
Photodermatology, Photoimmunology, and Photomedicine	471	50

(Data from *Journal Citation Reports on CD-ROM:JCR*, Science ed. Philadelphia, Institute for Scientific Information, 2000.)

CLINICAL DERMATOLOGY

1 Urticarial and Atopic Disorders

Methotrexate-Responsive Chronic Idiopathic Urticaria: A Report of Two Cases
Gach JE, Sabroe RA, Greaves MW, et al (Royal Berkshire and Battle Hosps, Reading, UK; St Thomas' Hosp, London)
Br J Dermatol 145:340-343, 2001   1–1

Background.—Chronic idiopathic urticaria (CIU) can be severe, and patients with this disorder can be difficult to treat. It is well known that about one third of patients with CIU have autoantibodies to the high-affinity IgE receptor or against IgE. Two patients who were responsive to methotrexate are discussed.

Case 1.—Woman, 42, sought medical attention for angioedema and severe urticaria beginning 1 week after a tetanus shot. Angioedema episodes occurred daily, with facial and throat swelling. Urticaria wheals lasted less than 24 hours and left no residual discoloration. Attacks of urticaria involved fever, bone pain, arthralgias, myalgias, eye soreness, breathlessness, and prostration. Her history included intermittent attacks of urticaria in childhood. The patient had no detectable autoantibodies, and administration of antihistamines was not effective. Other unsuccessful treatments included dapsone and doxepin. The CIU was controlled with methotrexate therapy.

Case 2.—Man, 37, reported an 8-month history of severe urticaria. Prednisolone, 50 mg daily, was necessary for symptomatic control. The patient had urticarial wheals daily, occurring at any site, lasting for 24 to 48 hours, and finally resolving with no discoloration. The urticaria was unresponsive to antihistamines, doxepin, and to a low salicylate, dye, and preservative-free diet. He had weekly attacks of lip swelling, yet he had no history of angioedema. No functional autoantibodies were detected. Methotrexate was required in addition to his other drugs to prevent relapse.

Conclusions.—These 2 patients with CIU had no detectable autoantibodies and were unresponsive to standard therapies. Control of disease was achieved ultimately with methotrexate.

▶ There never seem to be enough treatment alternatives for chronic idiopathic urticaria. Cyclosporine has been used for patients with autoantibodies against the high-affinity IgE receptor or against IgE. Neither of the 2 patients in the current report who responded to methotrexate had detectable autoantibodies.

B. H. Thiers, MD

Effect of Omalizumab on Symptoms of Seasonal Allergic Rhinitis: A Randomized Controlled Trial
Casale TB, for the Omalizumab Seasonal Allergic Rhinisitis Trial Group (Creighton Univ, Omaha, Neb; et al)
JAMA 286:2956-2967, 2001   1–2

Introduction.—Treatments currently available for seasonal allergic rhinitis include allergen avoidance, pharmacotherapy, and immunotherapy. For some patients, however, these therapeutic options fail to control symptoms. A recently developed recombinant humanized monoclonal anti-immunoglobulin (Ig)E antibody (omalizumab) blocks the binding of IgE to mast cells and basophils and lowers free IgE levels in the circulation. The efficacy of omalizumab was evaluated in a multicenter trial.

Methods.—A total of 536 of 959 screened patients from 25 centers throughout the United States met eligibility criteria and were randomly assigned to receive omalizumab (50, 150, or 300 mg) or placebo. Patients ranged in age from 12 to 75 years and had no or mild symptoms during the month before study entry but had at least a 2-year history of moderate to severe ragweed-induced seasonal allergic rhinitis. Baseline IgE levels ranged from 30 to 700 IU/mL. Doses of omalizumab or placebo were administered subcutaneously just before the start of ragweed season and repeated every 3 weeks (for a total of 4 treatments in patients with baseline IgE levels of 151 to 700 IU/mL) or every 4 weeks (for a total of 3 treatments in patients with baseline IgE levels of 30 to 150 IU/mL). Patients kept a daily diary to record symptom severity and duration scores. Rescue antihistamines could be used for severe symptoms, and patients were permitted limited use of decongestants and eye drops. Blood samples were obtained during and after treatment to measure IgE levels.

Results.—Patients who received 300 mg of omalizumab had significantly lower nasal symptom severity scores over the entire pollen season than those given placebo. Compared with the placebo group, patients in the 300 and 150 omalizumab groups had a significantly greater percentage of days with minimal nasal symptoms and required rescue antihistamine or concomitant medications on significantly fewer days. There was a significant association between IgE reduction and symptom improvement.

Conclusion.—For patients with seasonal allergic rhinitis, omalizumab lowered serum free IgE levels and consistently improved nasal symptom severity scores. The 300-mg dose of omalizumab was most effective.

▶ Omalizumab is a humanized monoclonal antihuman IgE antibody that binds specifically to the region of the IgE molecule that binds to the IgE receptor on mast cells or basophils. This interferes with binding of IgE to these cells and the concomitant release of pharmacologically active mediators. Casale et al report that administration of omalizumab to patients with allergic rhinitis decreased serum-free IgE levels and provided clinical benefit in a dose-dependent fashion. As noted in an editorial by Plaut that accompanied the article, the results provide strong evidence that IgE is essential to the pathogenesis of allergic rhinitis.[1] Hopefully, omalizumab will be used to explore the role of IgE in other diseases, eg, asthma and atopic dermatitis. Other biological agents under development for the treatment of allergic diseases include cytokine antagonists and molecules that block IgE antibody production.

B. H. Thiers, MD

Reference

1. Plaut M: Immune-based, targeted therapy for allergic diseases. *JAMA* 286:3005-3006, 2001.

Eradication of *Helicobacter pylori* and Improvement of Hereditary Angioneurotic Oedema

Farkas H, Füst G, Fekete B, et al (Semmelweis Univ, Budapest, Hungary; Hungarian Academy of Sciences, Budapest, Hungary; Natl Inst of Haematology and Immunology, Budapest, Hungary)

Lancet 358:1695-1696, 2001   1–3

Background.—A deficiency of C1-esterase inhibitor can lead to the development of hereditary angioneurotic edema. Various factors can trigger flares of the disease. *Helicobacter pylori* infection may be one of these factors. A screening program was developed to evaluate the frequency of *H pylori* infection in patients with hereditary angioneurotic edema. In addition, an attempt was made to correlate the occurrence of edematous episodes with the presence of this infection.

Methods.—In 65 patients with hereditary angioneurotic edema, the serum concentration of immunoglobulin G antibodies to *H pylori* was determined. All patients who had a positive *H pylori* result underwent the carbon-14–urease breath test. The infection was successfully eradicated in 18 patients.

Results.—*H pylori* infection was detected in 19 of the 65 patients, all of whom had a history of recurrent episodes of acute abdominal pain. Eleven of the 46 patients who were not infected also reported this history. Patients with the infection were significantly older than those not infected. The frequency of acute abdominal pain in infected patients was significantly higher than in noninfected patients after adjusting for age. After the infection was eradicated, only 1 patient in that group reported acute abdominal pain during the 2 to 25 months of follow-up. After eradication, the patients' C4- and C1-esterase inhibitor concentrations were significantly elevated.

Conclusion.—The presence of *H pylori* infection appeared to trigger exacerbations of acute hereditary angioneurotic edema. The mechanism may be activation of the humoral immune response against *H pylori*, which depletes C1-esterase inhibitor levels. The result may be uncontrolled activation of complement and other plasma enzyme systems. Thus, in patients with hereditary angioneurotic edema, screening for *H pylori* infection and its eradication may be justified.

▶ Infection with *H pylori* has been proposed as a causal factor for a number of dermatologic conditions including rosacea, urticaria, and atopic dermatitis.[1] A similar role has been suggested in patients with recurrent attacks of hereditary angioneurotic edema.[2] Although the findings of Farkas et al are far from definitive, screening for *H pylori* infection and eradication of the bacteria, if present, seem to be justified in patients with unexplained exacerbations of the disease.

B. H. Thiers, MD

References

1. Wedi B, Wagner S, Werfel T, et al: Prevalence of *Helicobacter pylori*-associated gastritis in chronic urticaria. *Int Arch Allergy Immunol* 116:288-294, 1998.
2. Rais M, Unzeitig J, Grant JA: Refractory exacerbations of hereditary angioedema with associated *Helicobacter pylori* infection. *J Allergy Clin Immunol* 103:713-714, 1999.

Prevalence of Atopic Dermatitis, Asthma, Allergic Rhinitis, and Hand and Contact Dermatitis in Adolescents: The Odense Adolescence Cohort Study on Atopic Diseases and Dermatitis

Mortz CG, Lauritsen JM, Bindslev-Jensen C, et al (Odense Univ, Denmark)
Br J Dermatol 144:523-532, 2001   1–4

Introduction.—Atopic diseases are common in children and adolescents, but epidemiologic knowledge is sparse regarding hand eczema and allergic contact dermatitis in these age groups. No population-based investigations have assessed the prevalence of atopic diseases and hand and contact dermatitis in the same group of adolescents. The prevalence of atopic dermatitis (AD), asthma, allergic rhinitis, and hand eczema was estimated in a cross-sectional investigation of an unselected population of adolescents in the Odense municipality of Denmark.

Methods.—A total 1501 eighth-grade students (ages 12-16 years) underwent interviews, clinical examinations, and patch testing.

Results.—The lifetime prevalence of AD was 21.3% (girls, 25.7%; boys, 17.0%; $P < .001$) according to the questionnaire-based criteria. The age at onset was less than 2 years in 45.4% of the children, between 2 and 5 years in 22.5%, and more than 5 years in 31.4% of the children. The 1-year period prevalence and the point prevalence (Hanifin and Rajka criteria) of AD were 6.7% and 3.6%, respectively. The lifetime prevalence of hand eczema based on the questionnaire was 9.2%, 1-year prevalence was 7.3%, and the point prevalence was 3.2%, with significant predominance in girls (4.2% vs 2.2%). A significant correlation was seen between AD and inhalant allergy and between AD and hand eczema according to lifetime prevalence measures. The point prevalence of contact allergy was 15.2% (girls, 19.4%; boys, 10.3%; $P < .001$). Present or past allergic contact dermatitis was identified in 7.2% (11.3% of the girls vs 2.5% of the boys). Positive tests were most frequently seen for nickel (8.6%) and fragrance mix (1.8%).

Conclusion.—Adolescent research subjects had a high prevalence of AD, hand eczema, and allergic contact dermatitis, and the diseases were closely related. A notable gender difference was observed for hand eczema and allergic contact dermatitis. Nickel allergy and perfume allergy were the main contact allergies.

▶ This study addresses the prevalence of AD, asthma, allergic rhinitis, hand dermatitis, and contact dermatitis in eighth grade students in the Danish community of Odense. A surprisingly high percentage (96%) of the 1501 eligible students and their parents agreed to participate in the study. The estimated lifetime prevalence of AD (21.3%) was comparable to that reported in other recent studies. The onset of disease occurred before the age of 5 years in two thirds of the students; other investigators have reported such early onset in a larger proportion of patients. The 1-year period prevalence of AD in these eighth graders was 6.7%. Many of the children with persistent AD also reported inhalant allergies.

This appears to be the first report of patch testing in a large number of unselected adolescents. Of the students tested, 7.2% had clinically relevant positive patch test results. Nickel and perfumes were the most common allergens, and significantly more girls than boys had positive test reactions.

S. Raimer, MD

Environmental Associations With Eczema in Early Life

Harris HM, Cullinan P, Williams HC, et al (Imperial College of Science and Technology, London; Queen's Med Centre, Nottingham, England)
Br J Dermatol 144:795-802, 2001   1–5

Introduction.—Family studies support a strong association between parental atopy and eczema, yet less is known about the influence of other factors such as diet and environment. A cohort of children recruited before birth was monitored for 2 years to determine the role of dietary and environmental factors in the development of atopic eczema.

Methods.—All newly pregnant women initially seen at 3 general practices in England between November 1993 and July 1995 were invited to participate. Information from either the first or second annual visit was available for 624 children (97% of the original cohort). A family history of allergic disease was recorded, and parents had skin prick tests to common aeroallergens performed. Home visits at 8 weeks included a collection of dust samples from the living room floor and the child's bed. Breast-feeding and infant feeding practices were also examined.

Results.—With the use of United Kingdom diagnostic criteria, the cumulative prevalence of atopic eczema by the age of 2 years was 14%. Almost half (45%) of mothers, however, reported that their child had ever had eczema, and the prevalence of maternally reported doctor-diagnosed eczema was 31%. Visible dermatitis was recorded for 69 children (11%) at either annual visit. Maternal associations were stronger than paternal for both parental history of allergic disease and parental atopy. There was a significant association between eczema in an older sibling and eczema in the study child. Rates of atopy and allergic history were found to increase with increasing maternal education and less crowding in homes, and these associations remained significant after controlling for other factors. Breast-feeding did not appear to protect against the development of eczema. Food intolerance was significantly more likely to be reported by mothers of children with visible dermatitis and maternally reported eczema.

Conclusion.—Environmental factors as well as family history influence the development of eczema in the first 2 years of life. Early exposure to infection, which occurs in more crowded houses with more older siblings, may offer protection against the development of eczema.

▶ Data from this large prospective study indicate that a child born to a well-educated mother and taken to live in an uncrowded home is disadvantaged, at least from the standpoint of being more likely to have atopic dermatitis (AD) develop. This is especially true for firstborn children. No protection from breast-feeding was noted and, somewhat surprisingly, children without eczema were actually exposed to higher concentrations of dust mites than those with the disease. The authors suggest that their data are compatible with the theory that frequent early infections, which are more likely to occur in crowded conditions, may offer some protection against the development of AD. Obviously, conclusive data to explain the increasing incidence of AD in industrialized countries are still lacking. Hopefully, future studies like this will help elucidate factors that aggravate AD, as well as those that may be protective against the development of the disease.

S. Raimer, MD

Exposure to Farming in Early Life and Development of Asthma and Allergy: A Cross-Sectional Survey
Riedler J, and the ALEX Study Team (Children's Hosp Salzburg, Austria; et al)
Lancet 358:1129-1133, 2001   1–6

Background.—Growing up on a farm has been reported to protect against allergic sensitization and the development of childhood allergic diseases. Whether increased exposure to microbial compounds must occur early in life to affect immune system maturation and reduce the risk for developing allergic diseases was investigated.

Methods.—A cross-sectional survey involving 3504 parents of 6- to 13-year-old children in rural Austria, Germany, and Switzerland was conducted. Seventy-five percent of the parents completed a standardized questionnaire on asthma, hay fever, and atopic eczema. Serum measurements of specific IgE antibodies to common allergens were taken from children from farming and nonfarming families who gave consent.

Findings.—Exposure to stables and consumption of farm milk among children younger than 1 year, compared with those aged 1 to 5 years, was associated with lower frequencies of asthma (1% and 11%, respectively), hay fever (3% and 13%, respectively), and atopic sensitization (12% and 29%, respectively). Continual long-term exposure to stables for children younger than 5 years correlated with the lowest frequencies of asthma (0.8%), hay fever (0.8%), and atopic sensitization (8.2%) (Table 3).

Conclusions.—These findings are consistent with previous reports of a lower frequency of asthma, hay fever, and atopic sensitization in children growing up on farms. Long-term, early-life exposure to stables and farm milk is associated with a strong protective effect against the development of these conditions.

▶ The authors present yet another bit of evidence that farm upbringing provides a measure of protection against allergic sensitization and development of childhood allergic diseases. Regular contact with farm animals has been shown to confer an important protective effect in such an environment.[1,2] It has been hypothesized that contact with endotoxins and other microbial compounds regulates various processes in the immune system, such as the production of interleukin 12 and interferon gamma. These factors might select against T-helper-2 cells and thus counteract allergic sensitization by leading to T-helper-1 cell dominance.

B. H. Thiers, MD

TABLE 3.—Frequency and Risk (Adjusted* Odds Ratio, 95% CI) of Asthma, Hay Fever, and Atopic Sensitization in Relation to Farming Activity of Pregnant Mothers in Farmers' Children Exposed to Stables and Farm Milk in the 1st Year of Life

	Pregnant Mother Active Daily on Farm (n=119)	Pregnant Mother Not Active Daily on Farm (n=58)	Pregnant Mother Not Active Daily on Farm and Child Not Exposed to Stable and Farm Milk in 1st Year (n=28)
Asthma diagnosis	0%	2% (1)	14% (4)
	..	0·02 (0·001-0·47)	Reference
At least one wheeze attack in past 12 months	1% (1)	3% (2)	7% (2)
	0·04 (0·001-1·30)	0·17 (0·01-2·51)	Reference
Hay fever	1% (1)	7% (4)	11% (3)
	0·07 (0·005-0·91)	0·43 (0·06-2·87)	Reference
Runny nose and itchy eyes in past 12 months	1% (1)	12% (7)	14% (4)
	0·04 (0·003-0·53)	0·61 (0·13-2·87)	Reference
Atopic sensitization†	8% (10)	19% (11)	39% (11)
	0·18 (0·06-0·56)	0·36 (0·12-1·08)	Reference

*Adjusted for age, sex, study area, parental education, family history of asthma and hay fever, and number of older siblings.
†Any reaction to inhalent allergens (house dust and storage mites, cat dander, grass and birch pollen, cow epithelium) of ≥3.5 kU/L.
(Courtesy of Riedler J, and the ALEX Study Team: Exposure to farming in early life and development of asthma and allergy: A cross-sectional survey. *Lancet* 358:1129-1133, 2001. Copyright by The Lancet, Ltd, 2001.)

References

1. Riedler J, Eder W. Oberfeld G, et al: Austrian children living on a farm have less hay fever, asthma and allergic sensitization. *Clin Exp Allergy* 30:194-200, 2000.
2. Von Ehrenstein OS, von Mutius E, Illi S, et al: Reduced risk of hay fever and asthma among children of farmers. *Clin Exp Allergy* 30:187-193, 2000.

Exposure to Endotoxin Decreases the Risk of Atopic Eczema in Infancy: A Cohort Study

Gehring U, Bolte G, Borte M, et al (Inst of Epidemiology, Neuherberg, Germany; Ludwig-Maximilians-Univ of Munich; Univ of Leipzig, Germany; et al)

J Allergy Clin Immunol 108:847-854, 2001   1–7

Background.—There has been a worldwide increase in the prevalence of asthma, with large regional differences. It has been suggested that hygiene standards in developed societies may be partially responsible for the increase in atopic disease in these populations. In studies that investigated this hypothesis, endotoxin was considered a potential marker for the level of hygiene. Previous studies have demonstrated that a protective effect accrues from early exposure to cats and dogs with respect to the development of atopic eczema, asthma, allergic rhinitis, and atopic sensitization later in life. This study investigated the association between bacterial endotoxin in house dust and atopic eczema, infections, and wheezing in the first year of life.

Methods.—The study group consisted of neonates from 2 large German cities (Munich and Leipzig). Data were analyzed from 1884 term and normal-weight neonates, including information regarding exposure to biocontaminants and confounding variables. Samples of house dust from the mattresses of the infants and their mothers were obtained 3 months after birth. A chromogenic kinetic limulus amoebocyte lysate test was used to quantify the endotoxin content.

Results.—The risk of atopic eczema was significantly decreased in the first 6 months of life by endotoxin exposure in dust from the mothers' mattresses in the fifth quintile. In contrast, the risk in the first 6 months of life for respiratory infections, bronchitis, or both, was increased. There was also a significant increase in the risk of wheezing in the first 6 months of life by endotoxin exposure in dust from the mothers' mattresses. These associations attenuated for the entire first year of life, with the exception of the risk of wheezing, which remained significant.

Conclusions.—These findings are supportive of the contention that exposure to high concentrations of endotoxins in the first months of life may provide protection against the development of atopic eczema and increase the prevalence of nonspecific respiratory diseases in the first 6 months of life.

▶ The results support those of other recent studies, suggesting that exposure to high concentrations of endotoxin very early in life might protect against the development of atopic dermatitis and that the hygiene standards of modern societies may be responsible, in part, for the increased incidence of atopic diseases in these populations.[1]

B. H. Thiers, MD

Reference

1. von Mutius E, Braun-Fahrlander C, Schierl R, et al: Exposure to endotoxin or other bacterial components might protect against the development of atopy. *Clin Exp Allergy* 30:1230-1234, 2000.

Probiotics in Primary Prevention of Atopic Disease: A Randomised Placebo-controlled Trial
Kalliomäki M, Salminen S, Arvilommi H, et al (Univ of Turku, Finland; Natl Public Health Inst, Turku, Finland)
Lancet 357:1076-1079, 2001   1–8

Introduction.—Proof of an inverse relationship between infections early in life and atopy has led to renewed interest in the hygiene hypothesis, which attributes an increase in the frequency of atopic diseases to reduced microbial exposure in early life. It may be that specific microbes in the commensal gut microflora are more important than sporadic infections in the prevention of atopic disease. Probiotics are cultures of potentially beneficial bacteria of the healthy gut microflora, including *Lactobacillus rhamnosus*. This strain has proved safe at an early age and effective in the treatment of allergic inflammation and food allergy. The effect of *Lactobacillus* GG given prenatally to mothers and postnatally for 6 months to their infants at high risk for atopic diseases was examined in a double-blind, randomized, placebo-controlled investigation.

Methods.—The only inclusion criteria was family history of atopic disease. Families were recruited from antenatal clinics between February 1997 and January 1998. One hundred fifty-nine females were randomly assigned to receive either 2 capsules of placebo (microcrystalline cellulose) or 1×10^{10} colony-forming units of *Lactobacillus* GG daily for 2 to 4 weeks before expected delivery. After delivery, breast-feeding mothers could take the capsules or children received capsule contents mixed with water and administered by spoon. Infants were evaluated during the neonatal period and at ages 3, 6, 12, 18, and 24 months. The outcome measure was atopic disease at age 2 years.

Results.—At age 2 years, 46 of 132 (35%) children had atopic eczema. Six of these children were diagnosed with asthma and 1 was diagnosed with allergic rhinitis. The incidence of atopic eczema in the probiotic group was half that of the placebo group (15/64, 23% vs 31/68, 46%; relative risk, 0.51 [95% CI, 0.32-0.84]); number needed to treat was 4.5 (95% CI, 2.6-15.6).

Conclusion.—Gut microflora have unique, although greatly unexplored, endogenous immunomodulatory properties. These properties may be indispensable in the fight against the increasing incidence of atopic, and perhaps other, immunologic diseases.

▶ Cultures of potentially beneficial bacteria of the gut microflora are referred to as probiotics. Kalliomäki and associates report that perinatal administration of a gram-positive probiotic, *Lactobacillus* GG, decreased by half the subsequent occurrence of eczema in at-risk infants. As discussed by Murch in a commentary that accompanied this article, several factors need to be considered.[1] The first is safety. Sporadic cases of septicemia have been reported, although these have occurred most often in immunodeficient patients.[2] Moreover, athymic nude mice given probiotics have experienced excess mortality compared with similarly treated immunodeficient adult mice.[3] Timing may also be an issue; in this study, the probiotic was given to the mothers for 2 weeks before delivery and then to the infants from birth for 6 months. This regimen likely increased concordance between infant and maternal flora. It has been shown that the first bacteria to colonize a previously sterile gut may establish a permanent niche, and while it is usually necessary in older children and adults to maintain chronic administration of probiotic organisms, intake from birth may induce long-term carriage at higher concentrations than if given later. Finally, it must be appreciated that eczema may result from a variety of causes, and it is unlikely that the regimen described here will be universally effective. The data presented by Kalliomäki and associates are truly exciting. The exact mechanisms by which probiotics may affect atopic disease remains speculative, and confirmatory data are anxiously awaited.

B. H. Thiers, MD

References

1. Murch SH: Toll of allergy reduced by probiotics. *Lancet* 357:1057-1059, 2001.
2. Salminen S, von Wright A, Morelli L, et al: Demonstration of safety of probiotics: A review. *Int J Food Microbiol* 44:93-106, 1998.
3. Wagner RD, Warner T, Roberts L, et al: Colonization of congenitally immunodeficient mice with probiotic bacteria. *Infect Immun* 65:3345-3351, 1997.

▶ This placebo-controlled study showed that perinatal administration of a gram-positive probiotic, *Lactobacillus rhamnosus* (*Lactobacillus GG*), halved the subsequent occurrence of eczema in at-risk infants. If confirmed by other studies, administration of probiotics in the perinatal period would represent an important advance in the prevention of this disease. The results were superior to those previously reported with administration of probiotics later in life. Larger studies to assess efficacy and safety issues will be required before these agents can be routinely used. Although probiotics generally have a favorable safety profile, there have been sporadic cases of adverse effects, such as septicemia and liver abscesses, in immunodeficient patients.[1]

The secret of successful immunotherapy for atopic dermatitis may rest in its timing. During the past century, there have been marked qualitative and quantitative changes in initial gut bacterial colonization, and real differences exist in intestinal flora between allergy-prone infants in the developed world and neonates in underprivileged countries. The dominance of bifidobacteria and lactobacilli in the initial flora of the infant in the developing world increasingly has been replaced by a variety of hospital-acquired organisms. It is notable that the first bacteria to colonize a previously sterile gut may establish a permanent niche and put later arrivers at a competitive disadvantage. Specific input from fecal flora to the neonatal immune system is essential for establishment and maintenance of mucosal immune tolerance.[2] Certain bacteria such as lactobacilli may induce enterocytes and immune cells to produce T-helper 1 (Th1) cytokines, which may in turn help to downregulate mucosal inflammatory responses.

A minority of patients with atopic dermatitis responds to dietary manipulation. It is not known whether the infants who responded to probiotics in this study represent a subgroup of the disease, or whether eczema in nonresponders evolves through a different pathogenetic mechanism. Further studies will be required to confirm the efficacy of probiotics, to determine the appropriate dosage and duration of treatment, and to determine whether single or multiple organisms should be given. If other studies prove this approach to be safe and effective, manipulation of initial gut bacterial colonization may be an important breakthrough in disease prevention.

S. Raimer, MD

References

1. Salminen S, von Wright A, Morelli L, et al: Demonstration of safety of probiotics—a review. *Int J Food Microbiol* 44:93-106, 1998.
2. Murch SH: The immunological basis for intestinal food allergy. *Curr Opin Gastroenterol* 16:552-557, 2000.

Double-blind Placebo-controlled House Dust Mite Control Measures in Adult Patients With Atopic Dermatitis

Gutgesell C, Heise S, Seubert S, et al (Univ of Göttingen, Germany)
Br J Dermatol 145:70-74, 2001   1–9

Introduction.—Evidence that eliminating house dust mites can reduce skin symptoms in patients with atopic dermatitis is limited, and the few published trials have yielded conflicting results. To further examine the issue, a house dust mite control study randomly assigned patients to placebo or an active treatment regimen.

Methods.—Participants were 11 women and 9 men aged 18 to 30 years. All had moderate to severe atopic dermatitis and sensitization to the house dust mite *Dermatophagoides pteronyssinus*. Excluded were patients with pets. Active treatment consisted of using polyurethane bed coverings that were allergen-impermeable and an acaricide spray. A water spray and allergen-permeable mattress coverings were provided to the control group. During the 12-month study, disease severity was scored every 2 months and eosinophil cationic protein in the serum determined by enzyme-linked immunosorbent assay. Patients used a visual analogue scale to assess daytime pruritus and pruritus-induced sleeplessness. Mattress dust samples were collected and analyzed for the house dust mite antigen Der p1.

Results.—Compared with the control group, the active treatment group showed a statistically significant reduction in Der p1 exposure at the end of the study. But as measured by SCORAD and serum eosinophil cationic protein, no statistically significant differences between active treatment and control groups were apparent in terms of change from the start to the end of the study. Some patients in the active treatment group reported a reduction in pruritus-induced sleeplessness.

Conclusion.—Among these young adult patients with atopic dermatitis, 1 year of house dust mite avoidance reduced allergen exposure but failed to improve overall disease activity. Patients likely continued to have contact with irritants and allergens other than house dust mites.

▶ Eedy has reviewed the controversy surrounding the role of house dust mites in the pathogenesis of atopic dermatitis.[1] A study of young children with extrinsic-type atopic dermatitis found that house dust mite allergen avoidance is associated with significant improvement in atopic dermatitis,[2] whereas another more recent study suggested that increased exposure to house dust mites early in life actually offers a protective effect against the disease (see Abstract 1–5). Other investigators have claimed that the introduction of house dust mite avoidance measures in the first months of life to children at risk helps prevent house dust mite sensitization and, especially, the development of asthma.[3,4]

B. H. Thiers, MD

References

1. Eedy DJ: What's new in atopic dermatitis? *Br J Dermatol* 145:380-384, 2001.
2. Ricci G, Patrizi A, Specchia F, et al: Effect of house dust mite avoidance measures in children with atopic dermatitis. *Br J Dermatol* 143:379-384, 2000.
3. Werfel T, Kapp A: Environmental and other major provocation factors in atopic dermatitis. *Allergy* 53:731-739, 1998.
4. Platts-Mills TAE: The role of allergens in allergic airway disease. *J Allergy Clin Immunol* 101:S364-S366, 1998.

Association Between Atopic Dermatitis and Insulin-Dependent Diabetes Mellitus: A Case-Control Study

Olesen AB, Juul S, Birkebæk N, et al (Univ of Aarhus, Denmark)
Lancet 357:1749-1752, 2001   1–10

Background.—Atopic dermatitis in childhood is characterized by a Th2 immune reactivity pattern, in which increased IgE production is associated with low production of interferon-γ and increased production of interleukin-4. In contrast, insulin-dependent diabetes mellitus (IDDM) appears to follow a Th1 immune reactivity pattern. It was postulated that atopic dermatitis and IDDM may have a reciprocal relationship, in that children with one condition would be unlikely to have the other. This hypothesis was tested in a case-control study.

Methods.—The case group consisted of 920 children aged 3 to 15 years with IDDM who were identified from the Danish Registry for Childhood Diabetes. The control group consisted of a random sample of 9732 children aged 3 to 15 years without diabetes who were registered in the Danish Medical Birth Registry. All patients and their families completed a questionnaire to ascertain the onset of IDDM and the incidence and onset of atopic dermatitis.

Results.—The cases were significantly less likely to have atopic dermatitis than were the controls (13.1% vs 19.8%). The incidence of atopic dermatitis in the controls was 1375 cases per 57,432 person-months. Among the cases, the incidence of atopic dermatitis before the development of IDDM was 73 cases per 5314 person-months, which was significantly lower than the incidence rate in controls (odds ratio, 0.49). Among cases who developed atopic dermatitis after their diagnosis of IDDM, however, the incidence rate did not differ significantly from that in controls (24 cases per 2956 person-months; odds ratio, 1.36).

Conclusions.—In children up to 15 years of age, the cumulative incidence of atopic dermatitis among children with IDDM was only about two thirds of that among nondiabetic control children. Differences in acquired or inherited reactivity patterns associated with atopic dermatitis and IDDM may help explain these findings.

▶ IDDM is thought to be a Th1-mediated disease. In contrast, atopic dermatitis displays a Th2 immune reactivity pattern. Because a reciprocal relation exists between Th1 and Th2 immune responses, the authors speculated that the 2 conditions are unlikely to coexist in the same person. Although the incidence of atopic dermatitis did appear to be decreased in children with IDDM, the 2 conditions were by no means mutually exclusive.

B. H. Thiers, MD

The Ascomycin Macrolactam Pimecrolimus (Elidel, SDZ ASM 981) Is a Potent Inhibitor of Mediator Release From Human Dermal Mast Cells and Peripheral Blood Basophils

Zuberbier T, Chong S-U, Grunow K, et al (Humboldt Univ, Berlin; Novartis Forschungs Institut, Vienna)

J Allergy Clin Immunol 108:275-280, 2001   1–11

Background.—Type I allergic diseases occur frequently in the general population, and their prevalence appears to be increasing. Mast cells and basophils are the primary effector cells in these diseases, and most therapeutic approaches have focused on antagonizing the effects of mast cell—derived mediators, particularly histamine. Cyclosporin A and tacrolimus have been described as having a direct inhibitory effect on mast cell mediator release at higher concentrations, but their pharmacologic profile limits their usefulness. The ascomycin macrolactam pimecrolimus has been developed as a new cell-selective inhibitor of inflammatory cytokine secretion. Pimecrolimus has fewer adverse effects than currently available drugs. The ability of pimecrolimus to directly inhibit in vitro mediator release from human skin mast cells and basophils was investigated in this study.

Methods.—Purified cutaneous mast cells or basophil-containing peripheral blood leukocytes were obtained from a group of healthy human donors. The samples were then preincubated with pimecrolimus in the absence or presence of its specific antagonist (rapamycin), cyclosporin A, or dexamethasone. The mast cells and leukocytes were then stimulated with anti-IgE or calcium ionophore A23187 plus phorbol myristate acetate. Cell supernatants were analyzed for histamine, tryptase, LTC4, and tumor necrosis factor (TNF)-α.

Results.—Pimecrolimus induced a strong, dose-dependent inhibition of anti-IgE–induced release of histamine from mast cells (maximally 73%) and basophils (maximally 82%) and of mast cell tryptase (maximally 75%), as well as a less-significant inhibition of LTC4 (maximally 32%) and strong inhibition of calcium ionophore plus phorbol myristate acetate–induced release of mast cell TNF-α (maximally 90% at 100 nmol/L pimecrolimus). In comparison, the maximal inhibition obtained during mast cell histamine release was 60% with cyclosporin A and only 28% with dexamethasone.

Conclusions.—Pimecrolimus was shown to have a significant inhibitory effect on mediator release from human mast cells and basophils, with a potency exceeding that of cyclosporin A and of dexamethasone. These findings suggest that pimecrolimus may be an effective treatment for patients with mast cell–dependent and basophil-dependent diseases.

SDZ ASM 981: An Emerging Safe and Effective Treatment for Atopic Dermatitis

Luger T, van Leent EJM, Graeber M, et al (Univ of Muenster, Germany; Univ of Amsterdam; Novartis Pharma AG, Basel, Switzerland; et al)
Br J Dermatol 144:788-794, 2001   1–12

Introduction.—The first ascomycin macrolactam derivative under development for the treatment of inflammatory skin diseases in SDZ ASM 981, a selective inhibitor of the production of pro-inflammatory cytokines from T cells and mast cells in vitro. High anti-inflammatory activity is observed in vivo with SDZ ASM 981 in mouse and pig models of allergic contact dermatitis after topical application. The efficacy and safety of 4 concentrations of SDZ ASM 981 cream were examined in the treatment of atopic dermatitis to ascertain the optimal concentration in terms of safety and efficacy.

Methods.—Two hundred sixty adult patients were recruited for this double-blind, randomized, parallel group, multicenter, dose-finding trial. Patients were randomly assigned to SDZ ASM 981 treatment with concentrations of 0.05%, 0.2%, 0.6%, 1.0% or matching vehicle cream, or the internal control of 0.1% betamethasone-17-valerate cream (BMV). Patients were treated twice daily for up to 3 weeks. Dermatitis was examined on days 1, 8, 15, and 22 with use of an adapted Eczema Area Severity Index (EASI). Pruritus was evaluated separately with use of a score ranging from 0 to 3 (none, 0; mild, 1; moderate, 2; and severe, 3).

Results.—Sixty-one patients discontinued treatment prematurely, mostly because of adverse events or lack of a therapeutic response. In 15 patients, treatment was ceased because of worsening of dermatitis at the treated area. The median EASI score diminished during treatment in the 0.2%, 0.6%, 1.0%, and BMV-treated groups (Fig 1). The greatest reduction was observed in patients treated with BMV, followed by the SDZ

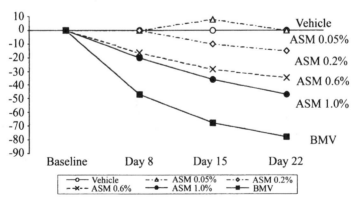

FIGURE 1.—EASI: median percentage change from baseline (intent-to-treat population). *Abbreviations: EASI*, Eczema Area Severity Index; *BMV*, 0.1% betamethasone-17-valerate cream. (Courtesy of Luger T, van Leent EJM, Graeber M, et al: SDZ ASM 981: An emerging safe and effective treatment for atopic dermatitis. *Br Dermatol* 144:788-794, 2001. Reprinted by permission of Blackwell Science, Inc.)

ASM 981 1.0% and 0.6% groups. Differences at the end point between vehicle and 1.0%, 0.6%, and 0.2% SDZ ASM 981 creams were significant (*P* = .008, .001, and .041, respectively). The 0.05% SDZ ASM 981 cream did not have a significant therapeutic effect. All treatments were less effective in patients with more severe disease. Pruritus was improved in all groups. Patients' assessment of their atopic dermatitis revealed that a higher proportion were moderately clear or better (greater than 50% improvement) in the SDZ ASM 981 1.0%, 0.6%, and 0.2% groups (53.3%, 54.8%, and 32.6%, respectively); for the BMV treatment group, this rate was 88.1%.

Conclusion.—Topical SDZ ASM 981 cream was well-tolerated and effective in improving atopic dermatitis.

First Experience of Topical SDZ ASM 981 in Children With Atopic Dermatitis

Harper J, Green A, Scott G, et al (Great Ormond Street Hosp for Children, London; Novartis Pharma AG, Basel, Switzerland; Novartis Research Centre, Horsham, England)
Br J Dermatol 144:781-787, 2001   1–13

Introduction.—The effectiveness and safety of newly developed SDZ ASM 981 cream has not been examined in the pediatric age group. This first pediatric open and noncontrolled trial of SDZ ASM 981 was designed to assess the systemic exposure to SDZ ASM 981 in young children with atopic dermatitis treated over extensive skin areas.

Methods.—Ten children aged 1 to 4 years with at least 10% of their total body surface area (BSA) affected by atopic dermatitis were treated twice daily for 3 weeks with 1% SDZ ASM 981 cream to all affected areas, including the head and neck. Oral or topical corticosteroids and emollients containing an active ingredient were not allowed. Patients were evaluated with use of the Eczema Area and Severity Index (EASI) on days 1, 4, 10, and 22 and 1 week after treatment completion.

Results.—The range of affected BSA was 23% to 69% at baseline. The EASI decreased a mean of 8.7 (*P* = .052). It improved by 8% to 89% from the baseline score at completion of 3 weeks of treatment, and a consistent recurrence was observed at the evaluation point 1 week after completing treatment. No serious adverse events occurred. Two patients discontinued treatment because of a flare of atopic dermatitis not controlled by the study medication. Of 63 SDZ ASM 981 blood concentrations assessed, 63% were less than 0.5 ng/mL; the maximum value was 1.8 ng/mL. No accumulation was observed between days 4 and 22.

Conclusion.—In young children with extensive lesions of atopic dermatitis treated twice daily for 3 weeks with 1% SDZ ASM 981 cream, blood concentrations of SDZ ASM 981 were consistently low, even in patients with the most extensive BSAs treated (up to 69%). The drug did not accumulate during the treatment period. No systemic effects were observed. The range of SDZ ASM 981 blood concentrations was comparable to that of adults.

▶ Hot on the heels of tacrolimus comes SDZ ASM 981. Indications from these 2 very short-term studies (Abstracts 1–12 and 1–13) suggest an efficacy comparable to a medium-strength topical steroid. Clearly, more data need to be obtained to determine its potential as a long-term treatment for atopic dermatitis.

B. H. Thiers, MD

Narrow-Band Ultraviolet B and Broad-Band Ultraviolet A Phototherapy in Adult Atopic Eczema: A Randomised Controlled Trial
Reynolds NJ, Franklin V, Gray JC, et al (Univ of Newcastle upon Tyne, England; Univ of Teesside, Middlesbrough, England; Newcastle Gen Hosp, England)
Lancet 357:2012-2016, 2001   1–14

Introduction.—Narrow-band ultraviolet B (UVB) is effective in the treatment of psoriasis. Open trials have indicated that this form of treatment may improve atopic eczema. The efficacy of narrow-band UVB and broad-band UVA as second-line, adjunctive treatments was assessed in adult patients with moderate to severe atopic eczema in a randomized, controlled, double-blind investigation.

Methods.—Between April 1995 and November 1997, 73 patients with ages ranging from 15 to 65 years were randomly assigned to 12 weeks of twice-weekly whole-body phototherapy with either narrow-band UVB, UVA, or visible fluorescent light. Treatment with very potent topical steroids was not allowed for 2 weeks before trial entry or during the evaluation period. However, patients were allowed to use emollients and moderate to potent topical steroids. The main end points were change in total disease activity and change in extent of disease from baseline to 24 treatments. Secondary end points included physician global evaluation, patient assessment of itch and loss of sleep, and quantities of topical steroid used.

Results.—The mean decreases in total disease activity over 24 treatments were 9.4 and 4.4 points, respectively, more than visible light for patients who received narrow-band UVB and UVA. Compared with visible light, the mean decreases in the extent of disease after 24 treatments were 6.7% for narrow-band UVB and −1.0% for those who received UVA. A small proportion of patients experienced erythema after phototherapy or had a flare in their eczema sufficient to withdraw from therapy.

Conclusion.—Narrow-band UVB phototherapy is effective and mostly well-tolerated as an adjunctive therapy for adults with moderate to severe atopic eczema.

▶ This study examined the usefulness of 2 forms of phototherapy, narrow-band UVB and broad-band UVA, as second-line adjunctive treatments for adult patients with moderate to severe atopic eczema. The improvement was modest, with narrow-band UVB being somewhat better than broad-band UVA. On a more positive note, improvements in physician global assessment and total disease activity were maintained 3 months after the discontinuation of phototherapy. Unfortunately, there was no significant reduction in the use of moderate to potent topical steroids with narrow-band UVB treatment.

B. H. Thiers, MD

▶ The effect of narrow-band UVB phototherapy in treating diseases such as psoriasis has been clearly demonstrated. In this study of patients with atopic dermatitis, the response to narrow-band UVB was better than that obtained with UVA phototherapy. The relative ease with which narrow-band UVB therapy can be administered (compared with PUVA) makes this a very appealing adjunct in the treatment of atopic dermatitis. Moreover, some patients now have access to home narrow-band UVB units, allowing treatment for those who live too far from a referral center to make hospital or office-based phototherapy a realistic option. The long-term safety profile of narrow-band UVB phototherapy for patients with atopic dermatitis still needs to be assessed.

K. Schwarzenberger, MD

Mycophenolate Mofetil Is Effective in the Treatment of Atopic Dermatitis
Grundmann-Kollmann M, Podda M, Ochsendorf F, et al (Johann Wolfgang Goethe-Univ, Frankfurt/Main, Germany)
Arch Dermatol 137:870-873, 2001   1–15

Background.—The current treatments for atopic dermatitis (AD) are not entirely satisfactory and are associated with severe adverse effects. A new agent, mycophenolate mofetil, was evaluated for its usefulness in managing moderate to severe AD.

Methods.—The 10 patients were treated in a university hospital dermatology department for moderate to severe AD that had been unresponsive to standard treatments. Mycophenolate mofetil, 1 g, was given orally 2 times each day for 4 weeks. Beginning with the fifth week, 500 mg was given twice a day through the eighth and final week. Follow-up extended for 20 weeks. Outcome was evaluated with the use of the subjective SCORing Atopic Dermatitis (SCORAD) index every 2 weeks.

Results.—Mycophenolate treatment markedly reduced the severity of AD within 4 weeks in all the patients evaluated. Before treatment, the mean SCORAD index was 49.2; after the full 8 weeks, it had decreased to 21.9. For the patients who completed the trial, the SCORAD index was reduced 74%. One patient discontinued therapy after 4 weeks because of the development of herpes retinitis, but the other patients had no adverse effects. During the course of the 20-week follow-up, 6 patients had no relapse.

Conclusions.—Mycophenolate is a highly effective treatment for moderate to severe AD that is unresponsive to standard therapy. Long-term effects remain to be evaluated.

▶ The authors assert that mycophenolate mofetil seems to have an improved risk-benefit ratio compared with the unwanted adverse effects associated with systemic steroids, azathioprine, or cyclosporine. While this may be true over the short-term, the long-term side effects of mycophenolate mofetil are still unknown. On a more positive note, remission in response to mycophenolate mofetil seemed to be long lasting, suggesting the possibility of intermittent rather than continuous therapy.

B. H. Thiers, MD

Systemic Ketoconazole Is an Effective Treatment of Atopic Dermatitis With IgE-Mediated Hypersensitivity to Yeasts
Lintu P, Savolainen J, Kortekangas-Savolainen O, et al (Univ of Turku, Finland)
Allergy 56:512-517, 2001   1–16

Background.—Yeasts have been associated with atopic dermatitis (AD), possibly acting as allergens or as triggering factors for elevated IgE antibody production and positive skin prick test reactions. Treatment for AD has involved the use of oral ketoconazole therapy to reduce the intensity of the disorder. The efficacy of antifungal treatment was assessed with the use of oral ketoconazole, with results monitored by measurement of yeast-specific IgE levels and saprophytic yeast growth.

Methods.—The AD patients chosen had positive radioallergosorbent (RAST)/skin prick tests for *Pityrosporum ovale* and/or *Candida albicans*. Either ketoconazole or placebo was given for 30 days and yeast growth on the skin and in the pharynx was monitored, along with total serum IgE levels and severity of the eczema. Follow-up testing was done 1 and 3 months after beginning treatment.

Results.—Of the 75 patients who completed the study, 74 had AD on the head, neck, or shoulder areas, 25 on the trunk, and 64 on the extremities. Those receiving ketoconazole had a statistically significant improvement from the first to the second visit. Specific parameters that improved included disease activity (erythema, papulation, excoriation, dryness, crusts, and lichenification), itching, and extent of dermatitis. No significant changes occurred in the placebo group. The extent of the dermatitis also decreased significantly in those receiving placebo. Those receiving ketoconazole and those receiving placebo had improved scores at the third visit, but the use of topical ketoconazole may have confounded the results. Women who had positive yeast cultures clearly benefited from therapy; men did not. Patients whose skin cultures grew *P ovale* at the beginning of the trial and who received ketoconazole had significant improvement; a less significant association was noted with *C albicans*. The eczema improved with ketoconazole significantly more than with placebo when total IgE levels were below 5000 kU/L; in patients with higher IgE levels, clinical parameters did not change significantly. Positive *P ovale* saprophytic cultures were significantly reduced when ketoconazole was used, but only a minor decrease was seen with placebo. Two months after treatment, the percentage of cultures that were positive for *P ovale* and *C albicans* returned to nearly pretreatment levels. No significant changes occurred in the yeast-RAST levels during the 3 months of treatment.

Conclusions.—Patients with AD who have positive yeast cultures and elevated IgE levels to yeasts may benefit from antifungal therapy, specifically ketoconazole. Significant improvement was seen during the course of 3 months of therapy.

▶ The role of microbial agents in causing and perpetuating AD has long been debated; in particular, the role of staphylococcal toxins has been extensively studied. This article attempts to characterize the role of IgE-mediated hypersensitivity to yeasts in patients with AD. The authors identified 80 patients with AD who showed evidence of IgE-mediated hypersensitivity to *C albicans* or *P ovale*. The patients were treated with ketoconazole or placebo, and a significant number in the treatment group showed clinical improvement. This would have been a more convincing study with an additional control group: patients with AD who had no evidence of yeast hypersensitivity.

K. Schwarzenberger, MD

2 Contact Dermatitis

Comparison of Patch Test Results With a Standard Series Among White and Black Racial Groups
Dickel H, Taylor JS, Evey P, et al (Rheinisch-Westfälische Technische Hochschule, Aachen, Germany; Cleveland Clinic Found, Ohio)
Am J Contact Dermatitis 12:77-82, 2001   2–1

Background.—Environmental, cultural, occupational, genetic, individual, and racial differences are important factors in the study of contact dermatitis. Some epidemiologic studies have compared overall sensitization rates among different racial groups, but similar data are lacking on individual allergens.

Objective.—Determine differences in sensitization rates between 2 racial groups in North America undergoing patch testing over a period of 4 years at the Cleveland Clinic Foundation (CCF), Ohio.

Methods.—Retrospective computer review of the standard screening tray results of 991 patients with an average age of 45.9 years consisting of 877 (88.5%) whites and 114 (11.5%) blacks.

Results.—Nickel sulfate and thiomersal (both 8.0%) and nickel sulfate and p-phenylenediamine (both 10.6%) were the 2 most common sensitizers among whites and blacks, respectively. There was a statistically significant difference ($P = .00599$) in the sensitization rate for p-phenylenediamine in blacks (10.6%) compared with whites (4.5%). There were also statistically significant differences in sensitization rates for p-phenylenediamine (21.2%; $P = .00005$) and imidazolidinyl urea in petrolatum (pet.) (9.1%; $P = .04103$) in black men compared with white men (p-phenylenediamine [4.2%] and imidazolidinyl urea [2.6% pet.]).

Conclusion.—The differences in sensitization rates, especially for p-phenylenediamine, may reflect variations in allergen exposure among racial groups or interindividual variations in the N-acetylation (N-acetyltransferase 1 [NAT1] and 2 [NAT2]) capacities of human skin for p-phenylenediamine.

▶ Does race have an effect on the development of allergic contact dermatitis? This retrospective study of almost 1000 patch-tested individuals showed a statistically significant higher sensitization rate for p-phenylenediamine in blacks than in whites. In addition, black men had slightly higher sensitization rates for imidazolidinyl urea than white men. The authors question whether these changes reflect differences in allergen exposure or, in the case of *p*-phenylenediamine, variations in the N-acetylation capacities of skin. This study failed to confirm several earlier reports that had suggested higher sensitivity rates to other allergens and also did not confirm an earlier study that suggested that white skin might be more susceptible to sensitization with less-potent allergens. What is quite interesting is that of the almost 1000 patients tested, the overwhelming majority, 88.5%, were white. It would be interesting to learn the racial mix of the clinic and whether black patients seen there had less allergic contact dermatitis or are simply patch-tested less frequently. Additional prospective studies might further our knowledge of this subject.

K. Schwarzenberger, MD

Patch Testing of Nickel Sulfate and Potassium Dichromate With a Standardized Ready-to-Use Test System Gives Highly Reproducibile Results: A Double-blind Multicentre Study
Brasch J, Henseler T, Aberer W, et al (Univ of Kiel, Germany; Univ of Graz, Austria; Univ of Göttingen, Germany; et al)
Acta Derm Venereol 81:122-124, 2001   2–2

Background.—Patch testing is the standard for the diagnosis of cutaneous delayed-type hypersensitivity, but questions remain about reliability and reproducibility. The intraindividual reproducibility of patch testing was evaluated using a commercially available system (TRUETest) with the use of a randomized, placebo-controlled, double-blind study design.

Study Design.—Thirteen centers contributed 589 patients with a history of nickel allergy, who were tested with nickel sulfate and potassium dichromate with the use of the TRUETest system. Each patient was tested simultaneously with 2 randomized strips. The patch test results were read on days 2 and 3 by members of the German Contact Dermatitis Research Group who were blinded as to patch test strip contents. Patch-test reproducibility and the reaction index (RI) were calculated.

Findings.—Of the 589 patients in the study group, 388 responded to nickel sulfate and 130 to potassium dichromate. The reproducibility of positive responses to nickel was 99.2%. For nickel sulfate the reaction index was 0.91, but it was only 0.23 for potassium dichromate, indicating many more questionable reactions.

Conclusions.—The findings of this study demonstrate that an appropriately standardized patch test system can deliver highly reproducible results. Nickel patch testing with the TRUETest system appears to be quite satisfactory, whereas the potassium dichromate patch test with the same system could be improved. Patch test reliability and reproducibility needs to be separately assessed for each allergen and test system.

Patch Testing Discordance Alert: False-Negative Findings With Rubber Additives and Fragrances
Sherertz EF, Fransway AF, Belsito DV, et al (Wake Forest Univ, Winston-Salem, NC; Fort Myers, Fla; Univ of Kansas, Kansas City; et al)
J Am Acad Dermatol 45:313-314, 2001   2–3

Background.—This report described false-negative readings occurring with fragrance mix, balsam of Peru, and the rubber additives, thiuram and carba mixes, when patch tests are performed with the TRUETest system (Glaxo Wellcome, Cary, NC).

Study Design.—From 1996 through 1998, the North American Contact Dermatitis Group examined 318 patients for suspected dermatitis by simultaneously patch testing with Hermal allergens using Finn Chambers (Epitest Ltd Oy, Tuusula, Finland) and the TRUETest allergen system. Patients were evaluated at 48, 72, 96, and 168 hours for patch test interpretation.

Findings.—There was a discrepancy between the results with the 2 patch test systems for screening allergens. This was most prominent with fragrance and rubber allergens. The Finn Chambers system was much more sensitive for the detection of sensitivity to balsam of Peru, fragrance, thiuram, and carba mix allergens.

Conclusion.—The findings indicate that use of the commercially available TRUETest system might lead to false-negative interpretations of allergen sensitivity, especially to balsam of Peru, thiuram, and carba mix allergens. When TRUETest patch screening results are negative and allergic contact dermatitis is suspected, a trial of allergen avoidance is probably still warranted. More extensive testing with the Finn Chambers technique should also be considered.

▶ For many years, standard patch testing involved the use of Finn Chambers, in which allergens were occluded on the skin by small metal chambers. The use of Finn Chambers was considered time consuming by many clinicians. In the past decade, a commercially available, ready-to-use test system, TRUETest, became available. With TRUETest, the allergens are prepared in a hydroxypropylcellulose gel base, which allows release of the allergen upon contact with the skin. The reproducibility of patch test results between these 2 systems has been questioned, as was the case in both studies (Abstracts 2–2 and 2–3) reviewed here. What can be concluded is that the reproducibility of patch test results between the Finn Chambers and the TRUETest systems varies depending on the allergen. The false-negative results reported for rubber additives and fragrances with the TRUETest system suggest that additional testing should be considered if clinical suspicion of allergy remains high despite negative testing.

K. Schwarzenberger, MD

Changing Frequency of Thiuram Allergy in Healthcare Workers With Hand Dermatitis

Gibbon K, McFadden JP, Rycroft RJG, et al (Whipps Cross Hosp, London; St Thomas' Hosp, London; King's College London)
Br J Dermatol 144:347-350, 2001   2–4

Background.—Hand dermatitis is seen among health care workers, with the use of natural rubber latex gloves acting as a major route by which these individuals become sensitized to rubber accelerators. Among the most common of these accelerators are the thiurams and the carbamates, which are often implicated in type IV reactions. Data were collected during a 16-year period to document the frequency of type IV thiuram allergy among health care workers with hand dermatitis.

Methods.—A retrospective analysis of the data showed that 1269 health care workers were tested, with 450 having primary hand dermatitis. Patients underwent patch testing to thiuram mix 1% in petrolatum to confirm the diagnosis, and their occupation was noted as a relevant factor. All were health care workers complaining of hand dermatitis. The frequency of thiuram-positivity in housewives having hand dermatitis was also assessed.

Results.—Of the 352 female and 98 male health care workers, 12% (56 patients) had a positive patch test for thiuram. A peak incidence of 27% was noted among the patients tested in 1994. Among health care workers who did not complain of hand dermatitis, thiuram-positive results were found in 3.6%. Of the 630 housewives with hand dermatitis, 7% had a positive patch test for thiuram, and the peak incidence was in 1988 (13%). The number of thiuram-positive results was significantly increased among those tested between 1989 and 1993. Among housewives, the number of thiuram-positive results tended to decrease with time but not at a significant rate. Because this trend was opposite to that noted in the health care workers, the increased numbers among health care workers are significant. In the later 1990s, the incidence of thiuram allergy declined. Only 5 health care workers had a positive reaction to 2-mercaptobenzothiazole (MBT), and 2 reacted positively to mercapto mix.

Conclusions.—More than 33% of the health care workers suffered hand dermatitis, and the number of positive results to thiuram testing tended to increase among health care workers while it decreased among housewives. Allergy to thiuram among health care workers with hand dermatitis increased to a significant degree, with a peak in the early 1990s.

▶ This interesting study documents the incidence of delayed-type hypersensitivity reactions to thiuram in health care workers with hand dermatitis during a long study period of 16 years. Gibbon et al demonstrates a significant increase in thiuram allergy with time, peaking in 1994. The incidence now appears to be declining. The authors speculate that the increasing incidence of thiuram allergy correlated with frequent use of powdered latex gloves in the 1980s and early 1990s, when universal precautions were adopted. It is interesting to note that while our awareness of latex allergy has, in general, increased during the past decade, the increased incidence of thiuram allergy may have gone unnoticed. This could become clinically relevant, as some institutions are minimizing their risk of latex allergy by switching to widespread use of nonlatex gloves. It is important to recognize that some synthetic rubber gloves, while free of natural latex rubber, may contain thiurams or other additives. Individuals with glove-related dermatitis might be best evaluated with both patch and prick testing.

K. Schwarzenberger, MD

Results of Evaluating Health Care Workers With Prick and Patch Testing
Holness DL, Mace SR (Univ of Toronto)
Am J Contact Dermatitis 12:88-92, 2001   2–5

Introduction.—Health care workers are exposed to many agents that are potential causes of irritant contact dermatitis (ICD), allergic contact dermatitis (ACD), and contact urticaria (CU). Few studies, however, have reported cases in which workers were assessed for these 3 problems simultaneously. The prevalence of ICD, ACD, and CU was examined in a retrospective chart review of health care workers referred for skin problems.

Methods.—Over the 2-year period from 1994 to 1996, 55 health care workers referred for work-related contact dermatitis were both patch tested and prick tested. Questionnaires completed at the time of patch testing provided information on demographic characteristics, medical history, use of gloves, symptoms, treatment, and workplace and other exposures.

Results.—The average age of the health care workers was 39; 86% were women and 45% were nurses. Glove use was almost universal at work, and approximately half of the group used gloves at home. Rubber gloves were the type most often worn at both work and home. The average duration of skin problems was 40 months. Common findings were itchy, red, scaly rashes on the hands. Prick testing with latex yielded a positive response in 27% of workers, and 51% had at least 1 positive response to patch testing. Final diagnoses (considered work-related in 95% of cases) were ICD in 61%, ACD in 31%, and CU in 27%; 11% of these health care workers had both ACD related to thiuram and CU related to latex. Individuals with a positive latex prick test had high rates of nasal (90%) and ocular (70%) symptoms and some (10%) experienced wheeze and systemic symptoms.

Discussion.—Health care workers with skin problems should undergo both patch testing and prick testing. In the group of workers reviewed here, 11% had both ACD and CU. Patients with CU sometimes described features typical of either an ICD or ACD, and these 2 conditions could not be differentiated by history alone. In testing for latex sensitivity, the possibility of inducing an anaphylactic response should be considered.

▶ Occupational skin disease, particularly contact dermatitis of the hands, is common in health care workers. Identifying the cause, particularly distinguishing between ACD and ICD, can be challenging. Dermatologists often offer patch testing to help identify ACD; however, this article suggests that prick testing should also be a standard part of the evaluation of workers who use latex products. Latex allergy, which often presents with immediate hypersensitivity, may be missed if patch testing alone is performed; likewise, contact allergies can be missed if only prick testing or serological testing for latex allergy is performed in individuals with hand or other dermatitis. Because many dermatologists do not perform prick testing, working closely with an allergist can enhance patient care.

K. Schwarzenberger, MD

A Preliminary Report of the Occupation of Patients Evaluated in Patch Test Clinics
Rietschel RL, Mathias CGT, Taylor JS, et al (Ochsner Clinic, New Orleans, La)
Am J Contact Dermatitis 12:72-76, 2001   2–6

Background.—The interplay between the occupational environment and worker's skin can result in contact dermatitis of both irritant and allergic types. Other forms of dermatitis can also be influenced by occupational exposures.

Objective.—The aim of this study is to compare the occupations and allergens of occupational contact dermatitis cases with nonoccupational contact dermatitis cases.

Methods.—Diagnostic patch testing with allergens of the North American Contact Dermatitis Group and occupational coding by the National Institute for Occupational Safety and Health methods.

Results.—Of 2889 patients referred for evaluation of contact dermatitis, 839 patients (29%) were found to have occupational contact dermatitis. Of the 839 cases deemed occupational, 455 cases (54%) were primarily allergic in nature and 270 cases (32%) were primarily irritant in nature. The remaining 14% were diagnoses other than contact dermatitis, aggravated by work. The occupation most commonly found to have allergic contact dermatitis was nursing. Allergens strongly associated with occupational exposure were thiuram, carbamates, epoxy, and ethylenediamine.

Conclusion.—Some contact allergens are more commonly associated with occupational contact dermatitis. Nursing and nursing support are occupations most likely to be overrepresented in contact dermatitis clinics.

▶ Who is at risk for contact dermatitis? This study suggests that nurses and nursing support staff are very likely to have dermatitis that results in their referral to a contact dermatitis clinic. Perhaps not surprisingly, mechanists and manual laborers also are at risk for occupationally related dermatitis. These patients were evaluated only by patch testing, and it might have been worthwhile to include prick testing to evaluate for latex allergy, particularly in those involved in nursing.

K. Schwarzenberger, MD

Dental Metal Allergy in Patients With Oral, Cutaneous, and Genital Lichenoid Reactions
Scalf LA, Fowler JF Jr, Morgan KW, et al (Univ of Louisville, Ky)
Am J Contact Dermatitis 12:146-150, 2001   2–7

Introduction.—Oral lichen planus (LP) is a well-recognized condition that is often considered to be idiopathic. Some studies have suggested that oral LP or lichenoid lesions (LL) in patients with allergy to dental metals improves significantly after their dental work is removed. Most of these reports have focused on allergy to mercury or gold salts. The role of dental metals in oral LP or LL was further investigated, evaluating a wider range of dental metals and including patients with cutaneous or genital LP.

Methods.—The study included 51 patients with a history of LP or LL (34 women, 17 men; mean age, 56). Thirty-four had oral LP; 13 had genital LP; and 35 had cutaneous LP, including 13 with isolated cutaneous disease. Mean duration of LP was nearly 9 years. The patients underwent patch-testing using allergens to a wide range of dental metals. After testing,

---

TABLE 1.—Positive Patch Test Results for the Entire Test Group

Positive Final Readings (n = 51)

	Percent (No.)	*P*-Value	NACDG Percent Allergic (1996-1998)
Potassium dichromate 0.25% pet.	9.8% (5)	0.028*	2.8%
Cobalt chloride 5% pet.	15.7% (8)	0.169	9.0%
Copper sulfate 2% pet.	3.9% (2)		NT
Gold sodium thiosulfate 0.5% pet.	19.6% (10)	0.041*	9.5%
Indium (III) sulfate 10.0% aq.	3.9% (2)		NT
Iridium (III) chloride hydrate 1.0% aq.	3.9% (2)		NT
Mercury 0.5% pet.	7.8% (4)		NT
Nickel sulfate hexahydrate 2.5% pet.	15.7% (8%)	0.896	14.2%
Palladium chloride 1% pet.	17.7% (9)		NT
Phenylmercuric acetate 0.05% pet.	27.5% (14)		NT
Silver nitrate 1% aq.	3.9% (2)		NT
Thimerosal 0.1% pet.	25.5% (13)	0.005†	10.9%
One or more mercury-containing compounds (mercury, phenyl-mercuric acetate, and/or thime-rosal)	49.0% (25)		Information not available

*P < .05
†P < .01
Abbreviations: NACDG, North American Contact Dermatitis Group; *pet*, in petrolatum; NT, not tested; *aq*, in water.
(Courtesy of Scalf LA, Fowler JF Jr, Morgan KW, et al: Dental metal allergy in patients with oral, cutaneous, and genital lichenoid reactions. *Am J Contact Dermatitis* 12:146-150, 2001.)

patients were offered the opportunity to replace their dental work. The 1-year follow-up results were evaluated by telephone survey.

Results.—About three fourths of patients with oral LP tested positive to 1 or more dental metals (Table 1). Comparison with patients patch-tested by the North American Contact Dermatitis Group found a higher prevalence of positive reactions to chromate, cobalt, gold, nickel, and thimerosal in patients with oral LP. The difference was significant for chromate, gold, and thimerosal. Patients with isolated cutaneous LP also had an increased incidence of positive reactions.

Nine patients with positive patch tests had their dental work replaced, and all demonstrated significant improvement in their LP at follow-up. In 24 patients not undergoing metal replacement, the improvement rate was 62.5%.

Discussion.—The prevalence of allergy to dental metals is greater in patients with oral, genital, or cutaneous LP or LL than in the general population. The results strengthen the hypothesis that dental metals may cause or trigger LP in sensitized patients. Replacement of dental metals may be beneficial in patients with chronic LP.

▶ A relatively small but significant body of literature links oral LP with dental metal allergy. Scalf et al evaluated a fairly large group of patients with cutaneous LP or mucosal lichenoid lesions for allergy to dental metals. A significant number had at least 1 positive reaction. The most common allergies detected were to mercury-containing compounds and metals, including gold, nickel, cobalt chloride, and potassium dichromate. Probably the most significant finding was that in all patients with a positive metal patch test LP improved after the metal was replaced. Long-term remission without further therapy would be significant and would likely justify replacing metals implicated in the cause of these lesions. In the patients with metal allergies who did not have the implicated metal replaced, there also was a fairly high rate of improvement; however, it is likely that these patients were undergoing treatment, and it would be interesting to determine their long-term prognosis. Not all of the allergens detected are found in the patch test kits generally available in the United States. Patch testing at a specialty center may be worthwhile if suspicion of allergy remains high despite negative initial testing.

K. Schwarzenberger, MD

3 Psoriasis

Contrasting Patterns of Streptococcal Superantigen-Induced T-Cell Proliferation in Guttate vs. Chronic Plaque Psoriasis

Davison SC, Allen MH, Mallon E, et al (King's College London; Chelsea and Westminster Hosp, London)

Br J Dermatol 145:245-251, 2001   3–1

Introduction.—Streptococcal throat infection may precipitate guttate psoriasis (GP) and may exacerbate chronic plaque psoriasis (CPP). The stimulus that causes accumulation of activated T cells in skin can be studied by analyzing the T-cell receptor (TCR) distribution. Superantigens activate T cells that express particular TCR Vβ chain families. The Vβ chain restriction seen in circulating peripheral blood lymphocytes in psoriasis resides within the cutaneous lymphocyte-associated antigen (CLA)-positive population. Superantigen-induced generation of CLA-positive lymphocytes in GP was compared with the same process in CPP.

Methods.—The eruption in 9 patients (5 women, 4 men; median age, 28 years) with GP was preceded by a sore throat associated with a positive swab for *Streptococcus pyogenes* and/or a raised antistreptolysin O (ASO) or antideoxyribonuclease B titer. A separate group of 7 patients (4 men; 3 women; median age, 32 years) had a previous history of GP that had completely resolved a minimum of 3 months earlier, and 11 patients (7 men, 4 women; median age, 39 years) had stable CPP. Six healthy volunteers were also evaluated. All 4 groups underwent determinations of peripheral blood lymphocyte (PBL) expression of CLA and T-cell receptor Vβ chain. The expression of superantigen-reactive Vβ families was compared with in vitro superantigen-induced peripheral blood mononuclear cell (PBMC) proliferation.

Results.—Compared with controls, the PBMCs from patients with active GP demonstrated a 2-fold increased proliferation after stimulation with streptococcal pyogenic toxin A (SPEA) and streptococcal pyogenic toxin C (SPEC) ($P > .01$). The response to the staphylococcal toxins and mitogenic stimulation was the same for all 3 groups. The PBLs from patients with active GP demonstrated increased use of the superantigen-reactive families Vβ2 ($P < .01$) and Vβ17 ($P < .01$). This was not observed in the other patient groups or controls. This pattern of Vβ expression was only seen in CLA-positive T cells. There was a positive association between

Vβ2 expression and enhanced proliferation after stimulation with SPEA ($r = 0.82$; $P < .01$) and SPEC ($r = 0.74$; $P < .05$) in active GP.

Conclusion.—In patients with GP, exposure to streptococcal superantigens may create a population of Vβ-restricted CLA-positive PBLs. The increased numbers of such cells could explain the increased proliferation to these superantigens. This process seems to be relatively superantigen specific.

▶ This elegant study was designed to elucidate the mechanisms underlying the increased lymphocyte proliferative response to streptococcal superantigens in patients with active GP. Populations of responding lymphocytes were characterized in terms of their TCR Vβ chains, which determine the nonantigen specific response of T cells to superantigens, and their expression of CLA, which is thought to play a role in T-cell homing to the skin. The results clearly showed that the enhanced response to SPEA and SPEC correlated with the expansion of T cells bearing the Vβ chains known to be bound by these superantigens, and that a large proportion of these T cells displayed CLA. These data strongly suggest that the association between streptococcal infection and GP reflects superantigen-driven proliferation of T cells that home to the skin.

G. M. P. Galbraith, MD

A Role for Mitogen-Activated Protein Kinase Activation by Integrins in the Pathogenesis of Psoriasis

Haase I, Hobbs RM, Romero MR, et al (Keratinocyte Lab, London)
J Clin Invest 108:527-536, 2001   3–2

Introduction.—In the normal epidermis, β1 integrin expression is restricted to the basal layer. In hyperproliferative epidermis, integrins are also expressed in the suprabasal layers. Attachment of basal keratinocytes to the basement membrane is facilitated by integrin receptors. The β1 integrins have an adhesive role and regulate keratinocyte differentiation.

Methods.—Suprabasal integrins were examined to determine if they contribute to epidermal hyperproliferation by activating mitogen-activated protein kinase (MAPK). Skin samples were obtained from: (1) psoriatic lesions from the upper leg of 9 untreated patients, (2) normal human skin from the upper leg, back, and cheek of 4 patients who underwent tumor excisions, and (3) the backs of transgenic mice expressing the human β1 integrin subunit or human α6β1 under the control of the involucrin promoter.

Findings.—Activation of MARK was observed in basal and suprabasal keratinocytes of human and transgenic mouse psoriatic lesions and healing mouse skins. Phenotypically normal human and transgenic mouse epidermis did not house activated MAPK. The transgene-positive keratinocytes generated more IL-1α than did controls. Keratinocyte MAPK could be activated by ligation of suprabasal integrins or treatment with IL-1α.

Constitutive activation of MAPK enhanced the growth rate of human keratinocytes and delayed onset of terminal differentiation. This recreated several of the histologic characteristics of psoriatic epidermis.

Conclusion.—It may be that activation of MAPK by integrins, either directly or through increased IL-1α production, is responsible for epidermal hyperproliferation in psoriasis and wound healing. The sporadic phenotype of transgenic mice may reflect the complex mechanisms by which IL-1 release and responsiveness are controlled in the skin.

▶ This study investigated the role of integrins in the epidermal proliferation that is characteristic of psoriasis. The authors examined not only human psoriatic tissue, but also transgenic mice expressing human β1 integrin, and keratinocyte cultures for expression of integrins, activation of MAPK, and production of proinflammatory cytokines. The results obtained, beautifully illustrated by the immunofluorescence photomicrographs in the article, indicated that β1 integrins were expressed in the suprabasal layer of the hyperproliferative epidermis, and that this correlated with MAPK activation. Furthermore, ligation of integrins with type IV collagen in keratinocytes derived from the transgenic mice resulted in increased expression of IL-1α. In separate experiments, IL-1α was shown to activate MAPK. The authors hypothesize that the epidermal proliferation in psoriasis results from MAPK activation by integrins, and that this may be mediated by IL-1α.

G. M. P. Galbraith, MD

Cytokine Gene Polymorphisms in Psoriasis
Craven NM, Jackson CW, Kirby B, et al (Univ of Manchester, England)
Br J Dermatol 144:849-853, 2001   3–3

Introduction.—Cytokine production is under genetic control. Certain allelic variants of cytokine genes are correlated with higher or lower cytokine production both in vitro and in vivo. Psoriasis is related to an overexpression in the involved skin of T-helper cell type 1 (Th1) cytokines (interferon [IFN]-γ and tumor necrosis factor alpha (TNFα) and relative underexpression of Th2 cytokines (interleukin [IL]-4 and IL-10). Eighty-four patients with psoriasis were evaluated to determine whether allelic variants of genes for a high production of Th1 cytokines or TNF-α or low production of Th2 cytokines represent a risk factor for the development of psoriasis.

Methods.—Genotyping for IFN-γ, TNF-α, IL-10, and IL-4 was performed for the 84 patients with psoriasis and was compared with control data on file. Polymerase chain reaction (PCR) amplification of the promoter regions of the genes was performed during genotyping by using specifically designed pairs of oligonucleotide primers. For IFN-γ, the microsatellite within the initial intron was amplified via PCR.

Results.—Genotyping frequencies demonstrated no differences between patients and controls for IFN-γ, TNF-α, or IL-4. For IL-10, patients with late onset psoriasis who were older than age 40 were more likely to be heterozygous at position -1082 ($P = .02$), corresponding to intermediate production of IL-10 both in vitro and in vivo.

Conclusion.—A genotype consistent with high production of Th1 cytokines or low production of Th2 cytokines does not characterize psoriasis. The Th1 cytokine profile seen in psoriatic plaques is most likely the result of local factors.

▶ It is now generally accepted that lesions of psoriasis are associated with a predominantly Th1 cytokine profile, with correspondingly reduced expression of Th2 cytokines such as IL-10. In their study, the authors determined the distribution of several cytokine gene polymorphisms, including a biallelic polymorphism at position -1082 of the IL-10 gene that has been associated with the level of gene expression. The results revealed an apparently significant increase in the heterozygous genotype in patients with late onset psoriasis when compared with control subjects; for IL-10, heterozygosity is associated with "intermediate" levels of cytokine production. No statistical corrections were made for multiple comparisons, the patient populations studied were small, and the authors themselves deemed the results spurious. It is hoped that this will not deter others from similar studies that attempt to determine the mechanisms underlying T-helper cell responses.

G. M. P. Galbraith, MD

Effects of Systemic Interleukin-10 Therapy on Psoriatic Skin Lesions: Histologic, Immunohistologic, and Molecular Biology Findings
Asadullah K, Friedrich M, Hanneken S, et al (Berlin Humboldt Univ)
J Invest Dermatol 116:721-727, 2001   3–4

Introduction.—Interleukin (IL)-10 is an important anti-inflammatory and immunosuppressive cytokine with significant impact on several immune reactions. IL-10 may represent a novel antipsoriatic drug. The histologic, immunohistologic, and molecular biology effects of systemic IL-10 therapy were evaluated.

Methods.—Serial biopsy specimens were obtained from 10 adult patients with moderate or severe chronic psoriasis receiving subcutaneous injections of recombinant IL-10 (either 8 µg/kg per day or 20 µg/kg 3 times a week [5 patients each, respectively]) over a period of 49 days. The treatment was well tolerated. Antipsoriatic effects were observed in 9 of 10 patients. The biopsy specimens underwent histologic and immunohistochemical analyses, molecular biology examination for cytokine mRNA expression, and quantification of gene expression via real-time polymerase chain reaction (PCR).

Results.—Histologic examination revealed a reduction in several parameters of psoriatic disease activity such as acanthosis and extension of the horny layer. Immunohistochemistry showed diminishing numbers of infiltrating T cells, dermal CD1a+ cells, and diminished proliferation of epidermal cells. The novel, quantitative reverse transcriptase-PCR approach identified a significant shift within the cytokine pattern. IL-10 therapy led to a reduction in cutaneous IL-8 and IL-10 mRNA expression. No significant changes in IL-6, tumor necrosis factor-α, and interferon-γ expression were observed. IL-4 was strongly upregulated, indicating a shift from a type 1 toward a type 2 cytokine pattern.

Conclusion.—Systemic IL-10 injection produced considerable effects on the skin immune system that may contribute to its antipsoriatic activity. It may be that IL-10 exerts its antipsoriatic activity by altering various immune cell populations within the skin and circulation, including T cells and antigen-presenting cells (APCs), and the interactions among them.

▶ As noted in this abstract, psoriasis is associated primarily with a Th1 cell-mediated immune response and relatively reduced expression of Th2 cytokines. The modulation of the Th1-Th2 balance therefore offers a possible therapeutic strategy. In this important study, 10 patients with chronic psoriasis were treated with IL-10 by repeated subcutaneous injections over a 7-week period. The majority of patients experienced significant clinical benefit, which correlated with histologic evidence of decreased psoriatic activity, including a reduction in infiltrating T cells and APCs. In addition, a marked shift in the Th1-Th2 balance was observed, as evidenced by increased IL-4 expression. Furthermore, IL-8 expression was significantly decreased, which may have contributed to the anti-inflammatory effect of the IL-10 therapy. Interestingly, treatment resulted in decreased IL-10 expression in the skin. The authors suggest that the response to IL-10 therapy in psoriasis is due to effects on T lymphocytes and APCs.

G. M. P. Galbraith, MD

Treatment of Chronic Plaque Psoriasis by Selective Targeting of Memory Effector T Lymphocytes

Ellis CN and Krueger GG, for the Alefacept Clinical Study Group (Univ of Michigan, Ann Arbor; et al)

N Engl J Med 345:248-255, 2001   3–5

Introduction.—Psoriatic plaques are infiltrated with CD45RO+ memory effector T lymphocytes. The recombinant protein alefacept binds to CD2 on memory effector T lymphocytes and restricts their activation. Because alefacept inhibits the activation of T cells and induces apoptosis in critical subgroups of T cells, the use of alefacept as an immunomodulatory therapy for psoriasis was assessed in a multicenter, randomized, placebo-controlled, double-blind investigation.

Methods.—The age range of the 229 patients with chronic plaque psoriasis involving 10% or more of the body surface was 18 to 70 years. Chronic psoriasis had been diagnosed a minimum of 12 months before enrollment, and patients had received previous systemic treatment or phototherapy or were candidates for such therapy. Patients were randomly assigned to treatment with either IV alefacept (0.025, 0.075, or 0.150 mg/kg body weight) or placebo weekly for 12 weeks. The follow-up period was an additional 12 weeks. At baseline, the median scores with the use of the psoriasis area-and-severity index (PASI) were between 14 and 20 in all groups (0 denotes no psoriasis and 72 the most severe disease possible). Other evaluations were conducted at weeks 1, 2, 4, 8, and 12. Patients were not allowed to receive systemic treatments, phototherapy, or potent topical medications between 4 weeks before baseline and 2 weeks after completion of therapy. The use of moderate-potency topical corticosteroids, keratolytics, coal tar, or calcipotriene was allowed for treatment of the groin, scalp, palms, and soles.

Results.—Alefacept was well tolerated and was not immunogenic. The mean decrease in the PASI score 2 weeks after completion of treatment with alefacept was greater (38%, 53%, and 53%, respectively, in the 0.025, 0.075, and 0.150 mg/kg groups) compared with placebo (21%; $P < .001$). At 12 weeks after completion of treatment, 28 patients who had received alefacept alone were clear or almost clear of psoriasis, versus 3 in the placebo group, all of whom had received additional systemic therapy. Alefacept decreased peripheral blood memory effector T lymphocyte (CD45RO+) counts. The decrease in the number of memory effector T lymphocytes was associated with improvement in psoriasis. Treatment was well tolerated, and no patients had any signs or symptoms suggestive of cytokine release or capillary leak syndromes.

Conclusion.—Treatment with alefacept for 12 weeks was correlated with improvement in chronic plaque psoriasis, with some patients experiencing a sustained clinical response after cessation of treatment. Alefacept selectively targets CD45RO+ memory effector T lymphocytes, indicating that they have a role in the pathogenesis of psoriasis.

▶ Clearly, a new era of psoriasis therapy is upon us, with the development of new agents to modify the immune response. The results described by the Alefacept Clinical Study Group could best be classified as modest, but combinations of alefacept with other therapies or modifications of the treatment protocol might increase its effectiveness. More agents that interfere with specific steps in the immunopathogenesis of psoriasis are certain to be introduced in the years to come.[1]

B. H. Thiers, MD

Reference

1. Granstein RD: New treatments for psoriasis. *N Engl J Med* 345:284-287, 2001.

The Treatment of Moderate to Severe Psoriasis With a New Anti-CD11a Monoclonal Antibody

Papp K, Bissonnette R, Krueger JG, et al (Probity Med Research Waterloo, Ont, Canada; Centre Hospitalier de l'Université de Montreal; Rockefeller Univ, New York; et al)
J Am Acad Dermatol 45:665-674, 2001

3–6

Background.—Anti-CD11a (hu1124) is a humanized monoclonal antibody directed against the CD11a subunit of LFA-1. This study investigated whether treatment with anti-CD11a antibody provides clinical benefit to patients with moderate to severe plaque psoriasis.

Methods.—This was a double-blind, placebo-controlled, phase II, multicenter study. In total, 145 patients with minimum Psoriasis Area and Severity Index scores of 12 and affected body surface area of 10% or more were sequentially enrolled into low-dose (0.1 mg/kg, n = 22) or high-dose (0.3 mg/kg, n = 75) groups. Within groups, patients were randomized to treatment or placebo (n = 48) in a 2:1 ratio. Drug was administered intravenously at weekly intervals for 8 weeks.

Results.—The percentage of subjects achieving more than 50% improvement in physician's global assessment at day 56 (1 week after final dose) was 15% and 48% for placebo and 0.3 mg/kg of drug, respectively (P = .002). A physician's global assessment of excellent (>75% improvement) was greater in the 0.3 mg/kg group versus placebo (25% vs 2%, P = .0003). Average Psoriasis Area and Severity Index scores at day 56 were 13.9 ± 7.5 (placebo) and 10.9 ± 8.4 (0.3 mg/kg) (P < .0001). Epidermal thickness was reduced in the 0.3 mg/kg group compared with the placebo group (37% vs 19%, P = .004). Treatment was well tolerated; mild to moderate flu-like complaints were the most common adverse events. White blood cell counts and lymphocyte counts transiently increased. Depletion of circulating lymphocytes did not occur.

Conclusions.—Anti-CD11a antibody administered intravenously in 8 weekly doses of 0.3 mg/kg was well tolerated and induced clinical and histologic improvements in psoriasis.

▶ As already stated for alefacept (Abstract 3–5), the therapeutic results reported thus far for the new biologic agents being developed to treat psoriasis have not been particularly impressive. However, T-cell inhibition as a therapeutic strategy for this disease has a proven track record (eg, cyclosporine) and certainly seems worth pursuing.

B. H. Thiers, MD

Improvement of Pyoderma Gangrenosum and Psoriasis Associated With Crohn Disease With Anti–Tumor Necrosis Factor α Monoclonal Antibody

Tan M-H, Gordon M, Lebwohl O, et al (New York Univ; Columbia Presbyterian Med Ctr, New York)
Arch Dermatol 137:930-933, 2001   3–7

Background.—Infliximab, an anti–tumor necrosis factor α monoclonal antibody, has been found to be effective in the treatment—and maintenance of remission—of active refractory Crohn disease and associated draining enterocutaneous fistulae. In studies of patients with rheumatoid arthritis, multiple infusions of infliximab have yielded promising results. However, the clinical experience with infliximab is limited, and there have been no published reports on its use in the treatment of cutaneous disorders. Experiences with 2 patients with Crohn disease and pyoderma gangrenosum and 1 patient with Crohn disease and psoriasis are reported. All three patients were treated with infliximab for recalcitrant Crohn fistulae, with concurrent improvement in their skin diseases.

Case 1.—Man, 39, with Crohn disease diagnosed in 1978 had a subtotal colectomy in July 1979 and had painful inflammatory skin lesions develop within 2 months and fistulae 2 years later. He received sulfasalazine and prednisone for treatment of Crohn disease as well as tacrolimus, metronidazole, mercaptopurine, total parenteral nutrition, and intralesional triamcinolone acetonide. Thalidomide was effective but was discontinued because of sensorimotor neuropathy. The patients had pustules and widespread ulcerations with violaceous undermined borders and purulence on the upper and lower extremities, chest, and back. He received 5 infusions of infliximab for recalcitrant rectal fistulae at 5 mg/kg over 12 months, with dramatic improvement in the pyoderma gangrenosum and fistulae. Most ulcers resolved completely within 1 week after the first infusion, with additional improvement 1 week after each subsequent infusion.

Case 2.—Woman, 50, with Crohn disease diagnosed in 1983 was treated with multiple ileocolic resections with ileostomy. Pyoderma gangrenosum and fistulae had been present in the perianal region, abdomen, and legs for 5 years. Previous treatments included intralesional triamcinolone acetonide, clobetasol propionate ointment, and various dressings. A variety of agents, including cyclosporine, prednisone, rifampin, and amoxicillin, were ineffective. Thalidomide was effective but was discontinued because of peripheral sensory neuropathy. Infliximab 5 mg/kg was infused in February 1999, and the lesions improved within 1 week, with complete and partial closure within 1 month. The effects lasted for 2.5 months, after which the lesions deteriorated. A second infusion was administered 3 months later, with similar results.

Case 3.—Man, 51, with refractory Crohn disease diagnosed in 1973 reported a long-standing, scaly, pruritic eruption diagnosed as psoriasis in 1987. He was seen in 1998 with increasing abdominal pain and fistula drainage, and treatment with infliximab was begun. Healing of the fistula began within 1 week, and complete closure was obtained within 2 days after a second infusion. There was also a slight improvement in psoriasis after the second infusion. After 3 infusions a year later for fistula recurrence, healing of the fistula was noted along with a decrease in scale, thickness, erythema, and pruritus of cutaneous lower limb plaques within 2 weeks, and almost complete clearance by 5 weeks.

Conclusions.—Infliximab, which has shown promising results in the treatment of refractory Crohn disease and fistulae, may also be effective in the treatment of pyoderma gangrenosum and psoriasis associated with Crohn disease.

▶ The usefulness of infliximab in the treatment of dermatologic diseases is the subject of intense investigation. As discussed elsewhere in this issue, significant benefits have already been observed in patients with psoriasis. More studies are undoubtedly forthcoming.

B. H. Thiers, MD

Treatment of Psoriatic Arthritis With Antitumour Necrosis Factor-α Antibody Clears Skin Lesions of Psoriasis Resistant to Treatment With Methotrexate
Ogilvie ALJ, Antoni C, Dechant C, et al (Univ of Erlangen, Germany)
Br J Dermatol 144:587-589, 2001   3–8

Background.—Keratinocytes and inflammatory cells produce great amounts of tumor necrosis factor (TNF)-α in inflamed skin. This cytokine has broad effects associated with inflammation. Therefore, an agent that blocks TNF-α may be effective in the treatment of inflammatory skin diseases. The efficacy of infliximab, an anti-TNF-α antibody, in the treatment of psoriatic arthritis was investigated.

Methods and Findings.—The study included 6 patients with progressive joint disease and psoriatic skin lesions that did not respond to methotrexate. Infusions of infliximab, 5 mg/kg, were given at week 0, 2, and 6. Before and 10 weeks after treatment initiation, the Psoriasis Area and Severity Index was recorded for each patient. All patients exhibited improvement in psoriatic skin lesions. Joint disease also markedly improved in all patients (Fig 1).

Conclusions.—Treatment with anti-TNF-α antibody is effective and well-tolerated for patients with psoriasis. Use of infliximab improves joint and skin symptoms in these patients. Further research is needed to verify these findings.

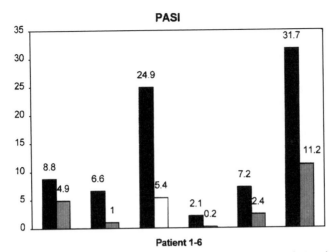

FIGURE 1.—Psoriasis Area and Severity Index (PASI) before (*black columns*) and 10 weeks after (*gray columns*) initiation of therapy with antitumour necrosis factor-α antibody in 6 patients suffering from severe psoriatic arthritis. (Courtesy of Ogilvie ALJ, Antoni C, Dechant C, et al: Treatment of psoriatic arthritis with antitumour necrosis factor-α antibody clears skin lesions of psoriasis resistant to treatment with methotrexate. *Br J Dermatol* 144:587-589, 2001. Reprinted by permission of Blackwell Science, Inc.)

Efficacy and Safety of Infliximab Monotherapy for Plaque-Type Psoriasis: A Randomised Trial

Chaudhari U, Romano P, Mulcahy LD, et al (UMDNJ-Robert Wood Johnson Med School, New Brunswick, NJ)
Lancet 357:1842-1847, 2001   3–9

Introduction.—The currently available treatments for patients with moderate to severe psoriasis are often either not completely effective or associated with serious toxic effects. Because tumor necrosis factor α (TNF-α) has a potential role in both of the major pathologic changes observed in psoriasis (epidermal hyperproliferation with abnormal differentiation and inflammatory cell infiltration of the epidermis and dermis), blockade of TNF-α activity may prove to be beneficial. The clinical efficacy and safety of infliximab, a monoclonal antibody against TNF-α, were examined in a randomized trial.

Methods.—All 33 patients were adults in generally good health, and all had failed to respond to topical steroid therapy. In a block-of-six randomization scheme, patients were assigned to receive placebo or infliximab, 5 or 10 mg/kg, at weeks 0, 2, and 6, in a 1/1/1 fashion. All investigators and patients were blinded to treatment assignment during the first 10 weeks of the study. Only nonmedicated emollients and nonprescription shampoos were allowed during the study period. Patients were assessed for response and monitored for adverse events. The primary efficacy end point was the Physician's Global Assessment (PGA) at week 10.

Results.—Three patients, 1 from each group, withdrew during the course of the study. The PGA rating of good, excellent, or clear was achieved in 82% of the patients in the infliximab 5 mg/kg group, 91% of those in the infliximab 10 mg/kg group, and 18% of those in the placebo group (Fig 5; see color plate III). In both active treatment groups, the median time to response was 4 weeks. Infliximab was well tolerated, with no serious adverse effects reported. Patients in the infliximab 10 mg/kg group were more likely to experience headache than patients in the 2 other groups.

Conclusion.—Patients with moderate to severe plaque-type psoriasis received a high degree of clinical benefit from anti-TNF-α infliximab

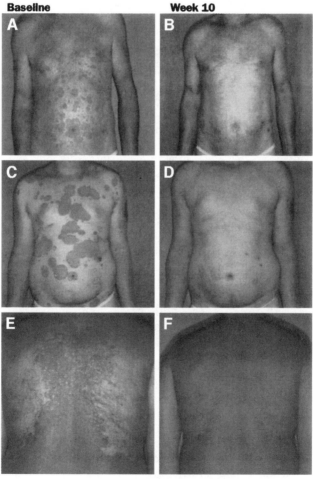

FIGURE 5.—Degree of improvement in psoriasis from baseline to week 10. **A** and **B**, Infliximab 5 mg/kg; **C** and **D**, infliximab 10 mg/kg; **E** and **F**, placebo. (Courtesy of Chaudhari U, Romano P, Mulcahy LD, et al: Efficacy and safety of infliximab monotherapy for plaque-type psoriasis: A randomised trial. *Lancet* 357:1842-1847, 2001. Copyright by The Lancet, Ltd, 2001.)

monotherapy. The time to response was rapid, and infliximab was well tolerated by all participants.

▶ The response to infliximab was similar to the response to cyclosporine in terms of the high proportion of patients who achieved clearance and the rapidity of the response. Moreover, the results are much better than those reported with etanercept, a soluble receptor fusion protein that inhibits TNF. In data published by Mease et al,[1] 26% of etanercept-treated patients achieved at least 75% improvement in the PASI score, compared with none of those receiving placebo. The more striking response with infliximab might be explained by several factors, including differences in the population of the patients studied, the route of infusion (IV for infliximab vs subcutaneous for etanercept), and the ability to obtain cell lysis.

B. H. Thiers, MD

Reference

1. Mease PJ, Goffe BS, Metz J, et al: Etanercept in the treatment of psoriatic arthritis and psoriasis: A randomised trial. *Lancet* 356:383-390, 2000.

Tuberculosis Associated With Infliximab, a Tumor Necrosis Factor α-Neutralizing Agent
Keene J, Gershon S, Wise RP, et al (Boston Univ; Food and Drug Administration, Rockville, Md)
N Engl J Med 345:1098-1104, 2001   3–10

Background.—Infliximab, a humanized antibody against tumor necrosis factor-α (TNF-α), is used to treat Crohn's disease and rheumatoid arthritis (RA). Although TNF-α has been found to have a protective effect against tuberculosis in animal models, no evidence of this effect has been found in humans. Tuberculosis in humans associated with the use of infliximab was investigated.

Methods.—All cases of tuberculosis after infliximab therapy reported to the MedWatch spontaneous reporting system of the Food and Drug Administration were analyzed. Reports received as of May 29, 2001, were included.

Findings.—Seventy cases of tuberculosis after infliximab treatment for a median 12 weeks were reported. Tuberculosis developed after 3 or fewer infusions in 48 patients. Disease was extrapulmonary in 40 patients. In 33 patients, the diagnosis was verified by biopsy. Sixty-four of the seventy reports were from countries with a low incidence of tuberculosis. The reported frequency of tuberculosis associated with infliximab treatment was much greater than that of other opportunistic infections. Also, the rate of reported cases among patients given infliximab was higher than the available background rates.

Conclusions.—Active tuberculosis can develop shortly after infliximab treatment is begun. Clinicians need to screen patients for latent tuberculosis infection or disease before prescribing infliximab.

▶ And now the bad news. Keane et al report an unusually high incidence of tuberculosis for patients treated with infliximab. Of special note is the fact that most of the 70 reported patients came from countries with a low incidence of tuberculosis. Equally disturbing was the high incidence of extrapulmonary disease in these patients, most of whom developed tuberculosis after 3 or fewer infusions. The incidence of other opportunistic infections was quite low. Clearly, screening for tuberculosis is indicated in any patient being considered for infliximab therapy. If latent infection is found, consideration should be given to prophylactic antibiotic therapy before infliximab is administered. Patients receiving infliximab should be advised to seek medical attention if they develop symptoms suggestive of tuberculosis. More recently, recurrence of another infectious granulomatous disease, histoplasmosis, has been reported after infliximab therapy.[1]

B. H. Thiers, MD

Reference

1. Nakelchik M, Mangino JE: Reactivation of histoplasmosis after treatment with infliximab. *Am J Med* 112:78, 2002.

Rapid Onset of Cutaneous Squamous Cell Carcinoma in Patients With Rheumatoid Arthritis After Starting Tumor Necrosis Factor α Receptor IgG1-Fc Fusion Complex Therapy
Smith KJ, Skelton HG (Natl Naval Med Ctr, Bethesda, Md; Lab Corp of America, Herndon, Va)
J Am Acad Dermatol 45:953-956, 2001   3–11

Introduction.—Tumor necrosis factor α (TNF-α) appears to be involved in the pathogenesis of synovitis and joint destruction in rheumatoid arthritis (RA). Treatment with etanercept, a recombinant human TNF-α receptor Fc fusion protein, has produced significant improvement in patients who have failed to respond adequately to methotrexate, sulfasalazine, or hydroxychloroquine. Etanercept appears to be safe and well tolerated, but systemic infections have occurred in a few patients. The 7 patients reported here experienced rapidly growing cutaneous squamous cell carcinoma (SCC) within 4 months of starting etanercept for RA.

Case Reports.—The patients, 4 women and 3 men, ranged in age from 53 to 72 years. All were taking or had previously received methotrexate before starting etanercept (25 mg subcutaneously, twice weekly). All showed improvement in RA, with no other side effects related to etanercept. Actinic damage was present in all patients, and 4 had a history of basal cell carcinoma. Nine SCCs were removed from areas of chronically exposed skin. Once the tumors appeared, growth was rapid. Histologic features were similar in all the SCCs. High-power views showed a mixed infiltrate with mononuclear cells and numerous eosinophils both surrounding and infiltrating tumor cells with areas of tumor cell necrosis.

Discussion.—Subclinical UV-induced tumors were probably present in these patients at the onset of etanercept therapy. After 1 year of follow-up, with continued etanercept treatment, no new SCCs have appeared. The therapy, through inhibition of a T_H1 cytokine pattern and inhibition of the direct and indirect cytotoxic effects of TNF-α, may initially decrease mechanisms for controlling subclinical tumors and contribute to the histologic features seen in these cases. It is also possible that prolonged TNF-α inhibition may have some antitumor effects.

▶ It is difficult to make generalizations from a small series such as this one, and the observations reported may represent coincidence rather than a pattern of acceleration of cutaneous carcinogenesis related to the drug, which recently has received an indication for the treatment of psoriatic arthritis. However, this report should serve to remind us that, like infliximab, etanercept and other biologic response modalities are new drugs whose complete side effect profile may not yet be evident.

B. H. Thiers, MD

Squamous-Cell Cancer of the Skin in Patients Given PUVA and Ciclosporin: Nested Cohort Crossover Study

Marcil I, Stern RS (Harvard Med School, Boston)
Lancet 358:1042-1045, 2001   3–12

Introduction.—Among patients who have had organ transplants, immunosuppressive treatment with cyclosporine is associated with an increased risk of squamous-cell carcinoma of the skin. There is concern that a similar risk may be present for patients with psoriasis who are taking cyclosporine and have had substantial exposure to psoralen and UV-A light (PUVA) or other carcinogenic treatments. The incidence of skin cancer before and after cyclosporine use was assessed in patients with psoriasis who were enrolled in a PUVA follow-up study.

Methods.—Data were available for 28 of 31 participants in the study. In addition, 1380 patients with psoriasis who had first been given PUVA in 1975 or 1976 were prospectively investigated. In the nested cohort crossover study, the 28 participants were compared for the frequency of squamous cell carcinoma before and after first use of cyclosporine. The large cohort was analyzed for the relationship between use of the drug and frequency of skin cancer.

Results.—Only 5 of the 28 patients who used cyclosporine underwent more than 30 PUVA treatments. Since enrollment in 1975, a total of 212 squamous cell carcinomas and 55 basal cell cancers were diagnosed in 14 (50%) cyclosporine users. After adjustment for amount of PUVA exposure and methotrexate use, the incidence of tumors was 7 times higher after the first cyclosporine use than in the previous 5 years. Among the 844 members of the large cohort with follow-up data, 26% had a total of 1736 squamous cell carcinomas diagnosed. There was a significant association between high-dose exposure to PUVA ($\geq$200 treatments) or methotrexate ($\geq$36 months of use) and risk of squamous cell carcinoma.

Conclusion.—Among patients from the PUVA study, those who had used cyclosporine for at least 3 months had more than 1 squamous cell carcinoma per person per year. This incidence is more than 100 times what would be expected in the general population. Basal cell carcinoma was also seen with increased frequency but to a far lesser degree. The carcinogenic potential of cyclosporine and other immunosuppressive agents should be carefully assessed in patients with psoriasis.

▶ The findings should come as no surprise, given the well-known association of both PUVA and cyclosporine with cutaneous squamous cell carcinoma. Dermatologists often consider combination therapy in patients with treatment-resistant psoriasis, but 1 combination that should be avoided is cyclosporine and PUVA. A more logical treatment would be so-called re-PUVA, in which a systemic retinoid, usually acitretin, is used in conjunction with the UV light treatment. A study done several years ago comparing the combination of cyclosporine and PUVA with rePUVA found the latter regimen to be more effective and associated with a more durable treatment response.[1] Moreover, the acitretin might exert a protective effect on the skin to counteract the damaging effects of the irradiation.

B. H. Thiers, MD

Reference

1. Koo J, Lebwohl M: Duration of remission of psoriasis therapies. *J Am Acad Dermatol* 41:51-59, 1999.

The Risk of Melanoma in Association With Long-term Exposure to PUVA

Stern RS, and the PUVA Follow up Study (Harvard Med School, Boston)
J Am Acad Dermatol 44:755-761, 2001   3–13

Introduction.—The risk of malignant melanoma increases beginning 15 years after initial treatment with oral methoxsalen (psoralen) and ultraviolet A radiation (PUVA), most notably in patients who have received 250 treatments or more. The risk of melanoma associated with long-term exposure to PUVA in 1380 patients who began PUVA treatment in 1975 and 1976 is reported.

TABLE 2.—Invasive and In Situ Cutaneous Melanoma: Number of, Time of Occurrence, and Incidence (per 100,000 Person-Years) for PUVA Cohort

Type of Tumor	Time Period			
	1975-1990	1991 to 2/29/96	2/29/96 to End	All Years
Invasive melanoma				
No.	4	7	7	18
Incidence	0.22	1.73	3.82	0.69
Melanoma in situ				
No.	0	3	4	7
Incidence	0	0.74	2.18	0.35
All melanomas				
No.	4	10	11	25
Incidence	0.22	2.47	6.00	1.04

Abbreviation: PUVA, Oral methoxsalen (psoralen) and ultraviolet A radiation.
(Courtesy of Stern RS, and the PUVA Follow up Study: The risk of melanoma in association with long-term exposure to PUVA. *J Am Acad Dermatol* 44:755-761, 2001.)

Methods.—The cohort has been prospectively followed since initial treatment with PUVA in 1975 and 1976. The occurrence of melanoma was documented. The observed and expected incidence is reported in this cohort, especially melanomas that developed since an earlier report, which included data through February 29, 1996.

Results.—Since 1975, 23 patients had 26 invasive or in situ cutaneous melanomas. In an average of 2.25 years since the last report, 7 additional invasive or in situ cutaneous melanomas have been identified (incidence rate ratio, 8.4; 95% CI, 2.4-17.3). This rate was more than double the number identified during the 15 years of follow-up from trial initiation in 1975 to the end of 1990 (Table 2). A noticeable difference in skin type was observed between patients who did and did not have melanoma. A higher frequency of Fitzpatrick skin types I and II was seen in those who had melanoma. Patients with types IV, V, or VI skin did not develop melanoma.

Conclusion.—Beginning 15 years after first exposure to PUVA, there is an increased risk of melanoma. This risk is greatest among patients exposed to high doses of PUVA, seems to increase with time, and should be considered in ascertaining the risks and benefits of this treatment approach. These data support the earlier observation of increased risk of melanoma in patients treated with PUVA.

▶ Stern et al report follow-up data to their previous article documenting an association between long-term exposure to PUVA and the risk of melanoma.[1] Their new data suggest that, with time, the dosage threshold at which this effect becomes manifest seems to be decreasing. It is possible that this increased risk will become even greater or will be exhibited in patients exposed to less PUVA after the passage of additional years. This can only be determined through a longer term prospective study.

B. H. Thiers, MD

Reference

1. Stern RS, Khanh TN, Vakeva LH: Malignant melanoma in patients treated for psoriasis with methoxsalen (psoralen) and ultraviolet A radiation (PUVA). *N Engl J Med* 336:1041-1045, 1997.

The Risk of Malignancy Associated With Psoriasis

Margolis D, Bilker W, Hennessy S, et al (Univ of Pennsylvania, Philadelphia)
Arch Dermatol 137:778-783, 2001   3–14

Introduction.—Patients with psoriasis appear to be at increased risk for the development of malignancy. Certain therapies, including systemic agents and psoralen with UV-A light treatment (PUVA), are associated with an increased incidence of cancer. The risk of malignancy for patients with psoriasis was compared with that for other patient groups in a retrospective cohort study.

Methods.—The cohort was drawn from participants in the Medicaid program of 3 large states from July 1992 to March 1996. Participants were classified into 1 of 5 study groups based on diagnosis and treatment: (1) severe psoriasis, (2) less severe psoriasis, (3) severe eczema, (4) heart, kidney, or liver transplants and treatment with immunosuppressive agents, and (5) essential hypertension (a reference group with a risk of cancer considered to be similar to that in the general population). The primary outcome was the first occurrence of a claim that included a diagnosis of any cancer at least 6 months after the patient was classified into a study group.

Results.—Most patients with severe psoriasis had received either methotrexate or etretinate therapy. Compared with patients with hypertension, those with severe psoriasis were more likely to receive a diagnosis of cancer (risk ratio, 1.78). The risk of malignancy in the severe psoriasis group approached that of patients in the organ transplant group (risk ratio, 2.12). Patients with severe eczema were least likely to receive a diagnosis of cancer. Compared with the reference group, the risk of malignancy was only slightly increased in the less severe psoriasis group (risk ratio, 1.13). Most of the increased cancer risk for both psoriasis groups was because of the incidence of lymphoma or nonmelanoma skin cancer among patients in these groups.

Conclusion.—After accounting for the effects of age and sex, patients with psoriasis requiring treatment with systemic agents are almost twice as likely as patients with hypertension to receive a subsequent diagnosis of cancer. The increased risk among patients with severe psoriasis is mainly for lymphoproliferative disorders and nonmelanoma skin cancers.

▶ In the 1970s, many dermatologists were of the opinion that patients with psoriasis had a decreased risk of skin cancer. The most popular treatment for severe psoriasis, the Goeckerman regimen, involved the use of 2 carcinogenic agents (tar and UV-B), yet it was somewhat unusual to see skin cancer in psoriasis patients treated in this manner. What has changed is not the disease itself but the methods we use to manage the disease. PUVA clearly increases the risk of skin cancer, and the systemic immunosuppressive therapies currently in use likely not only increase the risk of skin cancer, but the risk of lymphoproliferative disorders as well. Many of the new biologic therapies currently under investigation directly interfere with some aspect of the immune response, and treated patients will have to be monitored carefully for possible adverse long-term sequelae.

B. H. Thiers, MD

Mycophenolate Mofetil as a Systemic Antipsoriatic Agent: Positive Experience in 11 Patients
Geilen CC, Arnold M, Orfanos CE (Free Univ of Berlin)
Br J Dermatol 144:583-586, 2001   3–15

Introduction.—Mycophenolate mofetil (MMF) is a novel immunosuppressive drug that has a beneficial effect in patients with psoriasis and autoimmune dermatoses. It was initially used to prevent acute rejection after renal and cardiac transplantation. The efficacy and safety of oral MMF was examined in 11 patients with severe stable plaque-type psoriasis.

Methods.—The patients' ages ranged from 36 to 74 years. The patients had a mean Psoriasis Area and Severity Index (PASI) of 30.5 (range, 12 and 53). The PASI score was obtained at baseline and at 1, 2, 3, and 6 weeks of treatment. Patients received 1 g of oral MMF twice daily for 3 weeks, then 0.5 g 2 times daily for 3 weeks. No other topical or systemic antipsoriatic agent, including UV treatment, was allowed during the evaluation period.

Results.—Within 3 weeks of treatment, the mean PASI of the 11 patients was 15.6. There was a reduction in PASI of between 40% and 70% in 7 patients. Only 1 patient achieved a decrease in PASI of less than 25% from baseline. Decreasing MMF from 2 g daily produced slight additonal improvement in 6 patients during the following 3 weeks. In 4 patients, the PASI score rose during use of the lower dosage. The medication was withdrawn because of muscle pain in 1 patient whose symptoms abated within a few days of drug cessation. Other side effects, particularly gastrointestinal and hematologic toxicity, were not seen in any patients. The overall mean PASI after 6 weeks' treatment was 16.1.

Conclusion.—The use of MMF, 2 g daily, was effective and safe in the treatment of severe psoriasis.

▶ A number of articles have expounded the benefits of mycophenolate mofetil, not only for the treatment of psoriasis but for the treatment of several of the autoimmune blistering diseases as well. My own experience has been limited to patients with psoriasis, and I must admit that my results have not been nearly as good as those described in the literature.

B. H. Thiers, MD

Thioguanine for Refractory Psoriasis: A 4-Year Experience
Mason C, Krueger GG (Univ of Utah, Salt Lake City)
J Am Acad Dermatol 44:67-72, 2001   3–16

Background.—The therapies most effective for the treatment of psoriasis—methotrexate, cyclosporine, light-based therapies, and acitretin—have significant cumulative toxicity for the liver, kidneys, skin, and musculoskeletal system, respectively. There is a need for alternative therapies when the primary cumulative toxicity of a drug affects other organs, when the profile of acute side effects is different, and when efficacy for the treatment of psoriasis is comparable. In several studies, alleviation of psoriasis and psoriatic arthritis has been reported with the administration of thioguanine, an analogue of the natural purines hypoxanthine and guanine. The results of treatment of 21 patients with refractory psoriasis were reported.

Methods.—A retrospective review was conducted of the treatment courses of 21 patients with psoriasis who were treated with thioguanine. Both daily dosing and pulse dosing were used, ranging from 20 mg 2 times a week to 120 mg daily. All of the patients had previously been treated with other systemic therapies, and most of them (86%) had been treated with methotrexate.

Results.—The outcomes in patients were classified into 3 groups: those with more than 90% improvement, those with between 50% and 90% improvement, and those with less than 50% improvement. Outcome data were based on a subjective rating of disease severity by the patient before the start of thioguanine therapy and during the entire treatment course. Evaluation was possible in 18 of 21 patients, with 14 of 18 (78%) showing dramatic improvement (more than 90%), 3 of 18 (17%) showing lesser improvement (50% to 90%), and 1 of 18 demonstrating less than 50% improvement. The mean duration of treatment was 15.5 months. Myelosuppression, the primary side effect, was mild in 9 of 18 patients and severe in 1 of 18 patients.

Conclusions.—Thioguanine is an effective treatment for patients with severe recalcitrant psoriasis. Myelosuppression was found to be a significant but easily monitored side effect that can be more accurately predicted by the determination of thiopurine methyltransferase levels before the start of thioguanine therapy. Additional prospective studies are needed so that criteria that will maximize the efficacy and minimize the toxicity of thioguanine can be established.

▶ All currently available systemic therapies for psoriasis have recognizable side effects. Liver function is a concern with methotrexate, renal function and hypertension with cyclosporine, and hyperlipidemia with retinoids. With thioguanine, the concern appears to be myelosuppression. All of these potential adverse events can be easily monitored and a drug contraindicated for 1 patient may be perfectly suitable for another. Most patients with severe psoriasis can be significantly improved with carefully chosen therapies that may be combined or rotated. New biological therapies currently in testing may offer additional options in the future.

B. H. Thiers, MD

The Value of Amino-Terminal Propeptide of Type III Procollagen in Routine Screening for Methotrexate-Induced Liver Fibrosis: A 10-Year Follow-up
Zachariae H, Heickendorff L, Søgaard H (Marselisberg Hosp, Aarhus, Denmark; Univ of Aarhus, Denmark)
Br J Dermatol 143:100-103, 2001   3–17

Introduction.—The radioimmunoassay of amino-terminal propetide of type III procollagen (PIIINP) is not organ specific, but it can be used as a valuable noninvasive marker of liver fibrogenesis. It has also been evaluated as an indicator for the development of fibrosis in methotrexate (MTX)-treated patients with psoriasis. Trials have shown significantly higher levels of PIIINP in patients with fibrosis than in those with normal liver histology or steatosis alone. Seventy patients with psoriasis were retrospectively evaluated to determine whether normal serum levels of PIIINP indicated the absence of significant hepatic fibrosis, thus reducing the need for repeated liver biopsies in patients treated with MTX.

Methods.—All patients were taking MTX and had both a liver biopsy without fibrosis and a normal PIIINP in 1989 or 1990. Patients were monitored until they ceased taking MTX (range, 1-11 years; average, 4 years). All patients had at least 2 PIIINP analyses before or at the time of biopsy. The average cumulative MTX dose at the time of the latest biopsy was 3.5 g (range, 0.6-16.8 g).

Results.—Patients underwent 189 liver biopsies and 329 PIIINP analyses. There were 21 patients who had only 1 liver biopsy; all had at least 2 to 3 PIIINP samples, which were taken within a year around the time of the biopsy; at least 2 were obtained either before or at the time of biopsy. Each of the remaining patients underwent 2 to 7 liver biopsies and a total of 267 analyses of PIIINP. During the evaluation period, elevated serum PIIINP levels developed in 4 patients; each of them had hepatic fibrosis on biopsy. Two additional patients, 1 with psoriatic arthritis, had elevated PIIINP levels and normal liver biopsy findings. No liver fibrosis was found in the 63 patients who had consistently normal PIIINP levels.

Conclusion.—The fact that no liver fibrosis was missed in patients with consistently normal PIIINP levels supports the opinion that, as long as these levels remain normal, there appears to be only a minimal risk of substantial fibrosis.

▶ This is a follow-up study of patients reported by the same authors 10 years earlier.[1] They confirm the utility of monitoring serum levels of PIIINP in psoriasis patients receiving methotrexate therapy. Their data show that patients with normal serial PIIINP levels are highly unlikely to have hepatic fibrosis. Another group of investigators has recently examined the utility of serologic markers to predict liver fibrosis in patients with hepatitis C virus infection.[2]

B. H. Thiers, MD

References

1. Zachariae H, Aslam HM, Bjerring P, et al: Serum amino-terminal propeptide of type III procollagen in psoriasis and psoriatic arthritis: Relation to liver fibrosis and arthritis. *J Am Acad Dermatol* 25:50-53, 1991.
2. Imbert-Bismut F, Ratziu V, Pieroni L, et al: Biochemical markers of liver fibrosis in patients with hepatitis C virus infection: A prospective study. *Lancet* 357:1069-1075, 2001.

Childhood Psoriasis: A Clinical Review of 1262 Cases
Morris A, Rogers M, Fischer G, et al (Royal Alexandra Hosp for Children, Westmead, New South Wales, Australia)
Pediatr Dermatol 18:188-198, 2001   3–18

Background.—Clarification of the definition and natural history of psoriasis in children has been lacking. The results of 14 years' experience with childhood psoriasis in a tertiary pediatric dermatology service are reported.

Methods.—Data were collected from 1981 to 1995 on 1262 children (age range, 1 month to 15 years) diagnosed with psoriasis at the Royal Alexandra Hospital for Children, Sydney, Australia. Conventional terminology was used in describing the cases, with the type of psoriasis based on the dermatologist's findings at the time of presentation. Age, gender, family history in a first-degree relative, facial involvement, and history of psoriatic diaper rash were also recorded.

Results.—Sixteen percent of the participants were under age 1 year and 27% under age 2 years; there was a nearly equal distribution of girls (53%) and boys (47%). The highest incidence of disease was for the plaque type (Table 1). Facial involvement was noted in 38% of cases, including 40% of children who had plaque type and 40% of those with guttate psoriasis. Of those with facial involvement, the most common site was under the eyes. Four percent of the children studied had facial involvement as their only manifestation of psoriasis, with others having it as part of a more generalized rash. The most common diagnosis among children under age 2 years was psoriatic diaper rash with dissemination, found in 155 patients. Many of these patients who initially had diaper rash with dissemination subsequently developed other forms of psoriasis. It was noted that psoriatic diaper rash was brighter red, had better demarcation,

TABLE 1.—Type of Psoriasis

Type	Number	Percentage
Plaque	430	34.1
Psoriatic diaper rash with dissemination	161	12.7
Scalp	146	11.5
Anogenital	112	8.9
Guttate	81	6.4
Acropustulosis	60	4.7
Eczema-psoriasis overlap	55	4.3
Face plaque only	54	4.3
Palm and sole	50	3.9
Localized psoriatic diaper rash	45	3.6
Annular/nonpustular	26	2.1
Follicular/micropapular	24	2.1
Pustular	8	0.6
Nail	8	0.6
Erythrodermic	1	0.1
Linear	1	0.1
Total	1262	100

(Courtesy of Morris A, Rogers M, Fischer G, et al: Childhood psoriasis: A clinical review of 1262 cases. *Pediatr Dermatol* 18:188-198, 2001. Reprinted by permission of Blackwell Science, Inc.)

and was shinier than the rash of seborrheic dermatitis. Clinically, the plaques in children were noted to be smaller with a finer, softer scale than characterizes adult cases. Seventy-one percent of children whose family history was available had a first-degree relative with psoriasis. For 55 patients, both eczema and psoriasis were present; most of these individuals had a family history positive for atopic disease and psoriasis.

Conclusions.—The most common types of psoriasis found in this age group were plaque and scalp psoriasis if psoriatic diaper rash with dissemination was excluded. A positive family history for psoriasis and/or atopy was often found.

▶ This is an excellent review of the clinical findings in 1262 cases of childhood psoriasis observed by 2 pediatric dermatologists over a period of 14 years. The authors recognized an especially large number of children under age 2 who had well-demarcated diaper area involvement. Eyelid involvement may also be a clue to the diagnosis of psoriasis in young children.

S. Raimer, MD

Low Dose Cyclosporin A Treatment in Generalized Pustular Psoriasis
Kiliç SS, Hacimustafaoğlu M, Çelebi S, et al (Uludağ Univ, Bursa, Turkey; Kocaeli Univ, Bursa, Turkey)
Pediatr Dermatol 18:246-248, 2001   3–19

Background.—Rarely seen in children, generalized pustular psoriasis is characterized by a widespread eruption of sterile pustules. Childhood cases generally begin in the first year of life and tend to have a more benign course than adult cases. Boys are affected more often than girls, in a ratio of 3:2. No safe and effective treatment has been identified. Three patients with generalized pustular psoriasis occurring within the first 3 months of life who underwent successful treatment with cyclosporin A were described.

> *Case 1.*—Girl, 6 years, had psoriatic plaques from the age of 3 months that were resistant to treatment with topical and systemic steroids and methotrexate. Lesions were found over her trunk, gluteal region, scalp, and extremities and consisted of multiple erythematous and pustular plaques. She received cyclosporin A (2 mg/kg per day), then a 1 mg/kg per day suspension for 3 months. The psoriatic plaques and lymphadenopathy cleared within 2 weeks but reappeared when therapy was discontinued. A significant reduction in the psoriasis occurred when therapy was resumed for 9 months. No side effects of cyclosporin therapy were noted.
>
> *Case 2.*—Boy, 10 months, the brother of the girl in case 1, was resistant to topical steroid management of his generalized pustular psoriasis, which was present from the age of 2 months. He was given cyclosporin A (1 mg/kg per day) for persistent flares of fever and pustules, and control of his disease was achieved in 4 weeks. Continued therapy for 6 months produced a psoriasis-free result that has endured.
>
> *Case 3.*—Boy, 17 months, with generalized pustular psoriasis since birth, was resistant to topical steroids. After 2 weeks of therapy with cyclosporin A (1 mg/kg per day), his plaques disappeared. Therapy has continued beyond 5 months at last report.

Conclusions.—Response to cyclosporin A therapy occurred within 2 to 4 weeks in these 3 patients. One patient had a relapse of psoriasis when therapy was discontinued but responded to a resumption of therapy. Thus, low-dose cyclosporin A may be useful in limited courses for the treatment of severe episodes of generalized pustular psoriasis in children.

▶ In this report, 3 young children with generalized pustular psoriasis were treated for several months with low-dose cyclosporine, 1 to 2 mg/kg per day, with good results and without apparent side effects. Because generalized pustular psoriasis is a very painful and potentially life-threatening condition, treatment with low-dose cyclosporine, along with careful monitoring, appears to be a viable therapeutic option.

S. Raimer, MD

4 Bacterial Infections

Lyme Disease
Steere AC (Tufts Univ, Boston)
N Engl J Med 345:115-125, 2001   4–1

Background.—First described in 1977, Lyme disease is now the most common vector-borne disease in the United States, with about 15,000 cases reported each year. The epidemiology, clinical characteristics, diagnosis, treatment, and prevention of Lyme disease were reviewed.

Epidemiology.—Lyme disease is transmitted by ticks of the *Ixodes ricinus* complex that carry the spirochetes *Borrelia burgdorferi* (the only species found in the United States), and *B afzelii* and *B garinii* (the only species found in Asia, and the most common species found in Europe). Thus, the basic disease is similar around the world, but characteristics vary somewhat from region to region (Table 1).

Clinical Manifestations.—Early infection (stage 1) is characterized by a slowly expanding skin lesion (erythema migrans) at the site of the tick bite. Erythema migrans in Europe is often an indolent, localized infection, whereas in the United States it is associated with more intense inflammation and evidence of spirochete dissemination. Influenza-like symptoms often accompany the skin lesion and may be the presenting sign. Within days or weeks of infection, the causative organism becomes disseminated (stage 2) and causes neurologic abnormalities such as acute neuroborreliosis (which develops in about 15% of US patients), lymphocytic meningitis with headache and mild neck stiffness, subtle encephalitis accompanied by difficulty with mentation, cranial neuropathy, motor or sensory radiculoneuritis, mononeuritis multiplex, cerebellar ataxia, or myelitis. In children, inflammation or increased intracranial pressure can affect the optic nerve, which may lead to blindness. Within weeks to months, the acute neurologic abnormalities generally improve or resolve, even in untreated patients. However, *B burgdorferi* can cause chronic neuroborreliosis in up to 5% of untreated patients. Stage 3 begins weeks to months after onset of the disease. This stage is characterized by intermittent joint swelling and pain (in about 60% of untreated US patients) and cardiac involvement (in about 5% of untreated US patients).

Diagnosis.—Early in the illness, *B burgdorferi* infection can be definitively diagnosed by culturing samples from erythema migrans lesions (the most commonly sampled site) or plasma, or from cerebrospinal fluid in

TABLE 1.—Comparison of Lyme Disease in North America and Europe and Asia

Variable	North America (*Borrelia Burgdorferi*)	Europe and Asia (*B. Afzelii* or *B. Garinii*)
Skin		
Acute phase	Erythema migrans faster spreading, more intensely inflamed, and of briefer duration; frequent, possibly widespread hematogenous dissemination	Erythema migrans slower spreading, less intensely inflamed, and of longer duration; less frequent hematogenous dissemination, but possible regional or contiguous spread to other sites
Chronic phase	Acrodermatitis rarely reported	Acrodermatitis chronica atrophicans, caused primarily in *B. afzelii*
Nervous system		
Acute phase	Meningitis, severe headache, mild neck stiffness, less prominent radiculoneuritis	Severe radicular pain and pleocytosis; less prominent headache and neck stiffness, caused particularly by *B. garinii*
Chronic pulse	Subtle sensory polyneuropathy without acrodermatitis	Subtle sensory polyneuropathy within areas affected by acrodermatitis
	Subtle encephalopathy; cognitive disturbance, slight intrathecal antibody production	Severe encephalomyelitis, spasticity, cognitive abnormalities, and marked intrathecal antibody production, caused primarily by *B. garinii*
Cardiac		
Acute phase	Atrioventricular block and subtle myocarditis	Atrioventricular block and subtle myocarditis
Chronic phase	None reported	Dilated cardiomyopathy
Arthritis		
Acute phase	More frequent oligoarticular arthritis, more intense joint inflammation	Less frequent oligoarticular arthritis, less intense joint inflammation
Chronic phase	Treatment-resistant arthritis in about 10 percent of patients, probably due to autoimmune mechanism	Persistent arthritis rare, probably not due to an autoimmune mechanism
Asymptomatic infection	In about 10 percent of patients	In more than 10 percent of patients
Antibody response	Expansion of response to many spirochetal proteins	Expansion of response to fewer spirochetal proteins

TABLE 2.—Case Definition of Lyme Disease for National Surveillance*

Erythema migrans, observed by a physician. This skin lesion expands slowly over a period of days or weeks to form a large, round lesion, often with central clearing. To be counted for surveillance purposes, a solitary lesion must reach a size of at least 5 cm.
At least one subsequent manifestation and laboratory evidence of infection
    Nervous system: Lymphocytic meningitis, cranial neuritis, radiculoneuropathy, or rarely, encephalomyelitis, alone or in combination. For encephalomyelitis to be counted for surveillance purposes, there must be evidence in cerebrospinal fluid of the intrathecal production of antibody against *Borrelia burgdorferi*.
    Cardiovascular system: Acute-onset, high-grade (2nd- or 3rd-degree) atrioventricular conduction defects that resolve in days or weeks and are sometimes associated with myocarditis.
    Musculoskeletal system: Recurrent, brief attacks (lasting weeks to months) of objectively confirmed joint swelling in one or a few joints, sometimes followed by chronic arthritis in one or a few joints.
    Laboratory evidence: Isolation of *B. burgdorferi* from tissue or body fluid or detection of diagnostic levels of antibody against the spirochete by the two-test approach of enzyme-linked immunosorbent assay and Western blotting, interpreted according to the criteria of the Centers for Disease Control and Prevention and the Association of State and Territorial Public Health Laboratory Directors.†

*Adapted from recommendations made by the Centers for Disease Control and Prevention.
†In a person with acute disease of less than 1 month's duration, IgM and IgG antibody responses should be measured in serum samples obtained during the acute and convalescent phases. A Western blot for IgM antibodies is considered positive if 2 or more of the following 3 bands are present: 23, 39, and 41 kd. A blot for IgG antibodies is considered positive if 5 or more of the following 10 bands are present: 18, 23, 28, 30, 39, 41, 4, 58, 66, and 93 kd. Only the IgG response should be used to support the diagnosis after the first month of infection; after that time, an IgM response alone is likely to represent a false-positive result.
(Reprinted by permission of *The New England Journal of Medicine* from Steere AC: Lyme disease. *N Engl J Med* 345:115-125. Copyright 2001, Massachusetts Medical Society. All rights reserved.)

patients with meningitis. Later in the illness, polymerase chain reaction testing should be used to detect *B burgdorferi* in joint fluid samples. The Lyme urine antigen test is unreliable and should not be used. In the United States, diagnosis is based on the presence of the characteristic clinical findings, a history of exposure in an area in which Lyme disease is epidemic, and (for patients with stage 2 or 3 disease) enzyme-linked immunosorbent assay and Western blot evidence of an antibody response to *B burgdorferi* (Table 2). During the first several weeks of infection serodiagnostic tests are insensitive. Antibody titers slowly decrease after antibiotic treatment, but IgG and IgM responses may persist for years.

Treatment and Prevention.—Doxycycline is usually used for early localized or disseminated disease in nonpregnant patients aged 8 years or more (Table 3). More than 90% of patients with erythema migrans will respond to doxycycline, amoxicillin, or cefuroxime axetil. Patients with neurologic abnormalities require intravenous ceftriaxone. Even after treatment, symptoms of musculoskeletal pain or fatigue may persist for years. However, these symptoms of "chronic Lyme disease" may be no more common in patients who have had Lyme disease than in age-matched controls who have not. Measures to prevent Lyme disease include avoidance of tick-infested areas; use of protective clothing, repellents, and acaricides; checking for ticks; and modification of landscapes near residential areas. In addition, a recombinant OspA vaccine is available in the United States; booster injections of the vaccine may be needed every 1 to 3 years.

TABLE 3.—Treatment and Vaccination Regimens for Lyme Disease*

Variable	Regimen
Early infection (local or disseminated)	
Adults	Doxycycline, 100 mg orally twice daily for 14 to 21 days
	Amoxicillin, 500 mg orally three times daily for 14 to 21 days
	Cefuroxime axetil, 500 mg orally twice daily for 14 to 21 days
In case of doxycycline or amoxicillin allergy	Erythromycin, 250 mg orally 4 times a day for 14 to 21 days
Children	Amoxicillin, 250 mg orally 3 times a day or 50 mg per kilogram of body weight per day in 3 divided doses for 14 to 21 days
	Cefuroxime axetil, 125 mg orally twice daily or 30 mg per kg per day in 2 divided doses for 14 to 21 days
In case of penicillin allergy	Erythromycin, 250 mg orally 3 times a day or 30 mg per kg per day in 3 divided doses for 14 to 21 days
Neurologic abnormalities (early or late)	
Adults	Ceftriaxone, 2 g IV once a day for 14 to 28 days
	Cefotaxime, 2 g IV every 8 hr for 14 to 28 days
	Penicillin G sodium, 3.3 million U IV every 4 hr (20 million U per day) for 14 to 28 days
In case of ceftriaxone or penicillin allergy	Doxycycline, 100 mg orally 3 times a day for 30 days†
Facial palsy alone	Oral regimens may be adequate
Children	Ceftriaxone, 75 to 100 mg per kg per day (maximum, 2 g) IV once a day for 14 to 28 days
	Cefotaxime, 150 mg per kg per day in 3 or 4 divided doses (maximum, 6 g) for 14 to 28 days
	Penicillin G sodium, 200,000 to 400,000 U per kg per day in 6 divided doses for 14 to 28 days

Arthritis (intermittent or chronic)	Oral regimens listed above for 30 to 60 days or IV regimens listed above for 14 to 28 days
Cardiac abnormalities	
First-degree atrioventricular block	Oral regimens listed above for 14 to 21 days
High-degree atrioventricular block (PR interval >0.3 sec)	IV regimens listed above and cardiac monitoring‡
Pregnant women	Standard therapy for manifestation of the illness; avoid doxycycline
Vaccination	L-OspA in adjuvant, 30 µg intramuscularly, at 0, 1, and 12 months (or 0, 1, and 2 months)§

*The recommendations for antibiotics are based on the guidelines of the Infectious Diseases Society of America. The recommendations regarding vaccination are based on the results of a phase 3 efficacy and safety trial and on the recommendations of the Advisory Committee on Immunization Practices of the Centers for Disease Control and Prevention.

†This regimen may be ineffective for late neuroborreliosis.

‡Once the patient's condition has stabilized, the course may be completed with oral therapy.

§The third dose should be given in April. Booster injections may be necessary every 1 to 3 years to maintain protection. L-OspA is full-length OspA to which the lipid moiety has been added after translation.

Abbreviation: IV, Intravenously.

(Reprinted by permission of *The New England Journal of Medicine* from Steere AC: Lyme disease. *N Engl J Med* 345:115-125. Copyright 2001, Massachusetts Medical Society. All rights reserved.)

Prevention of Lyme Disease: A Review of the Evidence

Poland GA (Mayo Clinic, Rochester, Minn)
Mayo Clin Proc 76:713-724, 2001   4–2

Background.—Lyme disease is the most common tick-borne illness in the United States, with an incidence of 17.4 cases per 100,000 population between 1992 and 1996. One of the goals of the *Healthy People 2010* public health initiative is to effect a 44% decrease in the incidence of this disease. The evidence regarding the effectiveness of current preventive strategies for reducing the incidence of Lyme disease in the United States was reviewed.

Methods.—Bibliographic databases were searched for articles related to Lyme disease published between 1970 and September 2000. Data were extracted and analyzed according to 4 foci: risk assessment, environmental interventions targeting ticks or wildlife, behavioral interventions, and antimicrobial and vaccine prophylaxis.

Results.—Lyme disease is caused by spirochetes of the *Borrelia burgdorferi* genomic group borne by ticks of the *Ixodes ricinus* complex (*I scapularis* and *I pacificus* in the United States). The risk of Lyme disease is influenced by geography (region, climate, landscape) and the abundance of wildlife, ticks, and *B burgdorferi*. The density of *I ricinus* infestation correlates with the incidence of Lyme disease. Thus, most cases occur in areas known to contain *I scapularis*, in particular the northeast and north central regions. These ticks are most abundant in woodlands; tick density is lower among ornamental vegetation, in lawns, and in sandy areas. Nonetheless, despite these geographic predictors of Lyme disease, quantification of the risk of Lyme disease in humans is difficult because tick-human interactions cannot be predicted. Evidence suggests that both urban and rural outdoor workers are more likely than indoor workers to be seropositive for *B burgdorferi* antibody. However, reports of the correlation between outdoor activities and the risk of infection have been inconsistent. Preventive environmental interventions have included direct (toxins, biological control) and indirect (alteration of the landscape or wildlife population) methods. Efforts to alter the environment to decrease tick viability, such as burning or removing vegetation, the use of acaricides, and immunizing or eliminating deer, have reduced *I scapularis* populations by up to 94%. In addition, the application of acaricides to wildlife has decreased the nymphal *I scapularis* population by up to 80%. Reducing the population of infected ticks is likely to lower the risk of human infection, although the relationship between tick prevalence and risk has not been well defined. The reported effectiveness of preventive behavioral interventions, such as wearing protective clothing, avoidance of ticks, and use of insect repellant, to prevent Lyme disease has been inconsistent. Furthermore, fewer than half of the adults who are aware of Lyme disease take precautions against tick bites. No scientific evidence supports the use of antimicrobial prophylaxis of tick bites. In contrast, prophylaxis with vaccines containing recombinant OspA of *B burgdorferi* has been shown to be effective and well tolerated. One study also indicates that vaccination would be cost-effective at a societal level when the annual risk of Lyme disease is 1% or more.

Conclusions.—Environmental interventions can reduce the abundance of ticks, but practices such as vegetation removal or the treatment of deer can be labor-intensive and costly. Whether such practices help prevent Lyme disease remains to be determined. Personal protective strategies to prevent tick bites have largely proven ineffective in preventing the disorder. Vaccination is the only method that has been empirically demonstrated to prevent Lyme disease.

Prophylaxis With Single-Dose Doxycycline for the Prevention of Lyme Disease After an *Ixodes scapularis* Tick Bite
Nadelman RB, for the Tick Bite Study Group (New York Med College; et al)
N Engl J Med 345:79-84, 2001   4–3

Introduction.—Controlled treatment trials have failed to show the effectiveness of a 10- to 14-day course of antimicrobial therapy for the prevention of Lyme disease after *Ixodes scapularis* tick bites. A much shorter course of therapy, however, has been beneficial in treating other incubating spirochetal infections. The safety and efficacy of a single 200-mg dose of doxycycline in preventing Lyme disease after an *I scapularis* tick bite were examined in a randomized trial.

Methods.—Patients recruited for the trial had been bitten by an *I scapularis* tick in Westchester County, New York, and had removed the attached tick from their bodies within the preceding 72 hours. The active treatment group included 235 patients; 247 patients received placebo. All participants were interviewed and examined at baseline, 3 weeks, and 6 weeks and were given serum antibody tests and blood cultures for *Borrelia burgdorferi*. Ticks were examined for stage by a medical entomologist and classified as flat or partially engorged.

Results.—Twenty-eight participants had removed multiple ticks at the time of the bite that led to enrollment. Erythema migrans occurred at the site of the tick bite in 9 patients, 8 (3.2%) in the placebo group and 1 (0.4%) in the doxycycline group. The difference between the active treatment and placebo groups was significant. Skin cultures were positive for *B burgdorferi* in all 4 of the 9 patients with erythema migrans who underwent skin biopsy. No trial participants showed objective extracutaneous signs of Lyme disease, and no asymptomatic seroconversions occurred. In the placebo group, bites from nymphal ticks were significantly more likely to be associated with erythema migrans than were bites from adult ticks (5.6% vs 0%). In the 2 groups combined, nymphal ticks were nearly twice as likely as adult ticks to be partially engorged (59.8% vs 32.5%). Adverse effects, primarily nausea and vomiting, were more common in the doxycycline group (30.1%) than in the placebo group (11.1%).

Conclusion.—Antimicrobial prophylaxis with a single 200-mg dose of doxycycline administered within 72 hours after a bite from an *I scapularis* tick was highly effective in preventing the development of Lyme disease. The efficacy of doxycycline was 87%.

Two Controlled Trials of Antibiotic Treatment in Patients With Persistent Symptoms and a History of Lyme Disease

Klempner MS, Hu LT, Evans J, et al (Tufts Univ, Boston; Yale-New Haven Hosp, Conn; New York Med College, Valhalla; et al)
N Engl J Med 345:85-92, 2001   4–4

Introduction.—Antibiotic treatment is highly effective for the acute and late septic manifestations of Lyme disease, but some patients experience persistent fatigue, myalgias, arthralgias without arthritis, dysesthesias or paresthesias, or mood and memory disturbances after the standard course of antibiotics. These persistent symptoms have been reported both in patients who are seropositive and those who are seronegative for antibodies against *Borrelia burgdorferi*. Reported are findings from 2 randomized, placebo-controlled, double-blind trials of antibiotic therapy in patients who had chronic symptoms and were either seropositive or seronegative after treatment for Lyme disease.

Methods.—In 1 trial, 78 patients were seropositive for IgG antibodies to *B burgdorferi* at the time of enrollment; in the other trial, 51 patients were seronegative at enrollment. Patients were randomly assigned to treatment with either IV ceftriaxone, 2 g daily for 30 days, followed by oral doxycycline, 200 mg daily for 60 days, or matching intravenous and oral placebos. All patients had well-documented, previously treated Lyme disease and yet had persistent musculoskeletal pain, neurocognitive symptoms, or dysesthesias, frequently associated with fatigue. The main outcome measures were improvement on the physical and mental health component summary scales of the Medical Outcome Survey 36-Item Short-Form General Health Survey (SF-36) on day 180 of the investigation. Clinical and laboratory assessments were performed at baseline and on days 3, 5, 13, 21, 30, 45, 75, 90, and 180.

Results.—After a planned interim analysis, the data and safety monitoring board recommended that the trials be discontinued because data from the first 107 patients indicated that it was highly unlikely that a significant difference in treatment efficacy between the groups would be seen with the planned full enrollment of 260 participants. Baseline evaluations documented severe impairment in patients' health-related quality of life. In intention-to-treat analyses, there were no significant differences in outcomes with prolonged antibiotic treatment versus placebo among either seropositive or seronegative patients.

Conclusion.—Patients with chronic musculoskeletal pain, neurocognitive symptoms, or both that persist after antibiotic treatment for well-documented Lyme disease experienced considerable impairment in their health-related quality of life. Patients treated with IV and oral antibiotics had no significant treatment advanatage over those who received placebo.

▶ Steere and Poland (Abstracts 4–1 and 4–2) present nice reviews of Lyme disease and its prevention. In contrast to the results reported by Nadelman et al (Abstract 4–3), previous studies have shown no clear protection attributable to antimicrobial prophylaxis given after a tick bite.[1-3] Nadelman et al argue that their positive findings, demonstrating the efficacy of antimicrobial prophylaxis, probably relate to the size of their cohort, which provided the study with greater statistical power to show relatively small differences. The question that remains is: "Who should receive doxycycline for a tick bite?" As suggested by Shapiro[4] in an editorial that accompanied the article by Nadelman et al, candidates for antibiotic prophylaxis include persons bitten by ticks in areas where the incidence of Lyme disease is high, when the ticks are nymphal deer ticks that are at least partially engorged with blood. In the more common circumstance in which the bite occurs in a nonendemic area and the tick is not a nymphal deer tick, the species or stage of the tick is not known, or the tick is not at least partially engorged, the risk of Lyme disease is low enough that prophylaxis with doxycycline is not necessary. It should be noted that a Lyme disease vaccine is available and that vaccinated persons should also be at lower risk. The small minority of patients in whom Lyme disease does develop after a tick bite should be reassured that their prognosis is excellent. Unfortunately, as noted in the article by Klempner et al (Abstract 4–4), prolonged antibiotic therapy does not appear to improve symptoms that persist after the standard treatment of acute Lyme disease.

B. H. Thiers, MD

References

1. Costello CM, Steere AC, Pinkerton RE, et al: A prospective study of tick bites in an endemic area for Lyme disease. *J Infect Dis* 159:136-139, 1989.
2. Agre F, Schwartz R: The value of early treatment of deer tick bites for the prevention of Lyme disease. *Am J Dis Child* 147:945-947, 1993.
3. Shapiro ED, Gerber MA, Holabird ND, et al: A controlled trial of antimicrobial prophylaxis for Lyme disease after deer-tick bites. *N Engl J Med* 327:1769-1773, 1992.
4. Shapiro ED: Doxycycline for tick bites—Not for everyone. *N Engl J Med* 345:133-134, 2001.

Safety and Immunogenicity of a Recombinant *Borrelia burgdorferi* Outer Surface Protein A Vaccine Against Lyme Disease in Healthy Children and Adolescents: A Randomized Controlled Trial

Sikand VK, for the Pediatric Lyme Vaccine Study Group (Tufts Univ, Boston; et al)

Pediatrics 108:123-128, 2001

4–5

Background.—Lyme disease (LD), caused by *Borrelia burgdorferi*, accounts for more than 95% of all cases of vector-borne illness reported in the United States, having increased 25-fold since 1982. The vaccine for LD contains 30 µg of recombinant *B burgdorferi* lipidized outer-surface protein A and is licensed for use in individuals ages 15 to 70 years. This leaves children under 15 years vulnerable, although they account for almost 30% to 40% of cases. The safety and immunogenicity of LD vaccine for this population was assessed.

Methods.—From 17 sites in LD-endemic areas of the United States, 4090 healthy children were chosen to participate in a test of the LD vaccine for children ages 4 to 18 years. Children received either 30 µg of LD vaccine or placebo randomly in a 3:1 ratio according to a 0, 1, 12-month schedule. The data on immunogenicity were compared with those from an adult efficacy study. Three hundred one children participated in the analysis of immunogenicity. Safety was assessed based on both solicited events—local redness, swelling, or pain, or the generalized signs of fever, headache, fatigue, arthralgia, and rash—and unsolicited adverse events. Serum specimens were collected during the second month and at 6, 12, and 13 months at 2 study sites, and at baseline and during the second, 12th, and 13th months at a third site.

Results.—Children reported more local symptoms than general symptoms whether they received vaccine or placebo. Of those in the vaccine group, 78.2% reported local symptoms and 30.1% general ones; of those in the placebo group, 55.1% had local symptoms and 21.5% general ones. Most of these lasted 2 to 3 days and were of mild to moderate severity. At the 13th month, total immunoglobulin G anti-outer surface protein A geometric mean titer among the vaccine recipients was as good as and statistically greater than that noted among adults. The antibody concentration was more than the proposed seroprotective level in all the children, whereas only 90% of the adults achieved that level.

Conclusions.—The LD vaccine used was both safe and immunogenic in individuals ages 4 to 18 years. The side effects were mild to moderate, limited in duration, and generally well-tolerated. These children had a significantly more robust immune response than did the adults tested.

▶ This study suggests that a recombinant outer surface protein A vaccine is safe and effective in preventing Lyme disease in 4- to 18-year-old patients. Local and systemic side effects were mild and were generally well tolerated. The immune response was substantially more robust in children than in adults; thus, the vaccine appears to have the potential to contribute significantly to the prevention of Lyme disease in children.

S. Raimer, MD

Diagnostic Assessment of Haemorrhagic Rash and Fever

Nielsen HE, Andersen EA, Andersen J, et al (Gentofte Hosp, Hellerup, Denmark; Glostrup Hosp, Denmark; Holbæk Hosp, Denmark; et al)
Arch Dis Child 85:160-165, 2001   4–6

Introduction.—The combination of fever and hemorrhagic skin lesions in a child suggests the possibility of meningococcal disease (MD). The diagnosis is clear if nuchal rigidity or fulminant purpura and circulatory collapse are also present, but children with only small skin hemorrhages who are in relatively good general condition pose a diagnostic challenge. A large number of such children were studied prospectively to establish criteria for early distinction between MD and other conditions with similar clinical features, and to identify the etiology of disease when MD is ruled out.

Methods.—Five pediatric departments enrolled consecutive patients over a 24-month period. Those eligible ranged in age from 1 month to 16 years and had skin hemorrhages plus a rectal temperature above 38°C. All were considered to have illness clinically compatible with MD. The 264 patients were classified into 7 groups: confirmed MD (29 children; median age, 30 months); probable MD (10 children; median age, 26 months); invasive bacterial infection not MD (6 patients; median age, 14 months); enterovirus infection (18 patients; median age, 21 months); adenovirus infection (11 patients; median age, 22 months); no invasive bacterial disease (140 patients; median age, 27 months); and insufficient information (50 patients; median age, 18 months). Confirmed MD cases required culture of *Neisseria meningitidis* from blood and/or spinal fluid.

Results.—Etiologic agents were identified in only 28% of the children; 15% had confirmed or probable MD. The general condition was worse in the confirmed cases. Five clinical variables distinguished MD from other conditions on admission: skin hemorrhages of characteristic appearance (Fig 1; see color plate IV), universal distribution of skin hemorrhages, maximum diameter greater than 2 mm for at least 1 skin hemorrhage, poor general condition as determined by a standardized observation method, and nuchal rigidity. These variables had odds ratios of the same approximate magnitude. In the presence of 2 or more of the 5 clinical variables, the probability of identifying a patient with MD was 97%, and the false-positive rate was 12%.

Conclusion.—These simple clinical observations had a high discriminatory power for the diagnosis of MD. The algorithm was not useful, however, for the diagnosis of other invasive bacterial infections.

▶ In this prospective study of children with purpuric lesions and fever, the authors noted that 5 of the clinical signs investigated—appearance, generalized distribution, size of skin hemorrhages, poor general condition, and nuchal rigidity—were all independently predictive of the presence of meningococcal disease. If 2 or more signs were present, the probability of meningococcemia was very high. Three of the signs relate to the appearance

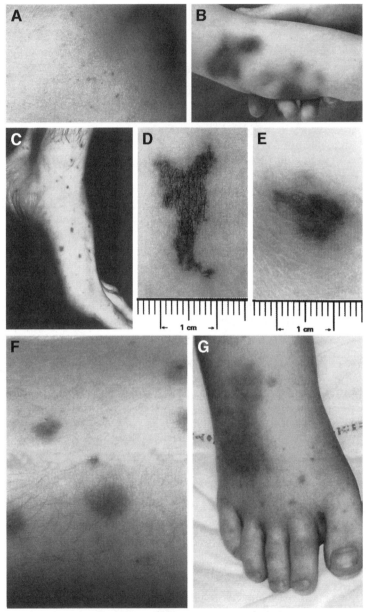

FIGURE 1.—Clinical photos on the study form. The photos are from patients with (**A**) micropetechiae, type 1; (**B**) thrombocytopenia, type 2; (**C-E**) meningococcal disease, types 3-5; (**F, G**) Henoch-Schönlein purpura, types 6 and 7. (Courtesy of Nielsen HE, Andersen EA, Andersen J, et al: Diagnostic assessment of haemorrhagic rash and fever. *Arch Dis Child* 85:160-165, 2001. Reprinted with permission from the BMJ Publishing Group.)

of the hemorrhagic skin lesions. Therefore, febrile children with suspicious lesions should be treated for meningococcemia pending the outcome of laboratory investigations.

S. Raimer, MD

Nasal Carriage as a Source of *Staphylococcus aureus* Bacteremia
von Eiff C, for the Study Group (Univ of Münster, Germany; et al)
N Engl J Med 344:11-16, 2001   4–7

Background.—One of the most common causes of both endemic and epidemic infections acquired in hospitals is *Staphylcoccus aureus.* Infection with this organism has resulted in substantial morbidity and mortality. Strategies for prevention are important, as the consequences of infection with *S aureus* can be severe. Isolates of *S aureus* from blood and from nasal specimens were examined to determine whether the organisms in the bloodstream originated from the patient's own flora.

Methods.—In a multicenter study, investigators obtained swabs for culture from the anterior nares of 219 patients with *S aureus* bacteremia immediately after the isolation of *S aureus* from the blood. A total of 723 isolates were collected and genotyped. Investigators also conducted a second study, in which 1640 *S aureus* isolates were collected from 1278 patients over 5 years and then compared with isolates from the blood of patients who subsequently had *S aureus* bacteremia.

Results.—In the first study, the blood isolates were identical to the isolates collected by nasal swab in 180 of 219 patients (82.2%). In the second study, in 14 of 1278 patients with nasal colonization with *S aureus*, *S aureus* bacteremia subsequently developed. In 12 of these 14 patients (86%), the isolates obtained by nasal swab were found to be clonally identical to the isolates obtained from blood 1 day to 14 months later.

Conclusion.—A significant proportion of *S aureus* bacteremia infections appear to derive from an endogenous source, originating from colonies in the nasal mucosa. These findings support strategies for prevention of systemic *S aureus* infections that are aimed at the elimination of nasal carriage of the organism.

▶ Previous studies have demonstrated an association between *S aureus* nasal colonization and skin infections and the value of mupirocin prophylaxis.[1,2] Unfortunately, the eradication by topical antibiotics is often temporary, and systemic antibiotics lead to the development of resistant organisms.[3] Von Eiff et al investigated the link between *S aureus* isolated from nasal specimens and *S aureus* isolated from blood. Three patterns of nasal carriage have been distinguished. First, approximately 20% of asymptomatic healthy people almost always carry a strain. Second, a large proportion of the population, approximately 60%, intermittently harbors *S aureus* and the strains change with varying frequency. The third pattern, involving approximately 20% of the population, includes people who almost never carry the organism.

Children more commonly are persistent carriers than are adults, and the carrier type often changes between the ages of 10 and 20 years. The key role the carriage of S aureus plays in the pathogenesis of infection has been convincingly demonstrated. An editorial that accompanies this article discusses strategies to reduce nosocomial S aureus infections.[3]

B. H. Thiers, MD

References

1. Doebbeling BN, Reagan DR, Pfaller MA, et al: Long-term efficacy of intranasal mupirocin ointment: A prospective cohort study of *Staphylococcus aureus* carriage. *Arch Intern Med* 154:1505-1508, 1994.
2. Raz R, Miron D, Colodner R, et al: A 1-year trial of nasal mupirocin in the prevention of recurrent staphylococcal nasal colonization and skin infection. *Arch Intern Med* 156:1109-1112, 1996.
3. Archer GL, Climo MW: *Staphylococcus aureus* bacteremia: Consider the source. *N Engl J Med* 344:55-56, 2001.

Necrotizing Fasciitis of the Head and Neck: An Analysis of 47 Cases
Lin C, Yeh F-L, Lin J-T, et al (Natl Yang-Ming Univ, Taiwan)
Plast Reconstr Surg 107:1684-1693, 2001   4–8

Introduction.—Necrotizing fasciitis is a severe acute inflammatory condition that usually affects the extremities, perineum, and abdominal wall. Patients are often elderly or immunocompromised, and mortality has been reported to be as high as 73%. Because only a few articles have discussed necrotizing fasciitis of the head and neck, 47 such cases treated over a 12-year period were analyzed.

Methods.—The 47 cases all met the clinical, pathologic, and CT criteria for necrotizing fasciitis of the head and neck. Cases were divided into 2 groups: survivors (35 patients) and nonsurvivors (12 patients). The 2 groups were compared for age, gender, smoking and drinking habits, underlying medical disease, operation/trauma history, hospital course, and outcome.

Results.—The median patient age was 63 (range, 5 months to 86 years). Thirty-eight patients were men, and 23 (48.9%) habitually smoked. Nearly half the patients were older than 65, and 89.4% had an underlying medical disease. Thirty-four patients (72.3%) had diabetes, and 17 (36.2%) had a history of minor trauma or operations. The most common lesion site was the anterior neck. Before antibiotic therapy, specimens were collected for bacterial culture. The total positive culture rate was 73%. Common pathogens (Fig 5) were *Klebsiella pneumoniae* (26% of cases), *Staphylococcus aureus*, and *streptococcus*. Seventeen patients required immediate resuscitation for shock, and 11 underwent endotracheal intubation or tracheostomy. All patients had surgical treatment within 48 hours after admission. The median duration of hospital stay was 21.5

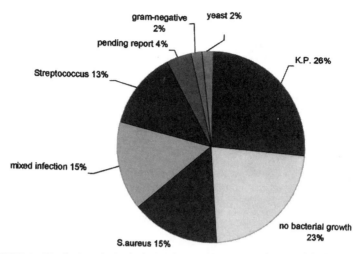

FIGURE 5.—Distribution of microbiologic infections in necrotizing fasciitis of the head and neck. *Abbreviation: K.P., Klebsiella pneumoniae.* (Courtesy of Lin C, Yeh F-L, Lin J-T, et al: Necrotizing fasciitis of the head and neck: An analysis of 47 cases. *Plast Reconstr Surg* 107:1684-1693, 2001.)

days. The only statistically significant factors associated with a poor prognosis were admission with septic shock and an underlying malignancy.

Discussion.—Because necrotizing fasciitis of the head and neck is uncommon, clinical detection may be difficult, but in all cases, there was marked swelling and erythema over the involved area, and 85% of patients experienced pain. The need for CT scans was not confirmed in this patient series, and demographics and laboratory findings did not predict outcome.

▶ Early diagnosis, aggressive surgical debridement, broad spectrum antibiotics, and intensive supportive care form the cornerstones of proper management for patients with necrotizing fasciitis of the head and neck.

B. H. Thiers, MD

Streptolysin S and Necrotising Infections Produced by Group G Streptococcus
Humar D, Datta V, Bast DJ, et al (Univ of California, San Diego; Mount Sinai Hosp, Toronto, Ont, Canada; Univ of Toronto; et al)
Lancet 359:124-129, 2002   4–9

Background.—Group G streptococci are part of the normal flora of human skin. This report describes 3 cases of severe necrotizing infections caused by β-hemolytic group G streptococcus. Because of the similarity between these infections and those of group A streptococcus, the group G β-hemolysin was identified and characterized to evaluate its contribution to pathogenesis.

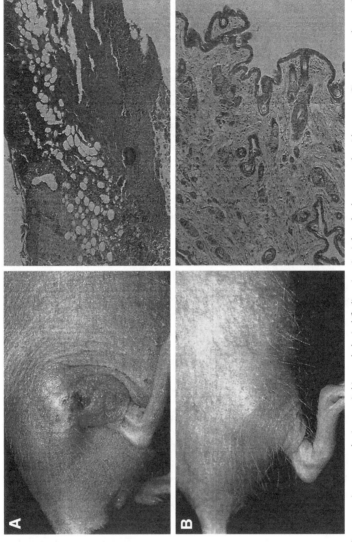

FIGURE 4.—Representative gross and microscopic histopathological findings in mice infected subcutaneously with a group G streptococcal necrotizing fasciitis clinical isolate (A) versus an isogenic streptolysin S–deficient mutant (B). Ulcer formation with necrotic tissue destruction, vascular thrombosis, and diffuse neutrophilic infiltrate are noted with the wild-type strain, whereas only minimal inflammatory changes are seen with the mutant. (Courtesy of Humar D, Datta V, Bast DJ, et al: Streptolysin S and necrotising infections produced by group G streptococcus. *Lancet* 359:124-129, 2002. Copyright by the Lancet Ltd, 2002.)

Case Report.—Man, 52, with type 2 diabetes mellitus, presented with a 6-day history of fever and swelling of the right leg. Erythema and edema extended from ankle to knee. The patient received antibiotics but remained febrile. Blood and blister fluid cultures were negative. Histopathology of surgical debridement samples revealed acute necrotizing inflammation and intravascular thrombosis. Debridement cultures grew group G streptococcus. Intravenous benzylpenicillin was initiated. The patient required further surgical debridement but improved and was discharged to a rehabilitation facility.

Methods.—Group G streptococcus was identified using the API 20 Strep identification system. Hemolytic titers were determined with a liquid-phase assay. The group G β-hemolysin gene was identified by dot-blot hybridization with a labeled group A *sag* (β-hemolysin streptolysin 5 [SLS]) probe. The identified group G DNA fragment was cloned and sequenced. A knockout plasmid was created from this clone and introduced into group G streptococcus by electroporation to evaluate its function by mutational analysis. Virulence was assessed with a mouse model of necrotizing fasciitis.

Results.—β-hemolytic group G streptococcus was the only microbe isolated from debrided necrotic tissue in each case. Each patient also had an underlying medical condition. A homologue of the group A streptococcus *sag* operon encoding the β-hemolysin SLS was identified in the group G streptococcus genome. Targeted mutagenesis of this gene eliminated β-hemolytic activity in group G streptococcus. Mice injected subcutaneously with wild-type group G streptococcus, but not bacteria mutated to remove the hemolytic activity, developed tissue necrosis (Fig 4).

Conclusions.—This report describes 3 patients with underlying medical conditions who had necrotizing soft tissue infections resembling those observed with group A streptococcus disease, but the only microbial isolate was group G streptococcus. The β-hemolytic phenotype of group G streptococcus is produced by a gene that is the functional homologue of the β-hemolysin of group A streptococcus, which is also responsible for necrotizing infections. The activity of β-hemolysin contributes to the pathogenicity of group G streptococcus infection. Neutralization of this activity would serve as a useful adjunct therapy for the treatment of streptococcal necrotizing infections.

▶ Microbiologically, human group G streptococcus isolates can be subdivided on the basis of colony size and hemolytic phenotype on sheep blood agar. Large colony isolates produce robust β-hemolysis and are morphologically very similar to the prominent pathogen, group A streptococcus. This study demonstrates that β-hemolytic group G streptococcus can produce necrotizing soft tissue infections similar to those produced by group A streptococcus and that the tissue damage appears to be mediated by the exotoxin SLS. Notably, in each of the patients reported by Humar et al, a significant underlying medical condition was present.

B. H. Thiers, MD

Gram-Negative Bacterial Toe Web Infection: A Survey of 123 Cases From the District of Cagliari, Italy
Aste N, Atzori L, Zucca M, et al (Cagliari Univ, Italy)
J Am Acad Dermatol 45:537-541, 2001   4–10

Background.—Foot intertrigo is mostly caused by dermatophytes and yeasts, less frequently by gram-positive and gram-negative bacteria. Nevertheless, the importance of polymicrobial infections and especially colonizations of *Pseudomonas aeruginosa* can cause therapy problems in relation to antibiotic resistance and the risk of potentially lethal complications.

Objective.—The aim of this study was to evaluate the main epidemiologic and clinical features of intertrigo from gram-negative bacteria, the function of promoting factors, and the measures taken to treat and prevent this disorder.

Methods.—Between 1989 and 1998, 123 cases of intertrigo from gram-negative bacteria were observed at the Cagliari University Dermatology Department. Routine clinical and blood examinations, repeated bacterioscopic and mycologic examinations, cultures aimed at identifying the responsible bacteria, and antibiograms were performed.

Results.—*P aeruginosa* was found to be the prevailing pathogen, both alone and associated with other gram-negative bacteria (such as *Escherichia coli, Proteus mirabilis, Morganella morganii*) and gram-positive bacteria. Clinical manifestations were similar in the majority of patients: erythema, vesicopustules, erosions, and marked maceration caused by abundant, malodorous exudate. Lesions affected the interdigital spaces of both feet and frequently extended to the planta and the back of the toes. Patients complained of burning and pain. Successful therapies were achieved with combined topical and systemic treatment; to avoid the risk of antimicrobial resistance, the choice of the active antibiotic was guided by antibiograms.

Conclusion.—In all symptomatic toe web infections, the presence of gram-negative germs, such as *P aeruginosa*, should be investigated to avoid the risk of treatment failures and more severe local or systemic complications.

▶ The authors are right on the mark. In my opinion, many patients with severe interdigital maceration fail to respond to antifungal agents because of overgrowth of gram-negative bacteria. I have found acetic acid soaks and topical gentamicin to aid immeasurably in the management of these patients.

B. H. Thiers, MD

The Pseudomonas Hot-Foot Syndrome

Fiorillo L, Zucker M, Sawyer D, et al (Univ of Alberta, Edmonton, Canada; Univ of Calgary, Alberta, Canada)
N Engl J Med 345:335-338, 2001   4–11

Background.—Folliculitis occurring in association with whirlpools, hot tubs, swimming pools, saunas, and hydrotherapy pools has been linked to *Pseudomonas aeruginosa*. An outbreak of a distinctive skin eruption on the soles of feet of children who frequented a community wading pool is described.

Methods.—The medical records of 40 children in whom the syndrome developed between March and May 1998 were reviewed; 1 other individual who used the pool had signs of pseudomonas folliculitis of the buttocks and trunk without plantar nodules, but was not included in the study. The authors treated 17 children, and advised the treating physicians of the other 23 children. Follow-up extended for up to 1 year.

Results.—The syndrome developed 10 to 40 hours after use of the wading pool; 34 cases were found in the first 9 days. The course was similar for all patients, consisting of initial intense pain in the soles of the feet, then marked swelling, redness, a hot sensation, and exquisite pain that kept the child from bearing weight on the affected areas. Physical examination showed a diffuse, dusky erythema and deep, extremely painful, red to purple nodules which measured 1 to 2 cm in greatest diameter and were concentrated on the foot's weight-bearing surfaces. Children with the most severe cases had fever (temperature, 37.7 to 38.8°C), malaise, and nausea. A painful nodule was present on the palmar aspect of 1 child's right middle finger; 1 had diffuse erythema over the palmar surfaces; and 3 had lymphangitic lines on the surface of the instep, but no palpable lymph nodes in either the inguinal area or the popliteal fossa. One patient had folliculitis of the buttocks along with the plantar nodules. After several days the affected areas looked bruised and desquamated. Treatment included general symptomatic therapy, cold compresses, analgesics, and elevation of the feet; 3 patients were given oral cephalexin. All signs and symptoms resolved in 1 to 14 days, and 88% of patients were free of problems in 7 days. Cultures from a skin nodule and the wading pool water yielded identical strains of *P aeruginosa*. The pool was closed on the ninth day after the outbreak began, the water was drained, and superchlorination was used. Over the next 2 weeks no samples yielded bacterial growth on culturing, and the pool was reopened. New cases were reported over the next 2 days, even with increased chlorine concentrations. The pool was closed for a second time when cultures again yielded *P aeruginosa*, and the floor, water pipes, and inlets were scrubbed with a quaternium ammonium compound followed by ozone treatment. No additional cases were reported.

Conclusions.—Superchlorination of pool water, reduced abrasiveness of the pool floor, and scrubbing of the floor, water pipes, and pool inlet surfaces with quaternium ammonium compounds along with ozone treatment were required to clear this wading pool of contamination with *P aeruginosa*. The outbreak may have been caused by inoculation of *P aeruginosa* into the soles of the feet as they rubbed against the pool's abrasive surface. The primary entity in the differential diagnosis of this disorder is recurrent idiopathic palmoplantar hidradenitis, but this is uncommon. Seventeen cases of suppurative panniculitis resulting from infection with *P aeruginosa* have been reported, but they differed in that they were sporadic, involved sepsis in most cases, and required antibiotic therapy along with incision and drainage of the nodules. In addition, the soles were spared; lesions instead occurred on the legs.

▶ The authors describe a novel manifestation of cutaneous pseudomonas infection. Pseudomonas hot-foot syndrome is characterized by painful cutaneous nodules on the feet. Fiorillo et al report 40 children who contracted the disease after wading in a pool with a constant water temperature of 33°C. *P aeruginosa* was cultured from the water. The most severely affected patients had fever, malaise, and nausea in addition to cutaneous lesions. Idiopathic palmoplantar hidradenitis can have a clinical appearance similar to pseudomonas hot-foot syndrome, but appears to be a different clinical entity. Idiopathic palmoplantar hidradenitis occurs sporadically and often involves the palms as well as the soles, and histologic analysis shows infiltrates of neutrophils confined to the eccrine apparatus.

S. Raimer, MD

Glanders in a Military Research Microbiologist
Srinivasan A, Kraus CN, DeShazer D, et al (NIH, Bethesda, Md)
N Engl J Med 345:256-258, 2001   4–12

Introduction.—Infection with *Burkholderia mallei* can produce a subcutaneous infection known as farcy. Its disseminated form is known as glanders and is characterized in humans by necrosis of the tracheobronchial tree, pustular skin lesions, and either a febrile pneumonia if inhaled or signs of sepsis and multiple abscesses if the skin is the port of entry. Described is the first case of human glanders in the United States in more than 50 years.

> *Case Report.*—Male, 33, with type 1 diabetes mellitus had tender left axillary adenopathy and fever develop in March 2000. He was a microbiologist for the US Army Medical Research Institute who had been investigating the basic microbiology of *B mallei* for 2 years. He did not routinely wear latex gloves. His fever and adenopathy were refractory to 10 days of treatment with a first-generation cephalosporin. The symptoms and adenopathy resolved in early April after 10 days of clarithromycin. He experienced a relapse 4 days after discontinuation of medication. He was hospitalized on May 2 with diabetic ketoacidosis. A CT scan revealed

multiple hepatic and splenic abscesses. On May 4, he required mechanical ventilation because of respiratory distress. Blood cultures and a fine-needle biopsy of a liver abscess grew an organism thought to be either *Pseudomonas fluorescens* or *P putida*. Gas-liquid chromatography of the cellular fatty acids definitively identified the organism as *B mallei*. Initial susceptibility testing revealed that the isolate was sensitive to imipenem, ceftazidime, and tetracycline. The patient's condition improved rapidly when he was treated with imipenem and doxycycline. The imipenem was replaced with azithromycin 2 weeks later, and the patient completed a 6-month course of azithromycin and doxycycline, after which a CT scan showed notable improvement in the liver and splenic abscesses. The patient was in good health at 1-year follow-up.

Conclusion.—This is the first case of glanders in a human reported in the English-language medical literature since 1949. It occurred within the context of research on agents of biological warfare.

▶ Infection with *B mallei* (formerly called *Pseudomonas mallei*) can cause a subcutaneous infection (farcy) or can disseminate (glanders). This zoonotic disease of horses and related animals was eliminated from the United States in 1934 and from other Western countries shortly thereafter. As a lethal, contagious disease, it was considered an ideal agent for biological warfare; in fact, it was used for this purpose by Germany in World War I. Re-emerging concern about bioterrorism has led to study of the disease in laboratories worldwide. As the events of the fall of 2001 have taught us, other long-forgotten infectious agents, such as the anthrax bacillus and the smallpox virus, might also be candidates for biological weapons programs.

B. H. Thiers, MD

Kif1C, a Kinesin-like Motor Protein, Mediates Mouse Macrophage Resistance to Anthrax Lethal Factor
Watters JW, Dewar K, Lehoczky J, et al (Harvard Med School, Boston; Whitehead Inst for Biomedical Research, Cambridge, Mass)
Curr Biol 11:1503-1511, 2001   4–13

Background.—Anthrax lethal toxin (LeTx), produced at high levels during systemic infection, mimics the lethal effects of systemic anthrax when administered in animal models. Inbred mouse strains differ significantly, however, in the susceptibility of their cultured macrophages to the effects of LeTx. Previous research has shown this difference in susceptibility to lie downstream of toxin entry into macrophages. A locus controlling this phenotype, *Ltxs1*, was previously mapped to chromosome 11. The identification of the *Ltxs1* gene as *Kif1C*, which encodes a kinesin-like motor protein of the UNC104 subfamily, was reported.

Findings.—*Kif1C* is the only gene in the *Ltxs1* critical interval that contains mutations between susceptible and resistant inbred strains. Multiple alleles of *Kif1C* determine the susceptibility or resistance of cultured mouse macrophages to LeTx. When resistant macrophages are treated with brefeldin-A, which alters the cellular localization of *Kif1C*, susceptibility to LeTx is induced. But ectopic expression of a resistance allele of *Kif1C* in susceptible macrophages results in a 4-fold increase in the number of cells surviving LeTx treatment. Resistant cells demonstrate cleavage of map kinase kinase 3, a target of LeTx proteolysis.

Conclusion.—Mutations of *Kif1C* appear to be responsible for the differences in susceptibility of inbred mouse macrophages to LeTx, and resistance to LeTx requires proper *Kif1C* function. Lethal factor is proteolytically active in the cytosol of resistant macrophages, indicating that *Kif1C* is not involved in LeTx uptake or activation and is likely to exert influence later in the intoxication pathway.

▶ The authors describe a gene, *Kif1C*, that renders mice resistant to a potent anthrax toxin. *Kif1C* codes a protein that appears to transfer other proteins, such as the anthrax toxin, within white blood cells. A change in the gene seems to determine either susceptibility or resistance to the toxin. Presumably, certain forms of the protein can carry the toxin to a place in the cell where it can be destroyed, whereas other forms of the protein lack this ability. Manipulation of the human equivalent to this gene (should one exist) ultimately might lead to new treatments for this deadly disease.

B. H. Thiers, MD

Candida Osteomyelitis and Diskitis After Spinal Surgery: An Outbreak That Implicates Artificial Nail Use

Parry MF, Grant B, Yukna M, et al (Stamford Hosp, Conn; Columbia Univ, New York)
Clin Infect Dis 32:352-357, 2001   4–14

Background.—Nosocomial infection of surgical sites by *Candida* species is uncommon but can occur when organisms are transferred from the hands of medical personnel or from point sources linked to medical devices that are excessively colonized. A cluster of wound infections found after surgery and caused by *Candida albicans* contaminating an operating room technician—specifically, her artificial fingernails—was reported.

Methods.—Surgical site infections caused by *C albicans* developed in 3 patients who had had lumbar laminectomy. Infection developed as long as 3 months after surgery, with isolates identified by surveying cultures in the microbiology laboratory. Laboratory records for the previous 10 years were reviewed retrospectively, but no similar infections were found. Control patients had no surgical site infection. Isolates were obtained from the 3 infected patients, a suspected health care worker, and random concurrent clinical isolates underwent pulsed-field gel electrophoresis with whole-cell DNA and *Sfi*I restriction endonuclease.

Results.—The 3 cases represented 11% of the spinal surgeries performed in the same time period. The pulsed-field gel electrophoresis analysis showed that the isolates from these 3 patients were identical and differed from the *C albicans* isolates obtained from 6 other patients. Exposure to 1 scrub technologist was the only risk factor occurring more commonly among these 3 cases than among control patients. During an interview, the technologist revealed that she had worn artificial fingernails during these patients' surgeries. The fingernails had been removed and were unavailable for culture, but throat cultures showed a few colonies of *C albicans*, although no clinical evidence of infection was found in samples taken from various sites (hand, fingernail, periungual, nares, or vaginal). The technologist was removed from duty and received oral fluconazole treatment for 14 days.

Conclusion.—The outbreak of three cases of *C albicans* infection at surgical sites appears to have been caused by infected artificial fingernails worn in the surgical area. This illustrates the need for a policy banning artificial fingernails in high-risk areas, which would include the operating room, the critical care unit, and the neonatal ICU.

Effect of Hand Cleansing With Antimicrobial Soap or Alcohol-Based Gel on Microbial Colonization of Artificial Fingernails Worn by Health Care Workers

McNeil SA, Foster CL, Hedderwick SA, et al (Ann Arbor Veterans Affairs Healthcare System, Mich; Univ of Michigan, Ann Arbor)
Clin Infect Dis 32:367-372, 2001   4–15

Background.—Hand cleansing, done correctly and thoroughly, has been seen as an effective way to prevent the transmission of nosocomial infections. The current trend of wearing artificial fingernails includes health care workers, and these artificial nails carry a significant load of potentially pathogenic organisms when compared with natural nails. The abilities of soap and alcohol-based gel to eliminate potentially infective organisms from natural and artificial fingernails worn by health care workers (HCWs) were compared.

Methods.—The 21 volunteers (15 nurses, 2 respiratory therapists, 2 technicians, 1 pharmacist, and 1 ward clerk) and 20 control subjects (13 nurses, 6 physicians, and 1 respiratory therapist) included workers from both inpatient and outpatient areas of the University of Michigan and the Veterans Affairs Medical Centers. The volunteers wore salon-applied, permanent polished acrylic artificial nails and the control subjects did not. Baseline samples were obtained, then the study group cleansed their hands as they normally did, using antimicrobial soap or alcohol-based gel. Cultures were repeated, with samples taken from the nail surfaces and subungual nail regions (all 5 fingers of the dominant hand). Comparison of the frequency with which organisms were isolated and of the quantity of the organisms was made between the 2 groups.

Results.—The control group's nails were shorter than the group with artificial nails. All HCWs wearing artificial nails, but no controls, wore nail polish. Baseline samples showed that those wearing artificial nails were more likely to have a pathogen isolated than were the control HCWs. Eighty-six percent of those cleansing with soap had a pathogen, compared with 35% of controls, and 68% of those cleansing with gel had a pathogen, compared with 28% of controls. The organisms found most often were *Staphylococcus aureus*, gram-negative bacilli, and yeasts. More organisms were found in the subungual region than on the surface in both groups. After cleansing with either gel or soap, 81% of the 21 HCWs wearing artificial nails had pathogens remaining; only 35% of the 20 controls had pathogens remaining. The number of workers wearing artificial nails who had yeasts or gram-negative bacilli was significantly higher compared with controls. Based on degree of nail colonization, the alcohol-based gel was better at removing pathogens than was the antimicrobial soap.

Conclusion.—Routine cleansing of hands with antimicrobial soap was unable to remove all pathogens from either artificial or natural fingernails, but the degree of colonization was significantly higher among those wearing artificial nails. These pathogens could be transmitted to patients, so the wearing of artificial nails by HCWs is an unsafe practice that should be eliminated from high-risk areas.

▶ These articles (Abstracts 4–13 and 4–14) add to the growing body of evidence, some of which was reviewed in the 2001 YEAR BOOK OF DERMATOLOGY AND DERMATOLOGIC SURGERY, that implicates artificial nails worn by health care workers in the pathogenesis of hospital-acquired infections.[1-3] Other factors, such as nail length, may also play a role. Indeed, in the study by McNeil et al, most volunteers in the control group wore their nails short and none wore nail polish, whereas all members of the artificial nail group wore their nails long and polished. The propensity of artificial fingernails to harbor pathogens may result from a combination of factors, including increased length, use of nail polish, and the presence of acrylic material. The Association of Operating Room Nurses maintains that the use of artificial fingernails by hospital workers may contribute to the transmission of pathogens to patients and advises that artificial fingernails not be worn in the operating room. Similar policies should be considered for other high-risk areas, including ICUs and neonatal nurseries.

B. H. Thiers, MD

References

1. Moolenaar RL, Crutcher JM, San Joaquin VH, et al: A prolonged outbreak of Pseudomonas aeruginosa in a neonatal intensive care unit: Did staff fingernails play a role in disease transmission? *Infect Control Hosp Epidemiol* 21:80-85, 2000.

2. Hedderwick SA, McNeil SA, Lyons MJ, et al: Pathogenic organisms associated with artificial fingernails worn by healthcare workers. *Infect Control Hosp Epidemiol* 21:505-509, 2000.

3. Foca A, Jakob K, Whittier S, et al: Endemic Pseudomonas aeruginosa infection in a neonatal intensive care unit. *N Engl J Med* 343:695-700, 2000.

Innate Antimicrobial Peptide Protects the Skin From Invasive Bacterial Infection

Nizet V, Ohtake T, Lauth X, et al (Univ of California, San Diego; Veterans Affairs San Diego Healthcare System, Calif; Massachusetts Gen Hosp, Boston)
Nature 414:454-457, 2001   4–16

Background.—Several mammalian gene families, such as the β-defensins and cathelicidins, encode peptides with antibacterial activity. These peptides are expressed on epithelial surfaces and in neutrophils and have been proposed to act as natural antibiotics to provide a first line of defense against infection. For example, the cathelicidins CRAMP and LL-37 are significantly increased in the skin after wounding because of their release from neutrophil granules and increased synthesis by keratinocytes. However, several peptides with antibacterial activity are easily inactivated and have other diverse cellular effects, findings that raise questions regarding their protective abilities. In this study the function of a specific antimicrobial peptide was investigated in a mouse model of cutaneous infection.

Methods.—A combined mammalian and bacterial genetic approach to the cathelicidin antimicrobial gene family was investigated by directly assessing the function of cathelicidins in vivo. Normal mice and mice null for *Cnlp* were used for the studies; the latter mice are CRAMP-deficient. A targeting vector was constructed in which exons 3 and 4, encoding the entire mature domain of *CRAMP*, were replaced with PGK-neo flanked 5' by a genomic Xba/R1 fragment and 3' by a 5.5-kilobase (kb) fragment of *Cnlp*. Group A *Streptococcus* was used in this model because the injury accompanying this pathogen results in a large increase in the local accumulation of CRAMP, and group A streptococci (GAS) are extremely sensitive to cathelicidin antimicrobial action. CRAMP-resistant mutants of GAS were compared with wild-type GAS for their ability to produce necrotizing cutaneous infection.

Results.—Mice infected with Tn917 mutant NZ131-CR or targeted mutant NZ131:*crg*R.KO had larger lesions of longer duration than mice infected with the parent GAS strain. Persistent infection was noted at day 7 in mice infected with the CRAMP-resistant mutants, compared with microbial clearing seen at this point with the CRAMP-sensitive parent GAS. *Cnlp*-deletion rendered mice more susceptible to severe GAS infection.

Conclusions.—This study provides in vivo evidence that endogenous expression of a mammalian antimicrobial peptide defends against invasive bacterial infection. These findings suggest that the specific antimicrobial activity of the cathelicidin is necessary for bacterial clearance and innate skin immunity.

Dermcidin: A Novel Human Antibiotic Peptide Secreted by Sweat Glands

Schittek B, Hipfel R, Sauer B, et al (Eberhard-Karls-Univ Tübingen, Germany; Univ of Tübingen, Germany)
Nat Immunol 2:1133-1137, 2001   4–17

Background.—The epithelium is the first line of defense against invading microorganisms. This report describes the isolation of a novel antimicrobial protein with no homology to known antimicrobial peptides. This protein is secreted in the sweat and may play a role in the regulation of human skin flora and the prevention of infection.

Methods and Results.—A subtracted cDNA library of primary melanoma and benign melanocytic nevus tissue was screened to identify a gene (*Dermicidin*[DCD]) with no homology to any previously published gene sequence. A dot blot with RNA from 50 different tissue types was screened with labeled DCD cDNA. There was no detectable response, indicating restricted expression. Reverse transcription–polymerase chain reaction was used to localize expression of DCD in skin, melanocytic nevus tissue, and cutaneous melanoma. In situ hybridization, immunohistochemistry, immunofluorescence, and immunoelectronmicroscopy were used to confirm the expression of DCD in eccrine sweat glands in the dermis of human skin. A 47–amino acid piece from the COOH-terminal of this protein (DCD-1) was detected in human sweat by high performance liquid chromatography. This peptide demonstrated dose-dependent antibacterial and antifungal activity in buffers that had a pH and ionic composition similar to human sweat.

Conclusion.—A gene encoding a novel antimicrobial peptide, DCD, has been identified. This protein is expressed in sweat glands. The petide DCD-1 is proteolytically processed from DCD and is secreted into the sweat. It possesses broad-spectrum antimicrobial activity under conditions similar to those found in human sweat. This peptide may play an important protective role at the skin surface.

▶ It is remarkable that skin and wound infections do not occur more frequently. Impetigo is relatively uncommon, especially in adults, and postsurgical wound infections are quite infrequent, especially considering that many office-based procedures are not done under strictly sterile conditions. The existence of innate antimicrobial peptides may explain the apparent resistance of the skin to infection. Defensins and cathelicidins are 2 classes of such antimicrobial peptides that previously have been identified. Dermcidin, which appears to be secreted by the sweat onto the skin, may be the first member of yet a third class.

B. H. Thiers, MD

Introduction of a Practice Guideline for Penicillin Skin Testing Improves the Appropriateness of Antibiotic Therapy
Forrest DM, Schellenberg RR, Thien VVS, et al (Univ of British Columbia, Vancouver, Canada)
Clin Infect Dis 32:1685-1690, 2001   4–18

Background.—Up to 10% of patients report a history of penicillin allergy, but only 10% to 30% of them have a positive result on penicillin skin testing. Penicillin skin testing can reliably distinguish between patients with IgE-mediated allergy and those without, with a negative predictive value of greater than 99%. Therefore, patients with a negative penicillin skin test can safely be treated with penicillin, and penicillin is generally cheaper, less toxic, and less likely to lead to the development of antibiotic resistance than alternative antibiotics. It was hypothesized that the introduction of a clinical practice guideline for penicillin skin testing would increase the appropriateness of skin testing and the use of penicillins, thereby reducing antibiotic costs for patients with a history of penicillin allergy who have infections that could be treated with penicillin or penicillin-like drugs.

Methods.—A clinical practice guideline for penicillin skin testing was developed by a multidisciplinary team. The guideline called for penicillin skin testing among inpatients reporting a history of penicillin allergy for whom a penicillin was the drug of choice based on the infecting organism. Because the cost of skin testing was about equal to the difference in cost between a 7-day course of vancomycin and a 7-day course of a penicillin, the guideline was applied only to inpatients who required treatment with an intravenous antibiotic for at least 7 days. The appropriateness of penicillin skin testing and daily antibiotic costs for the 3.5 years before the guideline was introduced and for the 2 years after its implementation were compared. The difference between the actual costs for patients who had negative results on skin testing and were treated with a penicillin instead of an alternative antibiotic, and the projected costs of continuing alternative antibiotics without skin testing, were calculated.

Results.—The proportion of eligible patients who underwent penicillin skin testing increased significantly after the guideline was implemented (from 17% before the guideline to 64% thereafter). The proportion of patients with negative skin test results who were switched to penicillin was greater after guideline implementation (93% vs 70%), but the increase in penicillin use was not statistically significant. Average daily costs did not differ significantly before and after guideline implementation, either for the cost of antibiotics alone ($37.24 before and $30.00 after) or for the cost of antibiotics, skin testing, and vancomycin ($39.84 before and $38.27 after). Among patients with a negative skin test result who were treated with a penicillin, actual costs of treatment did not differ significantly from projected costs had they not undergone skin testing.

Conclusions.—The use of a clinical practice guideline for penicillin skin testing in patients reporting a history of penicillin allergy dramatically increased the appropriate use of skin testing, and did so without increasing treatment costs.

▶ In the short term, no difference existed between the actual costs of treating penicillin-tested patients and the projected costs had they not been skin tested. However, since penicillin skin testing needs to be undertaken only once, significant savings might be realized in the care of patients who have recurrent infections. An additional benefit might be to allow for the use of penicillin or related narrow-spectrum antibiotics, which would be less likely to lead to antibiotic resistance than second-line broad-spectrum antibiotics.

B. H. Thiers, MD

Variation in Antibiotic Use in the European Union
Cars O, Mölstad S, Melander A (Uppsala Univ, Sweden; Swedish Inst for Infectious Disease Control, Stockholm, Sweden; Unit of Research and Development in Primary Health Care, Stockholm; et al)
Lancet 357:1851-1853, 2001   4–19

Introduction.—Antimicrobial resistance is thought to be related to increased antibiotic use, but few international comparisons of antibiotic sales have been made. The use of antibiotics in the 15 member states of the European Union (EU) was assessed and compared.

Methods.—Data for national sales of antibiotics in 1993 and 1997 for 13 countries of the EU were purchased from a private company (Institute for Medical Statistics). The National Corporation of Swedish Pharmacies and the Danish Medicine Agency provided data from Sweden and Denmark, respectively. Because hospital sales were obtained from only 9 countries, only nonhospital sales were used in the final analysis. The amount of antibiotic (in kilograms) was converted to oral defined daily dose where possible and this number was used for antibiotics with different routes of administration.

Results.—Between 1993 and 1997, 7 countries showed an increase of less than 4% in antibiotic use. Both Italy and Luxembourg had large increases (34% and 12%, respectively), whereas 5 countries recorded reductions in antibiotic use (ranging from 4% in Greece to 21% in Sweden). Overall, there was more than a 4-fold variation between countries in nonhospital use of antibiotics (Figure; see color plate V). Broad-spectrum penicillin was the most commonly used antibiotic in 11 of the 15 EU countries. This agent accounted for 56% of total sales in Spain. Narrow-spectrum penicillins accounted for 40% of total sales in Denmark and 36% in Sweden.

Conclusion.—The most important finding of this study was the great variation in outpatient antibiotic use among countries of the EU. Such differences are unlikely to result from differences in the frequency of bacterial infections but may be related to cultural and social factors,

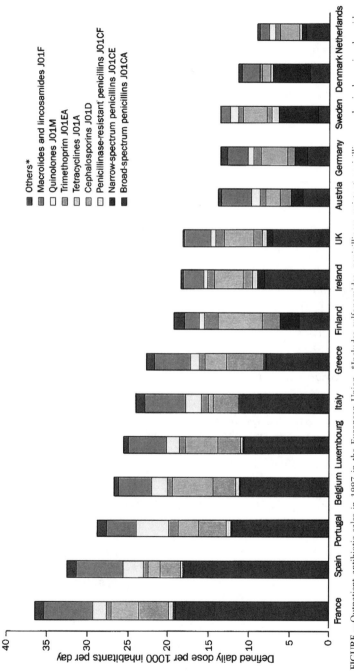

FIGURE.—Outpatient antibiotic sales in 1997 in the European Union. *Includes sulfonamides, penicillinase-resistant penicillins, amphenicols, aminoglycosides, and glycopeptides. (Courtesy of Cars O, Mölstad S, Melander A: Variation in antibiotic use in the European Union. *Lancet* 357:1851-1853, 2001. Copyright by The Lancet Ltd, 2001.)

disparities in health care systems, and patients' and physicians' attitudes. There is a need for more effective antibiotic use in member states of the EU.

▶ The variation in antibiotic prescribing habits between the countries is striking. This probably does not reflect differences in the frequency of bacterial infections in the different populations. Multiple factors may play a role. These factors include physician and patient attitudes toward antibiotics, historical backgrounds, cultural and social factors, marketing techniques by the pharmaceutical industry, and disparities in the health care systems. Appropriate antibiotic use is necessary to combat the threat of resistant organisms.

B. H. Thiers, MD

The Isolation of Antibiotic-Resistant Salmonella From Retail Ground Meats
White DG, Zhao S, Sudler R, et al (Ctr for Veterinary Medicine, Food and Drug Administration, Laurel, Md; Univ of Maryland, College Park)
N Engl J Med 345:1147-1154, 2001   4–20

Background.—The emergence of antimicrobial-resistant *Salmonella* spp has resulted from the use of antibiotics in food animals. Resistant bacteria can be transmitted to humans through foods, especially those of animal origin. Strains of *Salmonella* isolated from ground meats were identified and characterized.

Methods.—Samples of ground chicken, beef, turkey, and pork purchased at 3 supermarkets in the Washington, DC area were tested. *Salmonella* isolates were characterized using serotyping, antimicrobial-susceptibility testing, phage typing, and pulsed-field gel electrophoresis. Resistant integrins and extended spectrum β-lactamase genes were identified by the polymerase chain reaction and DNA sequencing.

Findings.—Twenty percent of 200 meat samples contained *Salmonella*. Thirteen serotypes were identified. Eighty-four percent of the isolates were found to be resistant to at least 1 antibiotic. Fifty-three percent were resistant to at least 3. Sixteen percent of isolates were resistant to ceftriaxone, which is the preferred drug for treating salmonellosis in children. Bacteriophage typing detected 4 *Salmonella enterica* serotype typhimurium definitive type 104 (DT104) isolates, 1 DT104b isolate, and 2 DT208 isolates. Five *Salmonella enterica* serotype agona isolates were resistant to 9 antibiotics. The 2 serotype typhimurium DT208 isolates were resistant to 12 antibiotics. Electrophoretic DNA patterns indistinguishable from one another were found repeatedly in isolates from different meat samples and stores. Eighteen isolates representing 4 serotypes had integrins with genes that conferred resistance to aminoglycosides, sulfonamides, trimethoprim, and β-lactams.

Conclusions.—Resistant strains of *Salmonella* were commonly found in the ground meats examined. Guidelines for the prudent use of antibiotics in food animals should be adopted. In addition, the number of pathogens present on farms and in slaughterhouses must be reduced. National surveillance for antimicrobial-resistant *Salmonella* needs to include retail meats.

Quinupristin-Dalfopristin-Resistant *Enterococcus Faecium* **on Chicken and in Human Stool Specimens**
McDonald LC, Rossiter S, Mackinson C, et al (Ctrs for Disease Control and Prevention, Atlanta, Ga; Univ of Maryland, Baltimore; Minnesota Dept of Health, Minneapolis; et al)
N Engl J Med 345:1155-1160, 2001   4–21

Background.—Late in 1999, the combination of the streptogramins quinupristin and dalfopristin gained US approval for treating vancomycin-resistant *Enterococcus faecium* infections. However, subtherapeutic concentrations of virginiamycin, another streptogramin, have long been used to enhance growth in farm animals. The frequency of quinupristin-dalfopristin-resistant *E faecium* was investigated.

Methods.—Samples from 407 chickens bought in 26 supermarkets in Georgia, Maryland, Minnesota, and Oregon between July 1998 and June 1999 were obtained for analysis and culture. In addition, 334 stool specimens from outpatients were obtained for analysis.

Findings.—Quinupristin-dalfopristin-resistant *E faecium* was isolated from 237 chicken carcasses and 3 stool samples. Resistant isolates from stool samples showed low levels of resistance. The resistant isolates from chickens, however, showed greater levels of resistance.

Conclusions.—Quinupristin-dalfopristin-resistant *E faecium* contaminated a large percentage of chickens sold in supermarkets in 4 different regions of the United States. The low prevalence and low levels of resistance of the strains found in human stool samples, however, suggest that the impact of virginiamycin use in animals is not great. Nevertheless, food-borne dissemination of resistance may increase with the increasing clinical use of quinupristin-dalfopristin.

Transient Intestinal Carriage After Ingestion of Antibiotic-Resistant *Entercoccus Faecium* **From Chicken and Pork**
Sørensen TL, Blom M, Monnet DL, et al (Statens Serum Institut, Copenhagen)
N Engl J Med 345:1161-1166, 2001   4–22

Background.—Antibiotic-resistant enterococci are commonly found in retail meat, but it remains unclear whether the ingestion of these contaminants results in sustained intestinal carriage. A randomized, double-blind study of the effects of such ingestion in healthy volunteers was performed.

Methods.—The study included 18 healthy volunteers who were divided into 3 equal groups. The subjects ingested a mixture either of 10^7 colony-forming units (CFU) of 2 glycopeptide-resistant strains of *Enterococcus faecium* from chicken bought at a grocery store, or 10^7 CFU of a strepto-gramin-resistant strain of *E faecium* obtained from a pig at slaughter, or 10^7 CFU of a glycopeptide-susceptible and streptogramin-susceptible strain of *E faecium* from chicken bought at a grocery store. Stool specimens were obtained from the participants before ingestion, daily for 1 week after ingestion, and at 14 and 35 days after ingestion. Selective culture techniques were used to identify resistant enterococci in the stool specimens.

Findings.—Before ingestion, none of the volunteers were colonized with glycopeptide-resistant or streptogramin-resistant *E faecium*. After ingestion, the strains ingested were isolated from the stools of all participants. The concentrations varied. The test strain was isolated in stool specimens from 8 of 12 participants on day 6 and from 1 participant on day 14. At day 35, all stool samples were negative.

Conclusions.—Ingesting resistant *E faecium* of animal origin results in detectable levels of the resistant strain in stools. These organisms, which remain detectable for up to 14 days after ingestion, survive gastric passage and multiply.

▶ This series of articles (Abstracts 4–20 to 4–22) presents more bad news on the spread of antibiotic resistant organisms. White et al (Abstract 4–20) purchased ground chicken, turkey, beef, and pork from supermarkets in the Washington, DC area. They found that 20% contained *Salmonella* spp of 13 different serotypes. Resistance to at least 1 antibiotic was found in 84% of the isolates, and more than half of them were resistant to 3 or more antibiotics. The high level of antibiotic resistance can best be attributed to widespread use of antibiotics in food animals.

McDonald et al (Abstract 4–21) studied resistance to quinupristin-dalfo-pristin, a combination of streptogramin antibiotics approved for the treatment of certain vancomycin-resistant *Enterococcus* infections. A related streptogramin has been used for decades as a growth promoter in farm animals. The investigators found quinupristin-dalfopristin-resistant entero-cocci in at least 17% of the chickens purchased in each state. It should be noted that the study was conducted in the United States before the approval of quinupristin-dalfopristin, suggesting that the resistant organisms were a likely consequence of the use of the related antibiotic in animals. The findings again emphasize that the widespread use of antibiotics in animals has potentially serious consequences for human health.

Sørensen et al (Abstract 4–22) showed that after ingestion of resistant enterococci, the organisms can survive gastric passage, multiply, and be passed in the stool for up to 2 weeks. This demonstrates that consumption of antibiotic-resistant enterococci in retail meats can lead to intestinal carriage of these organisms.

In an editorial that accompanied these articles, Gorbach[1] analyzed the data and concluded that it was time to stop routine use of antimicrobials in animal feed. He suggested that such drugs should be used only when prescribed by a veterinarian for an infected animal. Drugs that have important uses in humans, such as fluoroquinolones and third-generation cephalosporins, should be totally prohibited. Finally, he recommended that the use of sub-therapeutic doses of these antibiotics to promote growth and feeding efficiency should be banned. Implementing these suggestions would decrease the burden of antimicrobial resistance in the environment, and provide health-related benefits to both humans and animals.

B. H. Thiers, MD

Reference

1. Gorbach SL: Antimicrobial use in animal feed—time to stop. *N Engl J Med* 345:1202-1203, 2001.

5 Fungal Infections

***Trichophyton rubrum* Showing Deep Dermal Invasion Directly From the Epidermis in Immunosuppressed Patients**
Smith KJ, Welsh M, Skelton H (Natl Naval Med Ctr, Bethesda, Md; Univ of Alabama, Birmingham)
Br J Dermatol 145:344-348, 2001   5–1

Background.—*Trichophyton rubrum*, the most common dermatophyte infection, is usually considered exclusively keratinophilic and often leads

FIGURE 1

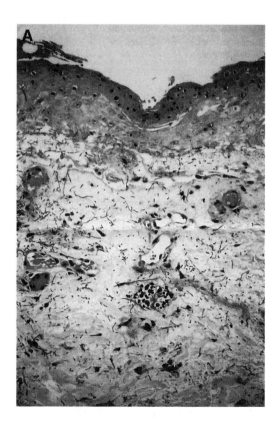

(*Continued*)

FIGURE 1 (cont.)

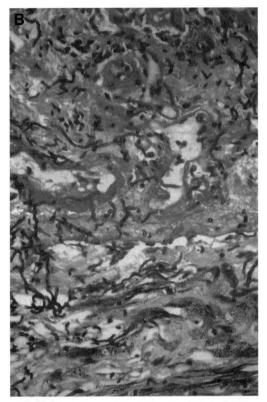

FIGURE 1.—A, Biopsy specimen from patient 1 showing epidermal parakeratosis with areas of epidermal necrosis and spongiosis. There is marked dermal edema and minimal mononuclear inflammatory infiltrate. In addition, there is some vascular thrombosis and fibrinoid surrounding vessels. Narrow, septate, branching hyphae are seen invading from the epidermis to the dermis and extending through the reticular dermis. Hematoxylin and eosin, original magnification × 100. B, Biopsy specimen from patient 2 showing narrow, septate, branching hyphae invading from the epidermis to the dermis with abundant fibrinoid around the dermal vessels. Periodic acid-Schiff reagent, original magnification × 600. (Courtesy of Smith KJ, Welsh M, Skelton H: *Trichophyton rubrum* showing deep dermal invasion directly from the epidermis in immunosuppressed patients. *Br J Dermatol* 145:344-348, 2001. Reprinted by permission of Blackwell Science, Inc.)

to chronic skin and nail infections, even in healthy persons. *T rubrum* infection occurring in immunosuppressed patients was discussed.

Methods and Findings.—Three patients with acute leukemias required treatment for ill-defined, pre-existing cutaneous eruptions. The patients were 2 men, aged 18 and 34 years, respectively, and 1 woman, aged 64 years. The skin lesions had been treated with potent topical corticosteroids without benefit. In all 3 patients, the cutaneous disease was shown to represent a deep dermal *T rubrum* infection. The fungus invaded directly from the epidermis, with no evidence of systemic spread (Fig 1; see color plate VI). Systemic amphotericin B was ineffective.

Conclusions.—Systemic pancytopenia associated with prolonged local immunosuppression may increase the risk for direct dermal invasion of dermatophyte infections. The risk of systemic spread, however, appears to be very low, even in immunosuppressed persons. Amphotericin B was ineffective in the treatment of these patients' dermatophyte infections.

▶ The findings emphasize the need to biopsy any unusual appearing lesion in an immunosuppressed patient. Another important observation is the relative ineffectiveness of systemic amphotericin B therapy despite an excellent in-vitro sensitivity profile. This may reflect the lack of diffusion of the intravenously administered drug to the outer layers of the skin. In contrast, systemic treatment with fluconazole or terbinafine appears to be effective.

B. H. Thiers, MD

Fungal Infection of the Diabetic Foot: Two Distinct Syndromes

Heald AH, O'Halloran DJ, Richards K, et al (Hope Hosp, Salford, England; North Manchester Gen Hosp, Manchester, England, Univ of Manchester, England; et al)
Diabetic Med 18:567-572, 2001

5–2

Introduction.—Diabetic foot ulceration may lead to complications that significantly increase the risk of amputation. Although the role of bacterial flora in the infective process is well described, no studies have examined the impact of fungal infection on the pathogenesis of diabetic foot lesions.

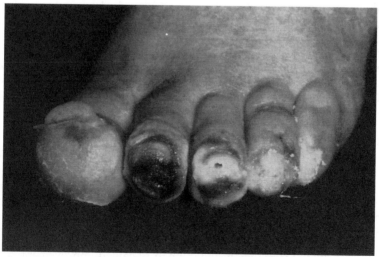

FIGURE 1.—An example of simultaneous multiple subungual and tip-of-the-toe ulcers with necrosis under the nail fold from which *Candida parapsilosis* and *C humicola* were grown. (Courtesy of Heald AH, O'Halloran DJ, Richards K, et al: Fungal infection of the diabetic foot: Two distinct syndromes. *Diabetic Med* 18:567-572, 2001. Reprinted by permission of Blackwell Science, Inc.)

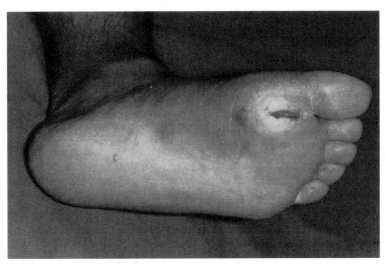

FIGURE 2.—Example of a single deep ulcer with heaps of macerated tissue along the margins from which *Candida parapsilosis* was grown. (Courtesy of Heald AH, O'Halloran DJ, Richards K, et al: Fungal infection of the diabetic foot: Two distinct syndromes. *Diabetic Med* 18:567-572, 2001. Reprinted by permission of Blackwell Science, Inc.)

Findings in the patients reported here suggest a role for *Candida* and dermatophyte infection in diabetic foot disease.

Methods.—The 17 patients had chronic foot ulcers from which *Candida* spp. were isolated or hyphae, sometimes with yeasts, were visualized in material from the ulcers or surrounding skin. Healing had failed despite intensive foot care. Broad spectrum antibiotics had been previously administered in 16 cases. Mycologic examinations were performed and ulcer swabs taken for microbial culture.

Results.—Patients were 11 men and 6 women with a median age of 66 years and a median duration of 11 years since diabetes diagnosis. All had peripheral neuropathy and 88% also had peripheral vascular disease. Multiple ulcers arising simultaneously were present in 10 patients (Fig 1; see color plate VII); 7 had single ulcers (Fig 2; see color plate VII) with markedly macerated margins. In a total of 9 patients, blisters preceded the development of ulcers.

Ten patients had clinical signs of necrosis under the nail fold (Fig 3) indicative of dermatophyte infection of the subungual space. *Candida* was grown from the ulcer in 12 cases, and more than 1 species was found in 5 cases. Osteomyelitis caused by *Candida* was proven in 1 case and clinically suspected in 2. Antifungal treatment was initiated in variable doses and for variable durations according to the clinical response. Oral systemic agents included flucytosine, fluconazole, itraconazole, and terbinafine. Six patients experienced complete healing, 9 had sustained improvement, and 2 relapsed after improvement when treatment was discontinued. Healing typically took from 3 to 6 weeks.

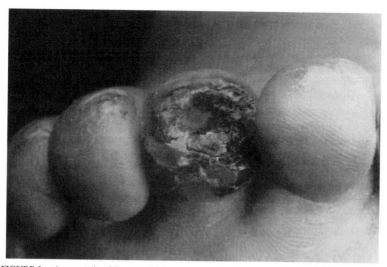

FIGURE 3.—An example of the typical appearance of ulceration caused by *Candida* spp which shows necrosis under the nail fold particularly well. *Candida albicans* was isolated from the bone of the distal phalanx of that toe following amputation. (Courtesy of Heald AH, O'Halloran DJ, Richards K, et al: Fungal infection of the diabetic foot: Two distinct syndromes. *Diabetic Med* 18:567-572, 2001. Reprinted by permission of Blackwell Science, Inc.)

Conclusion.—Two distinct patterns of protracted ulceration were seen in cases of fungal infection of the diabetic foot. Multiple simultaneous distal and subungual toe ulcers suggested the possibility of nonbacterial infection in 10 patients, whereas 7 patients had chronic single-site ulcers with macerated margins. The pathogenic role of *Candida* remains unclear.

▶ The question that remains, of course, is whether the isolated organisms were contaminants or bystanders or whether they were truly pathogenic. The improvement of many of the patients with systemic antifungal therapy suggests, but certainly does not prove, that infection rather than colonization occurred. All the patients reported in this study had received, and failed, antibiotic therapy. It is possible that such therapy allowed proliferation of *Candida* in ulcers, with subsequent local invasion of soft tissue and, in some cases, bone.

B. H. Thiers, MD

Efficacy of Itraconazole, Terbinafine, Fluconazole, Griseofulvin and Ketoconazole in the Treatment of *Scopulariopsis brevicaulis* Causing Onychomycosis of the Toes
Gupta AK, Gregurek-Novak T (Univ of Toronto; Sisters of Charity Clinical Hosp, Zagreb, Croatia)
Dermatology 202:235-238, 2001   5-3

Introduction.—Organisms causing onychomycosis include dermatophytes, *Candida* sp, and nondermatophyte molds. *Scopulariopsis brevicaulis* is a common nondermatophyte mold that has been linked to onychomycosis. The efficacy and safety of the oral antifungal agents griseofulvin, ketoconazole, itraconazole, fluconazole, and terbinafine in the treatment of *S brevicaulis* toenail onychomycosis were assessed in the first known comparative investigation of this kind.

Methods.—Patients with toenail onychomycosis caused by *S brevicaulis* sp were randomly assigned to treatment with 1 of the 5 aforementioned oral antifungal agents in a prospective, comparative, parallel-group, single-blinded, randomized, nonindustry-sponsored investigation. Patients were treated with either griseofulvin, 600 mg twice daily for 12 months; ketoconazole, 200 mg daily for 4 months; itraconazole pulse therapy for 3 pulses with each pulse consisting of 200 mg twice daily for 1 week with 3 weeks off between successive pulses; terbinafine, 250 mg daily for 12 weeks; or fluconazole, 150 mg daily for 12 weeks.

Results.—The mean age of the 48 men and 11 women was 35.6 years (range, 25-53 years). All patients had clinical evidence of distal and lateral onychomycosis and moderate to severe disease of the target nail. All treatment groups were similar in mean age and mean area of involvement with onychomycosis at baseline. Efficacy parameters were clinical cure (CC) and mycologic cure (MC). After 12 months of treatment, the response rates were as follows: griseofulvin, CC 3/11, MC 0/11, CC + MC 0/11; ketoconazole, CC 10/12, MC 8/12, CC + MC 8/12; itraconazole, CC 12/12, MC 12/12, CC + MC 12/12; terbinafine, CC 12/12, MC 11/12, CC + MC 11/12; and fluconazole, CC 8/12, MC 8/12, CC + MC 8/12. The adverse effects included the following: griseofulvin—gastrointestinal symptoms, allergic reaction, photodermatitis, hepatic and renal dysfunction in 11 patients, with discontinuation of treatment in 3 patients; ketoconazole—hepatic dysfunction but no symptomatic changes in 2 patients; terbinafine—taste disturbance in 2 patients and nausea in 3 patients; and fluconazole—severe gastrointestinal events in 5 patients. Treatment was not discontinued in any patients who received either ketoconazole, itraconazole, terbinafine, or fluconazole.

Conclusion.—Itraconazole and terbinafine were effective in many cases of *S brevicaulis* toenail onychomycosis. These agents seem to be safe and have a favorable benefit-to-risk profile.

▶ Data concerning the effectiveness of treatment options for onychomycosis caused by nondermatophyte molds is scarce. Gupta and Gregurek-

Novak show that itraconazole and terbinafine appear to be reasonable choices for the treatment of this condition.

B. H. Thiers, MD

Single-blind, Randomized, Prospective Study on Terbinafine and Itraconazole for Treatment of Dermatophyte Toenail Onychomycosis in the Elderly
Gupta AK, Konnikov N, Lynde CW (Univ of Toronto; New England Med Ctr, Boston; Toronto Gen Hosp)
J Am Acad Dermatol 44:479-484, 2001   5–4

Background.—Dermatophyte onychomycosis of the toe is most commonly treated with terbinafine (continuous) and itraconazole (pulse) therapy. Comparative studies have been performed to evaluate the efficacy of these 2 drugs in adults, but no studies have focused specifically on the subset of elderly adults. The efficacy and safety of terbinafine and itraconazole therapies were compared in the treatment of dermatophyte onychomycosis of the toe in the elderly population.

Methods.—A total of 101 elderly patients (60 years or older) with dermatophyte onychomycosis of at least 1 great toe were randomly assigned to receive either terbinafine (continuous), 250 mg/day for 12 weeks, or itraconazole (pulse), 200 mg twice a day for 1 week, given for 3 pulses. If there was less than 50% reduction in the affected nail plate area at 6 months of therapy compared with baseline, or if there was less than a 3 mm outgrowth of the unaffected nail plate as measured in midline, then patients who had been given terbinafine (continuous) therapy were given an extra 4 weeks of the drug, for a total of 16 weeks of therapy. Patients who had received itraconazole (pulse) therapy were given an extra, or fourth, pulse. Evaluation of patients occurred at 1.5, 3, 6, 12, and 18 months from the start of therapy. Measures of efficacy included the mycologic cure rate and clinical efficacy, which was defined as mycologic cure plus clinical cure or clinical improvement so that 10% or less of nail plate was clinically involved.

Results.—There were no significant differences between the groups in baseline age, percent of nail plate area involved, duration of onychomycosis, and number of nails involved. At month 6, 13 of 50 patients in the terbinafine (continuous) group and 23 of 51 patients in the itraconazole (pulse) group required additional treatment. The mycologic cure rate for the terbinafine group was 64%, and the clinical efficacy at 18 months was 62%. For the itraconazole group, the mycologic cure rate was 62.7% and the clinical efficacy at 18 months was 60.8%. Thus, no significant difference was observed between the 2 groups. No significant adverse effects were observed in either group.

Conclusions.—In the treatment of dermatophyte onychomycosis in elderly patients, terbinafine and itraconazole were found to be safe and effective and associated with high compliance.

▶ Reported response rates of onychomycosis patients to systemic antifungal therapy vary widely, a likely consequence of differences in patient selection, entry criteria, and dosing regimens. The recently reported association of systemic itraconazole therapy with congestive heart failure (Abstract 5–6) will probably limit its use in elderly patients with onychomycosis.

B. H. Thiers, MD

Long-term Efficacy of Antifungals in Toenail Onychomycosis: A Critical Review
Cribier BJ, Paul C (Clinique Dermatologique des Hôpitaux Universitaires, Strasbourg, France; Novartis Pharma AG, Basel, Switzerland; Hôpital du Moenschberg, Mulhouse, France)
Br J Dermatol 145:446-452, 2001   5–5

Introduction.—Numerous clinical trials have reported that 3 new drugs—terbinafine, itraconazole, and fluconazole—can achieve complete cure rates in a majority (up to 80% to 90%) of patients with fingernail or toenail onychomycosis. Cures are obtained after 3 to 6 months of treatment, but little is known about long-term outcome or whether one drug is superior to another in avoiding reinfection or recurrence. The long-term efficacy of antifungals in onychomycosis was examined through a critical review of the literature.

Methods.—A MEDLINE search identified 15 studies with results reported beyond 48 weeks. Two additional studies were included in the analysis: one dealing with nondermatophyte fungi and another using a combination of amorolfine and terbinafine. End points of the analysis were EP1 (the number of patients with negative mycology after follow-up, divided by the number of patients included at day 0) and EP2 (the number of patients with negative mycology after follow-up, divided by the number of patients with negative mycology at week 48). The clinical cure rate (EP*clin*) represented the number of patients clinically cured or with minimal residual lesions divided by the number of patients included at day 0.

Results.—The majority of available data concerned terbinafine, evaluated at periods ranging from 60 weeks to 4 years. There were also results documenting the efficacy of itraconazole after 2 years but none beyond 18 months for the other agents. Long-term cure rates obtained with terbinafine were high at 18 months, 2 years, and 4 years. Higher EP values confirmed the long-term superiority of terbinafine over itraconazole. At 18 months, EP1 was significantly higher with continuous terbinafine (66%) than with intermittent itraconazole (37%). And even after a longer duration of treatment, rates of mycological cure were substantially lower for fluconazole, ketoconazole, and griseofulvin.

Conclusion.—This analysis suggests that terbinafine achieves better long-term results than other agents (griseofulvin, ketoconazole, fluconazole, and itraconazole) in treating toenail onychomycosis.

▶ This article adds to the growing body of evidence supporting the relative superiority of terbinafine over competing drugs in the treatment of toenail onychomycosis. Like the landmark study by Evans et al, the current literature review was supported by Novartis Pharma AG, the manufacturer of terbinafine.[1] This being said, the weight of the evidence does in fact support the authors' conclusions. Nevertheless, it is hoped that our colleagues in the pharmaceutical industry will continue to search for drugs with a higher benefit/risk ratio for the treatment of this troublesome condition.

B. H. Thiers, MD

Reference

1. Evans EGV, for the LION Study Group. Double-blind, randomized study of continuous terbinafine compared with intermittent itraconazole in the treatment of toenail onychomycosis. *Br Med J* 318:1031-1035, 1999.

Congestive Heart Failure Associated With Itraconazole
Ahmad SR, Singer SJ, Leissa BG (Ctr for Drug Evaluation and Research, Food and Drug Administration, Rockville, Md)
Lancet 357:1766-1767, 2001

5–6

Introduction.—Itraconazole, a synthetic agent widely used for the treatment of localized and systemic fungal infections, may have negative inotropic effects. Investigators searched the Food and Drug Administration's Adverse Event Reporting System database to identify cases of congestive heart failure associated with oral and IV administration of itraconazole.

Methods.—Itraconazole was approved in the United States in September 1992. Between this date and April 2001, the FDA had received 58 reports of potential cases of congestive heart failure linked to itraconazole. The clinical details of these cases were summarized.

Results.—Complete data were not available for all 58 patients. The 50 patients whose ages were known ranged from 15 to 86 years (median, 57 years). Approximately two thirds of the patients were women. Indications for use of itraconazole were onychomycosis in 50% of 52 patients and systemic fungal infection in 29%. The median period between itraconazole administration and the onset of congestive heart failure was 10 days. The median drug dose was 300 mg/day. Twenty-eight patients were admitted to the hospital and 13 died. Because most patients who died were very ill and were taking many medications, a causal relationship between itraconazole and congestive heart failure was difficult to prove. In 2 survivors, however, symptoms were clearly related to the antifungal agent and withdrawal of itraconazole led to improvement.

Conclusion.—A search of the Adverse Event Reporting System yielded no cases of congestive heart failure in association with other azole antifungal drugs. The labeling of itraconazole has been revised and the drug is now contraindicated for treatment of onychomycosis in patients with evidence of ventricular dysfunction. Physicians should be aware of this rare but serious complication and weigh the benefits of itraconazole against its potential risks.

Terbinafine-Induced Subacute Cutaneous Lupus Erythematosus

Bonsmann G, Schiller M, Luger TA, et al (Univ of Münster, Germany)
J Am Acad Dermatol 44:925-931, 2001   5–7

Introduction.—Terbinafine, an oral antifungicidal agent widely used in the treatment of dermatophyte infections of the skin and nails, is considered to have an excellent safety profile. There have been isolated reports, however, of serious side effects, including the induction of subacute cutaneous lupus erythematosus (SCLE) and exacerbation of systemic lupus erythematosus (LE). The cases of SCLE reported here occurred in patients taking oral terbinafine for onychomycosis.

Methods.—Four of 21 consecutive patients with SCLE who were seen in a dermatology outpatient department over a 1-year period had terbinafine-induced disease. Patients were examined and photographed and their

TABLE 3.—Drugs Associated With Drug-Induced Lupus
Erythematosus Subacute Cutaneous

Thiazides*
Piroxicam*
D-Penicillamine*
Sulfonureas*
Procainamide*
Oxyprenolol*
Chrysotherapy*
Griseofulvin*
Naproxen*
Aldactone*
Diltiazem*
Cinnarizine
Captopril
Cilazapril
Verapamil
Nifedipine
Interferon beta
Ranitidine
Terbinafine†

*As reviewed by Provost TT, Watson R, Simmons-O'Brien E: Significance of the anti-Ro(SS-A) antibody in evaluation of patients with cutaneous manifestations of a connective tissue disease. *J Am Acad Dermatol* 35:147-169, 1996.
†Current cases.
(Courtesy of Bonsmann G, Schiller M, Luger TA, et al: Terbinafine-induced subacute cutaneous lupus erythematosus. *J Am Acad Dermatol* 44:925-931, 2001.)

laboratory test findings were reviewed. After terbinafine was discontinued, patients were followed at 4-week intervals until remission, then at 3- to 6-month intervals.

Results.—The 4 patients, all women, were being treated with 250 mg/ day terbinafine for suspected or culture-proved onychomycosis when they developed histologically confirmed LE. None had a personal or family history suggestive of photosensitivity, LE, or other collagen disease. All 4 women had high titers of antinuclear antibodies (ANA) with a homogeneous pattern and anti-Ro(SS-A) antibodies; 3 also had anti-La(SS-B) antibodies. Additional common findings were antihistone antibodies as in drug-induced lupus and the characteristic genetic association of SCLE with the HLA-B8,DR3 haplotype; HLA-DR2 was present as well in 2 patients. The ANA titers decreased when patients discontinued terbinafine and no relapse of SCLE occurred. A causal link between terbinafine and SCLE was suggested by the close temporal relationship, as eruptions appeared 4 to 7 weeks after the start of treatment.

Conclusion.—Terbinafine appears to be one of many drugs able to induce SCLE (Table 3). The patients reported here were genetically susceptible individuals with high titers of ANA and antihistone antibodies. A thorough history should be taken before the drug is prescribed, and its use should be avoided in those with known LE, a history of LE in a first-degree relative, known anti-Ro/anti-La antibodies, or significant ANA positivity.

Subacute Cutaneous Lupus Erythematosus Induced or Exacerbated by Terbinafine: A Report of 5 Cases
Callen JP, Hughes AP, Kulp-Shorten C (Univ of Louisville, Ky)
Arch Dermatol 137:1196-1198, 2001   5–8

Background.—Subacute cutaneous lupus erythematosus (SCLE) is a photosensitive cutaneous disorder that can be exacerbated by some drugs, most notably hydrochlorothiazide and calcium channel blockers. The oral antifungal agent terbinafine may also exacerbate SCLE, as described in 5 patients.

Case Reports.—Five patients (3 women and 2 men, 41-72 years of age) had SCLE within 4 to 8 weeks of starting terbinafine treatment for presumed onychomycosis. Three patients had a history of SCLE, 1 had a history of probable SCLE, and 1 had SCLE de novo. In addition, 2 patients had experienced a similar reaction after taking other drugs (hydrochlorothiazide or captopril). Annular lesions typical of SCLE were present in 3 patients, whereas an unusual gyrate erythema was present in the other 2 patients. Terbinafine therapy was discontinued in all patients; 3 also began oral prednisone therapy, and 1 began oral dapsone therapy. Erythema and lesions cleared within 6 weeks to 2 months after the last dose of terbinafine; however, 1 patient experienced a flare 3 weeks after discontinuing oral prednisone therapy.

Conclusions.—Terbinafine is generally considered to be a safe drug. However, there may be a link between terbinafine therapy and the onset or exacerbation of SCLE, particularly in patients with a history of SCLE or systemic lupus erythematosus.

▶ These articles (Abstracts 5–6 to 5–8) provide further evidence of the need for oral antifungal agents with an improved benefit:risk ratio. The package insert for itraconazole has been revised to state that the drug is contraindicated for the treatment of onychomycosis in patients with evidence of ventricular dysfunction. For patients with systemic fungal infections that are candidates for itraconazole treatment, the benefits and risks of the drug should be reassessed if signs or symptoms of congestive heart failure develop. The labeling for terbinafine likewise has been revised to stress the importance of monitoring liver function tests during the course of therapy.

B. H. Thiers, MD

Do Hair Care Practices Affect the Acquisition of Tinea Capitis? A Case-Control Study
Sharma V, Silverberg NB, Howard R, et al (Univ of Missouri, Kansas City; State Univ of New York, Brooklyn; Univ of California, San Francisco)
Arch Pediatr Adolesc Med 155:818-821, 2001   5–9

Introduction.—In the United States, most cases of tinea capitis (TC), a dermatophyte infection of the scalp and hair, occur in African American children. Some studies suggest that hairstyling practices may play a role in acquisition of the disease. Whether hair care practices are associated with TC in children was investigated in a case-control study.

Methods.—Findings from 134 children aged 12 years and younger were analyzed. Cases were enrolled from pediatric dermatology clinics and controls from general pediatric clinics. The 66 cases of TC all had positive culture results (65 for *Trichophyton tonsurans* and 1 for *T rubrum*). Controls were without known scalp disease and were age-, sex-, and race-matched to cases. Data were collected on hair care variables (including shampooing frequency, conditioner use, and types of hairstyles), history of exposure to TC, medical history of asthma or atopic dermatitis, and environmental variables.

Results.—The study population was 99% African American; 55% were boys. The mean age was 5.1 years for cases and 5.3 years for controls. Common symptoms recorded for cases were scaling (94%), alopecia (70%), and crusting (42%); erythema, pustules, and cervical lymphadenopathy each occurred in 33% of cases. In the final multivariate model, variables found to be significant for the development of TC were a history of exposure to TC and a history of having TC. The use of a conditioner was of borderline significance in exerting a protective effect.

Conclusion.—Hair care styling practices were not associated with the development of TC, but conditioners may have had a protective effect. Sharing combs and brushes was common in both groups and did not appear to increase the likelihood of TC. The most common mode of acquisition of the disease is probably infection, and reinfection, of persons within families, schools, and communities.

▶ To acquire an infection, one has to be exposed to the organism. Recruiting children of the same age and race may not make them an adequate control because most of these children likely would not have been exposed to the organism and, therefore, would have no chance of the disease developing. The incidence of TC does appear to be markedly higher in African American children than in those of other races. African Americans often shampoo once a week or less often because of hair styles and manageability of hair after shampoos. The answer to the question of whether hair care plays a role in the development of clinical infection could better be answered by manipulating the hair care routines of siblings of patients with TC who would have a high likelihood of exposure to fungal spores and assessing whether rates of clinical infection in these children differ from those using standard routines.

S. Raimer, MD

A Randomized Comparison of 4 Weeks of Terbinafine vs. 8 Weeks of Griseofulvin for the Treatment of Tinea Capitis

Fuller LC, Smith CH, Cerio R, et al (King's College Hosp, London; Univ Hosp Lewisham, London; Royal London Hosp; et al)
Br J Dermatol 144:321-327, 2001   5–10

Introduction.—Tinea capitis is a common childhood infection with a recently increased incidence in urban areas of Europe and the United States. The efficacy, safety, and tolerability of a 4-week course of oral terbinafine were compared with an 8-week course of griseofulvin in the treatment of children with tinea capitis. Cure rates and long-term (6-month) outcomes were compared in a prospective, open, randomized, parallel-group, multicenter trial involving 6 centers in the United Kingdom and funded by Novartis Pharmaceuticals UK Ltd.

Methods.—Patients were randomly assigned to either 4 weeks of treatment with oral terbinafine tablets (<20 kg, 62.5 mg daily; 20 to 40 kg, 125 mg daily; >40 kg, 250 mg daily) or 8 weeks of oral griseofulvin suspension (10 mg/kg^{-1} daily) (103 and 107 patients, respectively). Selenium sulfide shampoo was to be used at least twice weekly for the initial 2 weeks of treatment. Efficacy was evaluated in terms of clinical outcome and mycologic outcome. Follow-up was conducted for 24 weeks to ascertain short- and long-term efficacy and tolerability.

Results.—There were 147 evaluable patients (77 given terbinafine, 70 given griseofulvin). The 4-week course of terbinafine resulted in a trend toward more rapid clearance of tinea capitis. However, there were no significant differences between drugs at 4, 8, 12, or 24 weeks in terms of overall outcome or tolerability, with the exception of a subgroup of patients with *Trichophyton* infections who weighed more than 20 kg and responded better to terbinafine than to griseofulvin at 4 weeks. There was a better response to griseofulvin than to terbinafine in patients with *Microsporum audouinii* infections. The rates of "mycologic cure" at weeks 4, 8, 12, and 24 were 43%, 69%, 64%, and 70% in the terbinafine group; these rates for the griseofulvin group were 42%, 62%, 69%, and 72%, respectively. By 8 weeks of follow-up, desquamation and hair loss were rated as either absent or mild in nearly 90% of the children in both groups.

Conclusion.—The efficacy of 4 weeks of treatment with oral terbinafine was similar to that of 8 weeks of treatment with griseofulvin in children with tinea capitis.

▶ Foul! Although the authors concluded that 4 weeks of treatment with oral terbinafine is similar in efficacy to 8 weeks of treatment with griseofulvin, the dose of griseofulvin used (10 mg/kg/d) was much lower than the dose currently used by most dermatologists (20 to 25 mg/kg/d). As might have been predicted from previous studies, terbinafine was more effective for treating *Trichophyton* infections than *Microsporum* infections.

B. H. Thiers, MD

Therapeutic Options for the Treatment of Tinea Capitis Caused by *Trichophyton* Species: Griseofulvin Versus the New Oral Antifungal Agents, Terbinafine, Itraconazole, and Fluconazole
Gupta AK, Adam P, Dlova N, et al (Univ of Toronto; St Michael's Hospital, Toronto; Univ of Natal, Durban, South Africa; et al)
Pediatr Dermatol 18:433-438, 2001   5–11

Introduction.—Tinea capitis, a relatively common fungal infection in children, has long been treated with griseofulvin. Newer oral antifungal agents, however, are reported to be effective in treating the disease. Griseofulvin and the new oral antimycotic agents were evaluated in a prospective study carried out at centers in Canada and South Africa.

Methods.—Patients were randomly assigned to 1 of 4 study arms and evaluated in a single-blind manner. One group received griseofulvin (20 mg/kg/day) for 6 weeks. Terbinafine, itraconazole, and fluconazole were administered for an initial period of 2 weeks, and patients were reviewed at week 4. If clinical examination showed a need for further treatment, these 3 agents were given for an extra week (Table 1). Patients were re-evaluated at weeks 4, 8, and 12. Mycologic examination of scalp lesions were performed at baseline and at 4 and 12 weeks after the start of therapy. No topical therapies were allowed during the study period.

TABLE 1.—Treatment Regimens Used for Tinea Capitis

Drug	Dosage*	Duration	Extra Therapy
Griseofulvin	20 mg/kg/day	6 weeks	
Terbinafine	<20 kg, ¼ tablet (62.5 mg)	2 weeks	1 week†
	20–40 kg, ½ tablet (125 mg)		
	>40 kg, 1 tablet (250 mg)		
Itraconazole	5 mg/kg/day	2 weeks	1 week†
Fluconazole	6 mg/kg/day	2 weeks	1 week†

*The dosage was rounded up as necessary depending upon the amount of drug contained within the capsule/tablet.

†For terbinafine, itraconazole, and fluconazole, an extra week of therapy was administered at week 4 from the start of treatment, if clinically indicated.

(Courtesy of Gupta AK, Adam P, Dlova N, et al: Therapeutic options for the treatment of tinea capitis caused by *Trichophyton* species: Griseofulvin versus the new oral antifungal agents, terbinafine, itraconazole, and fluconazole. *Pediatr Dermatol* 18:433-438, 2001. Reprinted by permission of Blackwell Science, Inc.)

Results.—Each treatment group included 50 patients. At week 12, there were 46 evaluable patients in the griseofulvin group, 48 in the terbinafine group, 46 in the itraconazole group, and 46 in the fluconazole group. The causative organisms identified were *Trichophyton tonsurans* and *Trichophyton violaceum.* Treatment was judged effective in 92% of patients in the griseofulvin group, in 94% in the terbinafine group, in 86% in the itraconazole group, and in 84% in the fluconazole group. Gastrointestinal symptoms reported in 6 patients who received griseofulvin were the only adverse effects of treatment; 1 patient in this group discontinued the drug because of nausea.

Discussion.—The cure rates of griseofulvin, terbinafine, itraconazole, and fluconazole did not differ significantly in these children with tinea capitis, and each agent had a good safety profile. Griseofulvin has been considered the "gold standard" of therapy for 40 years, but the newer antifungal agents may be useful alternatives that allow a shorter duration of treatment.

▶ This study compared griseofulvin, 20 mg/kg/d for 6 weeks, with shorter regimens of some of the newer antifungals in the treatment of children with tinea capitis caused by *Trichophyton tonsurans* and *Trichophyton violaceum.* Efficacy was similar, and the incidence of side effects was low. The newer antifungal agents may need to be administered for a longer duration when treating *Microsporum canis* infections, and the effectiveness of terbinafine against this organism has been called into question.[1,2]

B. H. Thiers, MD

References

1. Hamm H, Schwinn A, Bräutigam M, et al: Short duration treatment with terbinafine for tinea capitis caused by *Trichophyton* or *Microsporum* species. *Br J Dermatol* 140:480-482, 1999.
2. Dragoš V, Lunder M: Lack of efficacy of 6-week treatment with oral terbinafine for tinea capitis due to *Microsporum canis* in children. *Pediatr Dermatol* 14:46-48, 1997.

6 Viral Infections (Excluding HIV Infection)

Cimetidine and Levamisole Versus Cimetidine Alone for Recalcitrant Warts in Children
Parsad D, Pandhi R, Juneja A, et al (Postgraduate Inst of Med Education and Research, Chandigarh, India; Himalayan Inst of Med Sciences, Jolly Grant, Dehradun, India)
Pediatr Dermatol 18:349-352, 2001   6–1

Introduction.—Cimetidine is a painless and relatively inexpensive treatment for warts, but studies of its effectiveness have yielded conflicting findings. The combination of cimetidine and levamisole, drugs with different target activities of immunomodulation, was examined for efficacy in a randomized trial that included 44 children with multiple recalcitrant warts.

Methods.—All children had been treated previously with at least 2 treatment modalities but had received no topical or systemic therapy for warts for at least 4 weeks before study entry. Randomization was to cimetidine, 30 mg/kg/d orally in 3 doses (group A), or to oral levamisole (2.5 mg/kg on 2 consecutive days per week), plus cimetidine, 30 mg/kg/d) for 12 weeks (group B). Group A children also received placebo on 2 consecutive days. Response was evaluated at 2-week intervals.

Results.—Nineteen group A and 20 group B patients could be evaluated. Complete resolution of warts occurred in 6 group A patients and 13 group B patients. Ten patients in group A, but only 4 in group B, showed no response. The difference between treatment groups in rates of marked to complete response was highly significant. Regression of warts was more rapid with the combination therapy (Fig 1). Side effects, mainly nausea, occurred only with levamisole therapy.

Conclusion.—The combination of levamisole and cimetidine was more effective than cimetidine alone for the treatment of recalcitrant warts in children. A synergistic effect may account for the superiority of the combined therapy.

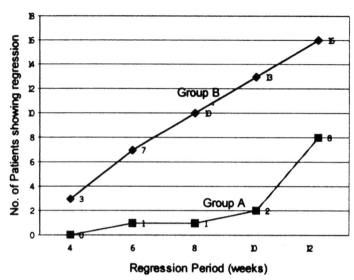

FIGURE 1.—Graphic comparison of regression of warts in groups A and B. (Courtesy of Parsad D, Pandhi R, Juneja A, et al: Cimetidine and levamisole versus cimetidine alone for recalcitrant warts in children. *Pediatr Dermatol* 18(4):349-352, 2001. Reprinted by permission of Blackwell Science, Inc.)

▶ A third group receiving double placebo therapy (in place of both cimetidine and levamisole) would have made this a better study. Unfortunately, at least as of this writing, levamisole is no longer available in the United States. A placebo-controlled double-blind study of cimetidine monotherapy showed it to be of little value in the treatment of warts.[1]

B. H. Thiers, MD

Reference

1. Yilmaz E, Alpsoy E, Basaran E: Cimetidine therapy for warts: A placebo controlled, double-blind study. *J Am Acad Dermatol* 34:271-272, 1996.

Effect of Condoms on Reducing the Transmission of Herpes Simplex Virus Type 2 From Men to Women
Wald A, Langenberg AGM, Link K, et al (Univ of Washington, Seattle; Chiron Corp, Emeryville, Calif; Westover Heights Clinic, Portland, Ore; et al)
JAMA 285:3100-3106, 2001   6–2

Background.—To date, no prospective study has shown that condom use reduces the transmission of herpes simplex virus type 2 (HSV-2). The risk factors for the acquisition of HSV-2 and the efficacy of condoms in preventing its transmission were reported.
Methods.—Data were obtained on 528 couples enrolled in a randomized, double-blind, placebo-controlled, 18-month follow-up trial of an ineffective candidate HSV-2 vaccine conducted from 1993 to 1996. The

couples were discordant for HSV-2 infection. Two hundred sixty-one men and 267 women were susceptible to HSV-2.

Findings.—Twenty-six women (9.7%) and 5 men (1.9%) acquired HSV-2 during follow-up. The rate per 10,000 sex acts for women and men were 8.9 and 1.5, respectively. A multivariate analysis showed that increased risk for HSV-2 acquisition was associated with younger age; seropositivity for HSV-1 and HSV-2, as opposed to HSV-2 alone in the source partner; and more frequent sexual activity. Condom use during more than 25% of sex acts protected women, but not men, from HSV-2 transmission but did not protect men. In the first 150 days, the risk of HSV-2 transmission was 8.5 per 100 person-years, declining to 0.9 in the final 150 days, concurrent with a decline in sexual activity and the proportion of sex acts taking place while the source partner had genital lesions.

Conclusion.—Condom use significantly protects susceptible women from HSV-2 transmission. Changes in sexual behavior after counseling to avoid sex in the presence of lesions were associated with a decrease in HSV-2 acquisition over time.

▶ Among monogamous couples with 1 partner who had known symptomatic HSV-2 infection and 1 who was susceptible to the infection, the rate of transmission from men to women was 8.9/10,000 sex acts, a rate similar to that seen with sexually acquired HIV infection.[1] Thus, the more frequent the sexual activity, the greater the risk. Condom use offered significant protection, at least for susceptible women.

B. H. Thiers, MD

Reference

1. Royce R, Sena A, Cates W, et al: Sexual transmission of HIV. *N Engl J Med* 336:1072-1078, 1997.

Application of a Topical Immune Response Modifier, Resiquimod Gel, to Modify the Recurrence Rate of Recurrent Genital Herpes: A Pilot Study
Spruance SL, Tyring SK, Smith MH, et al (Univ of Utah, Salt Lake City; Univ of Texas, Galveston; 3M Pharmaceuticals, St Paul, Minn)
J Infect Dis 184:196-200, 2001   6–3

Background.—Resiquimod (R-848) is a topically active immune response modifier that directly induces the endogenous production of interferon-α and interleukin-12, indirectly induces endogenous interferon-γ production, and enhances dendritic cell antigen presentation. Animal studies have shown that resiquimod decreases the recurrence rate of cutaneous herpes infection. Whether the application of topical resiquimod gel to recurrent genital herpes lesions would prevent subsequent recurrences in humans was determined.

Methods.—Participants were 52 patients aged 18 to 60 years with frequently recurrent genital herpes (at least 6 recurrences per year). Within 24 hours of lesion onset, patients were randomly assigned to begin 3 weeks of therapy with either vehicle gel (n = 18) or resiquimod gel in various combinations (0.01% gel twice [n = 9] or 3 times [n = 10] per week, or 0.05% gel once [n = 7] or twice [n = 8] per week). Patients were monitored for 6 months after treatment to determine recurrences.

Results.—During the follow-up period, patients using resiquimod gel had a significantly longer time to their first recurrence than did patients using the vehicle gel (median, 169 vs 57 days). The time to first recurrence was longest with the regimens of 0.01% resiquimod twice a week (median, 172.5 days) and 3 times a week (median, >195 days). The mean number of recurrences was also significantly lower with resiquimod (1.6 vs 3.1). Patients using resiquimod were also significantly more likely than those using vehicle gel to complete the entire follow-up period without a recurrence (32% vs 6%). The incidence of systemic adverse events or laboratory abnormalities did not differ between the 2 groups. However, dose-limiting inflammation at the application site was noted with resiquimod 0.05% administered twice weekly.

Conclusions.—The prompt application of topical resiquimod gel during a recurrence of genital herpes was associated with a delay in the time to the first subsequent recurrence and with a decrease in the total number of recurrences during 6 months of follow-up.

▶ The results are striking and hopefully will be confirmed in a larger study. The authors speculate that stimulation of herpes-specific cell-mediated immunity by resiquimod was a form of "endogenous vaccination" that may have helped control recurrences in the active treatment group.

B. H. Thiers, MD

Clinical Efficacy of Topical Docosanol 10% Cream for Herpes Simplex Labialis: A Multicenter, Randomized, Placebo-Controlled Trial
Sacks SL, for the Docosanol 10% Cream Study Group (Avanir Pharmaceuticals, San Diego, Calif; et al)
J Am Acad Dermatol 45:222-230, 2001   6–4

Background.—Recurrent herpes simplex labialis (HSL) occurs in 20% to 40% of the US population. Although the disease is self-limiting in persons with a healthy immune response, patients seek treatment because of the discomfort and visibility of a recurrent lesion.

Objective.—Our purpose was to determine whether docosanol 10% cream (docosanol) is efficacious compared with placebo for the topical treatment of acute HSL.

Methods.—Two identical double-blind, placebo-controlled studies were conducted at a total of 21 sites. Otherwise healthy adults, with documented histories of HSL, were randomized to receive either docosanol or polyethylene glycol placebo and initiated therapy in the prodrome or erythema stage of an episode. Treatment was administered 5 times daily until healing occurred (ie, the crust fell off spontaneously or there was no longer evidence of an active lesion) with twice-daily visits.

Results.—The median time to healing in the 370 docosanol-treated patients was 4.1 days, 18 hours shorter than observed in the 367 placebo-treated patients ($P = .008$; 95% confidence interval [CI]: 2, 22). The docosanol group also exhibited reduced times from treatment initiation to (1) cessation of pain and all other symptoms (itching, burning, and/or tingling; $P = .002$; 95% CI: 3, 16.5); (2) complete healing of classic lesions ($P = .023$; 95% CI: 1, 24.5); and (3) cessation of the ulcer or soft crust stage of classic lesions ($P < .001$; 95% CI: 8, 25). Aborted episodes were experienced by 40% of the docosanol recipients versus 34% of placebo recipients ($P = .109$; 95% CI for odds ratio: 0.95, 1.73). Adverse experiences with docosanol were mild and similar to those with placebo.

Conclusion.—Docosanol applied 5 times daily is safe and effective in the treatment of recurrent HSL. Differences in healing time compared favorably with those reported for the only treatment of HSL that has been approved by the Food and Drug Administration.

▶ The authors appear to be quite pleased that the mean time to healing (now, hold on to your hats, folks) was 18 hours shorter in docosanol-treated patients than in those treated with placebo. Perhaps they have cause to be giddy; the mean time to healing in patients treated with penciclovir, the only other prescription drug approved for topical treatment of herpes labialis, is only 12 hours less than placebo (another factoid not shared by your local drug rep)! I can think of better ways to put our health care dollars to work.

B. H. Thiers, MD

The Effectiveness of the Varicella Vaccine in Clinical Practice
Vázquez M, LaRussa PS, Gershon AA, et al (Yale Univ, New Haven, Conn; Columbia Univ, New York)
N Engl J Med 344:955-960, 2001   6–5

Introduction.—A varicella vaccine containing live attenuated virus (Oka strain) was created in Japan in the early 1970s. This vaccine was approved in the United States by the Food and Drug Administration in 1995 and is recommended for persons 12 months of age or older who are susceptible to chickenpox. Reported are findings from an ongoing case-control trial to examine the effectiveness of the vaccine as it is used in actual practice in the United States.

Methods.—Healthy children between the ages of 13 months and 16 years in whom chickenpox was suspected and who were from 15 participating pediatric practices were visited at home by a research assistant blinded to the vaccination status of each child. Children with chickenpox were ideally visited on day 3 of the illness and as late as day 5 when necessary. A parent was interviewed, and the severity of the illness was recorded. During the visit, a lesion was unroofed with a nonheparinized capillary tube into which vesicular fluid was collected to test for the presence of the varicella-zoster virus by means of the polymerase chain reaction (PCR). For every child with potential chickenpox, there were 2 controls matched for date of birth (within 1 month) and pediatric practice.

Results.—Between March 1997 and November 2000, data collection was completed for 330 patients with suspected chickenpox. Of these, 243 children (74%) had positive PCR tests for the varicella-zoster virus. Of the 56 vaccinated children with chickenpox, 86% had mild disease, compared with 48% of the 187 children who were not vaccinated ($P < .001$). Among the 202 children with PCR-verified varicella-zoster virus infection and their 386 matched controls for whom complete data were available, 23% of the children with chickenpox and 61% of the matched controls had been given the vaccine (vaccine effectiveness, 85%; $P < .001$). For moderately severe disease, the vaccine was 97% effective. The effectiveness of the vaccine was essentially unchanged (87%) after adjustment for potential confounders.

Conclusion.—The effectiveness of the varicella vaccine as used in actual practice in the United States is excellent in the short term. Nearly all of the vaccinated children in whom chickenpox subsequently developed (all of whom were infected with the wild-type virus) had very mild disease.

▶ This study demonstrates that varicella vaccine containing live attenuated virus is effective in markedly reducing the incidence of varicella as well as the severity of the disease should infection occur in vaccinated children. The duration of effectiveness of the vaccine remains a critical issue and will have to continue to be monitored. In Japan, where the vaccine was first introduced, protective concentrations of antibody have persisted for more than 20 years after immunization. This persistence, however, may be due to a booster effect from exposure to persons with varicella in a country where the vaccine is not widely used and the incidence of varicella remains high. There may be an additional benefit of the vaccine in addition to the prevention of varicella: by preventing infection with a wild strain of varicella virus, the incidence of severe painful zoster may be decreased.

S. Raimer, MD

Acute Pain in Herpes Zoster: The Famciclovir Database Project
Dworkin RH, Nagasako EM, Johnson RW, et al (Univ of Rochester, NY; Univ of Bristol, England; SmithKline Beecham Pharmaceuticals, Harlow, England)
Pain 94:113-119, 2001   6–6

Background.—Pain and dysesthesia are typical features of herpes zoster, and dermatomal pain often occurs before the characteristic rash. Postherpetic neuralgia (PHN) is the term used to identify pain that continues for at least 3 months after the rash has healed. Because PHN does not develop in all herpes zoster patients, factors have been sought that may lead to the development of PHN. Acute pain severity, demographic variables, and clinical features of the herpes zoster infection were evaluated to reveal any correlations that may carry prognostic significance.

Methods.—Four studies served as the database for the information assessed. All were randomized, multicenter, double-blind trials, and the 1778 individuals included were immunocompetent herpes zoster patients enrolled by their physicians or by referral. In 2 samples, follow-up extended for 6 months after the onset of the rash; in 2, it only continued through the acute phase of herpes zoster. Acute pain severity was rated by the patients as mild, moderate, or severe. Other variables were age, sex, presence of a prodrome, severity of the rash, duration of the rash, primary involvement of the trigeminal or other dermatomes, number of dermatomes involved, and involvement of nonadjacent dermatomes. Relationships were analyzed by variance analysis and χ-square tests.

Results.—There was a significant association between greater acute pain severity and increased age, female gender, more severe rash, presence of a prodromal phase, and primary involvement of nontrigeminal dermatomes. Older age, greater severity of rash, and presence of a prodrome were established as risk factors for PHN. These same factors were linked to more severe acute pain identified soon after the onset of the rash in these patients.

Conclusions.—Patients who were older, who had a more severe rash, and who reported a prodromal phase were more likely to have more severe acute pain within 72 hours of the rash developing and were more likely to have PHN develop. Thus, these patients should receive interventions to prevent PHN.

▶ Dworkin et al present data that indicate that the presence of a prodrome, the severity of the acute eruption, and older age are associated with increased acute zoster pain. This implies that patients seen with these criteria might be good candidates for systemic antiviral therapy, not only to decrease the acute pain, but also presumably to prevent PHN. However, another recent study suggests that the incidence of PHN in patients not treated with antiviral therapy may be less than previously thought.[1]

B. H. Thiers, MD

Reference

1. Helgason S, Petursson G, Gudmundsson S, et al: Prevalence of postherpetic neuralgia after first episode of herpes zoster: Prospective study with long term follow up. *BMJ* 321:794-796, 2000.

Correlation Between HHV-6 Infection and Skin Rash After Allogeneic Bone Marrow Transplantation

Yoshikawa T, Ihira M, Ohashi M, et al (Nagoya Univ, Japan; Fujita Health Univ, Toyoake, Japan; Japanese Red Cross Nagoya First Hosp, Japan)
Bone Marrow Transplant 28:77-81, 2001   6–7

Background.—Primary infection with variant B human herpesvirus 6 (HHV-6) is known to cause exanthem subitum, but the clinical features of variant A HHV-6 infection have not been fully elucidated. It is suspected that the virus latently infects the body after primary infection and then reactivates in an immunosuppressed host, as do other human herpesviruses. HHV-6 has recently been recognized as an opportunistic pathogen in transplant recipients and has been associated with fever and a skin rash that resembles graft-versus-host disease (GVHD), interstitial pneumonitis, encephalitis, and bone marrow suppression after bone marrow transplantation. The possibility of a causal relationship between HHV-6 and a skin rash resembling acute GVHD after bone marrow transplantation was investigated.

Methods.—The study was conducted using isolation of HHV-6 to monitor active HHV-6 infection. A total of 25 episodes of skin rash were analyzed in 22 recipients, all of whom were seropositive for HHV-6 before bone marrow transplantation. In group A, the onset of skin rash began sooner than 30 days after transplantation (15 of 25 cases). In the 10 group B cases, the onset of skin rash began more than 30 days after transplantation.

Results.—The HHV-6 genome was detected in 4 of 15 skin samples obtained from patients in group A but was not detected in any samples obtained from members of group B. HHV-6 was isolated from 11 of the 22 patients from 2 to 3 weeks after bone marrow transplantation. In 9 cases

TABLE 2.—Association Between the Results of Virologic Examinations and the Onset of Skin Rash

| | Onset of Skin Rash | | *P* Value |
	Days 0-30 (*n* = 15)	Days 31-201 (*n* = 10)	
HHV-6 DNA in skin tissue			
Positive	4	0	0.220
Negative	11	10	
Isolation of HHV-6 from PBMCs*			
Positive	9	0	0.008
Negative	6	10	
HHV-6 infection†			
Positive	11	0	0.001
Negative	4	10	

*HHV-6 was isolated within 10 days before or after the onset of skin rash.
†If HHV-6 DNA was detected in the skin tissue and/or virus was isolated from peripheral blood mononuclear cells between 10 days before or after the onset of skin rash, it was defined as HHV-6 infection.
(Courtesy of Yoshikawa T, Ihira M, Ohashi M, et al: Correlation between HHV-6 infection and skin rash after allogeneic bone marrow transplantation. *Bone Marrow Transplant* 28:77-81, 2001.)

in group A, HHV-6 was isolated within 10 days before or after onset of the skin rash (rash-related viremia) (Table 2). In contrast, no patient in group B developed skin rash-related viremia. Of the 4 patients in group A with positive detection of the HHV-6 genome in their skin tissue, 2 patients had HHV-6 viremia at the same time. HHV-6 viremia was found in 9 of 15 cases in group A (60%) but in none of the cases in group B. Overall, some evidence of HHV-6 infection was demonstrated in 11 of 15 cases in group A (73.3%) but in none of the 10 cases in group B.

Conclusions.—These findings suggest the involvement of HHV-6 in the development of skin rash in the first month after allogeneic bone marrow transplantation.

▶ The data suggest 3 possible pathologic mechanisms for developing acute GVHD or a skin rash after allogeneic bone marrow transplantation. One cause may be a simple viral exanthem secondary to HHV-6 infection. Second, HHV-6 infection could trigger acute GVHD. Third, acute GVHD might induce reactivation of latent HHV-6 infection. Elucidation of which mechanism applies in the individual patient is important. For example, the first 2 mechanisms suggest a role for antiviral therapy in patients receiving allogeneic bone marrow transplantation. On the other hand, if viral reactivation is induced by acute GVHD, anti-GVHD treatment would be the primary goal.

B. H. Thiers, MD

Lupus-like Presentation of Parvovirus B19 Infection

Narváez Garcia FJ, Domingo-Domènech E, Castro-Bohorquez FJ, et al (Delfos Med Ctr, Barcelona; Ciudad Sanitaria y Universitaria de Bellvitge, Barcelona)
Am J Med 111:573-575, 2001   6–8

Background.—Many clinical syndromes can be traced to human parvovirus B19, a small, single-stranded DNA virus. Various rheumatic diseases are the latest to be linked to parvovirus B19, especially systemic lupus erythematosus (SLE). Whether parvovirus B19 actually triggers SLE or produces a syndrome that mimics SLE is unclear, but a case is presented in which a self-limited disease mimicking SLE went into complete remission and attained normalization of the immunologic abnormalities.

> *Case Report.*—Man, 40, had a fever for 10 days; he also had malaise; myalgias; a maculopapular rash of the trunk, arms, and legs; and arthritis of the shoulders, wrists, knees, and metacarpophalangeal joints. Complete blood count and urinalysis were normal, as were other serum biochemical parameters. The erythrocyte sedimentation rate was 35 mm/h, and the test for rheumatoid factor was negative, although antinuclear antibody (ANA) testing was positive. The titer of anti-double-stranded DNA antibodies was 142 WHO-U/mL and anti-Sm antibody results were

negative. Complement levels were normal. Testing for parvovirus B19 was performed because the patient had been exposed to erythema infectiosum, and results were positive for immunoglobulin M (IgM) antibodies at a titer of 1:64; IgG antibodies were positive at a titer of 1:1024. Indomethacin treatment resulted in a resolution of symptoms within 6 weeks. On retesting 3 months later, ANA, anti-double-stranded DNA antibody, and parvovirus B19 results were negative.

Conclusions.—Several of the criteria set by the American College of Rheumatology to classify SLE were met and exposure to recent parvovirus B19 illness was present. Because of the complete resolution of symptoms and the return of laboratory results to normal values, it is speculated that parvovirus B19 produces an SLE-like illness rather than acting as a trigger for SLE itself. Thus, patients who present with SLE-like symptoms should have parvovirus B19 infection ruled out.

▶ Given the complete and rapid resolution of the observed clinical and laboratory abnormalities, the authors suggest that the parvovirus B19 infection triggered a lupus-like syndrome, rather than true SLE, in these patients. Other cases of parvovirus B19 infection mimicking SLE have previously been reported.[1,2] The clinical and immunologic similarities between the 2 conditions may make an accurate diagnosis at disease onset quite difficult. Contact with children with erythema infectiosum, a self-limited course, and the absence of serositis, neurologic, cardiac, or renal involvement, all suggest the possibility of parvovirus B19 infection with a lupus-like presentation.

B. H. Thiers, MD

References

1. Trapani S, Ermini M, Falcini F: Human parvovirus B19 infection: Its relationship with systemic lupus erythematosus. *Semin Arthritis Rheum* 28:319-325, 1999.
2. Moore TL, Bandlamudi R, Alam SM, et al: Parvovirus infection mimicking systemic lupus erythematosus in a pediatric population. *Semin Arthritis Rheum* 28:314-318, 1999.

7 Human Immunodeficiency Virus Infection

Feasibility of Postexposure Prophylaxis (PEP) Against Human Immuno-deficiency Virus Infection After Sexual or Injection Drug Use Exposure: The San Francisco PEP Study

Kahn JO, Martin JN, Roland ME, et al (San Francisco Gen Hosp; Univ of California, San Francisco; San Francisco Dept of Public Health)

J Infect Dis 183:707-714, 2001   7–1

Background.—The risk of acquiring HIV is significantly lessened if antiretroviral treatment is initiated immediately after perinatal or occupational exposure. The question arises as to whether postexposure prophylaxis (PEP) should be used for individuals exposed during sexual activity or injection drug use. The feasibility of providing PEP in light of these exposures was evaluated, and individual adherence to and side effects associated with a 4-week course of antiretroviral treatment were assessed.

Methods.—Subjects included individuals, at least age 13 years, who had been exposed to HIV infection through sexual activity or IV drug use 72 hours or less before coming for participation in the study. The exposures included intercourse without a condom or with a condom that failed to prevent exposure to genital fluids and sharing of equipment or other activities that exposed the individual to blood or genital fluid on either a mucous membrane or an area of broken skin. Each received 4 weeks of medications (zidovudine plus lamivudine given twice a day or didanosine plus stavudine given twice daily) and counseling regarding risk reduction and medication adherence (at baseline, after week 1, and after week 2). Evaluations were conducted 1, 2, and 4 weeks after exposure, with HIV antibody testing conducted 4 weeks and 6 months after exposure. Individuals were allowed to request repeated PEP for later exposures.

Results.—Four hundred one patients sought PEP, 94% of whom reported sexual exposure to HIV or suspected HIV. The sexual acts reported included receptive (40%) and insertive (27%) anal intercourse. The median number of hours between exposure and treatment was 33. Dual reverse-transcriptase inhibitors were used for 97% of participants; the 4-week program was completed by 78% of the subjects studied. HIV antibodies developed in none of the participants in the 6 months of the study. Twelve percent required a second course of PEP for a later exposure.

Conclusion.—Individuals receiving PEP within 72 hours of exposure to HIV or suspected HIV were effectively prevented from the development of detectable HIV antibodies within 6 months of exposure. This does not definitively represent efficacy, but it does indicate that PEP therapy can be used for persons at risk for HIV infection after sexual activity or injection drug use.

▶ Surprisingly, despite risk reduction counseling and medication adherence counseling, only 78% of participants completed the 4-week course of therapy. Moreover, a subsequent exposure necessitated a second course of PEP for 12% of the group.

B. H. Thiers, MD

Effect of Coinfection With GB Virus C on Survival Among Patients With HIV Infection

Xiang J, Wünschmann S, Diekema DJ, et al (Univ of Iowa, Iowa City; Helen C Levitt Ctr for Viral Pathogenesis and Disease, Iowa City, Iowa)
N Engl J Med 345:707-714, 2001   7–2

Introduction.—Persistent infection with GB virus C (GBV-C, also called hepatitis G virus) is reported in approximately 1.8% of healthy blood donors and at a rate as high as 35% in persons who are HIV positive. Previous research suggests that progression of HIV disease is delayed in patients coinfected with GBV-C. The effects of GBV-C coinfection on survival and on HIV replication in vitro were studied in a large population of patients with HIV infection.

Methods.—The study group included 362 patients with HIV infection; 144 were positive for GBV-C (39.8%), and 218 were negative for the virus. All patients provided blood samples for the investigation and had their demographic and clinical data prospectively entered into a relational database. The GBV-C–positive and GBV-C–negative groups were similar in the distribution of modes of HIV transmission (in each, sexual contact was the method of transmission in approximately three fourths of cases).

Results.—The mean duration of follow-up was 4.1 years. Forty-one patients with GBV-C viremia (28.5%) died during the follow-up period, compared with 123 patients (56.4%) who had tested negative for GBV-C RNA. In a Cox proportional hazards model, the adjusted relative risk of death was 3.7 in the GBV-C–negative group. The mortality rate was thus significantly lower for patients with HIV infection who were coinfected with GBV-C. Replication of HIV, as measured by detection of p24 antigen in culture supernatants, was inhibited by GBV-C coinfection in cultures of peripheral-blood mononuclear cells. In flow cytometry studies, coinfection did not alter the surface expression of HIV cellular receptors on peripheral-blood mononuclear cells.

Conclusion.—Among HIV-infected patients who were clinically comparable at baseline, the rate of mortality was significantly lower among those coinfected with GBV-C than among those without GBV-C coinfection. In a model of coinfection in cell cultures, GBV-C infection of peripheral-blood mononuclear cells inhibited HIV replication.

Infection With GB Virus C and Reduced Mortality Among HIV-Infected Patients
Tillmann HL, Heiken H, Knapik-Botor A, et al (Medizinische Hochschule, Hannover, Germany; Bayer Diagnostics, Emeryville, Calif)
N Engl J Med 345:715-724, 2001   7–3

Introduction.—A new virus identified in 1995, GB virus C (GBV-C), may have a beneficial effect when it appears as a coinfection in patients with HIV. Whether GBV-C viremia is beneficial in such patients, and whether any beneficial effect of GBV-C continues to be important after the introduction of highly active antiretroviral therapy, were examined prospectively. The correlation between the GBV-C load and the HIV load was also examined.

Methods.—The study enrolled 197 HIV-positive patients during 1993 and 1994. In this population, 33 (16.8%) tested positive for GBV-C RNA, 112 (56.9%) had detectable antibodies against the GBV-C envelope protein E2, and 52 (26.4%) had no marker of GBV-C infection and were considered unexposed. Cumulative survival and survival without progression to AIDS were calculated for each group.

Results.—Survival was significantly longer for patients who tested positive for GBV-C RNA, when calculated from the date of the first positive HIV test (Fig 2,A) and from the date of testing for GBV-C. The progression to AIDS was also significantly slower in this group, and GBV-C–positive patients survived longer after the development of AIDS (Fig 4,A). The association of GBV-C viremia with lower mortality remained significant after patients were stratified according to age and CD4+ cell count. The presence of GBV-C RNA remained predictive of longer survival in an analysis limited to the years after highly active antiretroviral therapy became available. Patients who were GBV-C positive had a lower HIV load than patients who were GBV-C negative, but the GBV-C load was not correlated with the CD4+ cell count.

Conclusion.—Coinfection with GBV-C was confirmed to have a beneficial effect on mortality among patients infected with HIV. The presence of GBV-C viremia was also associated with a slower progression to AIDS and a longer survival after the development of AIDS. GBV-C is not known to cause any disease, but its presence may lead to an inhibition of HIV replication.

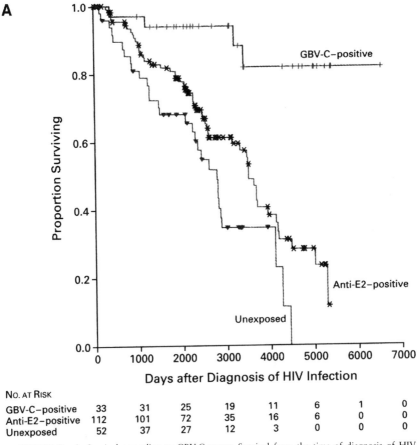

A

No. at Risk

GBV-C–positive	33	31	25	19	11	6	1	0
Anti-E2–positive	112	101	72	35	16	6	0	0
Unexposed	52	37	27	12	3	0	0	0

FIGURE 2.—A, Survival according to GBV-C status. Survival from the time of diagnosis of HIV infection is shown in relation to the GBV-C status. The patients who tested positive for GBV-C RNA had significantly better survival (P < .001 for the comparison with the unexposed group and with the anti-E2–positive group; P = .02 for the comparison between the anti-E2–positive group and the unexposed group). The tick marks on the curves indicate the last follow-up visits. (Reprinted by permission of *The New England Journal of Medicine* from Tillmann HL, Heiken H, Knapik-Botor A, et al: Infection with GB virus C and reduced mortality among HIV-infected patients. N Engl J Med 345:715-724. Copyright 2001, Massachusetts Medical Society. All rights reserved.)

▶ Xiang et al (Abstract 7–2) found evidence that HIV replication in cell cultures was inhibited by coinfection with GBV-C, a close relative of hepatitis C virus (HCV). Tillmann et al (Abstract 7–3) reported that coinfection with GBV-C was associated with improved survival in HIV-infected patients. This was true even after highly active antiretroviral therapy became available. These findings contrast to the situation with HCV coinfection, which is associated with poor survival. As noted by Stosor and Wolinsky,[1] clarification

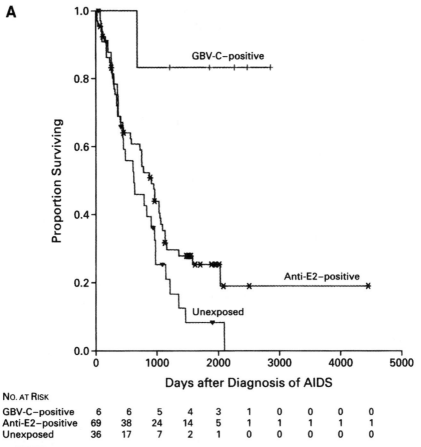

FIGURE 4.—A, Survival after the diagnosis of AIDS. From the time the diagnosis of AIDS was established, patients who tested positive for GBV-C RNA had better survival than those without GBV-C RNA ($P = .007$). The differences between the anti-E2–positive group and the unexposed group were not significant. The tick marks on the curves indicate the last follow-up visits. (Reprinted by permission of *The New England Journal of Medicine* from Tillmann HL, Heiken H, Knapik-Botor A, et al: Infection with GB virus C and reduced mortality among HIV-infected patients. *N Engl J Med* 345:715-724. Copyright 2001, Massachusetts Medical Society. All rights reserved.)

of the relation between GBV-C and HIV may have implications for the development of new treatments.

B. H. Thiers, MD

Reference

1. Stosor V, Wolinsky S: GB virus C and mortality from HIV infection. *N Engl J Med* 345:761-762, 2001.

Survival After AIDS Diagnosis in Adolescents and Adults During the Treatment Era, United States, 1984-1997

Lee LM, Karon JM, Selik R, et al (Ctrs for Disease Control and Prevention, Atlanta, Ga)

JAMA 285:1308-1315, 2001   7–4

Background.—Improvements in antiretroviral therapy and an increased proportion of patients receiving therapy are credited with producing the first decrease in the number of deaths from AIDS beginning in 1996. Trends in survival time among persons diagnosed with AIDS from 1984 to 1997 were assessed.

Methods.—Data were obtained from the national HIV/AIDS surveillance system of the Centers for Disease Control and Prevention and included both adolescents and adults whose AIDS was diagnosed between 1984 and 1997 and reported through December 1999. Deaths included took place through December 31, 1998, and were reported before December 31, 1999. The principal outcome sought was change in time from first AIDS-defining opportunistic illness (OI) to death. The months of survival after the AIDS diagnosis were compared by year of diagnosis.

Because the definition of an AIDS case was changed in 1993—which meant that immunologic criteria for the diagnosis were met at an earlier stage of HIV infection, before an OI developed—the survival time may appear to increase overall for persons whose diagnosis was based on immunologic criteria rather than on the development of an OI. This discrepancy was compensated for by focusing on cases reported in 1993 through 1997 categorized by initial diagnosis, whether immunologic or OI criteria.

Results.—The median survival time for the 394,705 individuals given a diagnosis between 1984 and 1997 improved from 11 months for diagnosis in 1984 to 46 months for diagnosis in 1995. Sixty-seven percent of patients with an OI diagnosis during 1996 and 1997 remained alive at least 36 months after diagnosis; 77% survived at least 24 months. For the 296,621 cases diagnosed between 1993 and 1997, immunologic criteria were the basis for 65% of the diagnoses; 35% were based on the presence of an OI. Survival probability for at least 24 months was 67% for those whose diagnosis rested on immunologic criteria in 1993; this rose to 90% in 1997. Twenty-four–month survival probability was 49% for those whose diagnosis was based on OI criteria in 1993; a rise to 80% was noted by 1997. The distribution among various groups was 80% for men, 42% for non-Hispanic blacks, 40% for non-Hispanic whites, 17% for Hispanics, 1% for Asians/Pacific islanders, and less than 1% for American Indians or natives of Alaska. With each year of diagnosis from 1984 to 1997, increased survival time was noted for black, white, and Hispanic groups. Patients receiving their diagnosis in 1995 and 1996 had the highest gains in annual survival.

Conclusion.—Whether the diagnosis was based on OI or immunologic criteria, the survival time after a diagnosis of AIDS increased with each subsequent year of diagnosis. All demographic groups revealed improvement, with the greatest annual survival gain made in patients given AIDS diagnoses in 1995 and 1996.

Expenditures for the Care of HIV-Infected Patients in the Era of Highly Active Antiretroviral Therapy

Bozzette SA, for the HIV Cost and Services Utilization Study Consortium (Univ of California, San Diego; et al)

N Engl J Med 344:817-823, 2001   7–5

Background.—Highly active antiretroviral therapy represents an expensive treatment regimen for patients with HIV infection. Questions have arisen concerning the relationship between expenditures for these drugs and total health care cost reductions. The expenditures over the course of 3 years for a sample of HIV-infected patients who were representative of the national spectrum for this disease were evaluated.

Methods.—A national probability sample representative of all adults with known HIV infection who made a minimum of 1 visit for health care was gathered. There were 2864 subjects. Interviews were conducted and follow-up extended for 36 months. Average expenditures for care per person per month were estimated on the basis of self-report of the care received.

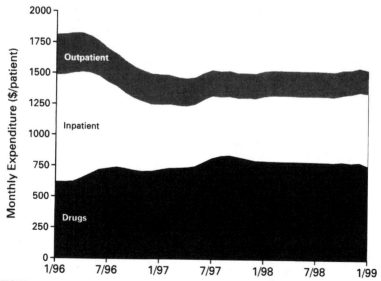

FIGURE 1.—Average monthly expenditures for the care of HIV-infected American adults (outpatient services, inpatient services, and drugs) between January 1996 and January 1999, adjusted for loss to follow-up and death. (Reprinted by permission of *The New England Journal of Medicine* from Bozzette SA, for the HIV Cost and Services Utilization Study Consortium: Expenditures for the care of HIV-infected patients in the era of highly active antiretroviral therapy. *N Engl J Med* 344:817-823, 2001. Copyright 2001, Massachusetts Medical Society. All rights reserved.)

Results.—The estimated total expenditure—adjusted for interview date, clinical status, and deaths—was $20,300 per patient in 1996. This declined to $18,300 per patient in 1998. The mean expenditure per patient per month was $1792 at baseline and fell to $1359 for survivors in 1997, with the reductions in hospital costs exceeding the increased pharmaceutical costs (Fig 1). An independent association was found between the use of highly active antiretroviral therapy and expenditure reductions. Those groups who were underserved—specifically blacks, women, and patients who did not have private insurance—had the lowest pharmaceutical costs and the highest hospital expenditures.

Conclusion.—The improved treatments available for retroviral illness have led to a marked decline in the total cost of hospital services used by patients with HIV infection. While the cost of highly active antiretroviral therapy remains high, as the treatment of HIV infection has improved, economic benefit is being realized. Thus, cost should not be the sole criterion on which treatment decisions are based.

The Cost Effectiveness of Combination Antiretroviral Therapy for HIV Disease
Freedberg KA, Losina E, Weinstein MC, et al (Harvard Med School, Boston; Boston Univ; Harvard School of Public Health, Boston; et al)
N Engl J Med 344:824-831, 2001   7–6

Background.—The current recommendation for the treatment of HIV disease is the use of a 3-drug antiretroviral regimen. Combining 3 drugs has benefited patients in terms of morbidity and mortality, but the expense of these costly antiretroviral agents is high. The clinical effect, cost, and cost effectiveness of combination antiretroviral therapy, relating expense to clinical benefit, were evaluated.

Methods.—A computer-based simulation model of HIV disease was used to compare various treatment strategies, including modifications in CD4 cell count, HIV RNA levels, development of opportunistic infections, adverse drug reactions, and death. Data were culled from the AIDS Clinical Trials Group 320 Study and several other major trials. The incremental cost-effectiveness ratio was calculated for the various alternative regimens to allow comparisons. The 3 categories of health and vital status—specifically, chronic illness, acute illness, and death—were stratified based on significant clinical parameters, as noted in the model. Antiretroviral therapy success was depicted as decreased HIV RNA levels that led to increased CD4 cell counts and a lessened probability that opportunistic infections or death would occur.

Results.—Patients whose disease course followed that of the model would have an increased quality-adjusted life expectancy of 1.53 to 2.91 years. With the 3-drug regimen, the lifetime cost of care per person was $77,300, compared with $45,460 when no therapy was used. In comparison with no therapy, the incremental cost per quality-adjusted year of life gained was $23,000. Depending on the data used, the cost-effectiveness ratio was between $13,000 and $23,000 per quality-adjusted year of life gained. The most important factors determining cost, clinical benefit, and cost effectiveness were initial CD4 cell count and cost of drugs.

Conclusion.—Combination antiretroviral therapy with the use of 3 drugs augmented the projected quality-adjusted life expectancy for the study population by 1.38 to 2.67 years. For each quality-adjusted year of life gained, the cost-effectiveness ratios were between $13,000 and $23,000, compared with the use of no therapy. The increased benefit noted with thrombolytic therapy for patients with suspected acute myocardial infarction is similar to the benefit in terms of life expectancy with the 3-drug regimen for HIV or AIDS treatment. Thus, this therapy is considered highly cost effective.

▶ Clearly, the survival time after AIDS diagnosis has increased dramatically since the early years of the epidemic. Despite the high cost of antiretroviral therapy, the study by Bozzette et al (Abstract 7–5) argues that the overall cost of caring for infected individuals has declined. Freedberg et al (Abstract 7–6) observed that the initial CD4 cell counts and drug costs were the most important determinants of overall costs, clinical benefits, and cost effectiveness. A thoughtful editorial accompanied the last 2 articles.[1]

B. H. Thiers, MD

Reference

1. Steinbrook R: Providing antiretroviral therapy for HIV infection. *N Engl J Med* 344:844-846, 2001.

Herpes Zoster as an Immune Reconstitution Disease After Initiation of Combination Antiretroviral Therapy in Patients With Human Immunodeficiency Virus Type-1 Infection
Domingo P, Torres OH, Ris J, et al (Universitat Autònoma de Barcelona)
Am J Med 110:605-609, 2001   7–7

Introduction.—Herpes zoster occurs frequently in patients at all stages of HIV-1 infection but tends to be a self-limited, dermatomal rash. In some patients with HIV-1 infection, a clinical syndrome with the appearance of herpes zoster occurs after administration of combination antiretroviral therapy. Patients in whom this syndrome developed were compared with a control group of matched patients with HIV-1 infection who did not have the syndrome.

Methods.—Cases of herpes zoster in patients with HIV-infection were collected prospectively over a 3-year period. Of 316 patients who began combination antiretroviral therapy, 24 (8%) were treated for herpes zoster within 17 weeks of starting the treatment. Controls were selected from a database of patients with HIV infection who were matched to cases by age, sex, baseline CD4 count, baseline plasma HIV-1 RNA concentration, and length of follow-up.

Results.—All 24 patients with herpes zoster had a typical dermatomal rash without dissemination, and all responded adequately to standard acyclovir therapy. Cases and controls were similar in history of HIV-1 infection, history of herpes zoster, and previous therapy. Cases, however, had a significantly greater mean increase in the number of CD8 cells (347/mL vs 54/mL in controls) after starting combination antiretroviral therapy. The only factor associated with the development of herpes zoster in multivariate analysis was the increase in CD8 cells from before the start of combination antiretroviral therapy to 1 month before development of herpes zoster.

Conclusion.—Patients with HIV-1 infection in whom herpes zoster was diagnosed after they started combination antiretroviral therapy had a greater mean increase in CD8 cell counts after starting the therapy than matched patients who remained free of herpes zoster. The incidence of herpes zoster in these patients was about 2 to 3 times greater than that reported among all HIV-infected patients.

▶ Martinez et al[1] also recognized the increased incidence of herpes zoster after initiation of protease inhibitor therapy and hypothesized that it might result from a disproportionate increase in CD8+ cells early in the course of treatment.

B. H. Thiers, MD

Reference

1. Martinez E, Gatell JM, Moran Y, et al: High incidence of herpes zoster in patients with AIDS soon after therapy with protease inhibitors. *Clin Infect Dis* 27:1510-1513, 1998.

Effect of Highly Active Antiretroviral Therapy on Frequency of Oral Warts
Greenspan D, Canchola AJ, MacPhail LA, et al (Univ of California, San Francisco)
Lancet 357:1411-1412, 2001   7–8

Background.—The oral lesions associated with HIV infection have been reported to decrease with highly active antiretroviral therapy (HAART). The pattern of oral lesions in patients with HIV was examined between 1990 and 1999 in 1280 patients with HIV-positive status.

Study Design.—One visit was randomly chosen for each patient per year, and the diagnosis and treatment of oral lesions was recorded. Immune status and HIV therapy were also assessed.

Findings.—Over the 9 years of this study, the incidence of oral candidiasis, hairy leukoplakia, and Kaposi sarcoma decreased markedly; however, the incidence of aphthous ulcers did not change, and the incidence of salivary gland disease and oral warts increased. The incidence of oral warts was higher among patients receiving HAART and increased with increasing CD4+ counts.

Conclusions.—An increase in oral warts was detected among patients with HIV who underwent HAART and who had increased CD4+ counts. This suggests that the increase in oral warts detected in these patients may be a complication of HAART. These warts present management challenges, as no effective treatment is available.

► The increase in oral warts contrasted sharply with the significant decreases in oral candidiasis, hairy leukoplakia, and Kaposi sarcoma. This could reflect a functionally incomplete reconstitution of the immune system, leading to a "blind spot" for certain opportunistic infections. Other opportunistic infections, including tuberculosis and cytomegalovirus retinitis, have been reported among patients receiving HAART, even as HIV viral loads fall and CD4+ cell counts improve.

B. H. Thiers, MD

HIV-1 Infection and Risk of Vulvovaginal and Perianal Condylomata Acuminata and Intraepithelial Neoplasia: A Prospective Cohort Study

Conley LJ, Ellerbrock TV, Bush TJ, et al (Ctrs for Disease Control and Prevention, Atlanta, Ga; New York City Dept of Health; Columbia Univ, New York)

Lancet 359:108-113, 2002   7–9

Background.—Invasive cervical cancer is an AIDS-defining disorder in women. A prospective cohort study was performed to identify other gynecologic disorders associated with HIV-1 infection.

Study Design.—From 1991 to 1998, 481 HIV-positive women, 437 HIV-negative women, and 7 women with unknown HIV status were enrolled in a trial in the New York City area. At enrollment and every 6 months for a median of 3.2 years, study participants were interviewed, submitted to CD4 T-lymphocyte counts, and had a gynecologic examination. Vulvar and perianal lesions were examined by colposcopy. Abnormalities were biopsied. Cervicovaginal lavage was performed and assayed for human papillomavirus DNA. Univariate and multivariate analyses of associations between lesions and risk factors were performed with the use of Cox's proportional hazards model.

Findings.—Vulvovaginal and perianal condylomata acuminata or intraepithelial neoplasia were present in significantly more HIV-positive than HIV-negative women. Risk factors for lesions included HIV-1 infection, human papillomavirus infection, lower CD4 lymphocyte count, and a history of use of injectable drugs.

Conclusion.—These findings indicate that women infected with HIV-1 are at increased risk for development of invasive vulvar and perianal carcinoma. Therefore, it is recommended that HIV-positive women have regular gynecologic examinations, including thorough inspection of the vulva and perianal region. Abnormalities should be evaluated by colposcopy and biopsy so that invasive disease can be detected at an early stage.

▶ It has long been known that women infected with HIV-1 are at an increased risk for development of cervical carcinoma, and in 1993 that tumor was designated an AIDS-defining disorder. This study shows that these women are at an increased risk for the development of invasive vulvar carcinoma as well.

B. H. Thiers, MD

8 Infestations

High-Magnification Videodermatoscopy: A New Noninvasive Diagnostic Tool for Scabies in Children
Lacarrubba F, Musumeci ML, Caltabiano R, et al (Univ of Catania, Italy; Northwestern Univ, Chicago)
Pediatr Dermatol 18:439-441, 2001   8-1

Introduction.—Scabies is usually diagnosed by microscopic examination of scales obtained by skin scraping. Because repeated tests might be needed, this technique can cause fear and pain in young children. High-magnification (HM) videodermatoscopy, a noninvasive method that allows a detailed inspection of the skin, was used to examine 100 young patients with suspected scabies.

Methods.—Patients were 57 girls and 43 boys with a mean age of 7.5 years. All had pruritus for at least 1 week and skin lesions suggestive of scabies. Skin videodermatoscopy was performed with low magnification (approximately 100×) for an overall view of affected areas, followed by higher magnification (up to 600×) for closer examination (Fig 4; see color plate VII) of burrows and mites. Images were stored on a personal computer or a video recorder. Antiscabies topical therapy (benzyl benzoate

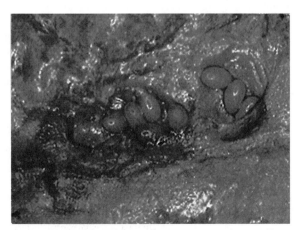

FIGURE 4.—Mite eggs at high magnification (600×). (Courtesy of Lacarrubba F, Musumeci ML, Caltabiano R, et al: High-magnification videodermatoscopy: A new noninvasive diagnostic tool for scabies in children. *Pediatr Dermatol* 18:439-441, 2001. Reprinted by permission of Blackwell Science, Inc.)

20% solution) was applied daily for 1 week if findings were positive. Scabies-negative patients were examined again after 2 weeks to confirm the absence of scabies infestation.

Results.—Videodermatoscopy identified mite migration burrows, eggs, and feces in 62 children; 56 exhibited complete clearing after 1 week of treatment and 6 required additional treatment. None of the 38 scabies-negative patients showed signs of infestation at the 2-week follow-up evaluation.

Conclusion.—High-magnification videodermatoscopy is a noninvasive, rapid, and accurate technique for the identification of scabies infestation. It is useful for primary diagnosis, follow-up, and screening of the patient's family members.

▶ The low morbidity of this procedure makes it especially appealing for pediatric patients. An added advantage is the ability to examine multiple sites without repeated scrapings.

B. H. Thiers, MD

Cutaneous Larva Migrans: Clinical Features and Management of 44 Cases Presenting in the Returning Traveller
Blackwell V, Vega-Lopez F (Univ College London)
Br J Dermatol 145:434-437, 2001   8–2

Introduction.—Cutaneous larva migrans (CLM) occurs after contact with soil or sand contaminated by stool from animals infected with intestinal parasites. Larvae hatched from nematode eggs passed with the stool can penetrate the human epidermis, causing a characteristic creeping eruption. At risk for CLM are travelers to the Caribbean, Africa, and other tropical climates. The clinical records of 44 cases of CLM were reviewed.

Methods.—Records were obtained from the database at the Hospital for Tropical Diseases, London, for the period between December 1997 and December 1999. Data examined were patient characteristics, source of infection, source of referral, clinical features, treatment, and outcome.

Results.—Most infections were acquired in Africa (32%), the Caribbean (30%), and Southeast Asia (25%), and 95% of patients reported beach exposure. The most common sites affected were the feet (39%), buttocks (18%), and abdomen (16%). No patients had laboratory abnormalities. Twenty-eight patients were cured by a single course of treatment, 11 required 2 courses, and 1 was treated 3 times; 4 patients needed no treatment. The cure rate for oral albendazole, 400 mg daily for 3 to 5 days, was 77%. Four of 5 patients who received 10% thiabendazole cream topically for 10 days were cured. Oral thiabendazole was less effective.

Conclusion.—The diagnosis of CLM is often missed, and many of the patients in this series had chronic disease. Recommended treatments include 10% thiabendazole cream, oral albendazole, 400 mg daily for 3 days; and single-dose ivermectin.

▶ Ivermectin has recently been shown to be effective in the treatment of CLM. A single dose of ivermectin, 12 mg, appeared to be more effective than a single dose of albendazole, 400 mg, in an open randomized study of 21 patients.[1] In that study, each of the 10 patients treated with ivermectin was cured without relapse.

B. H. Thiers, MD

Reference

1. Caumes E, Carriere J, Datry A, et al: A randomized trial of ivermectin versus albendazole for the treatment of cutaneous larva migrans. *Am J Trop Med Hyg* 49:641-644, 1993.

Maggot Débridement Therapy in Outpatients
Sherman RA, Sherman J, Gilead L, et al (Univ of Calif, Irvine; Hadassah Med Ctr, Jerusalem; Kiriat Menachem, Jerusalem; et al)
Arch Phys Med Rehabil 82:1226-1229, 2001   8–3

Introduction.—Outpatient wound care has a number of advantages over in-hospital care, including lower costs. Maggot debridement therapy appears well-suited for outpatient care because it is inexpensive and requires no specialized equipment or training. Within the past decade, maggot therapy with live fly larvae has come back into use as an alternative to conventional wound care. Practitioners of maggot therapy were surveyed about the benefits, risks, and problems associated with outpatient maggot wound care.

Methods.—Seventeen practitioners were identified and 7 submitted evaluations of 21 eligible patients (14 were diabetic) treated with maggot therapy between 1991 and 1997. Disinfected larvae were placed onto the wounds and contained within gauze wrap or cage-like dressings. The species *Phaenicia sericata* was used in 6 cases and the species *Neobellieria bullata* in 1 case. Maggot dressings were removed after 24 to 72 hours.

Results.—More than 95% of practitioners and 90% of their patients expressed satisfaction with outpatient maggot debridement therapy. The method completely or significantly debrided 18 (86%) wounds, 11 of which healed with no additional surgical procedures. Eight of the patients had been advised to undergo amputation or major surgical debridement; 2 needed amputation despite successful debridement and 1 did not complete maggot therapy and had his foot amputated. Patients expressed concern about the maggots escaping, but this rarely happened. Pain, reported by 8 patients, was treated with oral analgesics.

Conclusion.—Maggot therapy, commonly used in the first half of the 20th century, has more recently been limited to salvage therapy for the severely ill. But this safe and effective therapy should be considered for home-bound patients, those in rural communities, and individuals unable to afford the cost or inconvenience of hospitalization.

▶ Physicians are familiar with the common practice of pharmaceutical companies, including those manufacturing wound dressings, to host meal functions to promote their products. If maggot therapy is ever marketed by one of the bigger players, perhaps some day we'll have maggot dinners!

B. H. Thiers, MD

9 Acne

A Clinical and Therapeutic Study of 29 Patients With Infantile Acne
Cunliffe WJ, Baron SE, Coulson IH (Leeds Gen Infirmary, England; Burnley Gen Hosp, England)
Br J Dermatol 145:463-466, 2001   9–1

Background.—Infantile acne is relatively uncommon, with the clinical aspects and treatment forming the focus of most of the available literature. Follow-up from age of presentation until clearing of the lesions has not been reported previously. Twenty-nine children were studied over 25 years from presentation until resolution of their infantile acne.

Methods.—This retrospective case review focused on 29 consecutive patients (24 boys) seen in the dermatology department of the Leeds General Infirmary.

Results.—The mean age at onset of the acne was 9 months (range, 6 to 16 months), with 15 cases developing at 6 to 9 months, 11 at 11 to 13 months, and 3 at 14 to 16 months. The face, usually the cheeks, was affected in all patients. Two patients had lesions on the trunk. No other signs or symptoms of hyperandrogenism were present, and the children were otherwise healthy. Topical treatment was used exclusively in 7 patients with mild acne. Moderate acne (18 patients) was treated with topical plus oral therapy, using a pediatric suspension of erythromycin 125 mg twice a day. When no response occurred in 2 patients with erythromycin-resistant *Propionibacterium acnes*, treatment was changed to trimethoprim 100 mg twice a day with good response. In the 4 patients with severe acne, 1 was given 250 mg erythromycin twice a day, 1 received 375 mg erythromycin twice a day, 1 with *P acnes* resistant to erythromycin was switched to trimethoprim 100 mg twice a day, and 1 was given oral isotretinoin 0.5 mg/kg/d to treat localized persistent cheek acne with very deep palpable lesions. From 6 to 40 months of treatment was required for complete resolution of the acne, with mild cases and half of the moderate cases responding within 18 months, 9 with moderate and 2 with severe disease requiring over 24 months, and the infant receiving isotretinoin having treatment for 4 months. With topical therapy, mild irritant dermatitis developed but was managed by adjusting the frequency of application. With oral therapy, no obvious side effects developed. When patients required oral antibiotics for intercurrent infections, oral acne therapy was suspended. Cryotherapy was used for 2 patients with persistent inflammatory nodules. One patient with mild acne and the 4 with severe acne had facial scarring.

Conclusions.—The treatment of acne in infants is similar to the therapy in adolescents, but oral tetracycline is not used. Most cases cleared by 18 months; more severe disease required up to 40 months for the lesions to clear. Therapy was tolerated well with few adverse effects. Scarring is reduced when treatment is both early and effective.

▶ In this series of patients with infantile acne, most infants responded to a regimen of topical benzoyl peroxide, erythromycin, and/or retinoids; oral erythromycin was used when a systemic agent was needed. From 6 to 40 months of treatment were necessary for clearing. Four patients required oral trimethoprim, and 1 required isotretinoin. The isotretinoin capsules were opened and their contents mixed with margarine, then given to the infant on a small piece of toast. This was done in the dark, as vitamin A is fat soluble and light sensitive.

Hormone profiles in children with infantile acne have consistently been normal. In this study, as is generally recognized, there was male predominance. In both male and female infants, the neonatal adrenal gland has an enlarged androgen-producing area, the zona reticularis. In childhood, this area gradually decreases in size, beginning at about 1 year of age. At birth and in the first 6 to 12 months of life, boys have early pubertal levels of luteinizing hormone and, consequently, of testosterone, which likely contributes to the development of infantile acne in certain individuals. Therapy in these children is worthwhile as infantile acne may result in scarring.

S. Raimer, MD

Epidemiology of Acne in the General Population: The Risk of Smoking
Schäfer T, Nienhaus A, Vieluf D, et al (Technical Univ of Munich; Univ of Hamburg, Germany; Fachklinikum Borkum, Germany)
Br J Dermatol 145:100-104, 2001   9–2

Background.—Smoking may be correlated with acne. The prevalence of and demographic factors associated with acne in a general population were investigated, and the relationship of smoking to acne was determined.

Methods.—The study included 896 residents of Hamburg, Germany, who underwent dermatologic assessments. Study participants were aged from 1 to 87 years (median, 42 years).

Findings.—Acne was observed in a total of 26.8% of the participants, affecting 29.9% of men and 23.7% of women. The prevalence of acne followed a significant linear trend over age, peaking between 14 and 29 years. The reported age at onset in women was significantly lower than that in men. Multiple logistic regression analysis indicated that the prevalence of acne was significantly higher in active smokers than in nonsmokers, with an odds ratio of 2.04. Acne prevalence was significantly, linearly related to the number of cigarettes smoked per day. Linear regression analysis demonstrated a significant dose-dependent relationship between acne severity and daily cigarette consumption.

Conclusions.—These data suggest that smoking is a risk factor for acne. The underlying mechanism of this relationship, however, requires clarification.

▶ This is an interesting observation of marginal significance. If the threat of lung cancer, skin cancer, and wrinkles has not stopped people from smoking or sunbathing, the same can very likely be said of acne. The role, if any, that smoking might play in the pathogenesis of acne remains uncertain.

B. H. Thiers, MD

Hyperandrogenemia in Patients Presenting With Acne
Slayden SM, Moran C, Sams WM Jr, et al (Univ of Alabama, Birmingham)
Fertil Steril 75:889-892, 2001   9–3

Introduction.—Reports of elevated androgen levels in women with acne have often included both hirsute and nonhirsute patients, and there are few controlled studies of androgen levels in nonhirsute women with acne. The hypothesis that acne without hirsutism is frequently related to hyperandrogenemia, regardless of patient age, was tested.

Methods.—The prospective study included 30 consecutive unselected postmenarchal patients with acne without hirsutism and 24 eumenorrheic healthy control subjects matched by age and body mass index. Control subjects were free of acne and had no personal or family history of hirsutism or endocrine disorders. Serum samples were obtained for measurements of total and free testosterone, sex hormone-binding globulin (SHBG) and DHEAS levels. Nineteen patients also agreed to undergo an acute 60-minute corticotropin-(1-24) stimulation, measuring the 17-hydroxyprogesterone response to exclude 21-hydroxylase-deficient nonclassic adrenal hyperplasia (NCAH).

Results.—Compared with controls, the nonhirsute patients with acne had significantly lower levels of SHBG and higher free testosterone and DHEAS levels. Nineteen (63%) of these patients had at least 1 androgen value above 95% of controls. Younger patients (12-18 years) were more likely than older patients (19-43 years) to have at least 1 increased androgen value (88% and 55%, respectively), but the difference between age groups was not significant. One patient had 21-hydroxylase-deficient NCAH.

Conclusion.—Hyperandrogenemia was a common finding in nonhirsute acne patients, regardless of age. Measurement of circulating androgens may be indicated in nonhirsute women with acne, as androgen suppression may be useful in their treatment.

▶ In this series, 63% of 30 consecutive nonhirsute patients with acne had evidence of hyperandrogenemia; the prevalence was somewhat higher among adolescents (88%) than among adult women (55%). The presence or severity of hyperandrogenemia did not appear to be related to the severity of acne or the existence of menstrual dysfunction. Studies are needed to investigate the role of hormone suppression in the treatment of acne patients with excess circulating androgens. It is possible that hyperandrogenemic patients are more refractory to conventional therapies and may require drugs that suppress androgen production (such as metformin) or end-organ responsiveness (such as spironolactone).

B. H. Thiers, MD

A Randomized, Controlled Trial of a Low-Dose Contraceptive Containing 20 μg of Ethinyl Estradiol and 100 μg of Levonorgestrel for Acne Treatment
Thiboutot D, Archer DF, Lemay A, et al (Pennsylvania State Univ, Hershey; Eastern Virginia Med School, Norfolk; Centre Hospitalier Universitaire de Québec, Canada; et al)
Fertil Steril 76:461-468, 2001   9–4

Background.—Oral contraceptives (OCs) reduce circulating total androgens and the amount of bioavailable (free) testosterone by increasing sex hormone binding globulin. The efficacy of a low-dose OC containing 100 μg of levonorgestrel (LNG) and 20 μg of ethinyl estradiol (EE) was compared with that of placebo in patients with moderate acne.

Methods.—Three hundred fifty girls and women, aged 14 years or older, seen at dermatology clinics were enrolled in the multicenter, randomized, double-blind study. Two hundred twenty-six completed the 6-cycle study.

Findings.—Compared with placebo, LNG/EE given for 6 menstrual cycles was associated with significantly lower inflammatory, noninflammatory, and total lesion counts. Patients in the LNG/EE group had significantly better clinical global and patient self-assessment scores than those given placebo. The 2 groups had similar weight change from baseline at all times measured.

Conclusions.—A low-dose OC containing 20 μg of EE and 100 μg of LNG is effective and safe for treating moderate acne in girls and women with normal menstrual cycles. Patients given OCs had a significant reduction in lesion counts and better clinician global assessment scores than those given placebo.

▶ As in previous controlled trials[1,2] of another OC in the treatment of acne, a high rate of placebo response was observed. The available evidence suggests that OCs are at best modestly effective for treating acne in girls and women. In this study, no effort was made to screen patients for hormonal abnormalities. Perhaps in that subset of patients, hormonal treatment might produce more striking results.

B. H. Thiers, MD

References

1. Redmond GP, Olson WH, Lippman JS, et al: Norgestimate and ethinyl estradiol in the treatment of acne vulgaris: A randomized, placebo-controlled trial. *Obstet Gynecol* 89:615-622, 1997.
2. Lucky AW, Henderson TA, Olson WH, et al: Effectiveness of norgestimate and ethinyl estradiol in treating moderate acne vulgaris. *J Am Acad Dermatol* 37(5 Pt1):746-754, 1997.

Oral Contraceptives and the Risk of Myocardial Infarction

Tanis BC, van den Bosch MAAJ, Kemmeren JM, et al (Leiden Univ, The Netherlands; Univ Med Ctr, Utrecht, The Netherlands)
N Engl J Med 345:1787-1793, 2001
9–5

Introduction.—The few studies directly comparing third- and second-generation progestagens, while examining the association between oral contraceptives and myocardial infarction, have yielded conflicting results. A nationwide, population-based case-control study assessed the effect of low-dose combined oral contraceptives on the risk of myocardial infarction.

Methods.—Subjects were 248 women aged 18 through 49 years who had had a first myocardial infarction between 1990 and 1995; 925 control women without a myocardial infarction were matched to subjects for age, calendar year of the index event, and area of residence. Both groups completed questionnaires on oral contraceptive use and major cardiovascular risk factors. Consent to undergo DNA analysis for factor V Leiden and the G20210A mutation in the prothrombin gene was given by 88% of subjects and 82% of controls.

Results.—Compared with controls, subjects had a higher prevalence of major risk factors for cardiovascular disease, including current smoking and a lower level of education. After adjustment for age, calendar year, and area of residence, the risk of myocardial infarction was twice as high among users compared with nonusers of any type of oral contraceptive. The adjusted odds ratio was higher among users of second-generation oral contraceptives compared with third-generation users (2.5 and 1.3, respectively). Factor V Leiden or a G20210A mutation in the prothrombin gene was detected in a similar proportion (8%) of subjects and controls. Among users of oral contraceptives, the odds ratio was 2.1 for those without a prothrombotic mutation and 1.9 for those with a mutation. The risk for myocardial infarction was highest among users of oral contraceptives with the cardiovascular risk factors of smoking, diabetes, and hypercholesterolemia (odds ratios, 13.6, 17.4, and 24.7, respectively).

Conclusion.—The use of currently available combined oral contraceptives increased the overall risk for a first myocardial infarction. Odds ratios did not differ significantly among age categories or among doses of estrogen, but the risk appears to be lower with third-generation oral contraceptives.

▶ The authors report that the use of oral contraceptives increases the overall risk for a first myocardial infarction except for women 18 to 24 years old. The risk was greatest in women using first- and second-generation oral contraceptives, but the findings in women using third-generation oral contraceptives were inconclusive. Not unexpectedly, the risks were highest among users of oral contraceptives who smoked, who had diabetes, or who had hypercholesterolemia; they were not affected by prothrombotic gene mutations. Although the risk for myocardial infarction in users of oral contraceptives is admittedly small in absolute terms, it is still significant in that 35% to 45% of women of reproductive age use these drugs. The results are of importance to dermatologists in that oral contraceptives are increasingly being promoted for the treatment of acne in the female population. Moreover, the FDA wants all female isotretinoin patients to take oral contraceptives. Has anyone calculated the risk:benefit ratio of this mandate?

B. H. Thiers, MD

Third Generation Oral Contraceptives and Risk of Venous Thrombosis: Meta-analysis
Kemmeren JM, Algra A, Grobbee DE (Univ Med Centre Utrecht, The Netherlands)
BMJ 323:131-134, 2001   9–6

Background.—Increased risks of venous thrombosis were reported in 1995 and 1996 among women using "third-generation" oral contraceptives compared with users of second-generation oral contraceptives, with odds ratios reported to range from 1.5 to 2.2. Some investigators suggested that confounding, bias, or both accounted for the findings. The studies comparing effects of second- and third-generation oral contraceptives on the risk of venous thrombosis were quantitatively evaluated.

Methods.—A meta-analysis was performed of cohort and case-control studies assessing risk of venous thromboembolism among women who used oral contraceptives before October 1995. The data were evaluated by pooled adjusted odds ratios calculated by a general variance-based random effects method. Two-by-two tables were extracted and combined by the Mantel-Haenszel method whenever possible.

Results.—From an analysis of 7 studies, the overall adjusted odds ratio for third-generation versus second-generation oral contraceptives was 1.7. Similar risks were identified when oral contraceptives containing desogestrel or gestodene were compared with oral contraceptives containing levonorgestrel. For patients who were first-time users, the odds ratio for third-versus second-generation preparations was 3.1. For short-term users, the odds ratio was 2.5, compared with 2.0 for longer-term users. Studies funded by the pharmaceutical industry yielded an odds ratio of 1.3, while the odds ratio was 2.3 in other studies. Differences in age and certainty of diagnosis of venous thrombosis did not affect the results.

Conclusions.—The findings of this meta-analysis support the assertion that third-generation oral contraceptives are associated with an increased risk of venous thrombosis compared with second-generation oral contraceptives. This increase is not explained by several potential biases.

▶ As noted earlier (Abstract 9–5), oral contraceptives are increasingly being prescribed by dermatologists for the treatment of acne. As this article again demonstrates, these drugs are not without significant potential adverse effects.

B. H. Thiers, MD

Interpretations of a Teratogen Warning Symbol
Daniel KL, Goldman KD, Lachenmayr S, et al (Ctrs for Disease Control and Prevention, Atlanta, Ga; City Univ of New York; New Jersey Dept of Health and Senior Services, Lebanon)
Teratology 64:148-153, 2001   9–7

Introduction.—The teratogen warning symbol, used since 1988 to identify medications known to cause birth defects, appears on isotretinoin (Accutane) and thalidomide packaging. Yet patients do not always receive adequate counseling about such medications, and studies of isotretinoin use indicate a low rate (32%-38%) of compliance with pregnancy prevention measures. Interviews were conducted with a group of women of childbearing age to determine how the teratogen warning symbol is interpreted.

Methods.—Ninety-seven interviews were conducted at 10 sites including a well-baby clinic, an HIV/AIDS treatment clinic, and a shopping mall. Locations were chosen so that participants would vary in race, age, ethnicity, and education level. Participants were shown the warning symbol in its actual size and in a slightly enlarged version. After responses were recorded, the interviewer explained the concept of teratogens and asked participants how the symbol might be improved to communicate its message.

Results.—Only 21% of women correctly interpreted the warning symbol as meaning that they should either not take the medication if they are pregnant or not get pregnant while taking the medication. Twenty-seven percent initially thought that the symbol meant the package contained birth control medication, 24% said it indicated that the package contained drugs or medicine, and 7% replied that they did not know the symbol's meaning. As to the question of whether medications should be shared (posed to 61 women), 39% said it was never okay, and 39% gave circumstances in which sharing prescription drugs would be acceptable.

Conclusion.—The warning symbol used on teratogenic medications does not adequately communicate the risk for birth defects. Without education or counseling, many women thought that the symbol meant that the medication prevented pregnancy. A more effective warning symbol is needed, and patients must be better educated about teratogenic risks and counseled not to share medications with others.

▶ More than 2000 pregnancies were reported between 1982 and March 2000 in American women taking isotretinoin. As part of the Accutane Pregnancy Prevention Program, the teratogen warning symbol is placed on every capsule in the blister pack distributed to patients. As demonstrated by Daniel et al, this teratogen warning symbol can easily be misinterpreted. In their study, more than 25% of the 97 women surveyed thought the graphic meant that isotretinoin was a form of birth control, and only 21% understood the warning. This study did not include women who used or considered using isotretinoin, emphasizing the importance of pregnancy prevention counseling, including an explanation of the meaning of the warning symbol, for every female patient.

B. H. Thiers, MD

Ocular Side Effects Possibly Associated With Isotretinoin Usage
Fraunfelder FT, Fraunfelder FW, Edwards R (Oregon Health Sciences Univ, Portland, Ore; World Health Organization, Uppsala, Sweden)
Am J Ophthalmol 132:299-305, 2001   9–8

Background.—Isotretinoin has long been the treatment of choice for severe recalcitrant nodular acne. It has also been used to treat various other skin disorders. Ocular side effects that may be associated with the use of this agent were assessed.

Methods.—Data obtained from 1741 case reports received from spontaneous reporting systems were reviewed in concert with data obtained from the Drug Safety Section of Roche Pharmaceuticals. In addition, the worldwide literature on suspected ocular reactions to isotretinoin usage was reviewed.

Findings.—Thirty-eight signs or symptoms of ocular effects associated with isotretinoin use were classified as certain, probable, possible, unlikely, or conditional. Certain adverse ocular effects include abnormal meibomian gland secretion, blepharoconjunctivitis, corneal opacities, reduced dark adaptation, reduced contact lens tolerance, decreased vision, increased tear osmolarity, keratitis, meibomian gland atrophy, myopia, ocular discomfort, ocular sicca, photophobia, and teratogenic ocular abnormalities. Probable effects include decreased (but reversible) color vision and permanent loss of dark adaptation. Possible adverse effects include permanent keratoconjunctivitis sicca (Table 7).

TABLE 7.—Adverse Ocular Effects in Patients on Isotretinoin

Certain
  Abnormal meibomian gland secretion
  Blepharoconjunctivitis
  Corneal opacities
  Decreased dark adaptation
  Decreased tolerance to contact lens
  Decreased vision
  Increased tear osmolarity
Probable/likely
  Decreased color vision (reversible)
Possible
  Corneal ulcers
  Diplopia
  Eyelid edema
  Idiopathic intracranial hypertension with
    optic disk edema
Unlikely
  Activation of herpes simplex virus
  Corneal vascularization
  Exophthalmos
  Glaucoma
Conditional/unclassifiable
  Cataracts
  Cortical blindness
  Decreased accommodation
  Iritis

Keratitis
Meibomian gland atrophy
Myopia
Ocular discomfort
Photophobia
Ocular sicca
Teratogenic ocular abnormalities

Permanent loss of dark adaptation

Optic neuritis
Permanent sicca-like syndrome
Subconjunctival hemorrhage

Keratoconus
Limbal infiltrates
Pupil abnormalities
Vitreous disturbance

Peripheral field loss
Retinal findings
Scleritis

(Courtesy of Fraunfelder FT, Fraunfelder FW, Edwards R: Ocular side effects possibly associated with isotretinoin usage. *Am J Ophthalmol* 132:299-305, 2001. Copyright 2001 by Elsevier Science Inc.)

Conclusions.—Thirty-eight different signs or symptoms of ocular abnormalities associated with isotretinoin use were identified and classified. However, the association of ocular adverse effects with isotretinoin is controversial, and further research is needed.

▶ The authors nicely document the assortment of ocular abnormalities that can be seen in patients receiving isotretinoin. Most disconcerting is the "probable/likely" association of isotretinoin with permanent loss of dark adaptation and the "possible" association with permanent keratoconjunctivitis sicca.

B. H. Thiers, MD

An Analysis of Reports of Depression and Suicide in Patients Treated With Isotretinoin

Wysowski DK, Pitts M, Beitz J (Food and Drug Administration, Rockville, Md)
J Am Acad Dermatol 45:515-519, 2001
9–9

Background.—Isotretinoin (Accutane) is used in the treatment of severe recalcitrant nodular acne. The US Food and Drug Administration (FDA) has received reports of adverse psychiatric events, most notably depression and suicide, in patients treated with isotretinoin. As a result, in 1998 the manufacturer alerted physicians about a new warning in the approved labeling, indicating that Accutane may cause depression, psychosis and, in rare instances, suicidal ideation, suicide attempts, and suicide, and that the discontinuation of therapy may not ameliorate these side effects. Additional reports of depression and suicide in patients treated with isotretinoin have surfaced since this warning was issued. This study details all the cases of depression and suicide reported to the FDA in users of isotretinoin in the United States and analyzes the potential association between depression and isotretinoin use.

Methods.—Voluntary reports of depression, suicidal ideation, attempted suicide, and suicide among patients treated with isotretinoin were analyzed. The cases were reported to the FDA and the manufacturer from 1982 to May 2000 and were entered in the FDA's Adverse Event Reporting System database.

Results.—A total of 431 US patients treated with isotretinoin during this period were reported to the FDA as experiencing adverse effects such as depression and suicide. There were 37 reports of patients who committed suicide. Approximately 110 isotretinoin users were hospitalized for depression, suicidal ideation, or suicide attempts from 1982 to May 2000, and an additional 284 patients with nonhospitalized depression were reported. The factors identified as suggesting a potential association between isotretinoin and depression include a temporal association between the use of isotretinoin and depression, positive dechallenges, positive rechallenges, and possible biologic plausibility. Isotretinoin ranked among the top 10 drugs in number of reports of depression and suicide among all drugs in the FDA's Adverse Event Reporting System database to June 2000.

Conclusions.—There have been reports to the FDA of depression, suicidal ideation, attempted suicide, and suicide in patients taking isotretinoin. Further studies are needed to determine whether isotretinoin causes depression and to develop methods for identifying persons who might be susceptible to depression resulting from isotretinoin therapy. Physicians are advised to inform patients and parents as necessary of the potential for the development or worsening of depression with isotretinoin use and to warn them to immediately report mood swings and symptoms suggestive of depression for possible discontinuation of the drug and referral to psychiatric care.

▶ The jury is still out regarding the alleged association between isotretinoin and depression and suicide. The authors concede that there are anecdotal reports and studies that suggest a relationship between skin disorders and decreased self-esteem, anxiety, depression, and suicide. They then offer the dubious assertion that "the purported relationship between acne and depression would not fully explain the link between isotretinoin and depression since a positive disposition would be expected after efficacious isotretinoin treatment," yet offer no data to support that claim. I personally remain unconvinced of any association between the drug and depressive symptoms, although many dermatologists whose opinions I trust and respect believe otherwise.

B. H. Thiers, MD

A Randomized Trial of the Efficacy of a New Micronized Formulation Versus a Standard Formulation of Isotretinoin in Patients With Severe Recalcitrant Nodular Acne

Strauss JS, Leyden JJ, Lucky AW, et al (Univ of Iowa, Iowa City; Univ of Pennsylvania, Philadelphia; Dermatology Research Associates, Cincinnati, Ohio; et al)
J Am Acad Dermatol 45:187-195, 2001   9–10

Background.—Isotretinoin is very frequently the drug of choice for the management of severe recalcitrant nodular acne. Recently, a new micronized and more bioavailable formulation of isotretinoin has been developed that permits once-daily administration in lower doses than are usually used with standard isotretinoin (Accutane), regardless of whether it is taken with or without food.

Objective.—Our purpose was to determine whether micronized isotretinoin and standard isotretinoin are clinically equivalent.

Methods.—In this multicenter, double-blind, double-dummy study, 600 patients with severe recalcitrant nodular acne were treated with either 0.4 mg/kg of micronized isotretinoin once daily without food (n = 300) or 1.0 mg/kg per day of standard isotretinoin in two divided doses with food (n = 300). Lesion counts were monitored over 20 weeks.

Results.—Both treatment groups in this well-controlled clinical trial experienced an equivalent reduction in the number of total nodules (facial plus truncal). In addition, an equivalent proportion of patients achieved 90% clearance of the total number of nodules. Both formulations had similar results for other efficacy variables.

Conclusion.—Once-daily use of the micronized and more bioavailable formulation of isotretinoin under fasted conditions is clinically equivalent to the standard twice-daily formulation under fed conditions in the treatment of severe recalcitrant nodular acne.

Safety of a New Micronized Formulation of Isotretinoin in Patients With Severe Recalcitrant Nodular Acne: A Randomized Trial Comparing Micronized Isotretinoin With Standard Isotretinoin

Strauss JS, Leyden JJ, Lucky AW, et al (Univ of Iowa, Iowa City; Univ of Pennsylvania, Philadelphia; Dermatology Research Associates, Cincinnati, Ohio; et al)
J Am Acad Dermatol 45:196-207, 2001   9–11

Background.—Isotretinoin is a very effective drug for treating severe recalcitrant nodular acne. A new micronized formulation of isotretinoin has been shown to be clinically equivalent to standard isotretinoin with improved bioavailability and minimal food effect. The safety profile of the micronized formulation has not been described previously.

Objective.—The objective of this article is to report the incidence and intensity of adverse events found in a comparative, double-blind efficacy study that showed clinical equivalence of the new micronized formulation of isotretinoin and the standard isotretinoin formulation (Accutane).

Methods.—Six hundred patients with severe recalcitrant nodular acne were treated with micronized isotretinoin (n = 300) under fasted conditions or standard isotretinoin (n = 300) under fed conditions. One cohort received single daily doses of 0.4 mg/kg of micronized isotretinoin without food and the other cohort received 1.0 mg/kg per day of standard isotretinoin in two divided doses with food. Adverse events were monitored during 20 weeks of drug therapy.

Results.—The proportion of adverse events in most body systems was generally lower in patients receiving micronized isotretinoin than in those receiving standard isotretinoin.

Conclusion.—Micronized isotretinoin appears to have a safety profile similar to that of standard isotretinoin and to carry a lower risk of mucocutaneous events and hypertriglyceridemia.

▶ With a certainty approaching that of night following day, patent expiration of a previously proclaimed "miracle drug" sends shutters down the spine of its manufacturer and unleashes a curiously predictable scenario. This includes the introduction of a new and supposedly better formulation of the existing drug, along with subtle (and sometimes not so subtle) product bashing directed against the earlier version. We have seen this all too often, not only in dermatology, but in other fields of medicine as well. Prilosec/Nexium, Nizoral/Sporanox, Zovirax/Valtrex, and Sandimmune/Neoral are just a few examples. So let it be with isotretinoin. Only time will tell whether the new micronized product offers any real benefits. Interestingly, although psychiatric disorders were relatively uncommon adverse events, they occurred in 3.7% in the micronized group versus 0.3% in the group treated with the standard isotretinoin formulation. Given the estimated 10% prevalence of psychiatric disorders that occurs in the general population over the course of 1 year, the authors concluded that the notably low incidence in the standard isotretinoin group was attributable to chance.

B. H. Thiers, MD

Photodynamic Therapy of Acne Vulgaris With Topical δ-Aminolaevulinic Acid and Incoherent Light in Japanese Patients
Itoh Y, Ninomiya Y, Tajima S, et al (Natl Defense Med College, Saitama, Japan)
Br J Dermatol 144:575-579, 2001   9–12

Introduction.—Isotretinoin is extremely effective in the treatment of intractable acne, but it is not approved in Japan because of its potential for teratogenicity. The use of δ-aminolevulinic acid (ALA)–based photodynamic therapy (PDT) may be beneficial in the treatment of localized persistent acne in patients who are unable to tolerate isotretinoin because of side effects. The effect of ALA-PDT with polychromatic visible light was examined in 13 patients with intractable acne vulgaris.

Methods.—Twenty percent ALA in an oil-in-water emulsion was applied to lesions for 4 hours with the use of a light-shielding dressing. The lesions were exposed to polychromatic visible light at 600 to 700 nm with the use of a halogen light source with an energy intensity of 17 mW cm^{-2} and a total energy dose of 13 J cm$^{-2.}$

Results.—All patients experienced apparent improvement in facial appearance and a decrease in new acne lesions at 1, 3, and 6 months' follow-up. Adverse effects included discomfort, burning and stinging during irradiation, edematous erythema for 3 days after PDT, epidermal exfoliation on days 4 through 10, irritation and hypersensitivity to physical stimulation for 10 days after PDT, and pigmentation or erythema after epidermal exfoliation. The treated area returned to normal within 1 month.

Conclusion.—The ALA-PDT approach is effective for acne and may be used in patients with pigmented skin types. Polychromatic visible light is better than laser light for use in patients with acne because it is less expensive and produces uniform illumination of large areas of the skin surface.

▶ A previous study by the same author described the treatment of acne with ALA and 630-nm laser light.[1] Hongcharu et al[2] used broad-band light (550 to 700 nm), an approach similar to that followed in this study. Both of these earlier reports were reviewed in the 2001 YEAR BOOK OF DERMATOLOGY AND DERMATOLOGIC SURGERY. The broad-band approach offers some advantages, including cost effectiveness, uniform illumination, and a shortened time period to complete the irradiation. However, both methods cause a brisk inflammatory reaction that would be poorly tolerated by some patients; thus, considerable "tweaking" of the treatment protocol will be necessary before ALA-PDT becomes a viable treatment option for acne vulgaris.

B. H. Thiers, MD

References

1. Itoh Y, Ninomiya Y, Tajima S, et al: Photodynamic therapy for acne vulgaris with topical (δ-aminolevulinic acid. *Arch Dermatol* 136:1093-1094, 2000.

2. Hongcharu W, Taylor CR, Chang Y, et al: Topical ALA-photodynamic therapy for the treatment of acne vulgaris. *J Invest Dermatol* 115:183-192, 2000.

Association Between Sciatica and *Propionibacterium acnes*

Stirling A, Worthington T, Rafiq M, et al (Univ Hosp, Edgbaston, Birmingham, England; Aston Univ, Aston Triangle, Birmingham, England)
Lancet 357:2024-2025, 2001   9–13

Background.—Patients with sciatica have an area of inflammation surrounding the nerve root, which may be the result of microbial infection, possibly with organisms of low virulence, as noted in prosthetic hip infections. This study was undertaken to test the hypothesis that infection with *Propionibacterium acnes* may cause the inflammation noted in sciatica.

Methods.—A newly developed serologic (ELISA) test was used to investigate deep-seated infections caused by gram-positive microorganisms of low virulence, such as coagulase-negative staphylococci and propionibacteria, in 140 patients with sciatica. Originally set to be controls for a study of spondylodiskitis, 43 of these 140 patients had elevated serum IgG titers to the lipid S antigen. None had experienced any infection in the previous 6 months. Thirty-six additional patients with severe sciatica underwent clinical assessment and lumbar MRI, which revealed diskogenic radiculitis for which microdiskectomies were performed for pain relief. The disk tissue removed was evaluated for microorganisms.

Results.—Nineteen patients had positive culture results within 7 days of incubation of their tissue samples, and *P acnes* (84% of samples), coagulase-negative staphylococci (11% of cases), and *Corynebacterium propinquum* (5% of cases) were isolated. In 15 cases, blood samples were obtained for lipid S antibody estimation; 47% had positive results. Sixteen of the 17 patients who had negative culture results had negative results on lipid S antigen testing. There were more patients with positive culture results who had positive serologic test results than there were who had negative culture results. Concurrent examination of tissue obtained by diskectomy from 14 patients with other spinal disorders showed no positive culture results after long incubation times. Patients with sciatica had positive tissue culture results in 53% of cases; controls had positive tissue culture results in 0% of cases. No microorganisms were isolated from 11 gram-stained thin sections assessed using direct microscopy, so the number of microorganisms must have been small.

Conclusions.—Elevated concentrations of a specific serum antibody to lipid S, an exocellular bacterial cell wall component, were found in a significant number of patients with sciatica. In addition, there were microorganisms of low virulence, usually propionibacteria, found in a large percentage of these patients.

▶ A little respect for *P acnes*! In recent years, commensal organisms that populate the skin, such as coagulase-negative staphylococci and propionibacteria, have increasingly been recognized as agents of infection rather than simply contaminants. For example, both types of organisms have been found in prosthetic joints studied at revision arthroplasty.[1] Nevertheless, the exact role of *P acnes* in the pathogenesis of sciatica, as well as acne, remains to be elucidated.

B. H. Thiers, MD

Reference

1. Tunney MM, Patrick S, Gorman SP, et al: Improved detection of infection in hip replacements. *J Bone Joint Surg Br* 80:568-572, 1998.

10 Hair Disorders

Control of Hair Growth and Follicle Size by VEGF-Mediated Angiogenesis

Yano K, Brown LF, Detmar M (Harvard Med School, Boston)

J Clin Invest 107:409-417, 2001

10–1

Background.—The cycle of expansion and regression that murine hair follicles undergo requires changing degrees of vascular support. An important mediator of angiogenesis is vascular endothelial growth factor (VEGF), which acts during development as well as in various disease states associated with neovascularization. This study attempted to quantify the changes in vascularization that occur during the hair cycle and to explore the role of VEGF in hair growth and angiogenesis.

Methods.—The hair cycle was induced in the back skin of adult mice by depilation, which led to the synchronized development of anagen hair follicles. Samples obtained represented the cycle from the early anagen to the telogen phase. VEGF transgenic mice were established. Treatment was carried out with anti-VEGF antibody, and Miles vascular permeability assays were done.

Results.—The vascular remodeling that takes place during the hair cycle was found to be marked, with perifollicular vessel size increasing nearly 4-fold during anagen and declining rapidly during the catagen and telogen phases. Changes in follicle size were paralleled by changes in vessel size. Both in terms of time and location, perifollicular angiogenesis correlated with the upregulation of VEGF messenger RNA expression by the follicular keratinocytes found in the outer root sheath. When VEGF expression was exaggerated transgenically in the outer root sheath keratinocytes, vascularization was enhanced, hair regrowth after depilation was accelerated, and the vibrissa follicles, hair follicles, and hair shafts all were larger. When systemic treatment with anti-VEGF antibody blocked VEGF expression, hair growth was stunted and hair follicles were smaller.

Conclusion.—VEGF appears to play an important role in hair development and cycling. A paracrine mechanism was found by which the hair follicle compartment characterized by proliferative epithelium stimulates the increased vascular support needed to nourish follicles during the anagen phase. Normal growth of hair and size of hair follicles depend on the perifollicular angiogenesis induced by VEGF.

▶ The results provide evidence that follicle vascularization promotes hair growth and increases hair follicle and hair size and that these effects are mediated, at least in part, by VEGF. Improved vascularization has been thought by some investigators to underlie the mechanism by which topical minoxidil promotes hair growth.

B. H. Thiers, MD

---

p53 Involvement in the Control of Murine Hair Follicle Regression
Botchkarev VA, Komarova EA, Siebenhaar F, et al (Boston Univ; Univ of Illinois, Chicago; Johannes Gutenberg-Univ, Mainz, Germany)
Am J Pathol 158:1913-1919, 2001   10–2

Introduction.—A variety of biological responses are mediated by the transcription factor p53, including apoptotic cell death. p53 was recently shown to control hair follicle apoptosis that was induced by ionizing radiation and chemotherapy. Its role in apoptosis-driven physiologic hair follicle regression (catagen) has yet to be determined. During the cellular reaction to stress, p53 alters expression of multiple p53-responsive genes (Fas, Fas-ligand, Bax, bcl-2, insulin-like growth factor binding protein-3, insulin-like growth factor 1 receptor), the activity of which causes either cell survival or apoptotic death. Of note, proteins whose transcription is encoded by the aforementioned genes are expressed in the hair follicle during anagen-catagen transition. The distribution of p53 and its co-localization with apoptotic markers during catagen were examined in C57BL/6 mice. The dynamics of apoptosis-driven hair follicle regression was examined in wild-type and p53 knockout mice.

Findings.—Strong p53 protein expression and co-localization with apoptotic markers were seen in the regressing hair follicle compartments during catagen. Contrasted to wild-type mice, p53 knockout mice demonstrated significant retardation of catagen accompanied by a significant reduction in the number of apoptotic cells in hair matrix. The p53 null hair follicles were characterized by alterations in the expression of markers encoded by p53 target genes and implicated in the control of catagen (Bax, bcl-2, insulin-like growth factor binding protein-3).

Conclusion.—It is likely that p53 is involved in the control of apoptosis in the hair follicle during physiologic regression. Thus, the p53 antagonists may be helpful in the management of hair growth disorders characterized by premature entry into catagen, including androgenetic alopecia, alopecia areata, and telogen effluvium.

▶ Apoptosis defines the process of programmed cell death. The authors present data suggesting that p53 fosters apoptosis during physiologic regression of the hair follicle. They then argue that p53 antagonists may be useful for the management of disorders of hair growth characterized by premature entry into catagen, including androgenetic alopecia, alopecia areata, and telogen effluvium.

B. H. Thiers, MD

Prevention of Chemotherapy-Induced Alopecia in Rats by CDK Inhibitors
Davis ST, Benson BG, Bramson HN, et al (Glaxo Wellcome Research and Development, Research Triangle Park, NC)
Science 291:134-137, 2001   10–3

Background.—It is common for alopecia to occur when cytotoxic anticancer agents are used. The state of proliferation of the hair follicle cells makes them vulnerable to these anticancer agents, which are selectively toxic to cells undergoing division. The cytotoxic activity of cell cycle-active agents is diminished by inhibiting cell cycle progression. A key role in the orderly movement from late G_1 to late G_2 phase is ascribed to the protein cyclin-dependent kinase 2 (CDK2). The theory that inhibiting CDK2 may control cell division, thereby preventing chemotherapy-induced alopecia (CIA), was evaluated.

Methods.—Various synthetic CDK inhibitors were prepared and labeled compounds 1 through 4. Among them, compound 4 was found to be a potent and selective inhibitor of CDK2. A cell-based assay was used to assess the effects of compound 4 on cell cycle progression by blocking the movement from late G_1 to S phase. In vivo efficacy was studied with the use of a rat model of CIA. Etoposide and cyclophosphamide-doxorubicin were the drugs used to induce alopecia.

Results.—Topical application of compound 4 to the scalp hair of rat pups before the administration of etoposide protected scalp hair (but not body hair), and was completely effective in 50% of those treated and partially effective in 20%. The number of viable hair follicles was increased as was the number of dermal papilla; the level of inflammation, degree of cellular epithelial damage, epidermal thickening, and number of apoptotic cells in the hair follicle matrix were all decreased. Similar efficacy was demonstrated when 29 structural analogues of compound 4 were tested. Hair loss was prevented in 33% of the rats who received cyclophosphamide-doxorubicin.

Conclusion.—Based on these results, it would seem prudent to assess the effects of compound 4 and its analogues on cancer patients. The prevention of CIA by inhibiting CDK2 seems potentially achievable.

▶ One of the least recognized side effects of cancer therapy is the loss of self image associated with CIA. The pathogenesis of CIA is quite simple: antineoplastic drugs target rapidly-dividing cancer cells; unfortunately, as a consequence, rapidly dividing normal cells, such as those in the hair matrix, are killed as well. Davis et al used a new drug that targets an enzyme, CDK2, which drives a key step in the cell-division cycle. The hope was that inhibiting this step in the cell-division cycle would protect these cells from chemotherapeutic agents. Other researchers are studying the use of CDK inhibitors in an attempt to develop agents that block the growth of cancer cells. Fortunately, Davis et al could find no evidence that their drug interfered with the ability of chemotherapeutic agents to kill cancer cells, at least in animal tumor models.

B. H. Thiers, MD

The *Hairless* Gene Mutated in Congenital Hair Loss Disorders Encodes a Novel Nuclear Receptor Corepressor
Potter GB, Beaudoin GMJ III, DeRenzo CL, et al (Johns Hopkins Univ, Baltimore, Md)
Genes Dev 15:2687-2701, 2001   10–4

Background.—The first recognition of a mutation of the murine *hairless* (*hr*) gene occurred more than 75 years ago. The human ortholog was subsequently determined to be associated with alopecia universalis, papular atrichia, and other congenital hair disorders. Multiple murine and human alleles have been characterized. All of these alleles share a distinctive phenotype in which hair growth is normal initially, but hair does not regrow after shedding. The exact role of the *hr* gene in hair-follicle biology is not known, but it is known that this gene plays an important role in the brain, and some neurologic deficits are sometimes correlated with the hair loss phenotype that is typical of *hr* mutants. There are multiple cases in which mental retardation has been observed concurrent with the hair loss phenotype of *hr* mutants. It has been shown that the protein encoded by *hr* (called Hr) interacts directly and specifically with thyroid hormone receptor (TR), a transcription factor that represses transcription through interaction with corepressors such as nuclear receptor corepressor.

Methods.—Hr domains that specify TR interaction were identified to determine whether Hr is a corepressor.

Results.—A coimmunoprecipitation assay confirmed that Hr interacts directly and specifically with TR in vivo. Specifically, TR binding is mediated at two independent regions of Hr, and this interaction requires a cluster of hydrophobic residues that are similar to the binding motifs that have been proposed for nuclear receptor corepressors (N-CoR and SMRT). Hr was also shown to mediate transcriptional repression by unliganded TR. In the presence of Hr, transcriptional activity in the absence of TH is reduced five-fold only for the TH-responsive reporter gene. The interaction of Hr with histone deacetylases (HDACs) was also investigated, and it was shown that Hr interacts with HDACs and is localized to matrix-associated deacetylase (MAD) bodies. This finding indicates that the mechanism of Hr-mediated repression is likely through associated HDAC activity. It would appear, therefore, that Hr is a component of the corepressor machinery with a remarkably conserved mode of action despite its lack of sequence identity with previously described corepressors.

Conclusions.—Hr most likely defines a new class of nuclear receptor corepressors. These findings provide a molecular basis for specific murine and human hair loss syndromes.

▶ This important and fascinating article describes the elucidation of the *hr* gene product as a transcriptional corepressor. The *hr* gene is well known to dermatologists because its mutation in both mouse and human is associated with congenital hair loss and, occasionally, neurologic defects. The Hr protein interacts with the TR which, in the absence of thyroid hormone, acts as a repressor of target genes. The authors present convincing evidence that Hr interacts with the receptor in the absence of thyroid hormone and at the hormone binding site and mediates the repression of gene transcription by the receptor. Furthermore, Hr interacted and colocalized with HDACs in the nucleus, a characteristic of nuclear receptor corepressors. These data provide the first vital step in understanding the biologic function of the *hr* gene and the consequences of its mutation.

G. M. P. Galbraith, MD

High-Dose Pulse Corticosteroid Therapy in the Treatment of Severe Alopecia Areata
Seiter S, Ugurel S, Tilgen W, et al (Saarland Univ, Homburg/Saar, Germany)
Dermatology 202:230-234, 2001   10–5

Introduction.—The pathogenesis of alopecia areata (AA) is not known, but there is increasing evidence that a reversible tissue-restricted autoimmune process may be the causative mechanism. The efficacy of IV high-dose methylprednisolone pulse therapy in 30 patients with severe AA was assessed.

Methods.—Thirty patients (ages 14-56 years) were treated with methylprednisolone (8 mg/kg body weight) IV on 3 consecutive days at 4-week intervals for a minimum of 3 courses. Eight patients received a second series of 3 courses of IV pulse therapy with methylprednisolone because of a clinical relapse after initial regrowth of hair (7 patients with plurifocal AA and 1 patient with ophiasic AA).

Results.—More than 50% regrowth of hair was observed in 67% of the patients with AA plurifocalis. No patients with AA totalis or universalis and 1 patient with ophiasic AA had a therapeutic response. Among patients with AA plurifocalis, higher response rates were seen in those who had long-term disease than in those treated during their first episode of AA (73% vs 57%). In the group that received a second series of treatments, 1 had a complete response and 2 had a prolonged stable remission.

Conclusion.—High-dose methylprednisolone pulse therapy was effective and well tolerated in patients with severe AA plurifocalis. It may be less helpful in patients with ophiasic AA, AA totalis, or AA universalis.

▶ Most studies of treatment for AA have shown that patients with severe disease of long duration are least likely to respond. In this study, it was somewhat surprising that patients with long-term multifocal AA had a higher response rate than patients treated during their first episode, although more long-term patients experienced relapse. A truly effective treatment for this condition awaits more detailed elucidation of its pathogenesis.

B. H. Thiers, MD

The Use of Topical Diphenylcyclopropenone for the Treatment of Extensive Alopecia Areata
Cotellessa C, Peris K, Caracciolo E, et al (Univ of L'Aquila, Italy)
J Am Acad Dermatol 44:73-76, 2001   10–6

Background.—For more than a decade topical immunotherapy has been used for the treatment of severe alopecia areata (AA), and various contact allergens such as dinitrochlorobenzene and squaric acid dibutylester have enhanced regrowth of hair in patients with AA. Diphenylcyclopropenone (DPCP) has been described as a potent contact allergen in both humans and animals. The effectiveness of topical immunotherapy with DPCP in the treatment of AA has been demonstrated in several reports; however, the response rates in these reports have varied greatly from 4% to 85%. The efficacy and tolerability of DPCP as the treatment of chronic extensive alopecia areata were evaluated, and the long-term overall benefit of treatment was assessed.

Methods.—An open-label clinical trial involving 56 patients with chronic, extensive alopecia areata was conducted. The 30 men and 26 women ranged in age from 18 to 50 years, with a mean of 23 years. The patients were sensitized with 2% DPCP, and progressively higher concentrations, beginning at 0.001%, were then applied weekly for 6 to 12 months to 1 side of the scalp. When unilateral regrowth was noted, bilateral application was initiated.

Results.—The therapy was completed by 52 of the 56 patients. Total regrowth of terminal hair (initially unilateral) was achieved in 25 of the 52 patients (48%) at 6 months. An additional 6% of the patients experienced growth of terminal hair after 12 months of therapy. The most frequent side effect was an eczematous reaction that was observed at the site of application. A persistent response was observed in 60% of the 25 responding patients for 6 to 18 months after therapy.

Conclusions.—Topical treatment with DPCP was found to be effective and well tolerated and provided long-lasting therapeutic benefits.

▶ Experience teaches us that the response of extensive alopecia areata to topical sensitizers or, indeed, to any therapy depends on the extent and duration of disease. The results reported by Cotellessa et al are somewhat better than my own experience and those reported by Pericin et al.[1] It is not clear whether patients who obtained a grade 4 response ("regrowth of terminal hair on the whole scalp") had a truly acceptable cosmetic response. I personally have become less enthusiastic about topical sensitizers for alopecia areata. I have found that most of my patients who respond well initially will, with time, often become less reactive to the sensitizer. Many of them become increasingly refractory to therapy and eventually lose their early regrowth.

B. H. Thiers, MD

Reference

1. Pericin M, Trüeb RM: Topical immunotherapy of severe alopecia areata with diphenylcyclopropenone: Evaluation of 68 cases. *Dermatology* 196:418-421, 1998.

Predictive Model for Immunotherapy of Alopecia Areata With Diphencyprone

Wiseman MC, Shapiro J, MacDonald N, et al (Univ of British Columbia, Vancouver)
Arch Dermatol 137:1063-1068, 2001   10–7

Introduction.—Diphencyprone has been used extensively as immunotherapy for alopecia areata (AA), but reported response rates vary considerably. A large patient cohort was studied retrospectively to determine the efficacy of diphencyprone for AA, to identify patient and treatment factors predictive of success, and to develop a model for predicting patient response.

Methods.—The medical records of 148 consecutive patients treated with diphencyprone were reviewed. At the initiation of therapy, the mean patient age was 36.3 years and the mean disease duration was 9.6 years. For each patient, half of the scalp was assigned to treatment and the contralateral half served as an untreated control. The control side was selected for sensitization, with 2.0% diphencyprone applied to a 4-cm diameter circular area at the initial visit. Weekly applications were started with a 0.0001% concentration used on the treatment side of the scalp. The concentration of diphencyprone was titrated upward to produce a mild inflammatory response. Only 1 patient required more than 2% diphencyprone. A clinically significant response was defined as a cosmetically acceptable result or more than 75% terminal hair regrowth.

Results.—According to survival analysis, the cumulative patient response to diphencyprone immunotherapy was 77.9% at 32 months. The median time required to achieve significant regrowth was 12.2 months. Variables independently associated with clinically significant regrowth were older age at onset of AA and a more limited extent of disease. A cosmetically acceptable end point was achieved by all patients with 25% to 49% AA but by only 17.4% of those with alopecia totalis/universalis. Approximately two thirds of patients with significant regrowth experienced relapse. The median time to relapse was 30.7 months.

Conclusion.—The primary response rate to diphencyprone therapy is excellent for patients with AA, but relapse is common. Both the baseline extent of disease and age at AA onset are predictive of response. A prolonged course of immunotherapy with diphencyprone might be necessary.

▶ The findings reflect my own experience with diphencyprone immunotherapy for AA. Older patients with limited disease of short duration fair better. Although most patients do respond, relapses are common.

B. H. Thiers, MD

Biochemical Roles of Testosterone and Epitestosterone to 5α-Reductase as Indicators of Male-Pattern Baldness

Choi MH, Yoo YS, Chung BC (Bioanalysis and Biotransformation Research Ctr, Seoul, Korea; Sungkyunkwan Univ, Suwon, Korea)
J Invest Dermatol 116:57-61, 2001   10–8

Background.—The form of hair loss known as male pattern baldness (MPB) is linked to the interactions between androgen receptors, 5α-reductase, and dihydrotestosterone (DHT). These are all found clustered about the hair follicle. Androgen activity is enhanced when testosterone reacts with 5α-reductase and is converted to DHT. Blocking the enzyme 5α-reductase lowers DHT levels; this is the basis for drugs used to treat MPB. The conversion of testosterone to DHT may be suppressed with epitestosterone, which also can inhibit 5α-reductase activity. Clarification of the roles of testosterone and epitestosterone in hair growth and as indicators of MPB was investigated.

Methods.—Nineteen balding fathers, ranging in age from 28 to 55 years, and 16 of their sons, who were between 8 and 16 years of age, were compared with 55 age-matched subjects (fathers and sons) who were not balding. The 100-mg hair samples obtained included only the tip of the hair and were taken (when possible) from all areas of the scalp. The levels of testosterone, epitestosterone, and DHT were correlated with 5α-reductase by means of gas chromatography-mass spectrometry.

Results.—DHT levels were significantly higher among balding fathers than among nonbalding men; the levels in the balding fathers' sons were 0.02 to 0.14 ng/g, while DHT levels were absent among all but 2 of the nonbalding mens' sons. Epitestosterone levels differed only slightly between the 2 groups. A significantly greater ratio of testosterone to epitestosterone was found among the balding fathers and their sons than among the nonbalding control group (Fig 2). The balding fathers had a ratio 5

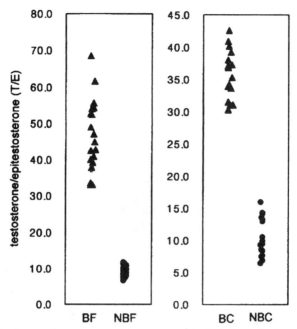

FIGURE 2.—Comparative testosterone-epitestosterone ratios in hair samples between the groups studied. The testosterone-epitestosterone ratio was significantly elevated (3 to 5 times; $P < .001$) in balding cases. *Abbreviations: BF*, Balding fathers; *NBF*, nonbalding fathers; *BC*, balding fathers' children; *NBC*, nonbalding fathers' children. (Courtesy of Choi MH, Yoo YS, Chung BC: Biochemical roles of testosterone and epitestosterone to 5α-reductase as indicators of male-pattern baldness. *J Invest Dermatol* 116:57-61, 2001. Reprinted by permission of Blackwell Science, Inc.)

times that of the nonbalding fathers. The sons of balding men had a ratio 3 times that of the nonbalding sons. Elevated ratios resulted from a significant decrease in epitestosterone and a slight increase in testosterone.

Conclusion.—It would seem possible to predict the development of MPB in young men based on a high DHT level and an increased testosterone-epitestosterone ratio. Thus, the possibility of hair loss can be foreshadowed by measuring steroid levels in hair. It is notable that these levels make their appearance early in the male's life, which could present the opportunity for interventions to prevent MPB by manipulating the steroid hormone balance.

▶ If confirmed, the results have significant implications for the management of patients with MPB. First, the findings demonstrate that analysis of terminal hair may provide the basis for predicting (and, hopefully, preventing) baldness when the subject is young. Second, they provide a rationale for manipulating the steroid hormone balance to prevent and treat this condition.

B. H. Thiers, MD

The Prevalence of Upper Lip Hair in Black and White Girls During Puberty: A New Standard

Lucky AW, Biro FM, Daniels SR, et al (Children's Hosp Med Ctr, Cincinnati, Ohio; Univ of Cincinnati, Ohio)
J Pediatr 138:134-136, 2001   10–9

Background.—Uncertainty exists among primary care physicians and specialists about when they should be concerned about excessive facial hair, especially in young girls. The Ferriman and Gallwey score of hair distribution at various sites is a frequently used assessment tool. However, this tool is based, in large part, on data from women 18 to 38 years of age, does not include data on African American women, and has no information on girls who have not yet entered puberty or on those who have just recently entered it. Subsequent studies of hair distribution in female research subjects have included only adolescents and adults. The distribution of upper lip hair in a population of more than 800 girls aged 9 to 19 years was evaluated.

Methods.—A total of 856 black and white girls were followed annually for more than 9 years, beginning at the ages of 9 and 10 years, as part of the National Heart, Lung, and Blood Institute Growth and Health Study. A total of 4693 observations were made. The girls were divided into 3 groups according to pubertal stage: group 1, premenarchal; group 2, less than 2 years postmenarchal; and group 3, 2 years or more postmenarchal. The premenarchal girls were all within 2 years of menarche. Scoring of upper lip hair was done according to the Ferriman and Gallwey method. Acne lesions were scored yearly, and serum levels of sex steroid hormones and sex hormone binding globulin were measured biannually.

Results.—Up to 2 years after menarche, 90% of girls had no upper lip hair. In those girls who did have small amounts of lip hair 2 years after menarche, 48.4% were black and 9% were white. A positive association was noted between upper lip hair scores and the severity of comedonal and inflammatory acne in group 3 ($P < .008$, Mantel-Haenszel chi-square test). No positive associations were found between laboratory abnormalities body mass index and the amount of upper lip hair.

Conclusion.—These data provide appropriate standards for distribution of upper lip hair in girls who have not yet entered puberty and in those who have just recently entered it. Hirsutism of lesser degrees in young girls may be more important clinically because most girls in this age group do not have any upper lip hair. The presence of current or future underlying hormonal abnormalities should be considered when upper lip hair is detected in an adolescent girl and appears to be excessive for that girl's degree of pubertal maturation and ethnic group.

▶ The authors performed yearly examinations from age 9 years to age 19 years on more than 800 girls and concluded that the presence of excessive hair on the upper lip is unusual, especially in whites. When upper lip hair is detected in an adolescent girl and appears excessive for the girl's degree of pubertal maturation and ethnic group, evaluation for hormonal abnormalities should be considered.

S. Raimer, MD

Polycystic Ovaries in Hirsute Women With Normal Menses
Carmina E, Lobo RA (Columbia Univ, New York)
Am J Med 111:602-606, 2001   10–10

Background.—Hirsute women with normal ovulation commonly are diagnosed as having idiopathic hirsutism. A group of hirsute ovulatory women were studied to determine whether they had a subtle form of polycystic ovary syndrome (PCOS) and any of the metabolic abnormalities associated with classic PCOS.

Methods.—The study included 62 hirsute women who were assessed prospectively. Baseline hormonal profiles, ovarian responses to gonadotropin-releasing hormone agonist, and ovarian morphology on US in the hirsute women were compared with those in 2 nonhirsute ovulatory control groups. One control group comprised 10 women matched for body mass index (overweight), and the other control group comprised 30 women with normal weight.

Findings.—Only 13% of the 62 hirsute ovulatory women had normal androgen levels and were judged to have idiopathic hirsutism. Thirty-nine percent had characteristic polycystic ovaries and/or an exaggerated 17-hydroxyprogesterone response to leuprolide, suggesting ovarian hyperandrogenism and the diagnosis of mild PCOS. The remaining 48% of the women in this group were considered to have unspecified hyperandrogenism. The hyperandrogenic subgroups had similar age, body weight, and androgen levels. Compared with normal and overweight control subjects and with patients with idiopathic hirsutism, the women with mild PCOS had greater fasting insulin levels, lower glucose-insulin ratios, higher low-density lipoprotein cholesterol levels, and lower high-density lipoprotein (HDL) cholesterol levels. Compared with patients with unspecified hyperandrogenism, these women had higher fasting insulin concentrations, lower glucose-insulin ratios, and decreased HDL cholesterol levels.

Conclusions.—Mild PCOS appears to be more common than idiopathic hirsutism. Subtle metabolic abnormalities were associated with mild PCOS.

▶ Hirsute women with normal ovulatory cycles and normal circulating androgen levels are traditionally classified as having "idiopathic" hirsutism. Carmina and Lobo demonstrate that some of these women may have characteristic polycystic ovaries on US examination, an exaggerated 17-hydroxyprogesterone response to a gonadotropin-releasing hormone agonist test (leuprolide acetate 1 mg administered subcutaneously), or both, suggesting ovarian hyperandrogenism and the diagnosis of mild PCOS. These findings are significant because of the other metabolic abnormalities found in these women, including decreased insulin sensitivity (based on higher fasting insulin levels) and lower glucose-insulin ratios. In addition, they tended to have lipoprotein profiles associated with a higher risk of development of cardiovascular disease.

B. H. Thiers, MD

11 Vitiligo

Narrow-Band Ultraviolet B Is a Useful and Well-Tolerated Treatment for Vitiligo

Scherschun L, Kim JJ, Lim HW (Henry Ford Health System, Detroit)

J Am Acad Dermatol 44:999-1003, 2001   11–1

Background.—Among the nonsurgical treatments for vitiligo are corticosteroids, oral or topical psoralens plus ultraviolet (UV) A, and narrow-band UVB therapy. The results of and experience with narrow-band UVB treatment at the Henry Ford Hospital in Detroit were reviewed.

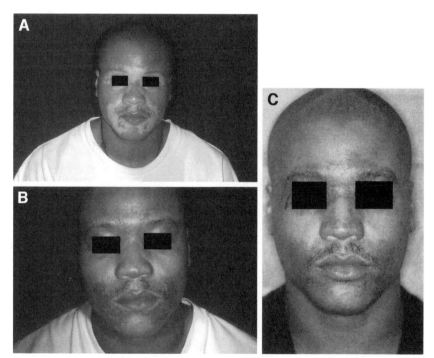

FIGURE 1.—**A,** Pretreatment photograph of a 25-year-old African American man with a 3-year history of vitiligo. Note depigmentation at periorbital and perioral areas. **B,** Complete repigmentation after 19 treatments, with darker color compared with the surrounding skin. **C,** Normalization of color intensity of the repigmented areas after 26 treatments. (Courtesy of Scherschun L, Kim JJ, Lim HW: Narrow-band ultraviolet B is a useful and well-tolerated treatment for vitiligo. *J Am Acad Dermatol* 44:999-1003, 2001.)

Methods.—Five women and 6 men, ranging in age from 19 to 59 years, were evaluated retrospectively. All had narrow-band UVB therapy as monotherapy 3 times a week over the course of 12 months. Results were assessed by physical examination and documented by lesional photography.

Results.—After losing 4 patients to follow-up, the remaining 7 patients, who either completed therapy or were still receiving it, were evaluated. Over 75% repigmentation after a mean of 19 treatments was achieved in 5 of the patients, whose mean duration of disease was 13 months (Fig 1; see color plate VIII). One patient had 50% repigmentation (46 treatments) and 1 had 40% repigmentation (48 treatments); these patients' mean duration of disease was 132 months. Results were maintained in 4 patients, with 1 still completely repigmented 11 months after therapy was discontinued. Two patients lost repigmentation with the discontinuation of therapy, but when therapy recommenced at 3 times a week, repigmentation recurred. Minimal adverse effects were noted, specifically mild erythema and pruritus.

Conclusion.—Narrow-band UVB appears to be both efficacious and well tolerated for the treatment of vitiligo. Rapid repigmentation was achieved with thrice weekly therapy and maintained in several patients.

▶ Although the study is small, the results are encouraging and appear to be at least as good as those achieved with photochemotherapy. Not surprisingly, those patients with the shortest duration of disease appeared to respond best.

B. H. Thiers, MD

Topical Calcipotriol as Monotherapy and in Combination With Psoralen Plus Ultraviolet A in the Treatment of Vitiligo
Ameen M, Exarchou V, Chu AC (Imperial College of Science, Technology and Medicine, London)
Br J Dermatol 145:476-479, 2001   11–2

Introduction.—Topical corticosteroids and phototherapy, the mainstays of treatment for vitiligo, carry potential risks for skin atrophy and carcinogenesis. The observation that hyperpigmentation occurred after topical calcipotriol and phototherapy were applied to psoriatic plaques prompted several studies of calcipotriol in the treatment of vitiligo. Topical calcipotriol, alone and in conjunction with psoralen plus ultraviolet A (PUVA), was evaluated in an open study of 26 patients with vitiligo.

Methods.—Patients were 22 Asians and 4 whites ranging in age from 5 to 61 years. The mean duration of vitiligo was 3.8 years. Widespread disease was present in 5 patients and the face was affected in 8. Topical or oral 8-methoxypsoralen PUVA had been ineffective in 4 patients, and 11 had not responded to past treatment with moderately potent or potent corticosteroids. Response to therapy was evaluated at 3-month intervals.

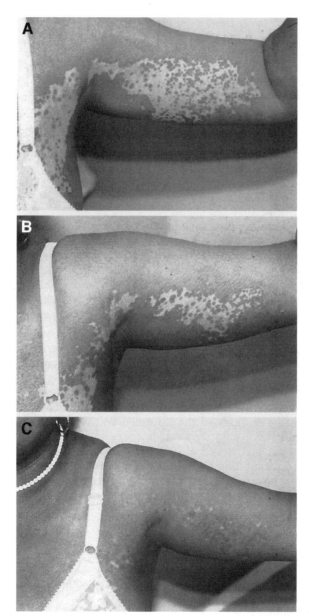

FIGURE 1.—A 49-year-old Asian woman had had vitiligo on the arms and trunk for 3 years. **A,** Treatment with topical psoralen plus ultraviolet A (PUVA) produced 10% improvement after 9 months. **B,** Patient after 3 months of dual therapy with calcipotriol and topical PUVA, showing 30% improvement. **C,** Patient after 9 months of treatment, showing greater than 90% improvement. (Courtesy of Ameen M, Exarchou V, Chu AC: Topical calcipotriol as monotherapy and in combination with psoralen plus ultraviolet A in the treatment of vitiligo. *Br J Dermatol* 145:476-479, 2001. Reprinted by permission of Blackwell Science, Inc.)

Results.—Treatment was well tolerated, with no reports of adverse effects. After a mean duration of therapy of 6 months, 17 of 22 patients (77%) treated with twice-daily topical calcipotriol monotherapy showed improvement ranging from 30% to 100%. Only 1 of 4 patients receiving dual therapy failed to respond; in 1 case (Fig 1; see color plate IX), more than 90% improvement was observed after 9 months. Improvement occurred in all responders during the first 3 months of treatment. Better responses were seen in those with less extensive disease (less than 10%) and with vitiligo of less than 5 years' duration.

Conclusion.—Topical calcipotriol was well tolerated and effective in treating patients whose vitiligo had failed to respond substantially to topical corticosteroids or PUVA. Topical calcipotriol may be useful as a first-line treatment for vitiliginous lesions and appears to be safe when combined with PUVA.

Is the Efficacy of Psoralen Plus Ultraviolet A Therapy for Vitiligo Enhanced by Concurrent Topical Calcipotriol? A Placebo-controlled Double-blind Study

Ermis O, Alpsoy E, Cetin L, et al (Akdeniz Univ, Antalya, Turkey; Antalya State Hosp, Turkey)
Br J Dermatol 145:472-475, 2001   11–3

Background.—Although its pathogenesis is not known, the characteristics of vitiligo include melanocyte destruction and loss of pigmentation. The most effective choice for treatment has been systemic and topical psoralen plus ultraviolet A (PUVA) therapy. Calcium ion regulation may be important in the etiology of the disease. Keratinocytes and melanocytes from vitiliginous skin samples have defective calcium ion transport. With decreased intracellular levels of calcium ion, the levels of reduced thioredoxin increase, inhibiting tyrosinase activity and melanin synthesis. Calcipotriol, an analogue of vitamin D, may be involved in calcium ion regulation and may increase the effectiveness of PUVA treatment for vitiligo.

Methods.—Twenty-seven patients (18 men and 9 women; mean age, 29.8 years) with generalized vitiligo were studied. Reference lesions meeting the study criteria were symmetrical, similar in size, showed no evidence of spontaneous repigmentation, and were located on the arms, legs, or trunk. One hour before PUVA treatment was begun, calcipotriol (0.05 mg/g cream) or placebo was applied to the reference lesions. Treatments were administered twice a week, and patients were assessed weekly. The mean number of sessions and the cumulative ultraviolet A (UVA) dosage for initial repigmentation and for complete return of pigment was evaluated.

Results.—For initial repigmentation, the mean cumulative UVA dose and number of UVA exposures were 52.52 J/cm and 9.33 for the patients receiving calcipotriol. The values at initial repigmentation for the placebo group were 78.20 J/cm and 12.00, respectively. For complete return of pigment, those receiving respective calcipotriol had values of 232.70 J/cm and 27.40; those receiving placebo had values of 259.93 J/cm and 30.07. The calcipotriol and PUVA combination produced significantly higher percentages of repigmentation at both points, with 81% having initial repigmentation and 63% having complete repigmentation. The values for placebo and PUVA were 7% and 15%.

Conclusion.—Combining calcipotriol with PUVA produced a safe, effective treatment of vitiligo in these patients.

▶ The hypothesis underlying the possible benefit of topical calcipotriol (calcipotriene) in the treatment of vitiligo is based on a possible role for calcium ion regulation in the etiology of the disease.[1-3] Lebwohl et al have reported that ultraviolet A degrades calcipotriol and have advised that when used in conjunction with PUVA, the compound be applied after UVA exposure.[4] Thus, although Ermis et al (Abstract 11–3) did find application of calcipotriol cream 1 hour before PUVA treatment to be more effective than PUVA alone, a more logical approach might be to apply the calcipotriol after the phototherapy has been administered.

B. H. Thiers, MD

References

1. Schallreuter-Wood KU, Pittelkow MR, Swanson NN: Defective calcium transport in vitiliginous melanocytes. *Arch Dermatol Res* 288:11-13, 1996.
2. Schallreuter KU, Pittelkow MP: Defective calcium uptake in keratinocyte cell cultures from vitiliginous skin. *Arch Dermatol Res* 280:137-139, 1988.
3. Schallreuter KU, Wood JM: Treatment of vitiligo with a topical application of pseudocatalase and calcium in combination with short term UVB exposure. *Dermatology* 190:223-229, 1995.
4. Lebwohl M, Hecker D, Martinez J: Interactions between calcipotriene and ultraviolet light. *J Am Acad Dermatol* 37:93-95, 1997.

12 Collagen Vascular and Related Disorders

A Candidate Gene Analysis of Three Related Photosensitivity Disorders: Cutaneous Lupus Erythematosus, Polymorphic Light Eruption and Actinic Prurigo
Millard TP, Kondeatis E, Cox A, et al (St Thomas' Hosp, London; King's College, London; Univ of Sheffield, England)
Br J Dermatol 145:229-236, 2001   12–1

Introduction.—The cutaneous forms of lupus erythematosus (LE), subacute cutaneous LE (SCLE) and discoid LE (DLE), as well as actinic prurigo (AP), may be associated with polymorphic light eruption (PLE). These 4 photosensitivity disorders may share a common pathologic basis, which was examined in an evaluation of specific candidate genes for shared susceptibility alleles between these related phenotypes.

Methods.—Eighty-five white patients with annular SCLE or DLE and 102 first-degree relatives underwent detailed interviews and clinical examination to ascertain the prevalence of PLE. Eighty-five patients with PLE and 59 with AP were also evaluated. Candidate genes were assessed by typing of single nucleotide polymorphisms of IL10 (-1082 G/a and -819 C/T), FCGR2A (131 R/H), SELE (128 S/R), ICAM 1 (241 G/R and 469 E/K), IL1A ($+4845$ G/T), IL1B (-511 C/T and $+3954$ C/T), IL1RN ($+2018$ T/C), and tumor necrosis factor (TNF) (-208 G/A) using polymerase chain reaction (PCR) with sequence-specific primers and 5'-nuclease PCR.

Results.—A significant correlation was observed between SCLE and the rare TNF -308 A allele compared with patients with DLE ($P = .043$), PLE ($P = .001$), AP ($P < .0010$, and healthy controls ($P < .001$). Strong linkage disequilibrium was identified between TNF -308 A and the HLA A*01, B*08, DRB1*0310 haplotype. A negative correlation was observed between SCLE and the IL1B $= 3954$ allele ($P = .039$); significance was lost on correction for multiple testing.

Conclusion.—A correlation was established between SCLE and the rare TNF -308 A allele, which could be pathogenic, or alternatively, a marker allele for the extended HLA A*01, B*08, DRB1*0301 haplotype that is associated with several autoimmune conditions. Many of the other evaluated loci failed to show an association; nevertheless, a candidate gene approach continues to be the most logical and most likely approach to yield positive results.

▶ The objective of this study was to determine the distribution of selected gene polymorphisms in photosensitivity diseases and to seek allele associations common to these diseases. The major finding was a significant association between the uncommon A allele of the single nucleotide polymorphism of the TNF gene at position −308 and SCLE. This is interesting because the TNF-α^{-308} A allele is a so-called "high producer"; subjects who possess the allele produce more cytokine in response to a given stimulus than those who lack the allele, and increased production of TNF may be involved in the pathogenesis of SCLE. However, the A allele is known to be in significant linkage disequilibrium with the ancestral 8.1 MHC haplotype that includes DR3, and it was not possible to determine from this study whether the association found was independent of that haplotype.

G. M. P. Galbraith, MD

Phototesting in Lupus Erythematosus Tumidus—Review of 60 Patients
Kuhn A, Sonntag M, Richter-Hintz D, et al (Heinrich-Heine-Univ, Düsseldorf, Germany; Univ of Witten-Herdecke, Wuppertal, Germany)
Photochem Photobiol 73:532-536, 2001   12–2

Background.—Lupus erythematosus is often characterized by photosensitivity. Lupus erythematosus tumidus (LET) is a less common form of lupus erythematosus, and its association with photosensitivity is not well understood. Phototests were performed on 60 patients with LET to determine the association between LET and photosensitivity.

Study Design.—Areas of uninvolved skin were irradiated with single doses of ultraviolet A (UV-A) and/or ultraviolet B (UV-B) daily for 3 consecutive days. Skin biopsy specimens were taken from primary lesions and from photo-induced lesions. Lupus autoantibodies were assayed using standard immunologic techniques.

Findings.—Patients with LET were photosensitive, with characteristic photo-induced skin lesions appearing in 72%. Of these, 50% reacted to UV-A and 48% to UV-B. Twenty-nine patients were aware of their photosensitivity, but 22 additional patients with photosensitive reactions were not. There was a positive correlation between antinuclear antibodies and positive phototest responses.

Conclusion.—The phototest is effective for identifying photosensitivity in patients with lupus erythematosus, especially LET, which a is highly photosensitive variant of the disorder. Patients with LET should be advised to avoid sun exposure.

▶ The authors reported a strong correlation between positive phototest responses and the presence of antinuclear antibodies. However, the discordance between patient reports of photosensitivity and the results of phototesting was striking. Many patients who claimed to be photosensitive had negative phototesting results and vice versa. Traditionally, LET has not been thought to be a condition exacerbated by exposure to UV light. Perhaps the results of this study should change our thinking.

B. H. Thiers, MD

Epidermal Grafting for Depigmentation Due to Discoid Lupus Erythematosus

Gupta S (Postgraduate Inst of Medical Education and Research, Chandigarh, India)
Dermatology 202:320-323, 2001   12–3

Introduction.—Long-standing lesions of chronic discoid lupus erythematosus (DLE) may heal with thin, white, scarred areas that are difficult to treat. Epidermal grafting was successfully used in 4 patients reported here.

Methods.—Patients were 3 men and 1 woman with facial DLE scars of 4 to 13 years' duration. Except for a small area of activity in 1 patient, all

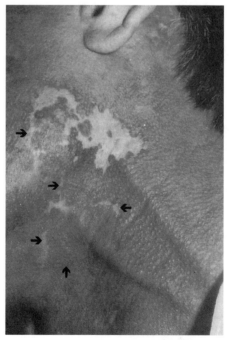

FIGURE 2.—More than 75% pigmentation in a depigmented lesion of old, quiescent discoid lupus erythematosus 6 months after the epidermal grafting. The depigmented area prior to grafting is marked by *arrows*. (Courtesy of Gupta S: Epidermal grafting for depigmentation due to discoid lupus erythematosus. *Dermatology* 202:320-323, 2001. Reproduced with permission from S Karger AG, Basel.)

DLE lesions were inactive. Previous treatment had consisted of antimalarials and topical steroids with sun protection. The patients received prophylactic antimalarials for at least 1 week before surgery and for 6 months postoperatively. Suction blisters were raised on the lateral aspect of the upper third of the thigh, and the roof of the blisters then transferred to the dermabraded recipient area. Donor and recipient sites were dressed with nonadherent tulle. The dressings were removed after 8 days.

Results.—The graft take was 100% in all patients, and none had recurrence of disease during a follow-up period of 6 months to 1 year. Pigmentation achieved was more than 100% of the grafted area (due to peripheral spread of the pigmentation) and more than 75% of the depigmented area (Fig 2; see color plate X). Not all depigmented areas could be grafted in a single session. Donor sites healed completely in 7 days.

Discussion.—Depigmentation or hypopigmentation is common after remission of localized DLE lesions, and scars that do not respond to topical steroids and antimalarials are difficult to manage medically. Epidermal grafting offers a cosmetically acceptable treatment for the leukodermic scars of healed inactive DLE lesions.

▶ The depigmentation that accompanies DLE can have devastating social and psychological consequences, especially in darkly pigmented patients. In this small series, suction blisters were successfully used as a source of melanocytes to repigment depigmented patches in patients with DLE. Suction blisters were used rather than punch grafts as the latter often result in a cobblestone appearance. Moreover, to promote spreading of the pigment, punch grafts require therapy with psoralen plus ultraviolet A, which is contraindicated in patients with DLE. The author emphasizes that to increase the likelihood of success, before any surgical procedure is undertaken the disease should be quiescent, the patient should be receiving antimalarial therapy, and sun exposure should be avoided.

P. G. Lang, Jr, MD

Peripheral Gangrene During Infancy: A Rare Presentation of Systemic Lupus Erythematosus
Shetty VB, Rao S, Krishnamurthy PN, et al (Univ Med Centre, Karnataka, India)
Arch Dis Child 85:335-336, 2001   12–4

Background.—Systemic lupus erythematosus (SLE) is rarely seen in children aged less than 5 years, although 20% of cases begin in childhood. Digital gangrene may occur in adults and children with SLE, but peripheral gangrene in an infant with SLE is exceedingly rare. This case report details such an occurrence in an 11-month-old boy with SLE.

Case Report.—Boy, 11 months, was well until that age, when he developed fever, breathlessness, and loose stools. In 4 days, he exhibited erythematous skin discoloration of both legs, and both feet were swollen. Six days later blisters formed over these areas. When examined 15 days after becoming ill, he was pale, had fever, and exhibited respiratory distress. Bluish-black skin lesions were noted with both macules and papules over the dorsal aspect of the left hand and the dorsum of both feet. A skin swab grew *Staphylococcus aureus,* and he was treated with ceftazidime. The fever resolved after 2 days on antibiotics, but the skin lesions worsened, with more vesicles. His extremities were cold and cyanotic, and no pulses could be felt in the posterior tibial and dorsal pedis arteries and left radial artery. Four days after admission, the tips of all 10 toes and the fingers of the left hand showed gangrene and extreme tenderness. Oral prednisolone (2 mg/kg per day) was started; the next day, gangrenous changes were observed on scrotal skin. No rheumatoid factor was detected, but nuclear antibody testing was positive at 18.32 arbitrary units (AU)/mL (normal upper range, 14 AU/mL). In addition, antibodies to double-stranded DNA were positive at 39.12 AU/mL (normal upper range, 26 AU/mL). Negative or normal results occurred with Ro and La antibody testing, anticardiolipin antibody determination, and measurement of C3 levels. SLE was diagnosed. Gangrene involved the entire left hand during the second week after hospitalization. Fifteen days after admission, a line of demarcation was noted, and the gangrenous tissue was excised with the boy under general anesthesia. Recovery began in the third week after admission, and the boy was discharged on oral prednisolone. Prednisolone use was tapered, then discontinued after 6 months when testing for nuclear antibodies and antibodies to double-stranded DNA yielded negative results (age of infant, 18 months). No symptoms are currently present in the 2-year-old boy, and results of testing for nuclear antibodies and antibodies to double-stranded DNA continue to be negative.

Conclusions.—Fever in a child with SLE generally indicates infection rather than active lupus, a fact that was true in this case. The development of gangrene of the extremities is extremely rare, especially when the lower extremities are affected. Judging by the child's recovery, steroids are effective treatment for vasculitis of the type noted in this case.

▶ Gangrene has been described as a complication of many collagen vascular diseases. Although rare in infants, this case illustrates that SLE should be included as a possible cause of gangrene in young patients. Endarteritis, a vasculopathy that affects the digital arteries, is an unusual but important complication of SLE. Poor perfusion leads to ischemia that can result in necrosis and infarction. The diagnosis can be confirmed by angiography, which shows loss of perfusion and narrowing of the radial or ulnar arteries and loss of flow to the digital arteries.

S. Raimer, MD

Combined Treatment With Calcipotriol Ointment and Low-Dose Ultraviolet A1 Phototherapy in Childhood Morphea

Kreuter A, Gambichler T, Avermaete A, et al (Ruhr-Univ Bochum, Germany)
Pediatr Dermatol 18:241-245, 2001   12–5

Background.—Morphea can be either generalized or localized, with signs such as circumscribed plaques, linear bands, areas of subcutaneous infiltration, en coup de sabre lesions, or facial hemiatrophy. It is more common in women, but approximately 15% of cases occur in children. Among the treatments are various pharmacologic options, but these have been largely ineffective. The use of a combination of low-dose UV-A1 plus twice daily calcipotriol ointment was evaluated for morphea in children.

Methods.—For each of the 19 children with morphea who participated (12 girls; age range, 3 to 13 years; mean, 8.5 years), a complete disease history was obtained. Clinical criteria provided the basis for diagnosis. The disease had been present for 9 to 69 months (mean, 29.5 months) and was generally of the plaque type or linear morphea (Table 1). For 10 weeks, patients received an exposure of UV-A1 of 20 J/cm^2 4 times each week as well as local therapy with calcipotriol ointment 0.005% twice daily (morning and evening) without occlusion. Emollient applications were permitted but not within 2 hours of phototherapy.

Results.—All patients completed the 10-week protocol without side effects except for mild skin irritation from the calcipotriol ointment in 2 children. The mean clinical score at the beginning of therapy was 7.3. On palpation and inspection after 10 weeks, all patients showed softening and repigmentation of the affected skin areas for a highly significant decline in the mean clinical score to 2.4. Thus, the relative reduction was 67.1% by the end of the study. Improvement in 4 patients was confirmed via US. A better outcome was found in patients with linear morphea than among those with plaque morphea. At least 1 year of improvement was maintained in all patients.

Conclusions.—Combining low-dose UV-A1 phototherapy with topical calcipotriol effectively addressed the problem of morphea in these children. Significantly, linear morphea responded to a greater extent than plaque morphea. The improvement was maintained for at least 1 year, and side effects were absent or minimal.

▶ Although this was an uncontrolled study, the fact that all patients improved within 10 weeks suggests that a combination of calcipotriol ointment and low-dose UV-A1 irradiation may be a promising therapeutic option for children with morphea. It is particularly encouraging that linear morphea, which is notoriously difficult to manage, responded well to treatment.

S. Raimer, MD

TABLE 1.—Summary of Clinical Data of Patients With Morphea Organized by Subtypes (n = 19)

Patient No.	Age/Sex	Subtype	Localization	Duration of Disease (Months)	Treatment Before Therapy	Clinical Score Before Therapy	Clinical Score After Therapy
1	13/F	HF	Right side of the face	41	Penicillin IV, Bath-PUVA	6	2
2	9/M	HF	Right side of the face	69	Penicillin IV	7	5
3	7/F	HF	Right side of the face	12	—	7	3
4	6/M	LM	Left leg	40	Penicillin IV	8	2
5	10/F	LM	Right sole	22	Bath-PUVA	9	2
6	11/F	LM	Left leg	34	Topical corticosteroid	8	2
7	11/F	LM	Forehead	19	Topical corticosteroid	7	3
8	8/M	LM	Right leg	15	Penicillin IV	8	1
9	7/F	LM	Left arm	44	Bath-PUVA	8	1
10	6/F	PM	Right leg	45	Penicillin IV	8	3
11	8/F	PM	Left arm	37	Penicillin IV	6	4
12	7/F	PM	Left breast	17	Penicillin IV	7	2
13	12/F	PM	Right arm and leg	24	—	5	2
14	5/M	PM	Back	48	Topical corticosteroid	8	3
15	11/F	PM	Chin	32	Penicillin IV	8	3
16	13/F	PM	Chin	11	—	6	2
17	8/M	PM	Right arm and leg	9	—	7	2
18	3/M	SM	Right leg	28	—	7	2
19	7/M	SM	Right leg	14	—	8	2
Mean						7.3	2.4*

*P < .001.
Abbreviations: M, Male; F, female; HF, facial hemiatrophy; LM, linear morphea; PM, plaque-type morphea; SM, subcutaneous morphea.
(Courtesy of Kreuter A, Gambichler T, Avermaete A, et al: Combined treatment with calcipotriol ointment and low-dose ultraviolet A1 phototherapy in childhood morphea. *Pediatr Dermatol* 18:241-245, 2001. Reprinted by permission of Blackwell Science, Inc.)

Lack of Relationship Between Functional Ability and Skin Score in Patients With Systemic Sclerosis

Herrick A, Rooney B, Finn J, et al (Univ of Manchester, England)
J Rheumatol 28:292-295, 2001   12–6

Background.—Problems with upper limbs account for much of the functional disability associated with systemic sclerosis (SSc). The authors recently developed an 11-question, SSc-specific index of functional status, focusing on upper limb function and muscle weakness. Skin thickening can have an important role in limitation of limb function. The correlation between the new SSc functional ability score and skin score was investigated.

Methods.—The study consisted of 140 patients seen at English SSc clinics: 114 women, 26 men; median age, 52 years; median duration of disease, 6 years. Cutaneous involvement was limited in 106 patients and diffuse in 34. All patients were evaluated with the 11-item functional questionnaire. The skin score was assessed using a modified Rodnan technique, evaluating 17 sites with a maximum score of 3 per site. Correlations between these scores were assessed.

Results.—The study sample had a median functional score of 6 and a median skin score of 7, with no significant correlation between the 2 scores. This also was so even on separate analyses restricted to upper limb and digital skin involvement.

Conclusions.—The skin score in patients with SSc cannot predict functional ability, at least as assessed by a new 11-item questionnaire. The findings suggest that skin score is not strongly related to ability to perform everyday activities in patients with SSc, despite its prognostic significance.

▶ It may be logical to assume that skin score and functional ability in patients with scleroderma might be related, as the indirect results of skin thickening, such as contractures and ulceration, restrict limb function. This article challenges that assumption. One explanation might be that the 2 parameters used, skin score and functional index, do not accurately measure the factors they were created to represent.

B. H. Thiers, MD

Decreased Susceptibility to Fas-Induced Apoptosis of Systemic Sclerosis Dermal Fibroblasts

Santiago B, Galindo M, Rivero M, et al (Hosp 12 de Octubre, Madrid)
Arthritis Rheum 44:1667-1676, 2001   12–7

Introduction.—The initial events in systemic sclerosis (SSc) resemble the normal process of wound healing: vascular damage, inflammatory cell infiltration, and fibroblast activation. But fibrosis progresses in SSc, perhaps because of an imbalance between fibroblast proliferation and apoptotic cell death. Skin biopsy samples from 9 patients with diffuse SSc were examined for the pattern of apoptosis regulation in fibroblasts.

Methods.—In addition to the samples from patients with SSc, investigators obtained skin samples from age- and sex-matched healthy individuals and from patients with nonfibrotic inflammatory autoimmune skin diseases (5 with cutaneous lupus lesions and 5 with dermatomyositis). The samples were used to establish fibroblast cultures and were examined histologically. Apoptosis was examined in skin sections using the TUNEL technique, and proliferation was assessed by immunostaining for proliferating cell nuclear antigen. The susceptibility of fibroblasts to apoptosis induced in vitro by different stimuli was studied by TUNEL. Western blot analysis was used to study expression of Bcl-2, Bcl-x, and Bax proteins in cultured fibroblasts.

Results.—Proliferation of dermal fibroblasts was observed in the skin samples from patients with SSc and other inflammatory skin diseases but not in normal skin. The fibrotic skin lesions of SSc did not exhibit apoptosis of fibroblasts. SSc fibroblasts were specifically resistant in vitro to apoptosis induced by Fas receptor stimulation, but these fibroblasts exhibited normal susceptibility to apoptosis induced by nonspecific stimuli (protein kinase inhibition or serum withdrawal). The decreased susceptibility to Fas stimulation was not the result of decreased levels of surface Fas receptor. Quiescence induced by confluence and serum starvation in the SSc fibroblasts was followed by an abnormal down-regulation of proapoptotic Bax protein. The susceptibility of SSc fibroblasts to Fas-mediated apoptosis was restored by up-regulation of the Bax:Bcl-2 ratio by Bcl-2 antisense oligonucleotides.

Conclusion.—Abnormal apoptotic regulation in fibroblasts may contribute to the pathogenesis of progressive fibrosis in SSc. Antifibrotic therapies for SSc and chronic fibrotic diseases might involve modulation of Bcl-2-related proteins.

▶ Apoptosis, or programmed cell death, is an important homeostatic mechanism that limits the life cycle of an individual cell. Under physiologic conditions, both proliferation and apoptosis of dermal fibroblasts are absent in normal adult skin, suggesting a very low rate of cell renewal. In contrast, during normal or pathologic wound healing and in inflammatory diseases such as SSc, both proliferation and apoptosis of fibroblasts occur, and the rate of fibroblast growth seems to be a function of both processes. The lack of fibroblast apoptosis observed in SSc skin (in contrast to related inflammatory diseases) suggests that defective elimination of these cells may explain their persistence and resulting progressive fibrosis. Santiago et al also observed abnormal down-regulation of the proapoptotic Bax protein in SSc and found that up-regulation of the Bax:Bcl-2 ratio restored the susceptibility of SSc fibroblasts to Fas-mediated apoptosis. This suggests that modulation of Bcl-2-related proteins by antisense oligonucleotides may be a potential therapeutic strategy for the development of apoptosis-based antifibrotic treatments.

B. H. Thiers, MD

Iloprost Suppresses Connective Tissue Growth Factor Production in Fibroblasts and in the Skin of Scleroderma Patients

Stratton R, Shiwen X, Martini G, et al (Univ College London; FibroGen Inc, San Francisco, Calif)
J Clin Invest 108:241-250, 2001   12–8

Background.—Skin tightness is reduced in patients with scleroderma receiving Iloprost infusions for severe Raynaud's phenomenon. Thus, this synthetic prostacyclin analogue may inhibit skin fibrosis. Connective tissue growth factor (CTGF) is involved in the fibrosis occurring in patients with scleroderma. This profibrotic cytokine acts downstream, in concert with tumor growth factor beta (TGF-β), to stimulate the fibrotic process. The effect of Iloprost on TGF-β-stimulated collagen and CTGF production was studied in cultured human skin fibroblasts obtained from patients with scleroderma and from healthy persons.

Methods.—Scleroderma skin fibroblasts were derived from the affected skin of 6 patients with diffuse scleroderma. Skin blister fluid was also obtained from 6 patients with diffuse scleroderma and 6 with limited scleroderma.

Findings.—Iloprost blocked the CTGF induction and the increase in collagen synthesis observed in scleroderma fibroblasts exposed to TGF-β. The potency of Iloprost in suppressing CTGF far exceeded that of other prostanoid receptor agonists, suggesting that the prostacyclin receptor IP mediates its effect. Dermal interstitial fluid analysis showed greatly increased CTGF levels in the dermis of patients with scleroderma compared with that of healthy persons. Iloprost infusion markedly reduced dermal CTGF concentrations.

Conclusions.—Iloprost may decrease the level of a key profibrotic cytokine in patients with scleroderma. The endogenous production of eicosanoids may limit the fibrotic response to TGF-β.

▶ The beneficial effects of Iloprost infusions for patients with severe Raynaud's phenomenon in association with scleroderma have been attributed to its vasodilatory properties. Stratton et al demonstrate that the drug may also inhibit fibrosis.

B. H. Thiers, MD

Calcium-Channel Blockers for Raynaud's Phenomenon in Systemic Sclerosis

Thompson AE, Shea B, Welch V, et al (Univ of Western Ontario, London, Canada; Ottawa Hosp, Ont, Canada)
Arthritis Rheum 44:1841-1847, 2001   12–9

Background.—Scleroderma (systemic sclerosis or SSc) is a connective tissue disease that causes fibrosis. Most patients with SSc also have Raynaud's phenomenon (RP), defined as vasospasm of arteries or arterioles causing pallor with color change on reperfusion. This meta-analysis was performed to examine the usefulness of calcium-channel blockers for the treatment of RP associated with SSc. The primary outcome measures were frequency and severity of ischemic attacks.

Methods.—The Cochrane search strategy was used to find trials in all languages. All included studies were randomized controlled trials of more than 2 days duration with a dropout rate of less than 35%. Most trials included both primary RP and RP secondary to SSc.

Findings.—Eight studies with 109 total patients were eligible for inclusion in the meta-analysis. The meta-analysis demonstrated that calcium-channel blockers provided a significant, but moderate, reduction in the frequency and severity of ischemic attacks compared with placebo in patients with RP secondary to SSc.

Conclusion.—RP, a common complication of SSc, often is treated with calcium-channel blockers. This meta-analysis revealed that calcium-channel blockers moderately reduced both the frequency and severity of ischemic attacks in these patients. A larger, randomized, controlled, double-blind clinical trial with a parallel design would be useful to lend support to the findings of this meta-analysis. Data on quality of life and side effects would also be beneficial.

▶ In reporting only a modest benefit with calcium-channel blocker treatment of RP associated with SSc, Thompson et al confirm my own experience. Better treatments must await increased knowledge of mechanisms underlying the pathogenesis of this condition.

B. H. Thiers, MD

Phase I/II Trial of Autologous Stem Cell Transplantation in Systemic Sclerosis: Procedure Related Mortality and Impact on Skin Disease
Binks M, Passweg JR, Furst D, et al (Felix Platter Hosp, Basel, Switzerland)
Ann Rheum Dis 60:577-584, 2001   12–10

Introduction.—The mortality rate is high among persons with systemic sclerosis (SSc, scleroderma) in either the diffuse or the limited skin forms when vital organs are involved. There is no known treatment that influences outcome or significantly affects the skin score, despite the fact that several forms of immunosuppression have been tried. Recent developments in hemopoietic stem cell transplantation (HSCT) have allowed the use of profound immunosuppression followed by HSCT, or rescue, in autoimmune diseases, including SSc. Reported are findings for 41 patients included in a continuing multicenter open phase I/II trial in which HSCT was used to treat poor-prognosis SSc.

Methods.—Of 41 patients, 37 had a predominantly diffuse skin form of the disease and 4 had the limited form, with some clinical overlap. The median patient age was 41 years. There was a 5:1 female-to-male ratio. The skin score was more than 50% of maximum in 20 of 33 patients

(61%) with some lung disease attributable to SSc in 28 of 37 patients (76%). The forced vital capacity was less than 70% of predicted value in 18 of 36 patients (50%). Seven (19%) and 5 (14%) patients, respectively, had pulmonary hypertension or renal disease. The Scl-70 antibody was positive in 18 of 32 patients (56%). The anticentromere antibody was positive in 10% of the patients so evaluated. Peripheral blood stem cell mobilization was performed with cyclophosphamide or granulocyte colony stimulating factor, alone or in combination. Thirty-eight patients had ex vivo CD34 stem cell selection; 7 patients had additional T cell depletion. Seven conditioning regimens were used; 6 used hemoimmunoablative doses of cyclophosphamide ± antithymocyte globulin ± total body irradiation. The median duration of follow-up was 12 months (range, 3 to 55 months).

Results.—An improvement in skin score of more than 25% after transplantation was observed in 20 of 29 (69%) evaluable patients. There was no significant change in lung function after transplantation. One in 5 patients with renal disease deteriorated. There were no new occurrences of renal disease after HSCT. Pulmonary hypertension did not progress in evaluable patients. Disease progression was observed in 7 of 37 (19%) patients after HSCT at a median of 67 days (range, 49 to 255 days). There were 11 patients (27%) who had died at census and 7 (17%) whose deaths were considered to be related to the procedure (direct organ toxicity in 4, hemorrhage in 2, and infection/neutropenic fever in 1). The 1-year cumulative probability of survival was 73%.

Conclusion.—These phase I/II trials have shown an effect on skin progression and a trend toward stabilization of lung disease in patients with SSc. However, these appear to be significant treatment toxicity.

▶ Autologous stem cell transplantation has been used experimentally for patients with severe autoimmune diseases. When used for hemopoietic or other malignant diseases, it carries a substantially lower transplant-related mortality rate than allogeneic transplantation. In this study of patients with severe SSc, a higher procedure-related mortality rate was found from the procedure compared with patients with breast cancer and non-Hodgkin lymphoma. However, there appeared to be some benefits in the surviving patients, including a marked impact on skin score and a trend toward stabilization of pulmonary function. Further studies need to be performed to assess the utility of autologous stem cell transplantation in patients with severe SSc and other autoimmune conditions.

B. H. Thiers, MD

Surgery for Ischemic Pain and Raynaud's Phenomenon in Scleroderma: A Description of Treatment Protocol and Evaluation of Results
Tomaino MM, Goitz RJ, Medsger TA (Univ of Pittsburgh, Pa)
Microsurgery 21:75-79, 2001   12–11

Background.—The symptoms of Raynaud's phenomenon (digital ischemic pain, ulceration, cold intolerance, and skin discoloration) can be attributed to an interplay between the adrenergic nervous system, vasospasm, and vaso-occlusion. Palmar sympathectomy (PS) can improve these symptoms in patients with scleroderma. Nonetheless, the long-term effectiveness of PS in these patients remains unclear. Experience with scleroderma patients who underwent PS with or without vascular reconstruction was retrospectively evaluated.

Methods.—The subjects were 1 man and 5 women (average age, 45 years) with scleroderma who underwent PS because of increasing pain, Raynaud's phenomenon, or nonhealing digital ulcers between July 1995 and February 1997. Cold stress tests were not performed. Preoperative Allen testing revealed ulnar artery occlusion in 6 of the 8 hands and ulcerations involving 20 digits on 6 hands. Digital ulcerations were treated by debridement or amputation. Upper extremity arteriograms confirmed the ulnar artery occlusion in the 6 hands but showed a patent radial artery and deep arch in all hands. Digital blood flow was also evaluated preoperatively by digital plethysmography and digital blood pressure recordings. Four hands had satisfactory distal blood flow (including 2 hands with ulnar artery thrombosis), whereas the remaining 4 hands (all with ulnar artery thrombosis) had unsatisfactory distal blood flow. Vascular reconstruction was performed in the hands with ulnar artery thrombosis and inadequate digital blood flow. During surgery, the radial and ulnar arteries were exposed at the wrist. Peripheral nerve connections were divided before the adventitia were stripped. Decompression arteriolysis was performed over a 4-cm segment length. Then a transverse incision was made in the distal palmar flexion crease, and the adventitia were stripped as follows: the superficial palmar arch; the radial digital artery to the index finger; the common digital artery to the index-long, long-ring, and ring-small finger web spaces to the origin of the proper digital arteries; and the ulnar digital artery to the small finger. In addition, for occluded vessels, the incision for ulnar artery arteriolysis was extended distally into the interthenar skin and connected with the transverse incision in the palm. Results at short-term follow-up (6 months) were extracted from medical charts, and results at long-term follow-up (18 to 40 months; average, 2.5 years) were assessed by telephone interview.

Results.—At short-term follow-up, 4 patients (6 hands) were very satisfied and 1 patient (1 hand) was satisfied with the results of surgery. Ischemic digital pain improved significantly, and cold intolerance improved moderately. At long-term follow-up, 3 patients (4 hands) remained very satisfied and 2 patients (3 hands) were satisfied. The 1 patient who was dissatisfied with both short-term and long-term results reported no improvement in cold intolerance, but pain score (as measured by a 10-point visual analogue scale) improved from 10 preoperatively to 0 at short-term follow-up, then increased to 4 at long-term follow-up. After debridement or amputation, all digital ulcerations healed; however, 1 patient who smoked had recurrent ulcerations but did not require further surgery. After surgery, 4 patients were able to discontinue narcotic analgesics, and 2 patients (the dissatisfied patient and the patient with recurrent ulcerations) continued to use narcotics. Surgery had no effect on the use of vasodilator medications (used by 5 of the 6 patients). All but 1 patient reported a significant improvement in their quality of life after surgery, and said they would undergo the procedure again.

Conclusions.—PS in combination with radial and ulnar arteriolysis provided satisfactory long-term results and improvements in pain and cold tolerance in most of these patients with scleroderma. Vascular reconstruction should be performed when major inflow occlusion exists and digital blood flow is inadequate.

▶ Raynaud's phenomenon is notoriously refractory to pharmacologic therapy, although a number of different approaches have been suggested. Tomaino et al offer a surgical alternative for patients with recalcitrant disease. Their retrospective study found palmar sympathectomy in combination with radial and ulnar arteriolysis to be effective, with vascular reconstruction recommended when major inflow occlusion exists and digital blood flow is compromised.

B. H. Thiers, MD

Predicting Factors of Malignancy in Dermatomyositis and Polymyositis: A Case-Control Study
Chen Y-J, Wu C-Y, Shen J-L (Taichung Veterans Gen Hosp, Taiwan)
Br J Dermatol 144:825-831, 2001   12–12

Background.—There have been a number of reports in the literature of an association between dermatomyositis (DM)/polymyositis (PM) and cancer. For decades, the validity of extensive evaluation for cancer in these patients has been questioned. To date, only limited number of reports have been published regarding the signs of cancer and the prognostic factors in DM/PM. The potential risk factors of concomitant neoplastic diseases in patients diagnosed as having PM/DM were evaluated.

Methods.—The study group was composed of 147 patients in whom probable or definite DM/PM was diagnosed from April 1983 to June 1999. The data on these patients were retrospectively reviewed, and the patients were subgrouped as 1 of 4 main types: primary idiopathic DM, primary idiopathic PM, juvenile DM/PM, and amyopathic DM (ADM). Univariate analysis was performed with logistic regression for the evaluation of the possible predictive factors for cancer. These possible predictive factors included mean age at onset, gender, initial presentation, cutaneous manifestations, association with other connective tissue diseases, complications, and laboratory data. Logistic regression was then used to select the significant factors for multivariate analysis for determination of the independent risk factors of cancer in DM/PM patients.

Results.—Primary idiopathic DM was the most common subgroup, (64%), followed by ADM (14%), juvenile DM/PM (13%), and PM (10%). Overall, the mean age at onset was 42.4 years. Other connective tissue diseases were present in 22% of all patients, particularly PM (50%) and juvenile DM/PM (28%). Internal cancers were found in 13% of patients, and in most patients these cancers were associated with primary idiopathic DM. The most common tumors were nasopharyngeal carcinomas (NPCs). Patients had a greater chance of developing concomitant cancers if they had primary idiopathic DM, an older age at onset, higher serum creatine phosphokinase levels, and male gender. Patients with complications, especially interstitial lung diseases, had a lower risk of associated neoplasia. Multivariate analysis revealed that an older age at onset and male gender, but not primary idiopathic DM, were associated with greater risk of cancer.

Conclusions.—Older age at onset (more than 45 years) and male gender were found to be independent predictors of cancer in patients with DM/PM. Patients with primary idiopathic DM were found to have a higher risk of internal cancer, particularly NPC. However, primary idiopathic DM was not identified as an independent predictive factor for concomitant neoplastic diseases in multivariate analysis. A significantly lower frequency of cancer was noted in patients who had interstitial lung disease.

Cutaneous Leukocytoclastic Vasculitis in Dermatomyositis Suggests Malignancy

Hunger RE, Dürr C, Brand CU (Univ of Berne, Switzerland)
Dermatology 202:123-126, 2001   12–13

Background.—The rare connective tissue disease dermatomyositis (DM) is characterized by muscle and cutaneous involvement. The disease was described in the last century, but clearly defined diagnostic criteria were not available before 1975. The origin of DM is unknown, but in some patients the disease has been associated with cancer or connective tissue disease. An analysis of DM patients was conducted to evaluate the characteristics of cancer-associated DM and to determine whether vasculitis is linked to this form of DM.

Methods.—A retrospective review was conducted of files and histology reports for 23 patients who presented to a Swiss clinic from 1991 to 1998 and fulfilled the diagnostic criteria for DM. Clinical and laboratory data were analyzed, hematoxylin—eosin–stained skin sections were evaluated, and the observed number of cancer cases was compared with the number of cases expected on the basis of the sex- and age-specific incidence rates for the total Swiss population.

Results.—The median age at diagnosis was 48 years. Cancers were identified in 5 of 23 patients (22%). Features of DM were evident in the skin biopsy specimens of all patients. In 7 patients, a leukocytoclastic vasculitis was detected. In 4 of the 5 patients with an associated cancer, histologic evaluation demonstrated a vasculitis in lesional skin, compared with a finding of vasculitis in lesional skin in only 3 of 18 patients without cancer.

Conclusions.—These findings are suggestive of the predictive value of vasculitis in lesional skin biopsy specimens for the presence of underlying cancer in patients with dermatomyositis.

Frequency of Specific Cancer Types in Dermatomyositis and Polymyositis: A Population-Based Study
Hill CL, Zhang Y, Sigurgeirsson B, et al (Boston Univ; Landspitalinn, Reykjavik, Iceland; Karolinska Hosp, Stockholm; et al)
Lancet 357:96-100, 2001   12–14

Objective.—Epidemiologic studies have shown an association between dermatomyositis (DM) and polymyositis (PM) and certain types of cancer, but there have been too few cases to test any association with specific cancers. The risk for development of specific cancers after the diagnosis of myositis was investigated by pooled analysis of published national data from Sweden, Denmark, and Finland.

Methods.—All adults with DM and PM were identified from the Swedish National Board of Health discharge data (1964–1983), the Danish Hospital Discharge Registry (1977–1989), and the Finnish National Board of Health (1969–1985). The association between these 2 diagnoses and all cancer types combined and specific types of cancer individually was determined, and standardized incidence ratios (SIRs) were calculated and compared with rates calculated from national cancer registries.

Results.—Men and women with DM were respectively 3.3 and 2.8 times more likely to have cancer. These patients were at highest risk of ovarian, lung, pancreatic, stomach, and colorectal cancers. PM increased cancer risk by 30%, and specifically by 1.4 times for men and 1.2 times for women. These patients were at highest risk of non-Hodgkin lymphoma and lung and bladder cancer but were not at increased risk of ovarian, colorectal, stomach, or pancreatic cancer. Cancer risk was highest within the first year after myositis diagnosis. Risk returned to expected rates at 5 years for those with PM but not for those with DM.

Conclusion.—DM is strongly associated and PM is weakly associated with development of a variety of malignant diseases.

▶ These articles (Abstracts 12–12 to 12–14) attempt to assist the clinician in identifying dermatomyositis patients at risk for malignancy and the sites at which these tumors might develop. Chen et al (Abstract 12–12) found internal malignancies in 13% of patients, most of whom had dermatomyositis, as opposed to polymyositis. This represents a significantly higher risk for malignancy than is observed in the general population of Taiwan (0.19%). Nasopharyngeal carcinoma was the most common cancer, and likely reflects the high incidence of that tumor in Asian countries. In Western countries, relative to the general population, ovarian and breast carcinoma in women and lung and prostate carcinoma in men are highly associated with dermatomyositis and polymyositis. Hunger et al (Abstract 12–13) reported vasculitis in lesional skin biopsy specimens as a predictive factor for the presence of underlying malignancy; histopathologic observations were not included in the study by Chen et al. Prospective epidemiologic studies are needed to confirm this finding. The data reported by Hill et al (Abstract 12–14) come largely from a Scandinavian population. They found an underlying malignancy in 198 of 618 patients with dermatomyositis and 137 of 914 with polymyositis. Ovarian, lung, gastric, colorectal, and pancreatic cancers, as well as non-Hodgkin lymphoma, were the malignancies most strongly associated with dermatomyositis, whereas in patients with polymyositis, the risk of lung cancer, bladder cancer, and non-Hodgkin lymphoma was increased. The observation that dermatomyositis was strongly associated with cancer, whereas the association with polymyositis was only modest, is consistent with the data reported by Chen et al.

B. H. Thiers, MD

Risk of Cancer in Patients With Dermatomyositis or Polymyositis, and Follow-up Implications: A Scottish Population-based Cohort Study
Stockton D, Doherty VR, Brewster DH (Information & Statistics Division, Edinburgh, Scotland; Royal Infirmary of Edinburgh, Scotland)
Br J Cancer 85:41-45, 2001   12–15

Background.—The incidence of cancer is apparently increased in patients with dermatomyositis (DM). However, estimated risks reported in previous studies have varied widely. The risk of cancer in a population-based cohort of patients with DM or polymyositis (PM) in Scotland was investigated.

Methods.—A cohort of 705 patients hospitalized with a first diagnosis of DM or PM between 1982 and 1996 was studied retrospectively. Data were obtained from a combination of hospital discharge records, cancer registration, and death records.

Findings.—A first malignancy was diagnosed concurrently or subsequently in 50 patients with DM and in 40 with PM. The standardized incidence ratios (SIR) were 7.7 and 2.1, respectively. Patients with DM had a significantly increased risk of lung, cervix uteri, and ovarian cancer, whereas patients with PM were at significantly increased risk of Hodgkin's disease. The excess cancer risk was greatest at about the time of diagnosis. For patients with DM, the risk remained high for at least 2 years. Risks for both sexes were increased, but significantly so only in women. Risks were greatest for patients aged 45 to 75 years at diagnosis of DM and for patients aged 15 to 44 years at diagnosis of PM.

Conclusions.—The risk of cancer is increased after the diagnosis of DM and PM for patients aged 45 to 75 years at DM diagnosis and for patients aged 15 to 44 years at PM diagnosis. The risk is increased significantly for women for both PM and DM. This increased risk was evident within the first 3 months after a PM diagnosis and in the first 2 years after a DM diagnosis. Clinicians need to maintain a high index of suspicion for malignancy in such patients.

▶ These findings are similar to those reported by Hill et al (Abstract 12–14). In their study, the risk of cancer was highest within the first year of myositis diagnosis and dropped substantially afterward. For patients with polymyositis, the risk fell to expected rates 5 years after diagnosis, although the risk in dermatomyositis patients did not return to expected population values for most cancers.

B. H. Thiers, MD

Polymyositis and Dermatomyositis: Short Term and Longterm Outcome, and Predictive Factors of Prognosis
Marie I, Hachulla E, Hatron P-Y, et al (Centre Hospitalier Universitaire de Rouen-Boisguillaume, Rouen, France; Centre Hospitalier Universitaire de Lille, France)
J Rheumatol 28:2230-2237, 2001   12–16

Introduction.—Polymyositis (PM) and dermatomyositis (DM) are chronic idiopathic inflammatory disorders with high morbidity and mortality rates. Because few studies have analyzed long-term outcome and prognostic factors in PM/DM, a retrospective study examined both short- and long-term outcomes of these disorders and variables predictive of remission and survival.

Methods.—Seventy-seven consecutive patients were included in the study, 36 with DM and 41 with PM. Diagnosis was based on the criteria of Bohan and Peter as follows: symmetric muscle weakness, increased muscle enzymes, myopathic changes on electromyography, histologic findings on muscle biopsy, and dermatologic signs. Patients underwent a standardized evaluation of organ involvement and biochemical analysis. The minimum follow-up period was 18 months.

Results.—Common disease manifestations in these patients included pulmonary involvement (42%), antinuclear antibodies (47%), Raynaud's phenomenon (32%), and malignancy (22%). After treatment with high-dose steroid therapy and immunosuppressive agents, remission occurred in 31 patients (40%); 33 (43%) showed improvement, and 13 (17%) experienced a worsening of their clinical status. Short-term recurrences of PM/DM during tapering of therapy occurred in 36 patients; 9 had long-term recurrences after therapy was discontinued. Even among patients with remission, only 52% were able to return to normal activities. Seventeen patients (22%) died, most of cancer and lung complications. Factors associated with PM/DM remission were younger age and shorter duration of clinical manifestations before the start of therapy. Variables associated with poor outcome were older age, pulmonary and esophageal involvement, and cancer.

Conclusion.—Knowledge of the prognostic factors for the course of PM/DM appears to be essential to improving outcome, and prompt treatment is important. Patients treated at an early stage have a more favorable response, perhaps because the extent of irreversible histologic muscle damage is reduced. The risk of cancer should be recognized and esophageal involvement and ventilatory insufficiency investigated in the initial evaluation of these patients.

▶ This study emphasizes the chronicity of PM/DM, with only 40% of patients achieving remission. Relapses were common, and only 52% of patients considered to be in remission experienced a return to previous normal activities. Mortality was high. In addition to cancer, the main cause of death was lung complications, which could represent primary ventilatory insufficiency or aspiration pneumonia caused by esophageal dysfunction. Because of this, the authors recommend investigation for lung impairment and subclinical esophageal dysfunction as part of the initial PM/DM evaluation, with aggressive therapy and close follow-up for affected patients.

B. H. Thiers, MD

Incidence of Malignant Disease in Biopsy-Proven Inflammatory Myopathy: A Population-Based Cohort Study

Buchbinder R, Forbes A, Hall S, et al (Cabrini Med Centre, Malvern, Australia; Monash Univ, Melbourne, Australia; Melbourne Univ, Australia; et al)
Ann Intern Med 134:1087-1095, 2001   12–17

Background.—Polymyositis and dermatomyositis have been reported to be associated with malignancies, but the significance of this association is not clear. The risk of malignancy was examined in a group of 537 patients with biopsy-proven inflammatory myopathy in a population-based, retrospective cohort study.

Study Design.—The Victorian Neuropathology Service was used to identify all patients with biopsy-proven idiopathic inflammatory myopathy who were first diagnosed from 1981 through 1985. These records were matched to those of the Victorian State Cancer Registry and the National Death Index. Standardized incidence ratios were calculated to compare the incidence of malignant disease among these patients with that among the general population.

Findings.—Among the 537 patients with inflammatory myopathy in the study group, there were 116 malignancies in 104 patients. The highest risk of malignancy was associated with polymyositis, followed by dermatomyositis and inclusion-body myositis. The risk was highest in the first year after diagnosis and then diminished; however, it was still above baseline at 5 years.

Conclusions.—A population-based cohort study was performed to examine the association between idiopathic inflammatory myopathy and malignancy. The myositis type was defined by pathologic evaluation to ensure diagnostic accuracy. An increased malignancy risk was associated with polymyositis, dermatomyositis, and inclusion-body myositis. This risk was highest in the initial period after diagnosis but was still elevated at 5 years.

▶ Quite frankly, this article left me with more questions than answers. As in previous studies, the incidence of malignancy was increased in patients with dermatomyositis and, to a lesser extent, in those with polymyositis. The excess risk of malignant disease gradually diminished with time. Buchbinder et al also noted an increased risk of malignant disease in patients with inclusion-body myositis, a pathologic diagnosis for which they gave no clinical correlate. In addition, they criticize the criteria of Bohan and Peter as being unacceptable for distinguishing between polymyositis and dermatomyositis yet offer no alternative method for clinical classification. Instead, they state, "By classifying our patients on histologic grounds, we reduced the risk for misclassification of polymyositis and dermatomyositis." This is, in a sense, putting the cart before the horse, as most of us treat the clinical disease and not its histopathologic nuances.

B. H. Thiers, MD

Lipodystrophy in Patients With Juvenile Dermatomyositis—Evaluation of Clinical and Metabolic Abnormalities

Huemer C, Kitson H, Malleson PN, et al (Univ of British Columbia, Vancouver, Canada; Univ of Vienna)
J Rheumatol 28:610-615, 2001   12–18

Introduction.—The coexistence of juvenile dermatomyositis (JDM) and lipodystrophy, with or without diabetes mellitus (yet always with hyperinsulinemia), has been noted in several case reports. Lipodystrophy describes a clinical condition characterized by either generalized or localized partial loss of subcutaneous fat, hirsutism, and acanthosis nigricans that is associated with hepatomegaly, insulin-resistant diabetes mellitus, and hyperlipidemia. The prevalence of lipodystrophy and the extent of metabolic abnormalities associated with lipoatropic diabetes mellitus were examined in patients with JDM.

Methods.—Twenty patients with JDM and associated lipoatropic diabetes mellitus (Table 1) seen between January 1, 1981, and June 30, 1996, underwent clinical evaluation by a pediatric rheumatologist and a pediatric endocrinologist, laboratory investigations, and metabolic studies (including an oral glucose tolerance test, lipid studies, and determination of

TABLE 1.—Clinical Characteristics of Patients

Patient	Sex	Age at Diagnosis, Yrs	Age at Study, Yrs	Course of Disease	Active Muscle Disease at Study	Active Skin Disease at Study	Duration of Prednisone Treatment, Mo	Prednisone Dose at Study, mg/kg/day	Weight for Age, Percentile	Height for Age Percentile
Group 1										
1	F	8.3	13.5	REC	No	GLD, CAL, HIR	59	0.17	< 5th	< 5th
2	M	4.2	15.1	REC	No	PLD, A	23	0.37	25th	75th
3	M	10.8	13	REC	Yes	PLD, CAL, A	27	0.22	25th	< 5th
4	F	10.7	16.7	REC	Yes	PLD, HIR, A	65	0	50th	< 5th
Group 2										
5	F	11.2	12.5	MC	Yes	R	17	0.24	10th	< 5th
6	M	10	14.5	REC	Yes	R, CAL	60	0.21	75th	< 5th
7	F	4.9	5	NEW	Yes	R	1	i.v. 3× 30	50th	10th
8	M	12.9	14	MC	Yes	R	13	0.24	75th	< 5th
9	F	7.4	10.2	REC	Yes	R	34	0.47	75th	< 5th
10	F	6.2	10	MC, REM	No	No	1	0	95th	> 95th
11	F	14	14	NEW	Yes	R, GP	1	1.0	50th	50th
12	F	15.7	15.7	NEW	Yes	R	1	0.9	50th	10th
Group 3										
13	F	3.5	7.9	MC	No	R	1	0	50th	50th
14	M	12.2	18.1	REC	No	R	2	0	10th	25th
15	M	1.7	4	MC	Yes	R	22	0.36	< 5th	< 5th
16	F	14.7	26.2	REC, REM	No	No	73	0	ND	ND
17	M	1.2	3.1	REC	No	GP	23	0.06	95th	90th
18	F	9	10.3	REC	Yes	R, CAL	38	0.43	10th	10th
19	F	3.7	4	MC	No	R	1	0.9	90th	95th
20	M	3.2	8.1	MC, REM	No	No	20	0	25th	10th

Abbreviations: MC, Monocyclic course of disease; *REC,* recurrent or continuous course of disease; *NEW,* newly diagnosed; *REM,* remission; *GLD,* generalized lipodystrophy; *PLD,* partial lipodystrophy; *CAL,* calcifications; *HIR,* hirsutism; *R,* JMD rash; *GP,* Gottron's papules: *A,* acanthosis nigricans; *ND,* not done.
(Courtesy of Huemer C, Kitson H, Malleson PN, et al: Lipodystrophy in patients with juvenile dermatomyositis—Evaluation of clinical and metabolic abnormalities. *J Rheumatol* 28:610-615, 2001.)

insulin antibodies). All patients were initially treated with high-dose (30 mg/kg) IV methylprednisolone pulse therapy.

Results.—There was clinical evidence of lipodystrophy and lipoatrophic diabetes mellitus in 4 patients with JDM. Metabolic abnormalities associated with lipodystrophy were observed in 8 other patients. Patients were grouped as follows: group 1, 4 patients with lipodystrophy and either diabetes mellitus or impaired glucose tolerance (2 patients each, respectively); group 2, 8 patients with abnormal glucose and/or lipid studies and no lipodystrophy; and group 3, 8 patients with no abnormal glucose or lipid studies and no lipodystrophy.

Conclusion.—One quarter of patients with JDM have lipodystrophy and half have hypertriglyceridemia and insulin resistance at the time of their initial visit. Screening for metabolic abnormalities in JDM needs to be included in routine follow-up testing because of the influence of lipodystrophy on long-term prognosis.

▶ In this series of 20 children with JDM monitored and evaluated for 15 years, 4 had lipodystrophy develop and an additional 8 exhibited metabolic abnormalities known to be associated with lipodystrophy. The authors postulate that the muscle disease may be a major contributor to insulin resistance and abnormal glucose tolerance in children with JDM. Skeletal muscle is the principle site of insulin-mediated glucose disposal, and differences in the rate of insulin-stimulated glycogen synthesis in muscle account for most of the variation in insulin sensitivity among healthy subjects. Inflammatory muscle disease, rather than corticosteroid treatment, is the probable link to insulin resistance in children with JDM. Therefore, more aggressive treatment with steroids and other agents, rather than a decrease in steroid dosage, is warranted if insulin resistance develops in these patients.

S. Raimer, MD

The Arthritis of Inflammatory Childhood Myositis Syndromes
Tse S, Lubelsky S, Gordon M, et al (Univ of Toronto)
J Rheumatol 28:192-197, 2001   12–19

Background.—Arthritis has been reported in 23% to 64% of persons with juvenile dermatomyositis (JDM); 13% of patients with JDM have chronic polyarthritis that continues into adulthood. The degree to which JDM-associated arthritis contributes to morbidity has not been determined. The frequency, course, and clinical, immunologic, and radiographic features of arthritis in a large cohort of patients with JDM were investigated. In addition, the extent of disability conferred by the arthritis was determined.

Methods.—Data were gathered from all patients who had a primary diagnosis of idiopathic myositis (including JDM, juvenile polymyositis [JPM], amyopathic JDM, and overlap myositis syndrome), as determined by established criteria, who came for treatment to the Hospital for Sick

Children between 1984 and 1999. Of this total population, 80 patients with JDM, 5 patients with amyopathic JDM, 3 patients with JPM, and 6 with overlap myositis syndromes were studied. Since 1990, evaluations of patients were completed in a separate myositis clinic by certified pediatric rheumatologists, with physiotherapy assessments performed at each visit. The definition of arthritis used was swelling or joint effusion, or at least 2 of the following: heat, decreased range of motion, tenderness, or painful movement.

Results.—Among the patients with JDM, 61% had associated arthritis, which occurred at a median of 4.5 months after the diagnosis of JDM. Initially, articular involvement was polyarticular (affecting more than 4 joints) in 33% of patients and pauciarticular in 67%. Among those with pauciarticular findings, 58% had asymptomatic knee effusions; 18 of these cases occurred after beginning corticosteroid therapy, which may have contributed to the development of the effusions. In general, the arthritis was characterized as painful but not markedly limiting function. The arthritis responded to myositis therapy, remitting in a median of 2.0 months. When corticosteroid therapy was discontinued, arthritis recurred in 39% of patients despite the continuation of other therapeutic agents (9 patients taking a nonsteroidal anti-inflammatory drug [NSAID], 6 taking methotrexate, 4 taking hydroxychloroquine, 1 taking azathioprine, and 4 receiving intravenous immunoglobulin). Radiographs were obtained in 27 of the 49 patients with arthritis, and revealed no erosions in the shoulders, elbows, wrists, hands, hips, knees, ankles, or feet. None of the patients with JPM had arthritis, but 3 of 5 patients with amyopathic JDM had arthritis, with nonerosive polyarthritis of the small joints in 1 patient and the involvement of small and large joints in 2 patients. Nonerosive poly-arthritis affecting small and large joints was found in 4 of 6 patients with overlap myositis syndromes.

Conclusions.—JDM is frequently attended by a nonerosive arthritis similar to that noted in systemic lupus erythematosus. The arthritis occurs early in the course of JDM, and its distribution includes the fingers, wrists, elbows, and knees. This arthritis is responsive to treatment for JDM. Among the other treatments used for arthritis management were NSAIDs, methotrexate, and intra-articular steroid injections. In 39% of the cases studied, arthritis persisted even when JDM was in remission.

▶ In this retrospective study of 80 patients with JDM, articular involvement was noted in 49 (61%) of the patients. In 18 of these patients, asymptomatic knee effusions were the only presenting findings. In all but 1 patient, these effusions developed after the initiation of systemic corticosteroid therapy, and therefore may have resulted from the therapy. The nonerosive, painful arthritis present in most of the patients resolved with corticosteroid therapy but recurred in 39% of them as the corticosteroid dosage was tapered; this often occurred despite the fact that the myositis was in remission. In these patients, the authors were frequently able to manage the arthritis with agents other than corticosteroids. Three of 5 patients with amyopathic JDM had arthritis. Arthritis appears to be not simply an overlap feature but a true sign of JDM. It is frequently a clinically important problem even when the myositis is in remission.

S. Raimer, MD

New Insight Into Calcinosis of Juvenile Dermatomyositis: A Study of Composition and Treatment
Mukamel M, Horev G, Mimouni M (Schneider Children's Med Ctr of Israel, Petah Tiqva; Tel Aviv Univ, Israel)
J Pediatr 138:763-766, 2001   12–20

Introduction.—There is no universally accepted treatment for calcinosis of juvenile dermatomyositis (JDM), but some success with bisphosphonates has been reported. In the 2 children reported here, the development of calcinosis was accompanied by subcutaneous aseptic fluid deposits containing noncrystallized calcium compatible with the "milk of calcium" previously reported in JDM.

Case 1.—Boy, 14 years, had been treated with steroids since chronic JDM was diagnosed at age 10 years. In addition to mild calcinosis around a knee, a painful fluid collection developed on the left elbow. Surgical drainage yielded 20 mL of aseptic fluid containing noncrystallized calcium and phosphorus. Cellular analysis revealed macrophages exclusively. The cytokines interleukin (IL)-6 and IL-1β and tumor necrosis factor-α were detected in the fluid, and IL-1β and IL-6 were also present in serum. The patient required no further treatment for calcinosis.

Case 2.—Boy, 6 years, had the diagnosis of JDM established at age 3 years. Methylprednisolone pulses and methotrexate were used to control relapses of myositis. Widespread calcinosis, accompanied by fluid collections containing milk of calcium, started to develop when the boy was 3½, and he gradually lost all ability to move. The boy's condition continued to deteriorate despite treatment with oral calcium, vitamin α D₃, prednisone, methotrexate, and a 6-month trial of diltiazem. By age 6, the boy had limited mouth opening, difficulty breathing, and severe osteoporosis. The addition of alendronate, 10 mg/d, resulted in marked clinical improvement. One year later, the boy could run, swim, and dress unaided, and had gained 8 cm in height. Radiologic and laboratory findings returned to normal. Alendronate was tapered after 1 year with no adverse effects. Several calcium tumors that had extruded through the patient's skin were found to consist of calcium, oxalate, phosphate, uric acid, calcium oxalate, and a hydroxyapatite nucleus.

Discussion.—Activated macrophages appear to play an important role in the calcinosis of JDM, and alendronate appears to be a safe and effective treatment. The drug may act by inhibiting bone resorption, reducing calcium turnover, and inhibiting calcium accretion to the already-formed calcification.

▶ The authors studied 2 children with JDM. They collected fluid (referred to as milk of calcium) from joints with calcium deposits around them. The fluid contained macrophages and cytokines (IL-6, IL-1β, and TNF-α) produced by macrophages. One of the children had severe debilitating calcinosis cutis that markedly improved after initiation of treatment with alendronate, 10 mg/d, for severe osteoporosis. The child experienced marked improvement without any apparent side effects.

Activated macrophages may play an important role in the pathogenesis of the calcinosis of JDM. Bisphosphonates are known to cause selective destruction of macrophages and to inhibit macrophage proinflammatory cytokine production. Previous studies using bisphosphonates to treat the calcinosis associated with JDM have produced equivocal results. One group of investigators reported failure with etidronate,[1] while another reported rapid regression of calcinosis with pamidronate and diltiazem.[2] Experience with alendronate in children is limited. Cimaz et al administered alendronate to 43 pediatric patients with rheumatic diseases and found it to be safe and effective.[3] Because most patients with JDM will require treatment with oral corticosteroids, the initiation of alendronate treatment might prevent the development of not only osteoporosis but calcinosis cutis as well.

S. Raimer, MD

References

1. Metzger AL, Singer FR, Bluestone R, et al: Failure of disodium etidronate in calcinosis due to dermatomyositis and scleroderma. *N Engl J Med* 291:1294-1296, 1974.
2. Oliveri MB, Palezmo R, Mantalenri C, et al: Regression of calcinosis during diltiazem treatment in juvenile dermatomyositis. *J Rheumatol* 23:2152-2155, 1996.
3. Cimaz R, Falcini F, Bardare M, et al: Safety and efficacy of alendronate for the treatment of osteoporosis in pediatric rheumatic diseases. *Arthritis Rheum* 42:S400, 1999.

Treatment of Calcinosis in Juvenile Dermatomyositis With Probenecid: The Role of Phosphorus Metabolism in the Development of Calcifications

Harel L, Harel G, Korenreich L, et al (Tel Aviv Univ, Israel)
J Rheumatol 28:1129-1132, 2001   12–21

Background.—Juvenile dermatomyositis (JDM) is often complicated by calcinosis (30%-70% of cases), which is difficult to treat. Long-term disability can result from calcinosis, even after myositis remission. A consistent method for treating calcinosis has not been found, and immunosuppressive agents and corticosteroids do not reduce calcinosis. A case report of JDM with calcinosis treated with probenecid shows the metabolic consequences of treatment.

> *Case Report.*—Girl, 9 years, with JDM and extensive calcinosis since 4 years of age, underwent biochemical studies before and during probenecid treatment to determine changes in calcium and phosphorus metabolism. Her presenting symptoms at 4 years of age were rash and progressive, painful muscle weakness. At that time, she had a creatine kinase level of 12,000 U/L (normal range, 60-149). JDM was confirmed by electromyography and muscle biopsy. She had calcinosis develop in March 1996 with deposits in the skin, muscles, tendons of the lower extremities, abdomen, chest, arms, and neck. Impaired gait, fever, pain, cellulitis, and upper body venous congestion resulted. Probenecid therapy at progressively increasing doses was started in January 1998, and calcinosis began to resolve in June 1998. Relapse of the disease occurred in December 1998, yet calcifications were still markedly decreased. Remission of skin and muscle disease, markedly reduced calcinosis, and increased bone mineral content were noted in June 1999. Probenecid was not reported to cause any side effects.

Results.—Increased renal phosphate clearance and decreased serum phosphorus levels were noted during probenecid treatment and resulted in reduced calcifications during the 18-month course of therapy. Uric acid reabsorption in the proximal tubule also was inhibited by probenecid.

Conclusion.—Certain JDM patients may have calcinosis develop because of increased renal phosphate reclamation. These patients may be effectively treated with probenecid.

▶ Calcinosis in JDM can be extremely debilitating. Diltiazem has also been used with inconsistent results.[1] Unfortunately, aggressive therapy of the underlying muscle disease usually does not prevent the development of calcinosis.

B. H. Thiers, MD

Reference

1. Oliveri MB, Palermo R, Mautalen C, et al: Regression of calcinosis during diltiazem treatment in juvenile dermatomyositis. *J Rheumatol* 23:2152-2155, 1996.

Comorbidity and Lifestyle, Reproductive Factors, and Environmental Exposures Associated With Rheumatoid Arthritis
Olsson AR, Skogh T, Wingren G (Linköping Univ, Sweden; Univ Hosp, Linköping, Sweden)
Ann Rheum Dis 60:934-939, 2001   12–22

Background.—Rheumatoid arthritis (RA) is a disorder with an unknown etiology. The development of this disorder appears to be influenced by genetic, hormonal, and environmental factors. The effect of lifestyle, reproductive, and environmental factors on the development of RA was retrospectively examined.

Study Design.—The medical records of patients attending the Division of Rheumatology at the University Hospital in Linköping, Sweden from 1980 to 1995 were used to identify 422 patients, aged 25 to 75 years, with RA. For each patient, 2 control subjects matched for age and living in the same area were randomly enrolled. A questionnaire was mailed to all participants in 1996.

Findings.—There was a negative association between atopy and RA and a positive association between insulin use and RA. Women with a short fertile period had an increased risk for RA. Smoking also increased the risk. Education was inversely associated with RA. Increased risk was observed for men born into homes with private wells and exposed to mold or farm animals. Previous joint injury and exposure to hair dye was associated with increased risk for RA in women.

Conclusion.—RA, which involves a T-helper(Th) 1 immune response, was inversely associated with atopy, which is dominated by a Th2 immune response, and positively associated with Th1-dominated diabetes mellitus. Current and past smoking was associated with RA, as found in previous studies. Higher education appeared to have a protective effect, which may be lifestyle related. There was an increased risk for RA associated with long-term use of hair coloring products. Further studies are necessary to understand all the risk factors associated with the development of RA.

▶ Olsson et al report that women who use hair dyes for more than 20 years may nearly double their risk for development of RA. The increased risk prevailed even after adjustment for work as a hairdresser. This study confirms a previous report linking hairdressers with an increased risk for RA.[1] Lymphoma and other hematopoietic neoplasms have also been associated with working as a hairdresser and customer use of hair dyes.[2-4]

B. H. Thiers, MD

References

1. Lundberg I, Alfredsson L, Plato N, et al: Occupation, occupational exposure to chemicals and rheumatological disease. *Scand J Rheumatol* 23:305-310, 1994.
2. Miligi L, Seniori Costantini A, Crosignani P, et al: Occupational, environmental, and life-style factors associated with the risk of hematolymphopoietic malignancies in women. *Am J Ind Med* 36:60-69,1999.

3. Georgescu L, Paget SA: Lymphoma in patients with rheumatoid arthritis: What is the evidence of a link with methotrexate? *Drug Safety* 20:475-487, 1999.

4. Correa A, Jackson L, Mohan A, et al: Use of hair dyes, hematopoietic neoplasms, and lymphomas: A literature review. II. Lymphomas and multiple myeloma. *Cancer Invest* 18:467-479, 2000.

Treatment of Early Seropositive Rheumatoid Arthritis: A Two-Year, Double-blind Comparison of Minocycline and Hydroxychloroquine
O'Dell JR, Blakely KW, Mallek JA, et al (Univ of Nebraska, Omaha; Platte Valley Med Group, Kearney, Neb; Central Plains Clinic, Sioux Falls, SD; et al)
Arthritis Rheum 44:2235-2241, 2001   12–23

Background.—Early diagnosis and treatment of rheumatoid arthritis (RA) is essential, but the optimal treatment regimen remains controversial. Tetracyclines have been advocated as an early treatment for RA. The efficacy of the tetracycline, minocycline, was compared with that of a conventional disease-modifying antirheumatic drug, hydroxychloroquine, in patients with early seropositive RA in a 2-year, double-blind, randomized, controlled study.

Study Design.—This study was performed by members of the RA Investigational Network. The study group consisted of 60 adult patients with early, active RA who had not previously received disease-modifying therapy. Patients received minocycline or hydroxychloroquine, plus nonsteroidal anti-inflammatory drugs and prednisone (5-7.5 mg/d). Steroid dosage could be tapered after 1 year. Patients were assessed every 3 months. Any toxic effects were noted. If no improvement was detected at 12 months, the treatment was considered to be a failure. The primary end points were treatment response and steroid dosage at 2 years. Data were analyzed on an intent-to-treat basis.

Findings.—Patients with early, active RA treated with minocycline were more likely to achieve an American College of Rheumatology 50% improvement response and used less prednisone at 2 years compared with patients treated with hydroxychloroquine.

Conclusions.—Minocycline was more effective than conventional treatment with hydroxychloroquine for patients with early, active RA. Minocycline therapy should be considered for patients with early, active RA.

▶ Shortly after this study was published, we saw in clinic a minocycline-treated patient with RA who had significant, generalized pigmentation as a result of her minocycline intake. With the more widespread use of minocycline by rheumatologists, this phenomenon is likely to become even more prevalent.[1] Another question that will need to be answered is whether patients with RA are in any way predisposed to have the lupus-like syndrome associated with minocycline.[2]

B. H. Thiers, MD

References

1. Assad SA, Bernstein EF, Brod B, et al: Extensive pigmentation secondary to minocycline treatment of rheumatoid arthritis. *J Rheumatol* 28:679-682, 2001.
2. Elkayam O, Yaron M, Caspi D: Minocycline-induced autoimmune syndromes: An overview. *Semin Arthritis Rheum* 28:392-397, 1999.

Papulopustular Skin Lesions Are Seen More Frequently in Patients With Behçet's Syndrome Who Have Arthritis: A Controlled and Masked Study

Diri E, Mat C, Hamuryudan V, et al (Univ of Texas Southwestern Med Centre, Dallas; Univ of Istanbul, Turkey)

Ann Rheum Dis 60:1074-1076, 2001   12–24

Introduction.—Arthritis and papulopustular skin lesions are 2 significant manifestations of Behçet's syndrome (BS). There is no histologic difference between the papulopustular lesions in BS and ordinary acne. The prevalence of acneiform skin lesions (comedones, papules, and pustules) was evaluated in patients who have BS with arthritis in a controlled and masked protocol.

Methods.—Of 86 patients with BS, 44 had BS with arthritis (32 men, 12 women; mean age, 37.8 years) and 42 had BS without arthritis (31 men, 11 women; mean age, 35.5 years). Also evaluated were 21 patients with rheumatoid arthritis (5 men, 16 women; mean age, 48.8 years) and 33 healthy volunteers (28 men, 5 women; mean age, 40.1 years). All probands and controls were assessed by a rheumatologist and a dermatologist. If needed, an ophthalmologic evaluation was performed. Skin lesions, including comedones, papules, and pustules, were counted and rated as: 0, absent; 1, 1 to 5; 2, 6 to 10; 3, 11 to 15; 4, 16 to 20; and 5, more than 20 lesions.

Results.—There was no significant difference among the 4 groups in the prevalence of comedones. The number of papules and pustules was significantly higher among patients who had BS with arthritis ($P = .0037$ for papules and $P < .0001$ for pustules) compared with the other 3 groups.

Conclusion.—Acneiform skin lesions (papules and pustules) appear to be more common in patients who have BS with arthritis. The arthritis observed in BS may be linked to acne-associated arthritis.

▶ The authors report an association between arthritis and acneiform skin lesions in patients with BS, and propose a possible common pathogenetic mechanism. Unfortunately, they present no hard data to back up this assertion. Although arthritis and arthralgias can occur in patients with acne fulminans, the clinical presentation of both the skin and joint disease in BS is much different. Moreover, the acneiform lesions the authors describe in BS may not be true acne but rather a manifestation of the pathergy that characterizes the disease.

B. H. Thiers, MD

Remission of Behçet's Syndrome With Tumour Necrosis Factor α Blocking Therapy

Goossens PH, Verburg RJ, Breedveld FC (Leiden Univ, The Netherlands)
Ann Rheum Dis 60:637, 2001   12–25

Background.—Behçet's disease causes necrotic vasculitis of all sizes of arteries and veins, and requires immunosuppressive drugs for treatment. Because high serum levels of tumor necrosis factor (TNF) and soluble TNF receptors are associated with Behçet's disease, treatment with a monoclonal antibody that can neutralize the activity of TNF, specifically infliximab, seems logical.

> *Case Report.*—Man, 40, had painful nodules and skin ulcers on his foot. Based on results of a deep biopsy specimen, which showed obliteration of the vascular lumen and necrosis accompanied by lymphocytic infiltration into the vascular wall, polyarteritis nodosa was diagnosed. Initial treatment with 40 mg of prednisone daily was eventually supplemented with 150 mg/day of azathioprine and then 100 mg/day of cyclophosphamide. Periodic recurrences continued, and steroid dependence developed, with no response to either cyclophosphamide pulse treatment or thalidomide. Ulcers of his mouth, anus, and penis developed, for which he received 15 mg/day of prednisone and 15 mg/week of methotrexate. Foot ulcerations and retinal lesions compatible with vasculitis then developed, leading to the diagnosis of Behçet's disease. Treatment with infliximab was carried out, with 2 injections of 10 mg/kg (700 mg) at an interval of 1 month.

Results.—Significant reductions in the size of the ulcerations of the penis, anus, mouth, and skin were noted 2 weeks after the first injection, with complete resolution by the time of the second injection. The patient remains in remission 12 months after the second injection.

Conclusions.—Infliximab treatment brought about rapid improvement of long-standing symptoms in this patient with Behçet's disease. Based on the mode of action of infliximab, which binds with high affinity to the soluble and transmembrane forms of TNF, a central role for TNF in the pathogenesis of Behçet's disease seems highly likely. Thus, TNF blocking therapy appears to be effective treatment for Behçet's disease.

Effect of Infliximab on Sight-Threatening Panuveitis in Behçet's Disease
Sfikakis PP, Theodossiadis PG, Katsiari CG, et al (Athens Univ Med School, Greece)
Lancet 358:295-296, 2001   12–26

Background.—Relapsing ocular inflammation that can result in permanent vision loss develops in approximately 70% of patients with Behçet's disease, even with intensive, long-term immunosuppressive therapy. The cause of Behçet's disease is unknown, but increased serum concentrations of tumor necrosis factor (TNF) and soluble TNF receptors are noted in patients with active disease. This study evaluated the efficacy of treatment with infliximab, a monoclonal antibody to TNF, for patients with long-standing Behçet's disease and multiple episodes of uveitis.

Patients.—The 5 patients (4 men and 1 woman) ranged in age from 21 to 56 years and were enrolled within 48 hours of relapse. One had severe unilateral panuveitis, with visual acuity limited to hand motion only; this patient was taking 5 mg/kg of cyclosporin A and 2.5 mg/kg of prednisolone. While taking 2.5 mg/kg of cyclosporin A, the second patient had bilateral relapse with visual acuity of 0.4 in the right eye and 0.1 in the left. Unilateral relapse (visual acuity of 0.7) occurred in the third patient while taking 2 mg/kg of cyclosporin A and 0.6 mg/kg of azathioprine. These 3 patients received infliximab (5 mg/kg) and their current therapy was adjusted to maximum doses (for cyclosporin A, 5 mg/kg; for prednisolone, 0.5 mg/kg; and for azathioprine, 1.2 mg/kg). The fourth patient had a unilateral relapse with blurred vision and was taking 0.6 mg/kg of cyclosporin A and 1.2 mg/kg of azathioprine. The fifth was taking 3 mg/kg of cyclosporin A, 0.5 mg/kg of prednisolone, and 2 mg/kg of azathioprine and suffered a bilateral relapse, with visual acuities of 0.4 and 0.2. Based on the results in the first 3 patients, patients 4 and 5 were given infliximab without increasing their current therapy.

Results.—For the first 3 patients, the severity of the inflammation had subsided by over half on the first day and by over 90% by the fourth day. By the seventh day, all had complete resolution of retinal infiltrates and vasculitis. Improved visual acuity was noted within the first 24 hours. The first patient was able to count fingers, the second patient's acuities improved to 0.6 and 0.3, and the third returned to normal vision. Further improvements occurred in these 3 patients (for the first and second patients until day 14) and was maintained for 28 days. The other 2 patients also improved. The degree of inflammation seen in the fourth patient decreased within 24 hours and the panuveitis was almost completely resolved by the fourth day. On the first day, the fifth patient had noticeable remission of ocular inflammation and improved visual acuity, with remission of the panuveitis by the seventh day; by the 10th day, the right eye had normal visual acuity and the left had visual acuity of 0.7. These values stabilized until 28 days after infliximab was given. Two patients had concomitant oral aphthous ulcers with the ocular relapse, and these healed by the second day after infliximab administration. One had concomitant arthritis in the left knee and ankle, which subsided in 4 days. No patients had adverse side effects.

Conclusions.—The administration of infliximab to these patients with Behçet's disease produced prompt and effective suppression of their acute ocular inflammation. In addition, extraocular manifestations also resolved quickly.

▶ The results are remarkable, especially considering the durability of the clinical response after only 1 or 2 infusions of infliximab. The 2 patients in the report by Sfifakis and associates (Abstract 12–26) who had oral ulcers experienced rapid resolution of them. The length of remission will be important to monitor, as the long-term consequences of multiple infusions of infliximab may be significant.[1] Nevertheless, the results suggest that TNF has an essential role in the pathogenesis of Behçet's disease, and that TNF blockade is an effective therapeutic strategy.

B. H. Thiers, MD

Reference

1. Illei GG, Lipsky PE: Novel, non-antigen-specific therapeutic approaches to autoimmune/inflammatory diseases. *Curr Opin Immunol* 12:712-718, 2000.

Cryoglobulinemia: Study of Etiologic Factors and Clinical and Immunologic Features in 443 Patients From a Single Center
Trejo O, Ramos-Casals M, García-Carrasco M, et al (Univ of Barcelona; Benemérita Universidad Autonoma de Puebla, Mexico)
Medicine 80:252-262, 2001   12–27

Background.—Cryoglobulins are immunoglobulins that precipitate when serum is incubated below 37°C. The term *cryoglobulinemic syndrome* is applied when there are symptoms such as purpura, arthralgia, and weakness. Many cases of cryoglobulinemia are associated with hepatitis C virus (HCV) infection. The etiology, symptoms, and immunologic features of a large series of consecutive patients with cryoglobulinemia were analyzed.

Study Design.—The sera from 7043 patients were tested for cryoglobulinemia between 1991 and 1999 at a single institution. A cryocrit of at least 1% was detected in 443 patients. The clinical and serologic characteristics of these 443 patients were retrospectively analyzed. Enzyme-linked immunosorbent assay was used to identify viral infection. Essential cryoglobulinemia was diagnosed in those cases in which no infectious, autoimmune, or hematologic disease could be detected.

Findings.—Of the 443 patients with cryoglobulinemia, 258 were women and 185 were men. The average age at diagnosis was 54 years. Cryocrit levels were less than 5% in 84% of these patients, while only 9% had cryocrit levels over 20%. Patients with a mixed type of cryoglobulinemia had more cutaneous manifestations, peripheral neuropathy, and

TABLE 3.—Etiologic Factors in 443 Patients With Cryoglobulinemia

	No. of Patients (%)*
Infection	331 (75)
HCV	321/443 (73)
HBV	15/443 (3)†
HIV infection	29/153 (19)‡
Autoimmune disease	94 (24)
Primary Sjögren syndrome	40 (9)
Systemic lupus erythematosus	30 (7)
Polyarteritis nodosa	7 (2)
Systemic sclerosis	6 (2)
Primary antiphospholipid syndrome	3 (1)
Rheumatoid arthritis	2 (0.5)
Autoimmune thyroiditis	2 (0.5)
Horton arteritis	2 (0.5)
Dermatomyositis-polymyositis	1 (0.2)
Henoch-Schönlein disease	1 (0.2)
Hematologic disease	33 (7)
Non-Hodgkin lymphoma	16 (4)
Chronic lymphocytic leukemia	3 (1)
Multiple myeloma	3 (1)
Hodgkin lymphoma	2 (0.5)
Chronic myeloid leukemia	2 (0.5)
Myelodysplasia	2 (0.5)
Waldenström disease	1 (0.2)
Castelman disease	1 (0.2)
Thrombocytopenic thrombotic purpura	1 (0.2)
Other diseases	2 (0.5)
Essential cryoglobulinemia	49 (11)

*The numbers of each category may add up to more than 443 because of overlapping of different etiologies.
†Twelve of 15 patients with hepatitis B virus (*HBV*) infection showed hepatitis C virus (*HCV*) coinfection
‡Twenty-two of 29 patients with HIV showed HIV coinfection
(Courtesy of Trejo O, Ramos-Casals M, García-Carrasco M, et al: Cryoglobulinemia: Study of etiologic factors and clinical and immunologic features in 443 patients from a single center. *Medicine* 80(4):252-262, 2001.)

higher rheumatoid factor levels. Infectious disease was associated with cryoglobulinemia in 75%, autoimmune disease in 24%, and hematologic disease in 7% (Table 3). Only 11% of patients had no identifiable disease associated with their cryoglobulinemia. HCV antibodies were detected in 73% of patients, hepatitis B virus (HBV) in 19%, and HIV in 19%. Most patients with HBV or HIV infection also had HCV infection.

Patients with cryoglobulinemia associated with HCV infection had a lower prevalence of autoimmune and hematologic disease. Patients infected with HCV had a lower prevalence of articular involvement; cutaneous involvement; lymphadenopathy; fever; Raynaud's phenomenon; antinuclear antibodies; and anti-Ro/SS-A, anti-La/SS-B, and anti-dsDNA autoantibodies. Clinical manifestations of cryoglobulinemia were detected in 47% of patients. At onset, the most common manifestations were cutaneous involvement, articular involvement, renal involvement, and peripheral neuropathy (Table 5). Palpable purpura was the most common

TABLE 5.—Clinical Manifestations at Onset and During Disease Evolution in 206 of 443 Patients in Whom Cryoglobulinic Symptomatology Developed

	At Onset No. (%)	Cumulative No. (%)
Cutaneous involvement	105 (24)	112 (25)
Articular involvement	82 (19)	91 (21)
Renal involvement*	80 (18)	115 (26)
Weakness	38 (9)	45 (10)
Peripheral neuropathy	26 (6)	35 (8)
Temperature >37.5°C	19 (4)	21 (5)
Lymphadenopathy	16 (4)	22 (5)
Central nervous system involvement	8 (2)	11 (2)
Pulmonary involvement	6 (1)	9 (2)
Intestinal infarction	1 (0.2)	5 (1)

*Patients with lupus nephropathy were excluded.
(Courtesy of Trejo O, Ramos-Casals M, García-Carrasco M, et al: Cryoglobulinemia: Study of etiologic factors and clinical and immunologic features in 443 patients from a single center. *Medicine* 80(4):252-262, 2001.)

cutaneous manifestation (Table 6). Patients with a cryocrit of greater than 5% were more likely to have clinical manifestations.

Conclusion.—Infectious disease was associated with the majority of these cases, and autoimmune and hematologic disease were detected frequently as well. Essential cryoglobulinemia was only diagnosed in 11% of these patients. Clinical manifestations were detected in 47%. The most common were cutaneous, renal, or articular involvement or peripheral neuropathy. Clinical manifestations were associated with a higher cryocrit in patients with cryoglobulinemia.

▶ The high incidence of HCV infection, even in patients with underlying hemologic or autoimmune disorders, is striking. With the exception of HCV, HBV, and HIV infection, infectious disorders were notably absent. Of interest to dermatologists was the high incidence of cutaneous involvement (nearly 25%) at disease onset; in fact, skin signs were the most common presenting

TABLE 6.—Cutaneous Manifestations During Disease Evolution

	No. (%)
Purpura	67 (15)
Raynaud phenomenon	23 (5)
Skin rash	20 (5)
Supramalleolar ulcers	16 (4)
Distal ischemia/grangrenous changes	9 (2)
Livedo reticularis	5 (1)
Acrocyanosis	3 (1)

(Courtesy of Trejo O, Ramos-Casals M, García-Carrasco M, et al: Cryoglobulinemia: Study of etiologic factors and clinical and immunologic features in 443 patients from a single center. *Medicine* 80(4):252-262, 2001.)

complaint. Palpable purpura was the most common skin finding, with Raynaud's phenomenon and ulcers on the distal lower extremities (most often in the supramalleolar region) being seen in a significant number of patients as well. Arthritic complaints, renal involvement, and other nonspecific signs were also important features in cryoglobulinemic patients.

B. H. Thiers, MD

Risk Factors for Visual Loss in Giant Cell (Temporal) Arteritis: A Prospective Study of 174 Patients
Liozon E, Herrmann F, Ly K, et al (Dupuytren's Univ, Limoges, France; Univ Hosps of Geneva)
Am J Med 111:211-217, 2001
12–28

Background.—Patients with temporal or giant cell arteritis can have permanent visual loss, but the risk factors associated with this complication are not known. The relationship between thrombocytosis and visual loss was examined in a large group of patients with temporal arteritis.

Study Design.—The study group consisted 147 patients with biopsy-proven giant cell arteritis. At diagnosis, pretreatment clinical, laboratory, and pathology data were recorded. All patients were treated according to the same protocol. Only visual events that occurred either before or within 2 weeks after therapy initiation were included. Multivariate logistic regression analysis was used to explore the relationship between pretreatment characteristics and visual loss.

Findings.—Visual ischemic complications of giant cell arteritis developed in 28% of patients, and permanent visual loss occurred in 13%. Independent factors associated with an increased risk of permanent visual loss included transient visual ischemic symptoms and high platelet counts. Constitutional symptoms, polymyalgia rheumatica, and C-reactive protein level were associated with a decreased risk of permanent visual loss. No patients with upper limb artery involvement had permanent visual loss. Of the 87 patients with thrombocytosis, 37% had ischemic visual complications compared with 18% of those without thrombocytosis.

Conclusions.—A large group of patients with temporal arteritis were evaluated to identify prognostic factors for the development of permanent visual loss. An elevated platelet count was strongly associated with a risk of permanent visual loss in this group of patients. This suggests that standard treatment with glucocorticoids may not be sufficient for patients with giant cell arteritis and thrombocytosis. Further studies should be performed to examine whether additional therapy with anticoagulants or platelet inhibitor agents would be useful for these patients.

▶ The results suggest that systemic steroid treatment alone may be inadequate for patients with temporal arteritis and thrombocytosis. Studies need to be performed to demonstrate whether anticoagulants or platelet inhibitors might be helpful. Such studies would need to respect the possible cumulative toxic effects of nonsteroidal anti-inflammatory drugs when given together with systemic steroids.

B. H. Thiers, MD

Predictive Factors for Renal Sequelae in Adults With Henoch-Schönlein Purpura

García-Porrúa C, González-Louzao C, Llorca J, et al (Univ of Cantabria, Santander, Spain)

J Rheumatol 28:1019-1024, 2001   12–29

Background.—There has been extensive reporting of pediatric Henoch-Schönlein purpura (HSP), which is generally considered to be a self-limited and benign condition. However, little has been reported regarding adult HSP. The outcome and risk factors for renal sequelae in an unselected population of adults with HSP were examined.

Methods.—Twenty-eight patients (19 men) older than 20 years with biopsy-proved cutaneous vasculitis who received a diagnosis of HSP between 1984 and 1998 at a single center were retrospectively studied. Patients were included if their HSP was classified by means of proposed criteria, and if they were available for at least 1 year of follow-up. Patients with cutaneous leukocytoclastic vasculitis not related to HSP were excluded.

Results.—The mean follow-up period was 5.5 years, at which time 36% of patients (n = 10) showed renal sequelae and 7% (n = 2) had renal insufficiency. Other factors including gender, drug history, and age at disease onset did not correlate with permanent renal problems. Renal sequelae were found most frequently in patients who had hematuria at disease onset or renal involvement during the course of the disease ($P <$ .001). Those with renal sequelae were more likely to have disease onset during the summer ($P <$ .05) and were more likely to be anemic ($P =$ .05) at disease onset. Patients with relapses of HSP demonstrated a higher trend to develop renal sequelae ($P =$ .07). Permanent renal involvement was found in all patients who had at least 2 of these 5 risk factors. With this model, renal sequelae could be predicted in 8 of the 10 patients who had this complication. The Goodman-Kruskal gamma test yielded a value of 0.92 (95% confidence interval, 0.78-1.00).

Conclusion.—Renal sequelae are fairly common in adult patients with HSP. Predictive factors for developing renal involvement include hematuria at disease onset, ongoing renal manifestations, summer onset, anemia at disease onset, and disease relapse.

▶ The findings are not surprising. One would expect that the HSP patients most likely to have long-term renal sequelae would be those who have renal involvement at the time of diagnosis. Any patient with cutaneous vasculitis, especially with associated signs of renal involvement (hematuria, proteinuria, etc), needs to be monitored for evidence of continuing renal compromise.

B. H. Thiers, MD

Grading of Acute and Chronic Renal Lesions in Henoch-Schönlein Purpura
Szeto CC, Choi PCL, To KF, et al (Chinese Univ of Hong Kong, Shatin)
Mod Pathol 14:635-640, 2001   12–30

Introduction.—Primary immunoglobulin (Ig)A nephropathy and Henoch-Schönlein purpura (HSP) share many clinical and immunologic features, including an almost identical renal lesion, yet a possible link between the 2 disorders remains controversial. Thirty-four patients with HSP nephritis were assessed for renal outcome by means of a system used to classify primary IgA nephropathy to determine whether this system is applicable to HSP nephritis.

Methods.—Patients were identified through a review of renal biopsy cases beginning in 1984 in the files of the study institution. Selection criteria included a diagnosis of primary IgA nephropathy; a nonthrombocytopenic purpura; a minimum follow-up of 12 months; and 5 mm or greater of renal cortex, 10 glomeruli, and 3 arterioles on light microscopy. Features analyzed at the time of renal biopsy and during follow-up were patient age and sex and measurements of serum creatinine, proteinuria, and blood pressure. Biopsy sections were independently scored by 2 investigators.

Results.—The median follow-up period was 65 months. A correlation was found between renal survival and hypertension and serum levels of creatinine and proteinuria at the time of renal biopsy. Acute glomerular lesions were common; mesangial hypercellularity was observed in 41% of cases, endocapillary proliferation in 12%, necrosis in 50%, cellular crescents in 29%, and leukocyte infiltration in 32%. Only glomerular necrotizing lesions and cellular crescents correlated with renal survival. Evaluation of chronic renal lesions, based on a grading system applied to primary IgA nephropathy, was predictive of subsequent clinical events associated with disease progression, including impaired renal function, significant proteinuria, and development of hypertension.

Discussion.—Not all patients with HSP will experience significant renal symptoms or nephritis, but some will exhibit a slowly progressive course culminating in end-stage renal failure. The distinction between acute and chronic lesions of HSP nephritis is important for both management and prognosis. When chronic renal lesions are present, therapy designed to control hypertension and significant proteinuria should be initiated.

▶ This article attempts to correlate the histology of renal lesions with the prognosis of patients affected with HSP. Szeto et al found that all chronic renal lesions were predictive of renal outcome, and hence their presence was of prognostic significance. In contrast, of acute lesions, only glomerular necrosis and cellular crescents were associated with progressive nephritis and renal failure. Thus, the histologic distinction between acute and chronic lesions has implications for prognosis and management of the renal disease in patients with HSP. The frequency of renal disease in HSP, estimates of which have ranged from 25% to 85%,[1] was not addressed in this study, which included patients specifically selected for biopsy because of the suspicion of significant renal involvement.

B. H. Thiers, MD

Reference

1. Kaku Y, Nohara K, Honda S: Renal involvement in Henoch-Schonlein purpura: A multivariate analysis of prognostic factors. *Kidney Int* 53:1755-1759, 1998.

13 Blistering Disorders

Bullous Pemphigoid Therapy—Think Globally, Act Locally
Stern RS (Beth Israel Deaconess Med Ctr, Boston)
N Engl J Med 346:364-367, 2002   13–1

Background.—Bullous pemphigoid accounts for approximately 75% of cases of autoimmune blistering skin disease. Until recently, systemic immunosuppressive agents, particularly oral corticosteroids, have been the standard treatment for this disease. However, oral corticosteroids are responsible for much of the excess mortality and morbidity among patients treated for bullous pemphigoid, and a recent French study (Abstract 13–2) has supported the use of high-dose topical corticosteroids as safer and more effective than oral corticosteroids in the treatment of extensive bullous pemphigoid. This article reviews the clinical findings in bullous pemphigoid, the use of oral versus topical corticosteroids for treatment, and the differences between the American and European health care systems that mitigate against the widespread adoption of therapies that require extensive topical treatment.

Overview.—The criteria that differentiate bullous pemphigoid from other blistering skin diseases are the absence of atrophic scars, the absence of mucosal involvement, the absence of involvement of the head and neck, and age of more than 70 years (Table 1). Bullous pemphigoid is clinically and immunologically distinct from the pemphigus group of autoimmune interepidermal diseases. The significantly higher incidence of bullous pemphigoid among elderly persons differentiates it from most other autoimmune diseases. Mortality rates are significantly higher among these patients than among similar patients without bullous pemphigoid. Oral corticosteroid treatment is the standard but has been found to be responsible for much of the excess mortality and morbidity that accompanies this disease. Joly et al (Abstract 13–2) have reported that large quantities of high-potency topical corticosteroids applied to the entire body surface were safer and more effective in controlling extensive bullous pemphigoid than oral corticosteroids. Patients treated in this manner had shorter hospital stays, more rapid control of disease, fewer severe complications, and lower mortality rates than patients treated systemically with prednisone. There was a significant reduction in the incidence of severe adverse events likely related to corticosteroid use.

TABLE 1.—Clinical Features and Antigenic Targets of Autoimmune Blistering Skin Diseases*

Bullous Disease	Percentage of Cases	Characteristics of Patients	Clinical Features	Principal Target Antigens
Bullous pemphigoid	74	Elderly (>60 yr old)	Tense blisters, pruritic, involvement of trunk and proximal extremities, involvement of mucous membranes (20%), absence of scarring	BPAG1, BPAG2
Cicatricial pemphigoid	12	Elderly (>60 yr old), twice as common in women	Involvement of mucous membranes (especially oral cavity or conjunctiva) (95%), limited skin involvement, scarring	BPAG2, integrin β_4, laminin-5 or 6, type VII collagen
Herpes gestationis	4	Pregnant or post partum	Papulovesicular, pruritic, involvement of abdomen, self-limited	BPAG2
Linear IgA dermatosis	5	Adult	Heterogeneous, pruritic, involvement of extensor surface, involvement of mucous membranes (70%)	BPAG2, type VII collagen, LAD-1†
Chronic bullous disease of childhood	?	Child (<5 yr old)	Tense blisters, "cluster of jewels" appearance, perineal and perioral, involvement of mucous membranes (70%)	BPAG2, type VII collagen, LAD-1†
Epidermolysis bullosa acquisita	3	Adult, associated with inflammatory bowel disease	Tense blisters, noninflammatory, skin fragility, acral distribution, scarring, milia	Type VII collagen
Bullous systemic lupus erythematosus	2	History of systemic lupus erythematosus	Resembles epidermolysis bullosa acquisita, systemic lupus erythematosus	Type VII collagen

*BPAG1 denotes bullous pemphigoid antigen 1, and BPAG2 bullous pemphigoid antigen 2.
†LAD-1 is a 97-kD protein located in the lamina lucida, but it is uncertain whether it is a distinct antigen or is part of the extracellular portion of BPAG2.
(Reprinted by permission of *The New England Journal of Medicine* from Stern RS: Bullous pemphigoid therapy—think globally, act locally. *N Engl J Med* 346:364-367, 2002. Copyright 2002, Massachusetts Medical Society. All rights reserved.)

Conclusions.—Topical corticosteroids should now be considered the treatment of choice for patients with bullous pemphigoid. However, significant differences between the health care systems in the United States and Europe, where this study was conducted, may preclude the widespread adoption of topical therapy. Inpatient skin care is still widely available in Europe, but in the United States, access to and payment for long-term intensive nursing for skin diseases are limited.

A Comparison of Oral and Topical Corticosteroids in Patients With Bullous Pemphigoid

Joly P, for the Bullous Diseases French Study Group (Univ of Rouen, France; Univ of Paris XII; Bichat Univ, Paris; et al)
N Engl J Med 346:321-327, 2002

13–2

Introduction.—Systemic corticosteroids are considered the standard treatment for bullous pemphigoid, but these agents are poorly tolerated by the elderly patients in whom this autoimmune disease most often occurs. A multicenter trial was conducted to determine whether topical corticosteroids might be a safer, more effective means of controlling bullous pemphigoid.

Methods.—The 341 newly diagnosed patients enrolled in the prospective, randomized trial were drawn from 20 dermatologic centers in France. All were stratified according to disease severity and assigned to topical clobetasol propionate cream (40 g per day) or oral prednisone (0.5 mg/kg body weight per day for moderate disease; 1 mg/kg body weight per day for extensive disease). After disease control was achieved, the initial dose of prednisone was maintained for 15 days. The dose was then reduced by 15% every 3 weeks and stopped after 12 months. Patients were monitored for relapse and overall survival.

Results.—During the 1-year follow-up period, 107 patients died. The topical corticosteroid was superior to oral prednisone among the 188 patients with extensive bullous pemphigoid. Mortality in these patients was 24% in the topical corticosteroid group versus 41% in the oral prednisone group. In patients with moderate bullous pemphigoid, the rate of control at 3 weeks and the incidence of severe complications did not differ between topical and oral treatment groups. In these patients, the mortality rate was 30% in each treatment group. Severe complications were common overall but occurred at a higher rate among patients treated with oral prednisone (54%) than among those treated with topical corticosteroids (29%).

Conclusion.—Systemic corticosteroids cause numerous side effects when used to treat bullous pemphigoid in elderly patients. Clobetasol propionate cream proved an effective alternative to oral prednisone in patients with both moderate and extensive disease. For all outcomes examined (overall survival, disease control, severe side effects, and length of hospitalization), the topical corticosteroid was superior in treating patients with extensive bullous pemphigoid.

▶ In his editorial (Abstract 13–1) accompanying this article, Stern included a table summarizing the key clinical and immunologic features of the major blistering diseases (Table 1) and a diagram beautifully illustrating the immunopathology of the dermal-epidermal junction (Fig 1; see original article[1]). Also, he insightfully acknowledged that although the data presented by Joly et al suggest that topical steroids should be considered the treatment of choice for bullous pemphigoid, such a philosophy is unlikely to be adopted in the United States, where our social and health care systems are not supportive of such labor-intensive therapies.

B. H. Thiers, MD

Reference

1. Stern RS: Bullous pemphigoid therapy—Think globally, act locally. *N Engl J Med* 346:364-367, 2002.

Mast Cells Play a Key Role in Neutrophil Recruitment in Experimental Bullous Pemphigoid
Chen R, Ning G, Zhao M-L, et al (Univ of North Carolina, Chapel Hill; Med College of Wisconsin, Milwaukee; Univ of California, San Francisco)
J Clin Invest 108:1151-1158, 2001   13–3

Introduction.—Bullous pemphigoid (BP) is an acquired autoimmune inflammatory disease that is characterized by autoantibodies against 2 hemidesmosomal antigens, BP230 (BPAG1) and BP180 (BPAG2), and subepidermal blisters. Mast cell (MC) degranulation is a feature of BP. Chemoattractants from MCs, including eosinophilic/neutrophilic chemotactic factors and histamine, are observed in high concentrations in BP blister fluids. Similar skin lesions are present in the pregnancy-related nonviral disorder herpes gestationis. These findings suggest that MCs may have a role in blister formation. The role of MCs was examined in experimental BP with the use of mice genetically deficient in MCs.

Findings.—Wild-type mice injected intradermally with pathogenic anti-mBP180 IgG experienced extensive MC degranulation in skin, which preceded neutrophil infiltration and subsequent subepidermal blistering. Mice genetically deficient in MCs or MC-sufficient animals pretreated with an inhibitor of MC degranulation did not develop BP. In contrast, MC-deficient mice reconstituted in skin with MCs became susceptible to experimental BP. Despite the activation of complement to yield C3a and C5a, in the absence of MCs, accumulation of neutrophils at the injection site was blunted (Fig 2). The lack of response caused by MC deficiency was overcome by intradermal administration of a neutrophil chemoattractant, IL-8, or by reconstitution of the injection sites with neutrophils.

+/+   Mgf SI/Mgf SI-d

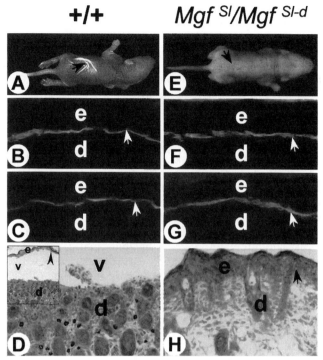

FIGURE 2.—Clinical and immunohistological analysis of neonatal MC-deficient and -sufficient mice injected with pathogenic anti-MBP180 IgG. The anti-MBP180 IgG (2.5 mg/g body weight) induced extensive blistering disease in MC-sufficient (+/+) mice (A). The skin of these animals showed linear deposition of rabbit IgG (B) and murine C3 (C) at the BMZ, as determined by direct IF. Toluidine blue-staining revealed epidermal-dermal separation with MC degranulation (D). In contrast, MC-deficient (MGf^{sl}/Mgfs^{sl-d}) mice injected intradermally with pathogenic IgG showed no evidence of skin disease (E). Direct IF demonstrated BMZ deposition of rabbit IgG (F) and murine C3 (G). Toluidine blue staining showed no epidermal-dermal separation and absence of MCs (H). *d*, dermis; *e*, epidermis; *v*, vesicle; *black arrow* in A and E, site of clinical blister; *white arrow*, site of antibody labeling; *black arrow* in D and H, site of BMZ. ×400. Inset in D is a lower-magnification micrograph showing the edge of a subepidermal vesicle. ×100. (Reprinted with permission of the *Journal of Clinical Investigation* from Chen R, Ning G, Zhao M-L, et al: Mast cells play a key role in neutrophil recruitment in experimental bullous pemphigoid. *J Clin Invest* 108:1151-1158, 2001. Reproduced by permission of the publisher via Copyright Clearance Center, Inc.)

Conclusion.—These findings offer the first direct evidence that MCs have an important role in neutrophil recruitment during subepidermal blister formation in experimental BP.

▶ Chen et al present evidence that the subepidermal blistering induced by pathogenetic anti-mBP180 antibodies depends on MCs, whose degranulation plays an essential role in recruiting neutrophils to the target tissue. MC products, including tumor necrosis factor-alpha and tryptase, have been linked directly to neutrophil influx, although it is still not known whether they play a key role in recruiting neutrophils in BP. Also to be determined is whether inhibition of MC degranulation could be an effective therapeutic strategy for controlling this disease.

B. H. Thiers, MD

Anti-epiligrin Cicatricial Pemphigoid and Relative Risk for Cancer

Egan CA, Lazarova Z, Darling TN, et al (NIH, Bethesda, Md)
Lancet 357:1850-1851, 2001   13–4

Introduction.—Patients with anti-epiligrin cicatricial pemphigoid (AECP) may have an increased risk of cancer, but the extent of this risk has not been determined. The incidence of cancer in a cohort of patients with AECP was compared with that of the general population.

Methods.—The 35 patients included in the study were assembled over a 12-year period; all met the case definition for AECP. Patients with this form of cicatricial pemphigoid have pathogenic IgG autoantibodies directed against laminin 5 ($\alpha3\beta3\gamma2$) in the epidermal basement membrane. The median age of the cohort was 65 years. Cohort entry was defined as either 12 months before the onset of AECP or at the date of blister onset. Controls were 100 normal volunteers, 130 patients with other immunobullous diseases, and 50 patients with solid cancers. Sera from patients and controls were obtained for indirect immunofluorescence microscopy and immunoprecipitation studies.

Results.—A solitary cancer developed in 10 patients (28.6%) with AECP during a median observation period of 2.67 years (with cohort entry calculated as 12 months before the onset of blisters). There were 3 lung, 3 stomach, 2 colon, and 2 endometrial cancers. The cancer was diagnosed in 8 patients after onset of AECP (6 within 1 year and 7 within 14 months). For 9 of the 10 patients, the time between blister onset and cancer diagnosis ranged from 14 months before to 14 months after the AECP diagnosis. Eight of the 10 patients with cancer died during the follow-up period, and all deaths were cancer related.

Conclusion.—Depending on the method of determining cohort entry date, the relative risk (RR) of development of cancer among these patients with AECP was 6.8 or 7.7. Their RR of cancer was similar to that for adults with dermatomyositis, and for both AECP and dermatomyositis the RR of cancer is particularly high in the first year of the disease. Drug treatment was not a likely cause of cancer in these patients with AECP.

▶ Patients with the anti-epiligrin variant of cicatricial pemphigoid represent a subset of patients with that disorder. Previous studies have suggested an association between cancer and bullous pemphigoid, particularly in seronegative patients with mucosal involvement. These reports date from a time when antiepiligrin cicatricial pemphigoid could not be differentiated from bullous pemphigoid, and it is possible that those cohorts included a disproportionate number of patients who were immunologically similar to those cited in the current study.

B. H. Thiers, MD

Antibodies to Desmogleins 1 and 3, but Not to BP180, Induce Blisters in Human Skin Grafted onto SCID Mice

Zillikens D, Schmidt E, Reimer S, et al (Univ of Würzburg, Germany; Univ of Frankfurt, Germany)
J Pathol 193:117-124, 2001   13–5

Introduction.—The autoimmune skin disease pemphigus is character-ized by the formation of intraepidermal blisters. In bullous pemphigoid (BP), a subepidermal blistering disease of the elderly, autoantibodies are directed against 2 hemidesmosomal proteins, BP230 and BP180. Because passive transfer models for pemphigus and BP have a number of disad-vantages, researchers used a different strategy and grafted human skin onto mice with severe combined immune deficiency (SCID). Purified IgG from well-characterized patients was then passively transferred into the human grafts.

Methods.—The sera studied were from 2 patients with pemphigus fo-liaceus (PF), 1 with pemphigus vulgaris (PV), 2 with BP, and 3 healthy control subjects. Three weeks after receiving grafts of human skin from adult and neonatal foreskins, the mice were injected with IgG, recombi-nant interleukin-8 (IL-8), and recombinant human C5a.

Results.—The injection of purified IgG fraction from the serum of patients with PF and PV resulted in subcorneal and suprabasal splits in the human grafts, and human IgG was deposited intercellularly in the upper and lower layers of the epidermis. The anti-BP180 autoantibodies purified from the serum of patients with BP and from a rabbit immunized with recombinant human BP180 strongly bound to the basement membrane zone of the grafts, fixed murine complement, and led to the recruitment of neutrophils to the upper dermis of the graft, but did not induce subepi-dermal blisters.

Conclusion.—In previous transfer neonatal mouse models for pemphi-gus and BP, disease developed in the murine host but not in human tissue. In the experimental model used here, acantholytic blisters were induced in human skin grafted onto SCID mice that were injected with antibodies to desmogleins (Dsg) 1 or 3 from patients with PF and PV, respectively.

▶ Hopefully, this new experimental model will be used to identify pathoge-netically relevant epitopes on human Dsg 1 and 3. This may lead to novel therapies for PF and PV. The inability of anti-BP180 autoantibodies to induce subepidermal blisters is curious, especially given their ability to bind to the basement membrane zone of the graft, fix murine complement, and recruit neutrophils to the upper dermis of the graft. Previous studies in neonatal mice have failed to show significant binding of human anti-BP180 autoantibodies to the basement membrane zone of the mice, which likely reflects the lack of crossreactivity of the anti-BP180 autoantibodies with antigens in the mouse basement membrane.

B. H. Thiers, MD

The Severity of Cutaneous and Oral Pemphigus Is Related to Desmoglein 1 and 3 Antibody Levels
Harman KE, Seed PT, Gratian MJ, et al (St Thomas' Hosp, London; Guy's Hosp, London; King's College, London)
Br J Dermatol 144:775-780, 2001   13–6

Introduction.—Pemphigus vulgaris (PV) and pemphigus foliaceus (PF) are characterized by autoantibodies to the desmosomal proteins desmoglein 3 (Dsg3) and desmoglein 1 (Dsg1), respectively. Earlier trials using indirect immunofluorescence (IIF) as a measure of pemphigus antibody levels have not consistently demonstrated a correlation between disease severity and IIF levels. Unlike enzyme-linked immunosorbent assays (ELISA), which use recombinant proteins, IIF is not capable of measuring Dsg1 and 3 antibodies separately. With the use of ELISA, the severity of oral ulceration and cutaneous involvement were independently compared with Dsg1 and 3 antibody levels in 104 patients with PV and PE.

Methods.—A total of 424 serum samples were analyzed from 80 and 24 patients with PV and PF, respectively. The presence of Dsg1 autoantibodies in PF and Dsg3 autoantibodies in PV were examined with the use of ELISA. The associated severity of skin and oral disease was graded from 0 to 3 (quiescent, mild, moderate, and severe) in all samples.

Results.—An association was shown between Dsg1 antibodies and skin severity to the degree that a 10-unit increase in the Dsg1 ELISA value was correlated with a 34% chance of having a higher severity score ($P < .0005$). This was seen in both PV and PF. A 10-unit increase in the Dsg3 ELISA value was correlated with a 25% chance of a higher oral severity score ($P < .0005$). A wide range of Dsg3 ELISA values were observed with each oral disease severity score. A general trend of increasing oral disease severity and rising Dsg3 ELISA value was observed. No consistent association between oral disease severity and Dsg1 ELISA values was observed, even after correction for the effect of Dsg3 antibodies. No association between Dsg3 antibodies and skin severity or between oral disease severity and Dsg1 ELISA values was found (Fig 1; see color plates X and XI).

Conclusion.—In pemphigus, skin disease severity is associated with Dsg1 antibodies; oral severity is associated with Dsg3 antibody levels. Any combination of clinical characteristics can generally be explained by levels of Dsg1 and 3 autoantibodies.

▶ This nicely done study is yet another in a series of articles that documents the importance of the desmosomal antibody profile in patients with PV and PF.[1-4] The Dsg1 antibody titer seems to correlate with the severity of skin

FIGURE 1

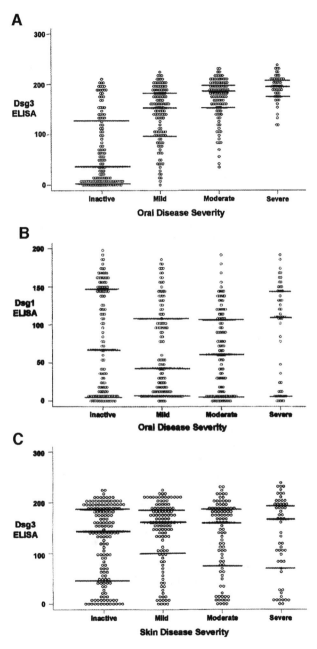

(*Continued*)

FIGURE 1 (cont.)

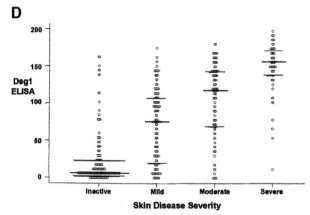

D

Dsg1 ELISA

Skin Disease Severity

FIGURE 1.—A, Oral disease severity in pemphigus vulgaris (PV) and pemphigus foliaceus (PF) plotted against desmoglein (Dsg) 3 antibody levels measured by enzyme-linked immunosorbent assay (ELISA). Median and quartile values are marked with red and green lines, respectively. A 10-unit increase in Dsg3 ELISA value was associated with a 25% greater chance of having a higher oral severity score [95% CI, 17%-33%, $P < .0005$]. B, Oral disease severity in PV and PF plotted against Dsg1 antibody levels. C, Skin disease severity in PV and PF plotted against Dsg1 antibody levels. A 10-unit increase in Dsg1 ELISA value was associated with a 34% greater chance of having a higher oral severity score (CI, 25%-45%, $P < .0005$). D, Skin disease severity in PV and PF plotted against Dsg3 antibody levels. (Courtesy of Harman KE, Seed PT, Gratian MJ, et al: The severity of cutaneous and oral pemphigus is related to desmoglein 1 and 3 antibody levels. *Br J Dermatol* 144:775-780, 2001. Reprinted by permission of Blackwell Science, Inc.)

disease, whereas the Dsg3 antibody titer seems to correlate with the severity of oral lesions. Antigen expression at various skin and mucous membrane sites also likely plays a role in determining the clinical phenotype.

B. H. Thiers, MD

References

1. Amagai M, Tsunoda K, Zillikens D, et al: The clinical phenotype of pemphigus is defined by the anti-desmoglein autoantibody profile. *J Am Acad Dermatol* 40:167-170, 1999.
2. Harman KE, Gratian MJ, Bhogal BS, et al: A study of desmoglein 1 autoantibodies in pemphigus vulgaris: Racial differences in frequency and the association with a more severe phenotype. *Br J Dermatol* 143:343-348, 2000.
3. Mahoney MG, Wang Z, Rothenberger K, et al: Explanations for the clinical and microscopic localisation of lesions in pemphigus foliaceus and vulgaris. *J Clin Invest* 103:461-468, 1999.
4. Wu H, Wang ZH, Yan A, et al: Protection against pemphigus foliaceus by desmoglein 3 in neonates. *N Engl J Med* 343:31-35, 2000.

Intravenous Immunoglobulin Therapy in the Treatment of Patients With Pemphigus Vulgaris Unresponsive to Conventional Immunosuppressive Treatment

Ahmed AR (Harvard Univ, Boston)
J Am Acad Dermatol 45:679-690, 2001   13–7

Background.—Severe pemphigus vulgaris (PV) is conventionally treated with high-dose oral prednisone, usually in combination with an immunosuppressive agent (ISA). Some patients experience significant side effects, which are sometimes fatal, from prolonged immunosuppression.

Objective.—Intravenous immunoglobulin (IVIg) was administered to 21 patients with severe cutaneous and mucosal PV who had not responded to the prolonged use of oral prednisone and multiple ISAs.

Methods.—A preliminary dose-determination study tested 7 additional volunteers to ascertain the optimal IVIg dose of 2 g/kg per cycle. Parameters to assess clinical outcome were recorded before and after IVIg therapy. Variables tested were highest dose, total dose, and duration of prednisone and ISAs, their side effects, frequency of recurrence and relapse, duration of IVIg therapy, clinical response, induction and duration of remission, number of hospitalizations, total days of hospital stay, and quality of life.

Results.—Use of IVIg monotherapy resulted in effective control of disease and produced a sustained remission in the 21 patients. The patients became free of lesions and remained so after finishing IVIg therapy. IVIg had a steroid-sparing effect and produced a high quality of life. Serious side effects from the use of IVIg were not observed. IVIg needs to be gradually withdrawn after achievement of clinical control.

Conclusion.—In patients with PV who do not respond to conventional immunosuppressants, IVIg appears to be an effective treatment alternative. Its early use is of significant benefit in patients who may experience life-threatening complications from immunosuppression. IVIg is effective as monotherapy.

▶ Assessment of the effectiveness of IVIg for treating various autoimmune and inflammatory diseases has been compromised by a lack of controlled studies. Nevertheless, the results reported by Ahmed certainly appear to be impressive and worthy of follow-up in controlled trials.

B. H. Thiers, MD

Toxic Epidermal Necrolysis Treated With Intravenous High-Dose Immunoglobulins: Our Experience

Stella M, Cassano P, Bollero D, et al (Trauma Centre, Torino, Italy)
Dermatology 203:45-49, 2001   13–8

Background.—Burn surgeons have become interested in the syndrome termed toxic epidermal necrolysis (TEN), whose clinical presentation is similar to that of extensive partial-thickness burns. The mortality rate of this severe acute exfoliative drug-induced skin and mucosal disorder averages 10% to 40%. Many different drugs have been identified as causative. The mechanism underlying TEN may involve changes in the control of keratinocyte apoptosis, which is mediated by the interaction of the cell surface death receptor Fas and its ligand, FasL (CD95L). Specifically, upregulation of keratinocyte FasL expression may act as a trigger for keratinocytic destruction in TEN. Treatment with IV immunoglobulins (IVIG), which inhibit Fas–FasL–mediated apoptosis, has proved effective. Treatment with high-dose IVIG and IV pulse methylprednisolone was evaluated.

Methods.—The 9 patients evaluated had been admitted to the Turin Burn Centre from January 1999 to October 2000. One was given a diagnosis of Stevens-Johnson syndrome and 8 of TEN. Each patient was treated with high doses (0.6 to 0.7 g/kg of body weight daily) of IVIG for 4 days and received IV methylprednisolone (250 mg) every 6 hours for the first 48 hours after admission. In addition, patients were given prophylactic low–molecular-weight heparin, H_2 antihistamines, and gastric protectors. Efficacy was assessed as time between the beginning IVIG therapy and cessation of further epidermal detachment and time needed for complete healing of the skin lesions.

Results.—The 9 patients had erythematous body surface areas of between 38% and 85% and dermoepidermal detachment of 4% to 37%. One patient died of septic shock and multiple organ failure. The 8 who were healed had further epidermal detachment cease an average of 4.8 days after beginning treatment with IVIG. After 12 days, on average, complete wound healing was accomplished. Three patients had acute respiratory failure that required mechanical ventilation; 1 had acute renal failure that responded to dialysis. Dyschromia and nail dystrophies were noted on long-term assessment. No hypertrophic scars occurred.

Conclusion.—IVIG with methylprednisolone appeared to halt the progression of TEN and decrease mortality. Thus, it may be considered effective treatment for this disorder.

▶ The title of the article is somewhat misleading; the treatment protocol used would more appropriately be characterized as high-dose IVIG *plus* IV pulse methylprednisolone rather than IVIG alone. The results are impressive, with an 89% survival rate. Unfortunately, it is unclear whether biopsy specimens were taken to confirm the diagnosis in any or all of the patients. The authors cite previous studies that suggest that upregulation of keratinocyte Fas ligand (FasL or CD95L) expression is the critical trigger for keratinocyte destruction in TEN[1] and speculate that naturally occurring Fas-blocking antibodies found in human immunoglobulin preparations may inhibit this process.

B. H. Thiers, MD

Reference

1. Viard I, Wehrli P, Bullani R, et al: Inhibition of toxic epidermal necrolysis by blockade of CD95 with human intravenous immunoglobulin. *Science* 282:490-493, 1998.

Mixed Immunobullous Disease of Childhood: A Good Response to Antimicrobials
Powell J, Kirtschig G, Allen J, et al (Oxford Radcliffe Hosps, England)
Br J Dermatol 144:769-774, 2001   13–9

Background.—The most common of the acquired immunobullous diseases noted in children is chronic bullous disease of childhood (CBDC), with cases of bullous pemphigoid (BP), epidermolysis bullosa acquisita (EBA), and cicatricial pemphigoid (CP) occurring rarely. Most often, 1 autoantibody isotype is detected in each patient; in CBDC, it is immunoglobulin (Ig)A, and in BP, EBA, and CP, it is IgG. Eight pediatric patients with a dual response involving both IgA and IgG were evaluated. The cases were compared on the basis of presentation, immunopathologic findings, severity, and disease outcome with those of 62 children who had a single autoantibody response.

Methods.—The 8 patients were ages 3 to 12 years when examined at or shortly after presentation. Direct and indirect IF were performed. Treatment involved the use of dapsone, prednisolone, sulphapyridine, and erythromycin, as appropriate. Follow-up extended for 6 months to 4 years after the onset of disease.

Results.—Widespread disease was present in the 8 patients with a dual response, with 6 having CBDC and the 2 others having either CBDC or BP. The dual response was detected on indirect immunofluorescence (IF) in 7 patients and direct IF in 3. In 5 patients, binding was confined to the epidermal side of the basement membrane zone, 2 had bindings on the epidermal and dermal sides, and 1 had an intraepidermal antigen detected with IgG and an epidermal antigen detected with IgA. All patients responded to treatment within 3 months, with dapsone being effective for 5 patients, sulphonamides for 2, and erythromycin for 1. When only systemic steroids were used, the response to therapy sometimes occurred after more prolonged disease activity. After 1 to 4 years, 5 patients remained in remission without further treatment.

Conclusions.—Whether there was a single or a dual antibody response made no difference in the target antigens identified on immunoblotting. Because the treatment response is similar between the 2 groups, the dual antibody response apparently has no effect on the course of the disease.

▶ Eight children seen with a bullous disease were noted by direct IF of skin biopsy specimens or indirect IF of serum samples to have both IgA and IgG autoantibodies to basement membrane zone target antigens. The presence of IgG did not appear to make the children less responsive to treatment. One of them cleared after treatment with oral erythromycin and topical cortico-steroids. Because sulfapyridine may be difficult to obtain, and dapsone may cause methemoglobinemia in children, an initial trial of erythromycin in children with a linear IgA bullous disease, with or without IgG, may be a reasonable therapeutic strategy.

S. Raimer, MD

Two-Year Effects of Alendronate on Bone Mineral Density and Vertebral Fracture in Patients Receiving Glucocorticoids: A Randomized, Double-blind, Placebo-controlled Extension Trial
Adachi JD, Saag KG, Delmas PD, et al (McMaster Univ, Hamilton, Ont, Canada; Univ of Iowa, Iowa City; Hosp Edouard Herriot, Lyon, France; et al)
Arthritis Rheum 44:202-211, 2001   13–10

Introduction.—Patients given glucocorticoids are at significantly in-creased risk for hip fracture. A recent meta-analysis found that bisphos-phonate therapy is more effective than calcium, vitamin D, or calcitonin in preventing bone loss in patients with corticosteroid-induced osteoporosis. Results were reported for a 12-month extension of a previously reported 48-week randomized placebo-controlled trial in which patients receiving glucocorticoids were given alendronate (ALN), a potent bisphosphonate.

Methods.—Patients eligible for the extension study were continuing treatment with at least 7.5 mg of oral prednisone or equivalent doses of other glucocorticoids daily. All patients continued to receive calcium and vitamin D supplements. The primary end point was the mean percentage change in lumbar spine bone mineral density (BMD) from baseline to 24 months. Patients were also observed for changes in hip and total body BMD, biochemical markers of bone turnover, radiographic evidence of joint damage to the hands, and the incidence of vertebral fractures.

Results.—Of the 560 patients initially enrolled in the trial, 208 contin-ued in the double-blind extension, and 166 completed 2 years of treat-ment. BMD of the lumbar spine, total hip, trochanter, and total body increased at 24 months after treatment with 5 or 10 mg ALN. The ALN-associated improvements were increased relative to both placebo group and baseline values and were greatest within the first year of ALN treatment. On average, 84% of patients given ALN gained spinal bone mass versus 45% receiving placebo. There was a significant decrease in bone turnover markers during ALN treatment. No new vertebral fractures occurred in patients who received any dose of ALN during the second year.

Conclusion.—In this heterogeneous group of patients receiving gluco-corticoids for a variety of diseases, ALN was an effective and well-toler-ated agent for the prevention and treatment of therapy-induced osteoporo-sis. Significant increases in BMD were recorded at all measured sites, and the incidence of new vertebral fractures was reduced.

▶ Over the past several years, the pharmaceutical industry has brought us drugs to enhance bone strength and decrease the incidence of bone fractures in patients receiving prolonged glucocorticoid therapy. It is essential that we consider the use of these drugs to decrease the incidence of osteoporosis and its attendant complications in patients with chronic steroid-responsive dermatoses (like the blistering disorders discussed in this chapter) in whom long-term glucocorticoid therapy is contemplated. ALN is a difficult drug to take, and esophageal irritation is a major problem. The recently described weekly dosing regimen might be an alternative for patients unwilling or unable to comply with daily dosing.[1,2] Note that all patients in the current study received calcium and vitamin D supplementation in addition to ALN.

B. H. Thiers, MD

References

1. Baran D: Osteoporosis: Efficacy and safety of a bisphosphonate dosed once weekly. *Geriatrics* 56:28-32, 2001.
2. Schnitzer T, Bone HG, Crepaldi G, et al: Therapeutic equivalence of alendronate 70 mg once-weekly and alendronate 10 mg daily in the treatment of osteoporosis. Alendronate Once-Weekly Study Group. *Aging* (Milano) 12:1-12, 2000.

14 Photobiology

Cutaneous Photoprotection From Ultraviolet Injury by Green Tea Polyphenols
Elmets CA, Singh D, Tubesing K, et al (Case Western Reserve Univ, Cleveland, Ohio; Univ of Alabama, Birmingham; Estee Lauder Companies Inc, Research Park, Melville, NY)
J Am Acad Dermatol 44:425-432, 2001   14–1

Background.—Overexposure of the skin to the ultraviolet (UV) component of solar radiation has a number of adverse effects, including sunburn, basal cell and squamous cell carcinoma, melanoma, cataracts, photoaging of the skin, and immune suppression. The alarming increase in the incidence of sunlight-related skin and eye disorders has prompted much attention in recent years. From 1960 to 1986, a 240% increase in the incidence of cutaneous squamous cell carcinoma was reported, and in certain areas of the United States there was a 400% increase in the incidence of melanoma. In animal models, green tea extracts have demonstrated impressive efficacy in reducing the severity of adverse effects of UV radiation. The use of green tea extracts and other natural products in sunscreens is increasingly being explored. The effect of polyphenols from green tea on parameters associated with acute UV injury was evaluated.

Methods.—In a group of normal volunteers, areas of skin were treated with an extract of green tea or one of its constituents. After 30 minutes, the treated sites were exposed to a dose of simulated solar radiation. The UV-treated skin was then clinically examined for UV-induced erythema, evaluated histologically for the presence of sunburn cells or Langerhans cell distributions, or evaluated biochemically for UV-induced DNA damage.

Results.—A dose-dependent inhibition of the erythema response evoked by UV radiation resulted from the application of green tea extracts. The constituents that most efficiently inhibited erythema were the (−)-epigallocatechin-3-gallate (EGCG) and (−)-epicatechin-3-gallate (ECG) polyphenolic fractions. The (−)-epigallocatechin (EGC) and (−)-epicatechin (EC) fractions demonstrated little effect. Histologic examination of skin treated with green tea extracts revealed a reduced number of sunburn cells. In addition, epidermal Langerhans cells were protected from UV damage. The DNA damage that formed after UV radiation was also reduced by green tea extracts.

Conclusions.—Polyphenolic extracts of green tea were found to be effective chemoprotective agents for many of the adverse effects of UV solar radiation. These extracts may be useful as a natural alternative for photoprotection.

▶ The green tea story continues to evolve and was initially reviewed in the 2001 YEAR BOOK OF DERMATOLOGY. Further testing is clearly necessary to define the role that green tea polyphenols and other natural chemopreventive agents will play in protection from UV radiation damage. Unlike sunscreens, the compounds discussed here do not appear to absorb significant amounts of UV radiation. This suggests that green tea polyphenols, when combined with traditional sunscreens, may have additive or synergistic photoprotective effects.

B. H. Thiers, MD

Inhibitory Effects of Orally Administered Green Tea, Black Tea, and Caffeine on Skin Carcinogenesis in Mice Previously Treated With Ultraviolet B Light (High-Risk Mice): Relationship to Decreased Tissue Fat
Lu Y-P, Lou Y-R, Lin Y, et al (Rutgers Univ, Piscataway, NJ; Univ of Medicine and Dentistry of New Jersey, New Brunswick)
Cancer Res 61:5002-5009, 2001   14–2

Background.—The most prevalent form of cancer in the United States and many other temperate areas of the world is sunlight-induced skin cancer. UVB light and, to a lesser extent, UVA light are responsible for the development of sunlight-induced cancer. It would appear that this form of cancer is increasing in incidence and that the trend will continue as recreational exposure increases and the stratospheric ozone layer is depleted. In an earlier study, SKH-1 mice were exposed to UVB twice a week for 22 weeks. The mice were tumor-free but had hyperplasia and were at a high risk for the development of skin tumors within several months despite no additional treatment with UVB. The inhibitory effects of orally administered green tea, black tea, and caffeine on skin carcinogenesis were studied in this animal model.

Methods.—Green tea, black tea, or decaffeinated tea was administered to UVB-pretreated SKH-1 hairless mice for 23 weeks.

Results.—With green tea or black tea, the number of tumors per mouse was decreased, as were the size of the parametrial fat pads and the thickness of the dermal fat layer away from the tumors and directly under the tumors (Fig 1; see color plates XII and XIII). When decaffeinated tea was administered, there was little or no effect on any of these parameters. The addition of caffeine to the decaffeinated tea in an amount equivalent to that found in the regular teas restored the inhibitory effects of the tea. When caffeine alone was administered, decreases were seen in the number of tumors per mouse, the size of the parametrial fat pads, and the thickness of the dermal fat layer away from the tumors and under the tumors. With

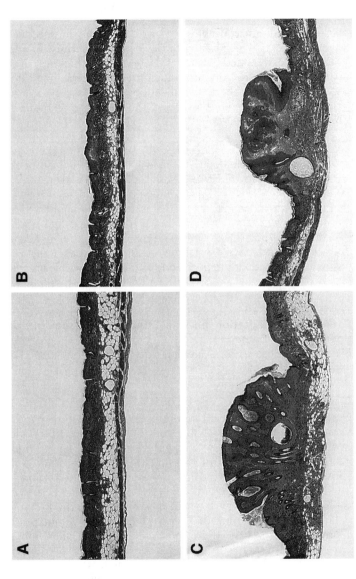

FIGURE 1.—Effect of oral administration of green tea to high-risk mice for 23 weeks on the dermal fat layer (histologic evaluation in representative mice). High-risk SKH-1 mice received water (*A and C*) or 0.6% green tea (*B and D*) as their sole drinking fluid for 23 weeks. The dermal fat layer was examined histologically (100-fold magnification) in areas of the skin away from tumors (*A and B*) and in areas under keratoacanthomas (*C and D*). (Courtesy of Lu Y-P, Lou Y-R, Lin Y, et al: Inhibitory effects of orally administered green tea, black tea, and caffeine on skin carcinogenesis in mice previously treated with ultraviolet B light (high-risk mice): Relationship to decreased tissue fat. *Cancer Res* 61:5002-5009, 2001.)

the use of data from individual mice and linear regression and correlation analysis, a highly significant positive correlation was found between the thickness of the dermal fat layer away from tumors and the number of tumors per mouse. However, the correlation between average tumor size per mouse and the thickness of the dermal fat layer away from tumors was weak.

Conclusions.—Oral administration of tea or caffeine may have reduced tumor multiplicity in part by decreasing fat levels in the dermis. In addition, it was found that caffeinated beverages decreased the thickness of the dermal fat layer under large tumors to a much greater extent than under small tumors. The results are the first indications of a close association between the inhibition of carcinogenesis and the lowering of tissue fat levels by a chemopreventive agent.

▶ The tea saga continues. Lu et al present data confirming the chemopreventive benefits of various caffeinated beverages in the pathogenesis of skin cancer. In addition, they note that these same substances decrease the thickness of the murine dermal fat layer, suggesting a close association between inhibition of carcinogenesis by a chemopreventive agent and the lowering of tissue fat levels. Whether this is a true "cause and effect" relationship is uncertain. The authors speculate that tea or caffeine-induced decreases in arachidonic acid levels in fat may result in decreased levels of prostaglandins, which are thought to play a role in the carcinogenic process.

B. H. Thiers, MD

Solar-Simulated Skin Adaptation and its Effect on Subsequent UV-Induced Epidermal DNA Damage
de Winter S, Vink AA, Roza L, et al (Leiden Univ, The Netherlands; TNO Voeding, Zeist, The Netherlands)
J Invest Dermatol 117:678-682, 2001   14–3

Background.—Many persons use tanning beds to increase their tolerance for UV radiation and erythema. But does the development of tolerance protect the skin against DNA damage? Using a UV lamp with a radiation spectrum similar to that of the sun, these authors studied the effects on DNA after a single UV exposure and after a simulated course of tanning.

Methods.—Two studies were performed; in both studies, the radiation source was a lamp that emits radiation in the UV range that simulates the spectrum of sunlight. In the first study, 25 white subjects (7 men and 18 women; mean age, 22 years) were divided on the basis of minimal erythema dose (MED) and pigmentation score into light-skinned (n = 9) and darker-skinned (n = 16) groups. At baseline, all subjects were challenged at 3 times their MED on a small area of the buttocks or lower back, then 15 minutes later, punch biopsy specimens were taken. The subjects then began a tanning course on the back skin, 3 days a week for 3 weeks.

After the final exposure, the 3-MED challenge was repeated and biopsy specimens were obtained. In the second study, 13 subjects (2 men and 11 women; mean age, 22 years) received a single dose of 1.2 MED on a previously unexposed area of the buttocks or lower back. Punch biopsy specimens were taken from both the exposed and unexposed (control) area at 15 minutes and 24, 48, 72, and 96 hours after exposure. Biopsy specimens were examined histologically to determine the thickness of the epidermis and stratum corneum. In addition, immunohistochemical staining was used to evaluate the expression of two markers of DNA damage: cyclobutane pyrimidine dimer (CPD; a DNA photoproduct) and (in the second study only) p53 protein.

Results.—At the end of 3 weeks of UV exposure, the skin of both groups was significantly darker. In addition, the epidermis was significantly thicker in both the light-skinned (by 36% ± 9%) and the darker-skinned (by 46% ± 6%) groups (between-group difference not significant). Most of this increase was attributable to a thickening of the stratum corneum. There was also a significant decrease in the sensitivity to erythema after the 3-week tanning course. MED increased by an average of 3.78 ± 0.44 units in the light-skinned group, and by 4.19 ± 0.40 units in the darker-skinned group (between-group difference, $P = .03$). At the end of the study, CPD formation was reduced by an average of 60% after the 3-MED challenge ($P < .0001$), with darker-skinned subjects having slightly (but not significantly) better protection against UV damage than the light-skinned group. In the second experiment, CPD expression became apparent as early as 15 minutes after a single UV exposure but was barely detectable at 72 hours. p53 expression peaked at 24 hours after exposure but returned to background levels by 72 to 96 hours.

Conclusions.—Repeated UV exposure protects against erythema and DNA damage, in that a 4-fold higher dose of UV radiation was needed to cause erythema and CPD formation was decreased by 60% after the 3-week course of tanning. After a single UV exposure, CPD and p53 expression return to baseline levels in 3 to 4 days. Thus, the authors recommend that, for persons who are intent on increasing their UV tolerance, only slightly erythematogenic UV doses should be used twice a week with at least 3 days between exposures.

▶ The authors show that skin adaptation to repeated UV irradiation provides some protection against UV-mediated DNA injury and that a single UV irradiation causes epidermal DNA damage that requires several days to be repaired. They then imply, without good supporting data, that allowing the skin to "rest" for a few days between UV exposures may constitute a less hazardous way of tanning.

B. H. Thiers, MD

Exposure to Ultraviolet Radiation: Association With Susceptibility and Age at Presentation With Prostate Cancer

Luscombe CJ, Fryer AA, French ME, et al (Keele Univ, Staffordshire, UK)
Lancet 358:641-642, 2001   14–4

Introduction.—Environmental factors, including latitude, are suspected in prostate cancer susceptibility. The relationship with latitude has been interpreted to indicate that ultraviolet radiation (UVR) protects against prostate cancer. UVR exposure was compared between 210 patients with sporadic prostate cancer and 155 patients with benign prostatic hypertrophy.

Findings.—A validated questionnaire was used to evaluate UVR exposure. A neutral script was used to guide questions. Cumulative lifetime exposure to UVR was determined for cases and controls (355 and 393 wks, respectively). Sun exposure was estimated with the use of weekday and weekend activity, including both occupational and recreational exposure. The UVR exposure had a significantly protective effect on cancer risk (Table 1). A comparison of the odds of having prostate cancer between the lowest and highest quartiles of exposure revealed a significant increase in protection with increased UVR. Childhood sunburn, regular foreign holidays, sunbathing score, and low exposure to UVR were correlated with the development of prostate cancer. Males with prostate cancer and low UVR exposure developed cancer at a younger median age compared with those with higher exposure (67.7 years vs 72.2 years; $P = .006$).

Conclusion.—These findings are compatible with UVR having a protective role against prostate cancer and agree with earlier reports predicting a protective effect of UVR on prostate cancer risk.

▶ Luscombe and associates present data suggesting that UV exposure may have a protective role against prostate cancer. Taking this 1 step further, one might assume that patients with nonmelanoma skin cancer (who presumably have had considerable UV exposure) should have a lower incidence of prostate cancer. The existing data are inconclusive. One report has shown that patients with basal cell carcinoma do in fact have a reduced risk of subsequent prostate cancer; however, other studies have shown that individuals with cutaneous squamous cell carcinoma have a higher than expected frequency of the disease.

B. H. Thiers, MD

TABLE.—Exposure to UV Light Derived From Questionnaire Responses

	BPH	Cancer	Odds Ratio (95% CI)	P
Chronic exposure				
Mean weeks cumulative exposure (SD)	393 (201)	355 (194)	0.998 (0.997-0.999)*	0.006
Lowest exposure quartile (%)	18.7	29.0	3.03 (1.59-5.78)	0.008
25-50% exposure quartile (%)	24.5	25.2	1.51 (0.83-2.76)	0.182
50-75% exposure quartile (%)	27.1	22.9	1.18 (0.65-2.16)	0.588
Highest exposure quartile (%)	29.7	22.9	1.00	
Living abroad in sunny country for >6 months (%)	32.9	31.0	0.71 (0.45-1.14)	0.161
Acute exposure				
Positive childhood sunburn (%)	21.9	4.3	0.18 (0.08-0.38)	0.0001
Mean sunbathing score (SD)	7.7 (2.8)	6.2 (2.8)	0.83 (0.76-0.89)†	0.0001
History of regular foreign holidays (%)	34.8	17.1	0.41 (0.25-0.68)	0.005
Mean weeks foreign holiday/year (SD)	1.05 (1.7)	0.56 (1.8)	0.85 (0.74-0.98)*	0.030

*Per week.
†Per unit score.

(Courtesy of Luscombe CJ, Fryer AA, French ME, et al: Exposure to ultraviolet radiation: Association with susceptibility and age at presentation with prostate cancer. Lancet 358:641-642, 2001. Copyright by The Lancet Ltd, 2001.)

Pseudoporphyria: A Clinical and Biochemical Study of 20 Patients
Schanbacher CF, Vanness ER, Daoud MS, et al (Mayo Clinic, Rochester, Minn)
Mayo Clin Proc 76:488-492, 2001   14–5

Background.—Pseudoporphyria, a dermatologic condition resembling porphyria cutanea tarda (PCT), is associated with various medications, such as nabumetone, naproxen, triamterene with hydrochlorothiazide, amiodarone, carisoprodol, furosemide, nalidixic acid, flutamide, tetracycline, and various nonsteroidal anti-inflammatory drugs; with UV-A radiation; and with hemodialysis. Normal or near-normal porphyrin levels are noted in the serum, urine, or stool in pseudoporphyria, differentiating it from PCT. The natural course, associated problems, and prognosis of pseudoporphyria were explored based on experience with 20 patients.

Methods.—A computerized search of the Mayo Clinic diagnostic database for all patients diagnosed with porphyrin metabolism abnormalities or pseudoporphyria was done to identify all possible cases of pseudoporphyria. Eliminating patients with noncutaneous porphyrias, well-documented PCT, and variegate porphyria left those who had cutaneous lesions resembling those of PCT but lacked the laboratory abnormalities of that disorder. The data obtained for the final population of 20 patients (13 women) included clinical, histologic, immunologic, and laboratory information, with follow-up review through visits and telephone calls.

Results.—The clinical features noted were characteristic of PCT, with 95% of patients having blisters, 70% having healed blisters with scar formation (Fig 1; see color plate XIV), 65% having photosensitivity, 65% with skin fragility, 40% having milia, 15% having hypertrichosis, and 5% with hyperpigmentation. Histologic features (gleaned from 17 patients) included subepidermal separation with classic festooning of the dermal

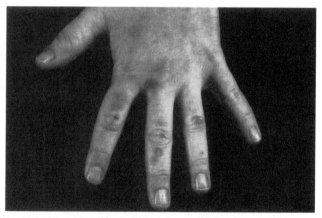

FIGURE 1.—Multiple excoriations and well-healed scars on the dorsum of the hand of a patient with pseudoporphyria. (Courtesy of Schanbacher CF, Vanness ER, Daoud MS, et al: Pseudoporphyria: A clinical and biochemical study of 20 patients. *Mayo Clin Proc* 76:488-492, 2001.)

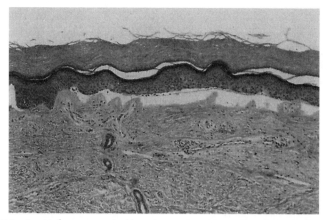

FIGURE 2.—Pauci-inflammatory subepidermal separation with prominent festooning in a patient with pseudoporphyria (hematoxylin-eosin, original magnification ×100). (Courtesy of Schanbacher CF, Vanness ER, Daoud MS, et al: Pseudoporphyria: A clinical and biochemical study of 20 patients. *Mayo Clin Proc* 76:488-492, 2001.)

papillae, minimal inflammatory infiltrates with some focal hemorrhaging in the papillary dermis in 71% of cases (Fig 2; see color plate XIV), and nonspecific findings in 5 specimens. Neither hepatitis B nor hepatitis C was found in any patient. Porphyrin profiles were not diagnostic. Persistent symptoms were noted in 11 of 16 patients during follow-up, with some extending as long as 2.5 years after assessment. Five patients had no further symptoms 1 week to 6 months after the presumed offending agent was discontinued.

Conclusions.—Normal or near-normal porphyrin levels were noted in serum, urine, or stool, but the cutaneous signs and symptoms of these patients with pseudoporphyria mimicked those of PCT. Even with discontinuation of the offending medication, symptoms persisted in several cases.

▶ Pseudoporphyria continues to be an enigma, and an identifiable inciting agent is often difficult to identify. When an offending drug is withdrawn, remission usually follows. In other cases, the cause may remain elusive, and the course may be chronic.

B. H. Thiers, MD

15 Genodermatoses

Absence of the Inferior Labial and Lingual Frenula in Ehlers-Danlos Syndrome
De Felice C, Toti P, Di Maggio G, et al (Univ of Siena, Italy)
Lancet 357:1500-1502, 2001   15–1

Background.—Various diagnostic signs have been described in patients with Ehlers-Danlos syndrome (EDS) including hyperelastic skin, hypermobile joints, tongue hypermobility, eyelid extensibility, dystrophic "cigarette paper" scarring, and postural acrocyanosis. EDS has no currently known congenital physical markers, which prevents diagnosis until clinical features develop later in life. Developmental abnormalities of the oral frenula, which is composed primarily of connective tissue, may be associated with EDS.

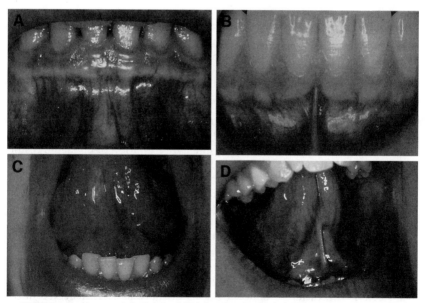

FIGURE.—**A**, Absence of the inferior labial frenulum in classical EDS; **B**, Normal inferior labial frenulum is shown for comparison; **C**, Absence of the lingual frenulum in hypermobility EDS; **D**, Normal inferior lingual frenulum is shown for comparison. *Abbreviation: EDS*, Ehlers-Danlos syndrome. (Courtesy of De Felice C, Toti P, Di Maggio G, et al: Absence of the inferior labial and lingual frenula in Ehlers-Danlos syndrome. *Lancet* 357:1500-1502. Copyright 2001, by The Lancet Ltd.)

Methods.—Twelve consecutive patients, aged 15 to 45 years (mean age, 29.7 years; 5 male), belonging to 7 unrelated families and fulfilling the clinical criteria for hypermobility EDS (n = 8) or classic EDS (n = 4), and 154 unrelated, age-matched and sex-matched controls were examined to determine whether their superior labial, inferior labial, and lingual frenula were normal or absent.

Results.—The inferior labial frenulum was absent in all 12 patients with EDS, and the lingual frenulum was also absent in 9 of these patients (Figure; see color plate XV). Of the 3 patients who did not have an absent lingual frenulum, 2 had classic and 1 had hypermobility EDS. All controls had a normal lingual frenulum, and all but one had a normal labial frenulum. The superior labial frenulum was normal in all patients and controls.

Conclusion.—Classic and hypermobility EDS was associated with absence of the lingual frenulum (71.4% sensitivity; 100% specificity) and of the inferior labial frenulum (100% sensitivity; 99.4% specificity).

▶ If confirmed, this observation would allow identification of patients with EDS at an early age, as most other clinical features develop later in life. To lessen the possibility of false-positive identifications, a family history of EDS should be elicited at the time of examination.

B. H. Thiers, MD

Adenoviral Gene Transfer Restores Lysyl Hydroxylase Activity in Type VI Ehlers-Danlos Syndrome

Rauma T, Kumpumäki S, Anderson R, et al (Univ of Oulu, Finland; Univ of Iowa, Iowa City)
J Invest Dermatol 116:602-605, 2001   15–2

Background.—Type VI Ehlers-Danlos syndrome (EDS VI) is a connective tissue disease caused by mutations in the lysyl hydroxylase 1 gene. These mutations lead to disturbed lysine hydroxylation of collagen, resulting in structurally weak collagen molecules. The skin of patients with EDS VI is hyperelastic; wounds heal poorly and are likely to leave scars. Given that EDS VI is a recessively inherited disease, it was hypothesized that transferring functional lysyl hydroxylase 1 (LH) genes into fibroblasts in and around wounds might improve local healing. The feasibility of gene transfer therapy in vitro into fibroblasts from a patient with EDS VI and in vivo into rat skin was tested.

Methods.—Human LH cDNA was cloned into a recombinant adenoviral vector (Ad5RSV-LH), and fibroblasts from a patient with EDS VI were transfected with different concentrations of the vector. Transfected fibroblasts and fibroblasts from a healthy control were cultured for 48 hours, at which time enzyme activity was measured as a percentage of hydroxylated lysine residues in protocollagen substrate, normalized for the cell lysate protein content. The vector was also injected into the abdominal skin of Sprague-Dawley rats, which have low endogenous skin LH activity. Animals were killed at 0, 2, 7, and 14 days after transfection (3 animals per group), and human mRNA levels, β-galactosidase expression, LH activity, and hydroxylysine levels were measured.

Results.—LH activity in the transfected fibroblasts from the patient with EDS VI increased as the concentration of Ad5RSV-LH increased. At the highest concentration of vector (100 pfu/cell), LH activity in the transfected fibroblasts was higher than that in the control fibroblasts. In the in vivo model, transfection of rat fibroblasts with Ad5RSV-LH resulted in the expression of human LH mRNA and β-galactosidase. LH activity increased by day 2 in all animals and at day 7 remained higher than at baseline. By day 14, LH activity remained elevated in 2 of the 3 animals but had returned to baseline in the third animal. The hydroxylysine content in rat skin did not increase significantly after transfection.

Conclusions.—In vitro tests showed that the transfection of skin fibroblasts from a patient with EDS VI with an adenoviral vector expressing human LH cDNA restored LH enzyme activity to normal or even higher than normal levels. In vivo tests in the rat showed that the intradermal injection of this vector into the abdominal skin resulted in human LH mRNA expression and increased LH activity. The lack of a significant increase in hydroxylysine content in rat skin may indicate that endogenous LH activity was sufficient to produce fully hydroxylated skin collagen. Thus, gene transfer therapy may help improve healing of skin wounds in patients with EDS VI.

▶ Most diseases of collagen metabolism are dominantly inherited conditions in which the defective structural protein disturbs the function of a product of a healthy allele. In contrast, EDS VI is a recessively inherited disorder in which the defective allele does not appear to interfere with the wild-type enzyme. Thus, EDS VI patients theoretically should benefit from therapeutic gene transfer. Unfortunately, the major signs and symptoms of most inherited connective tissue diseases, including EDS VI, arise because of events that occur during embryonic development, and thus curative treatment may not be possible in the newborn. However, the data presented by Rauma et al suggest that gene transfer may help alleviate the local symptoms of EDS VI.

B. H. Thiers, MD

A Recessive Form of the Ehlers-Danlos Syndrome Caused by Tenascin-X Deficiency
Schalkwijk J, Zweers MC, Steijlen PM, et al (Univ Med Ctr, Nijmegen, The Netherlands; Univ of California, San Francisco)
N Engl J Med 345:1167-1175, 2001   15–3

Background.—The Ehlers-Danlos syndrome, an inheritable connective-tissue disorder, is caused by defects in fibrillar-collagen metabolism. Type

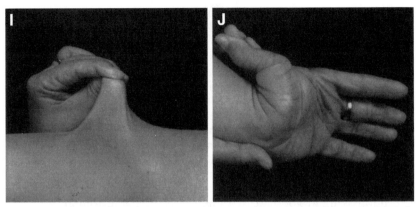

FIGURE 2.—Histopathologic findings in skin in patients with tenascin-X deficiency. **Panels I, J,** the skin and joints of a patient with the Ehlers-Danlos syndrome and tenascin-X deficiency. Note the skin hyperextensibility and joint hypermobility typical of tenascin-X-deficient patients with the Ehlers-Danlos syndrome. (Reprinted by permission of *The New England Journal of Medicine* from Schalwijk J, Zweers MC, Steijlen PM, et al: A recessive form of the Ehlers-Danlos syndrome caused by tenascin-X deficiency. *N Engl J Med* 345: 1167-1175, 2001. Copyright 2001, Massachusetts Medical Society. All rights reserved.)

V collagen gene mutations compose up to 50% of classic Ehlers-Danlos syndrome cases, many other cases being unexplained. Whether a deficiency in the tenascins, extracellular-matrix proteins expressed highly in connective tissues, is associated with the Ehlers-Danlos syndrome was investigated.

Methods.—Serum samples were obtained from 151 patients with classic, hypermobility, or vascular-type Ehlers-Danlos syndrome; 75 with psoriasis; 93 with rheumatoid arthritis (RA); and 21 healthy persons. Samples were analyzed for the presence of tenascin-X and tenascin-C by enzyme-linked immunosorbent assay (ELISA). The expression of tenascins and type V collagen in skin was studied by immunohistochemical techniques, and the tenascin-X gene was sequenced.

Findings.—Tenascin-X was found in serum of all healthy persons, all patients with psoriasis, all with RA, and 146 of 151 with Ehlers-Danlos syndrome. The 5 patients without tenascin-X were unrelated, had normal expressions of tenascin-C and type V collagen, and the symptoms of hypermobile joints, hyperelastic skin, and easy bruising without atrophic scarring (Fig 2). These 5 patients were found to have tenascin-X mutations. One had a homozygous tenascin-X gene deletion, 1 was heterozygous for the deletion, and 3 had homozygous truncating point mutations, which confirmed the causative role of tenascin-X and a recessive inheritance pattern.

Conclusions.—Tenascin-X deficiency underlies a clinically distinct, recessive type of Ehlers-Danlos syndrome. Thus, factors other than the collagens or collagen-processing enzymes can cause the syndrome. Tenascin-X appears to play a central role in maintaining the integrity of collagenous matrix.

▶ The authors show that factors other than the collagens or collagen-processing enzymes can cause a recessive form of Ehlers-Danlos syndrome. They suggest that tenascin-X plays an essential role in maintaining the integrity of the collagen matrix. A thoughtful editorial by Byers in the same issue of the journal puts this finding in perspective.[1]

B. H. Thiers, MD

Reference

1. Byers PH: An exception to the rule. *N Engl J Med* 345:1203-1205, 2001.

Clues to Epidermal Cancer Proneness Revealed by Reconstruction of DNA Repair-Deficient Xeroderma Pigmentosum Skin In Vitro
Bernerd F, Asselineau D, Vioux C, et al (Centre C Zviak, Clichy, France; Centre Hospitalo-Universitaire, Bab-El-Oued, Algeria; Centre National de la Recherche Scientifique Unité Propre de Recherche, Villejuif, France)
Proc Natl Acad Sci U S A 98:7817-7822, 2001   15–4

Background.—Both premature skin aging and the development of neoplastic lesions accompany exposure to UV radiation. Patients with xeroderma pigmentosum (XP) suffer exaggerated responses. XP is characterized by a severe deficiency of nucleotide excision repair (NER) of UV-induced DNA lesions. The development of an in vitro model of photosensitive human skin using cells from independent primary strains of epidermal keratinocytes and dermal fibroblasts from XP patients (taken from unexposed body areas) is reported. The resulting skin maintained the NER deficiency of the original XP skin.

Methods.—The primary XP keratinocytes and fibroblasts were cultured from skin biopsy specimens of XP patients. Reconstructed skin was then prepared.

Results.—Stratification was obtained, but epidermal differentiation products (for example, keratin K10 and loricrin) were delayed in expression and reduced in quantity. XP keratinocytes proliferated more rapidly than normal keratinocytes. In the basement membrane zone, the deposits of cell attachment proteins (α-6 and β-1 integrins) were increased. The expression of β-1 integrin, which is normally limited to basal keratinocytes, extended into a number of suprabasal cell layers. The XP skin that was reconstructed in vitro showed several proliferative epidermal invasions within dermal equivalents. The epidermal invasion and high proliferation rates resembled the early stages of neoplasia. All epidermal layers, including the basal layer where carcinoma develops, showed DNA repair deficiency, characterized by long-lasting persistence of DNA damage caused by UVB radiation.

Conclusions.—Keratinocytes and fibroblasts from the unexposed skin of individuals with XP were able to reconstruct XP skin (comprising full-thickness epidermis and a dermal equivalent) in vitro, retaining the

DNA repair deficiency that characterizes XP. This reconstructed skin may allow research into the effects of sunlight on aging and carcinogenesis, and may expand the use of tissue therapy.

▶ The availability of in vitro reconstructed XP skin may be an invaluable tool for studying the processes of DNA repair, photoaging, and photocarcinogenesis. It also may serve as a useful model for testing gene therapy approaches for inherited and acquired diseases of DNA damage.

B. H. Thiers, MD

Effect of Topically Applied T4 Endonuclease V in Liposomes on Skin Cancer in Xeroderma Pigmentosum: A Randomised Study
Yarosh D, for the Xeroderma Pigmentosum Study Group (Applied Genetics Incorporated Dermatics, Freeport, NY; King's College London; Cornell Univ, New York; et al)
Lancet 357:926-929, 2001   15–5

Introduction.—Patients with xeroderma pigmentosum (XP) have a genetic defect in DNA repair that results in higher rates of actinic keratosis and skin cancer than in the general population. Intracellular delivery of the bacterial DNA repair enzyme, T4 endonuclease V (T4N5), has increased the rate of repair of sunlight-induced DNA damage in human cells. A prospective study was conducted to evaluate the ability of T4N5 liposome lotion to reduce the rate of appearance of new actinic keratoses and basal cell carcinomas in patients with XP.

Methods.—Thirty patients who had a confirmed diagnosis of XP were enrolled in the multicenter double-blind study. The patients ranged in age from 2 to 65 years and had a history of actinic keratoses or skin cancer. Twenty were assigned to T4N5 liposome lotion and 10 to a placebo liposome lotion, to be applied daily for 1 year. Patients were seen at 3-month intervals for identification and removal of new actinic keratoses or basal cell carcinomas.

Results.—The active treatment and placebo groups were similar in demographic characteristics and initial assessment of disease severity. All patients used sunscreens with a protection factor of greater than 15, and all but 3 used sunscreens with a protection factor of 30 or greater. The annualized rate of new actinic keratoses was 8.2 among the patients randomly assigned to T4N5 liposome lotions and 25.9 among those randomized to placebo, a significant difference. The 2 groups also differed significantly in the mean rate of new basal cell carcinomas (5.4 vs 3.8 per patient per year in the placebo and T4N5 groups, respectively). For actinic keratoses, the treatment effect at 10 years of age was greater than at 18 years. Rates of development of squamous cell carcinoma and melanoma in the study population were not large enough for statistical analysis. No adverse effects were associated with treatment.

Conclusion.—In patients with XP, treatment with T4N5 liposome lotion lowered the rate of development of new actinic keratoses and basal cell carcinomas compared with placebo lotion. The treatment effect was observed within 3 months.

▶ This is an interesting preliminary study involving a small number of patients. More data are needed to quantitate the degree of protection conferred by this liposomal preparation, and it is uncertain whether the results can be extrapolated from patients with XP to individuals with normal DNA repair mechanisms. Interestingly, younger patients appeared to obtain the most significant benefit from the study lotion.

B. H. Thiers, MD

Diagnosis of Autosomal Recessive Lamellar Ichthyosis With Mutations in the TGM1 Gene
Cserhalmi-Friedman PB, Milstone LM, Christiano AM (Columbia Univ, New York; Yale Univ, New Haven, Conn)
Br J Dermatol 144:726-730, 2001   15–6

Background.—The disorder known as autosomal recessive lamellar ichthyosis (ARLI) is clinically and genetically heterogenous, with varying severity. Genetic heterogeneity has been confirmed by using linkage analysis, with the disease mapped to chromosome 14 and mutations noted in the transglutaminase 1 gene (TGM1). Other cases that are clinically indistinguishable from these TGM1 cases have been mapped to chromosome 2, and still others have shown linkage to chromosome 3p21 and 19p. The molecular basis of ARLI was investigated in 10 patients with the typical clinical presentation of the disorder to determine possible genotype-phenotype correlations in ARLI and to compare various diagnostic approaches.

Methods.—The 10 patients were studied with the use of DNA-based mutation analysis, immunofluorescence microscopy, and enzyme activity assay. Fifty unrelated, clinically unaffected persons served as controls. All patients were evaluated via polymerase chain reaction (PCR) and direct sequencing-based mutation screening; selected patients had TGM1 immunofluorescence microscopy and in vitro enzyme activity assays.

Results.—Fourteen mutations were identified in 7 patients; none were noted in 3 patients. Four had previously been reported, 4 were novel nonsense mutations or out-of-frame insertions or deletions, and 6 were novel missense mutations. Patients with nonsense mutations or out-of-frame insertions or deletions had negative immunofluoresence microscopy findings. With missense mutations or no mutations in the TGM1 gene, immunoflurorescence microscopy gave mixed results. The results obtained by using an enzyme activity assay were consistent with the mutation data.

Conclusions.—Only a blood sample is required for PCR and direct sequencing-based mutation screening, and the results are available quickly.

These are the least invasive methods and give the most information as a first step in evaluating patients believed to have ARLI.

▶ The authors used DNA-based mutation analysis, immunofluorescence microscopy, and an enzyme activity assay to investigate the molecular basis of ARLI in 10 new patients. They concluded that immunofluorescence microscopy (which requires a skin biopsy) and in vitro enzyme activity assays (which also require tissue) are very tedious and time-consuming to perform, and are unlikely to provide more information than can be obtained with PCR and direct sequencing-based mutation screening (which can be performed by using only a blood sample and provides a definitive result). The definitive molecular diagnosis of patients with TGM1 mutations obtained by mutation screening can be used directly for genetic counseling.

S. Raimer, MD

The RNA Component of Telomerase Is Mutated in Autosomal Dominant Dyskeratosis Congenita

Vulliamy T, Marrone A, Goldman F, et al (Hammersmith Hosp, London; Univ of Iowa, Iowa City; HGMP Resource Centre, Cambridge, England; et al)
Nature 413:432-435, 2001   15–7

Background.—Telomeres, the nucleoprotein caps at the ends of eukaryotic chromosomes, require the RNA-protein complex telomorase for maintenance. From an early age, patients with dykeratosis congenita, a syndrome characterized by progressive bone marrow failure, abnormal skin pigmentation, leukoplakia, and nail dystrophy, have much shorter telomeres than normal. Stem cell function may be affected by defects in ribosomal RNA synthesis or in telomere maintenance.

Methods.—Autosomal dominant, autosomal recessive, and X-linked inheritance of dyskeratosis congenita have been found in different pedigrees. Mutations of the long arm of the X chromosome, particularly mutations of the DKC1 gene in band 2, sub-band 8, cause the X-linked form of the disease. Specific residues of ribosomal RNA are pseudouridylated by the affected protein, dyskerin. Dyskerin is associated with the H/ACA class of small nucleolar RNAs as well as with telomerase RNA (hTR). An H/ACA consensus sequence is contained in hTR. The gene responsible for dykeratosis congenita was mapped in a family with autosomal dominant inheritance.

Results.—Family members with dyskeratosis congenita were found to have a chromosome 3q deletion of 821 base pairs that removed the 3' 74 bases of hTR. The hTR mutations were then found in 2 additional families with autosomal dominant dyskeratosis congenita.

Conclusion.—Dyskeratosis congenita in 3 families (autosomal dominant pedigrees) was likely caused by one mutated allele of the telomerase RNA component. A haplo-insufficiency or a dominant negative effect may have caused this. It is likely that defective telomerase activity is the cause of dyskeratosis congenita.

▶ The inheritance of dyskeratosis congenita can be either X-linked, autosomal recessive, or autosomal dominant. The mutated gene in the X-linked form of the disorder encodes dyskerin, a protein that affects the RNA part of telomerase, an enzyme that helps to maintain the ends of chromosomes (telomeres).[1] Vulliamy et al found that in the autosomal dominant form of the disease, mutations occur in the gene that encodes for the RNA part of telomerase itself. The telomerase defect may lead to poor chromosome maintenance and early cell senescence. Thus, both forms of dyskeratosis congenita might result from a defect in telomerase activity through 2 distinct mechanisms.

B. H. Thiers, MD

Reference

1. Mitchell JR, Wood E, Collins K: A telomerase component is defective in the human disease dyskeratosis congenita. *Nature* 402:551-555, 1999.

Safety and Efficacy of Recombinant Human α-Galactosidase A Replacement Therapy in Fabry's Disease

Eng CM, et al for the International Collaborative Fabry Disease Study Group (Mount Sinai School of Medicine, New York; et al)
N Engl J Med 345:9-16, 2001   15–8

Introduction.—Among patients with Fabry's disease, a deficiency of lysosomal α-galactosidase A activity leads to progressive microvascular disease of the kidneys, heart, and brain. Treatment has been limited to the management of pain and end-stage complications. A phase 1 and 2 open-label dose-escalation study found replacement therapy with recombinant α-galactosidase A to be safe and effective in clearing globotriaosylceramide, which accumulates in affected organs of patients, from plasma and tissue. This therapy was evaluated in a multicenter, randomized, double-blind, placebo-controlled trial and a subsequent open-label study.

Methods.—In the double-blind phase, 58 patients were randomly assigned to receive recombinant α-galactosidase A (1 mg/kg body weight) or placebo, administered IV every other week for 20 weeks. All patients received active treatment in the open-label study, but infusion rates were increased as tolerated. The primary efficacy end point was clearance of renal microvascular endothelial deposits of globotriaosylceramide.

Results.—Twenty of the 29 patients who received recombinant α-galactosidase A in the double-blind study had no microvascular endothelial deposits of globotriaosylceramide in renal biopsy specimens after 20 weeks of therapy. This response was not seen in any patients in the placebo group. Active treatment also significantly decreased the deposits of globotriaosylceramide in the skin and heart. There was a direct correlation between decreased plasma levels of globotriaosylceramide and clearance of the microvascular deposits. After 6 months of open-label treatment, all patients who had been randomly assigned to placebo and 98% of those randomly assigned to active treatment and who underwent biopsies had clearance of microvascular endothelial deposits of globotriaosylceramide. The infusions were generally well tolerated. Mild to moderate infusion-associated reactions occurred in 34 patients during the 2 phases of the study but were controlled by reducing the infusion rate, preventive medications, or both.

Conclusion.—A dose of 1 mg/kg or recombinant α-galactosidase A, administered to patients with Fabry's disease every other week for about 6 weeks to 1 year, was safe and effective in reversing the accumulation of microvascular endothelial deposits of globotriaosylceramide in the kidneys, heart, and skin.

Improvement in Cardiac Function in the Cardiac Variant of Fabry's Disease With Galactose-Infusion Therapy

Frustaci A, Chimenti C, Ricci R, et al (Università Cattolica del Sacro Cuore, Rome; Università La Sapienza, Rome; Mount Sinai School of Medicine, New York)
N Engl J Med 345:25-32, 2001   15–9

Introduction.—In the cardiac variant of Fabry's disease, an X-linked inborn error of glycosphingolipid catabolism caused by deficient activity of α-galactosidase A, involvement is primarily limited to the heart, but cardiac problems progress with age and lead to death. Results of a recent clinical trial suggest that enzyme-replacement therapy may be a safe and effective treatment, enhancing the residual activity of α-galactosidase A. A patient with end-stage hypertrophic cardiomyopathy was successfully treated with IV infusions of galactose.

Case Report.—Man, 55, had a 15-year history of cardiac problems but no family history of Fabry's disease or hypertrophic cardiomyopathy. An irregular rhythm, left ventricular hypertrophy, and nonspecific ST-T wave changes were observed, and global left ventricular function was depressed, with an ejection fraction of 31.5%. The patient was considered for cardiac transplantation. Morphologic, biochemical, and molecular studies, however, led to a diagnosis of Fabry's disease. Molecular analyses identified the α-galactosidase A G328R missense mutation in the patient; his sister and her 3 daughters were carriers.

When an initial infusion of galactose increased the α-galactosidase A activity in lymphocytes and in endomyocardial biopsy specimens, the patient was started on a regimen of galactose infusions (1 g/kg, given over a 4-hour period every other day). During more than 2 years of treatment, the patient's New York Heart Association functional status improved from class IV to class I and the mass of the left ventricle decreased by about 20%. The patient was able to perform activities involving moderate effort without chest pain or dyspnea.

Discussion.—Patients with the cardiac variant of Fabry's disease have little, if any, vascular involvement, and cardiac symptoms develop late in life. Galactose infusions in the patient reported here were well tolerated and brought about marked improvement, confirmed by 2-dimensional echocardiography and cardiac MRI studies. Patients with unexplained left ventricular hypertrophy or hypertrophic nonobstructive cardiomyopathy should be evaluated for Fabry's disease.

▶ Previous studies have demonstrated the safety and effectiveness of enzyme replacement therapy for patients with type I Gaucher's disease.[1,2] The article by Eng et al (Abstract 15–8) shows the feasibility of the same approach for classic Fabry's disease. As noted by Frustaci et al (Abstract 15–9), patients with the cardiac variant of Fabry's disease have residual α-galactosidase activity and do not have vascular endothelial cell accumulation of glycosphingolipid. In these patients, IV infusions of galactose may allow the molecule to enter the cells and increase the stability and activity of the residual enzyme. As noted in an editorial that accompanied these articles, the treatment of genetic diseases has truly entered a new era.[3]

B. H. Thiers, MD

References

1. Grabowski GA, Leslie N, Wenstrup R: Enzyme therapy for Gaucher disease: The first 5 years. *Blood Rev* 12:115-133,1998.
2. Mistry PK: Gaucher's disease: A model for modern management of a genetic disease. *J Hepatol* 30(Suppl 1):1-5,1999.
3. Gahl WA: New therapies for Fabry's disease. *N Engl J Med* 345:55-57, 2001.

Clinical and Molecular Genetic Features of Pulmonary Hypertension in Patients With Hereditary Hemorrhagic Telangiectasia

Trembath RC, Thomson JR, Machado RD, et al (Univ of Leicester, England; Univ of Cambridge, England; Univ of Auckland, New Zealand; et al)

N Engl J Med 345:325-334, 2001   15–10

Introduction.—In most cases of familial primary pulmonary hypertension, defects in the gene for bone morphogenetic protein receptor II (*BMPR2*), a member of the transforming growth factor β (TGF-β) superfamily of receptors, are identified. Pulmonary hypertension that is clinically and histologically indistinguishable from primary pulmonary hypertension may occur in patients with hereditary hemorrhagic telangiectasia, an autosomal dominant vascular dysplasia. The genetic basis of pulmonary hypertension was investigated in these patients.

Methods.—Members of 5 kindreds and 1 individual patient with hereditary hemorrhagic telangiectasia were evaluated. Ten cases of pulmonary hypertension were identified, with the diagnosis determined through clinical evaluation, chest radiography, ECG, Doppler echocardiography, right-heart catheterization, and histologic examination of tissue obtained by excision of a lung or at autopsy. Microsatellite markers were used in the 2 largest families to test for linkage to genes encoding TGF-β–receptor proteins, including endoglin and activin-receptor–like kinase 1 (*ALK1*), and *BMPR2*. In study subjects with hereditary hemorrhagic telangiectasia and pulmonary hypertension, *ALK1* and *BMPR2* were also scanned for mutations.

Results.—Analyses identified suggestive linkage of pulmonary hypertension with hereditary hemorrhagic telangiectasia on chromosome 12q13, a region that includes *ALK1*. Patients with clinical and histologic features indistinguishable from those of primary pulmonary hypertension were found to have inherited amino acid changes in activin-receptor–like kinase 1. In 4 study subjects and 1 control, immunohistochemical analysis revealed pulmonary vascular endothelial expression of activin-receptor–like kinase 1 in normal and diseased pulmonary arteries.

Conclusion.—Mutations in *ALK1* can be involved in the pulmonary hypertension that occurs in association with hereditary hemorrhagic telangiectasia. Among the various effects associated with these mutations are vascular dilatation (characteristic of hereditary hemorrhagic telangiectasia) and occlusion of small pulmonary arteries (typical of primary pulmonary hypertension).

▶ The findings suggest that the overlapping clinical features of hereditary hemorrhagic telangiectasia and primary pulmonary hypertension may originate in a common genetic defect on chromosome 12q13. Primary pulmonary hypertension is a progressive disease with a poor prognosis; untreated patients have a median survival of less than 3 years after diagnosis. Certainly, any patients with suspected hereditary hemorrhagic telangiectasia should be screened for pulmonary abnormalities.

B. H. Thiers, MD

A Microbiological Study of Papillon-Lefèvre Syndrome in Two Patients

Robertson KL, Drucker DB, James J, et al (Univ of Manchester, England; Univ of Queensland, Brisbane, Australia)
J Clin Pathol 54:371-376, 2001   15–11

Introduction.—Papillon-Lefèvre syndrome (PLS) is a rare autosomal recessive disease characterized by palmar-plantar hyperkeratosis. Early periodontal destruction of both the deciduous and permanent teeth also occurs, possibly because of the proliferation of certain periodontopathogens. Plaque samples from 2 patients with PLS were studied to identify the subgingival plaque microflora present and to assess the amounts of the periodontopathic bacteria, *Actinobacillus actinomycetemcomitans, Porphyromonas gingivalis*, and *Prevotella intermedia* with the use of a quantitative enzyme-linked immunosorbent assay (ELISA).

Methods.—A combination of commercial identification kits, traditional laboratory tests, and gas liquid chromatography was used to identify bacterial isolates. All isolates were Gram stained and tested for catalase, oxidase activity, aerobic growth, and anaerobic growth.

Results.—One hundred eight pure cultures of predominant organisms were obtained for identification. Most were capnophilic and facultatively anaerobic species, mainly *Capnocytophaga* species and *Streptococcus* species (including *S constellatus, S oralis*, and *S sanguis*). Other facultative bacteria belonged to the genera gemella, kingella, leuconostoc, and stomatococcus. The aerobic bacteria isolated were species of neisseria and bacillus; anaerobic species included *P intermedia, P melaninogenica*, and *P nigrescens*, in addition to *Peptostreptococcus* species. In 1 patient, ELISA detected *P gingivalis* in all sites that were sampled. In the other patient, *A actinomycetemcomitans* was detected in only 1 site. Both patients had only low numbers of *P intermedia*. Microscopy confirmed the occurrence of spirochetes in the plaque.

Conclusion.—A range of bacteria is found in the subgingival plaque of patients with PLS, but no particular periodontopathogen is invariably associated with the disease. Because the severity of periodontitis in patients with PLS is not explained solely by the presence of the identified bacteria, even the recognized periodontopathogens, host factors may determine a person's susceptibility.

▶ Patients with PLS have severe, early onset periodontal disease. Although numerous recognized periodontal pathogens were found by Robertson et al, none was present consistently, and the authors concluded that the severity of the periodontitis in these patients could not be explained by the microbiological findings alone. They argue that host factors, including the inherited immune and epithelial defects that have been documented in PLS, likely play a critical role.[1]

B. H. Thiers, MD

Reference

1. Velazco CH, Coelho C, Salazar F, et al: Microbiological features of Papillon-Lefèvre syndrome periodontitis. *J Clin Periodontol* 26:622-627, 1999.

16 Steroids and Nonsteroidal Anti-inflammatory Drugs

Risk of Hospitalization Resulting From Upper Gastrointestinal Bleeding Among Patients Taking Corticosteroids: A Register-based Cohort Study
Nielsen GL, Sørensen HT, Mellemkjoer L, et al (Aarhus Univ, Denmark; Inst of Cancer Epidemiology, Copenhagen; Internatl Epidemiology Inst, Rockville, Md; et al)
Am J Med 111:541-545, 2001   16–1

Background.—Corticosteroid therapy has been associated with several adverse effects, such as upper gastrointestinal (GI) bleeding, but it is unclear whether such effects result from the corticosteroids themselves, other medications taken (especially nonsteroidal anti-inflammatory drugs [NSAIDs]), or underlying disease. The risk of hospitalization for upper GI bleeding among patients taking systemic corticosteroids was determined, considering also the use of other drugs that may increase bleeding risk.

Methods.—The population-based cohort study was conducted in Denmark. Data on the use of corticosteroids, NSAIDs, aspirin, and anticoagulants between 1991 and 1995 were analyzed. Among 45,980 patients, 18,379 person-years of corticosteroid use were accumulated.

Findings.—Among corticosteroid users, 109 hospital admissions for GI bleeding occurred, compared with an expected 26. Thus, the relative risk was 4.2. This same risk was 2.9 among corticosteroid users who did not use other drugs associated with GI bleeding. When current corticosteroid use was compared with former use, the relative risk declined further to 1.9.

Conclusions.—Patients taking corticosteroids, especially those using other medications also, have an increased risk of hospitalization for upper GI bleeding. Underlying disease, however, may also have contributed to the observed increase in risk.

▶ The authors report a modest but definite increase in the absolute risk of upper GI bleeding associated with corticosteroid treatment. This risk appeared to be most pronounced among patients with a history of GI complaints and when corticosteroid treatment was combined with other drugs, especially aspirin or other NSAIDs.

B. H. Thiers, MD

Steroids and Risk of Upper Gastrointestinal Complications
Hernández-Díaz S, García Rodriguez LA (Harvard School of Public Health, Boston; Spanish Centre for Pharmacoepidemiologic Research (CEIFE), Madrid)
Am J Epidemiol 153:1089-1093, 2001   16–2

Background.—Numerous studies have shown that taking nonsteroidal anti-inflammatory drugs (NSAIDs) increases the risk of upper gastrointestinal complications. Whether the use of corticosteroids confers a similar risk independent from that associated with NSAIDs is not known. The risk of upper gastrointestinal complications related to steroid treatment, and the potential interaction between steroids and NSAIDs, were assessed in a nested case-control study.

Methods.—The UK General Practice Research Database was used to identify 2105 patients aged 40 to 79 years with upper gastrointestinal complaints (bleeding or perforation in the stomach or duodenum, or a bleeding peptic ulcer) and 11,500 age- and sex-matched controls without upper gastrointestinal complaints. The database was searched to determine the type of upper gastrointestinal complaint, the number of patients taking NSAIDs or steroids or both, and the frequency and dosage of NSAID and steroid therapy. Data were adjusted for age, sex, study year (it was a 5-year study), ulcer history, and smoking status.

Results.—Compared with nonusers, current oral steroid users were significantly more likely to have upper gastrointestinal complications (adjusted odds ratio [OR], 1.8). The association between upper gastrointestinal complications and current oral steroid use was stronger for gastric complications (adjusted OR, 2.4) than for duodenal damage (adjusted OR, 1.2), bleeding (adjusted OR, 1.8), or perforation (adjusted OR, 1.6). Higher doses of oral steroids were associated with a greater risk for upper gastrointestinal complications than were lower doses, although the difference was not statistically significant. Current NSAID users were also significantly more likely to have upper gastrointestinal complications compared with nonusers (adjusted OR, 4.3). Furthermore, the risk of upper gastrointestinal complaints was significantly higher in patients who used multiple NSAIDs (adjusted OR, 11.1) and in patients who switched NSAIDs (adjusted OR, 13.5) compared with nonusers. The simultaneous use of steroids with NSAIDs significantly increased the risk of upper gastrointestinal complaints compared with nonusers (steroid plus low- to medium-dose NSAID: adjusted OR, 4.0; steroid plus high-dose NSAID: adjusted OR, 12.7).

Conclusions.—The current use of steroids increased the risk of upper gastrointestinal complications by a factor of 1.8, whereas the current use of NSAIDs increased this risk by a factor of 4.3. When used in combination, steroids and high doses of NSAIDs increased the risk of upper gastrointestinal complications by a factor of 12.7. The number of NSAIDs being used and their dose markedly influenced the risk of upper gastrointestinal complaints as well. Thus, to reduce the risk of upper gastrointestinal complications, steroids and NSAIDs should be administered as monotherapy whenever possible, and at the lowest effective dose.

▶ Because both systemic steroids and NSAIDs are each associated with upper gastrointestinal complications, it is not surprising that simultaneous use of the 2 classes of drugs increases toxicity. The authors considered the possibility that the underlying diseases, rather than the drugs, might have increased the risk of bleeding. However, the decrease in risk after cessation of treatment and the observed dose-response suggests a drug effect.

B. H. Thiers, MD

Role of *Helicobacter pylori* Infection and Non-steroidal Anti-inflammatory Drugs in Peptic-Ulcer Disease: A Meta-analysis
Huang J-Q, Sridhar S, Hunt RH (McMaster Univ, Hamilton, Ont, Canada)
Lancet 359:14-22, 2002   16–3

Background.—Authorities continue to disagree on the association of *Helicobacter pylori* infection and NSAID use in the pathogenesis of peptic-ulcer disease. A meta-analysis was conducted to investigate this issue.

Methods.—Observational studies on the prevalence of peptic-ulcer disease in adults taking NSAIDs and on the prevalence of *H pylori* infection and NSAID use in patients with peptic-ulcer bleeding were identified in a literature review. Of 463 studies, 25 met the inclusion criteria for analysis.

Findings.—In 16 studies involving a total of 1625 NSAID users, uncomplicated peptic-ulcer disease was significantly more common in patients testing positive for *H pylori* than in those testing negative, with an odds ratio of 2.12. In 5 controlled studies, peptic-ulcer disease was significantly more common in NSAID users than in control subjects, regardless of *H pylori* infection. Compared with NSAID nonusers testing negative for *H pylori*, NSAID users testing positive for *H pylori* had a 61.1 risk of ulcer. The presence of *H pylori* infection increased the risk of peptic-ulcer disease by 3.53-fold in NSAID users in addition to the risk associated with NSAID use. In the presence of the risk of peptic-ulcer disease associated with *H pylori* infection, NSAID use increased the risk of peptic-ulcer disease 3.55-fold. The risk of peptic-ulcer disease was increased 1.79- and 4.85-fold by *H pylori* infection and NSAID use, respectively. When both factors were present, the risk of ulcer bleeding rose to 6.13.

Conclusions.—These data show that *H pylori* and NSAID use significantly, independently increase the risk of peptic ulcer and ulcer bleeding. A synergism exists between these variables for the development of peptic ulcer and ulcer bleeding. In NSAID nonusers without *H pylori* infection, peptic ulcer disease is rare.

Eradication of *Helicobacter pylori* and Risk of Peptic Ulcers in Patients Starting Long-term Treatment With Non-steroidal Anti-inflammatory Drugs: A Randomised Trial

Chan FKL, To KF, Wu JCY, et al (Chinese Univ of Hong Kong, Special Administrative Region of China)
Lancet 359:9-13, 2002   16–4

Background.—Debate continues about whether *Helicobacter pylori* infection increases the risk of ulcers for patients using NSAIDs. The value of eradicating *H pylori* as a means of decreasing the risk of ulcers for patients beginning long-term NSAID therapy was investigated.

Methods.—The study included 210 NSAID-naive patients with arthritis. After screening, 128 (61%) were found to be positive for *H pylori*, and 102 (80%) were finally enrolled. By random assignment, patients were given 1 week of omeprazole triple therapy (omeprazole with antibiotics) for eradication of the infection or omeprazole with placebo. Slow-release diclofenac, 100 mg daily, was given to all patients for 6 months.

Findings.—*H pylori* infection was eliminated in 90% of the eradication group and in 6% of the placebo group. Ulcers were documented in 5 of 51 patients in the eradication group and in 15 of 49 patients in the placebo group. The 6-month probability of ulcers in the 2 groups were 12.1% and 34.4%, respectively. The probabilities of complicated ulcers at 6 months were 4.2% and 27.1%, respectively.

Conclusions.—Screening and treatment for *H pylori* infection significantly decreased the risk of ulcers for patients beginning long-term NSAID treatment. These findings support the existing consensus recommendation to test for and eradicate this infection before NSAID therapy initiation.

▶ Huang et al (Abstract 16–3) report synergism for the development of peptic ulcer and upper gastrointestinal bleeding between *H pylori* infection and NSAID use. Chan et al (Abstract 16–4) found that screening and treatment for *H pylori* infection significantly reduced the risk of ulcers for patients taking NSAIDs. The results may have significant implications for patients in whom long-term NSAID use is contemplated. It should be noted, however, that some gastroenterologists believe that *H pylori* may exert a protective effect against gastroesophageal reflux disease and the development of lower esophageal adenocarcinoma.

B. H. Thiers, MD

Acetaminophen, Aspirin, and Chronic Renal Failure

Fored CM, Ejerblad E, Lindblad P, et al (Karolinska Inst, Stockholm; Huddinge Univ, Sweden; Internatl Epidemiology Inst, Rockville, Md; et al)
N Engl J Med 345:1801-1808, 2001   16–5

Introduction.—The use of analgesics containing acetaminophen or aspirin has been linked to chronic renal failure, but previous case-control studies have had methodologic limitations. A nationwide, population-based case-control study from Sweden was designed to overcome the shortcomings of earlier investigations.

Methods.—Face-to-face interviews were conducted with 926 patients with newly diagnosed renal failure and 998 controls. Patients were identified by physicians who treat patients with renal disease and controls by random selection throughout the 2-year ascertainment period from the Swedish Population Registry. Controls were frequency matched to patients by age (in 10-year groups) and sex. Logistic regression models were used to estimate the relative risks of disease-specific types of chronic renal failure associated with the consumption of various analgesics. Regular use of an analgesic was defined as use at least twice a week for 2 months; nonusers were those who reported taking fewer than 20 tablets during their lifetime.

Results.—Overall, 86% of patients and 75% of controls reported using nonnarcotic analgesics. Regular use of aspirin was reported by 37% of patients with renal failure and 19% of controls. Acetaminophen was used regularly by 25% of patients and 12% of controls. The regular use of either drug in the absence of the other was associated with an increase by a factor of 2.5 in the risk of chronic renal failure from any cause. Relative risks rose with increasing cumulative lifetime doses, increased more consistently with acetaminophen than with aspirin use, and were increased for most disease-specific types of chronic renal failure. These associations were altered only slightly when recent use of analgesics, prompted perhaps by symptoms linked to renal disease, were disregarded.

Conclusion.—As reported in previous studies, the regular use of either acetaminophen, aspirin, or both was associated in a dose-dependent manner with an increased risk for chronic renal failure. In general, this risk was not associated with the regular use of other nonnarcotic analgesics.

Cyclooxygenase Inhibitors and the Antiplatelet Effects of Aspirin

Catella-Lawson F, Reilly MP, Kapoor SC, et al (Univ of Pennsylvania, Philadelphia)
N Engl J Med 645:1809-1817, 2001   16–6

Introduction.—Aspirin use reduces the risk of myocardial infarction and stroke, but the effectiveness of traditional nonsteroidal anti-inflammatory drugs (NSAIDs) in preventing vascular events is not known. However, many patients take both aspirin and NSAIDs, and a competitive interaction between these drugs may exist. The potential interactions between aspirin and commonly prescribed arthritis therapies were investigated in a group of healthy individuals.

Methods.—Various combinations of drugs were administered to the group for 6 days: (1) aspirin (81 mg every morning) 2 hours before ibuprofen (400 mg every morning) and the same medications in the reverse order; (2) aspirin 2 hours before acetaminophen (1000 mg every morning) and the same medications in the reverse order; (3) aspirin 2 hours before the cyclooxygenase-2 inhibitor rofecoxib (25 mg every morning) and the same medications in the reverse order; (4) enteric-coated aspirin 2 hours before ibuprofen (400 mg 3 times a day); and (5) enteric-coated aspirin 2 hours before delayed-release diclofenac (75 mg twice daily). The first 3 combinations were given in a randomized crossover manner with washout periods of at least 14 days before the medication order was reversed. The last 2 combinations were taken in a parallel-group, randomized, open-label, 6-day design.

Results.—Levels of serum thromboxane B_2, an index of cyclooxygenase-1 activity in platelets, and platelet aggregation were found to be maximally inhibited 24 hours after aspirin administration on day 6 in participants who took aspirin before a single daily dose of any other drug. This effect was also noted in those who took rofecoxib or acetaminophen before taking aspirin. A single daily dose of ibuprofen, however, when taken before aspirin, blocked the inhibition of serum thromboxane B_2 and platelet aggregation by aspirin. This interaction also occurred when multiple daily doses of ibuprofen were taken after aspirin. The pharmacodynamics of aspirin were not affected by concomitant use of rofecoxib, acetaminophen, or diclofenac.

Conclusion.—The cardioprotective effects of aspirin in patients with increased cardiovascular risk may be reduced by concomitant administration of ibuprofen. Of the 4 commonly used analgesics tested, only ibuprofen antagonizes the irreversible platelet inhibition induced by aspirin.

▶ The article by Fored et al (Abstract 16–5) is of interest to dermatologists because of the high incidence of skin problems among patients with chronic renal failure. The authors could find no evidence that the renal failure itself influenced the consumption of analgesics. Acetaminophen is used more commonly than aspirin in dermatology patients, especially those undergoing dermatologic surgery. Although this may result in fewer problems with gastric irritation or postoperative bleeding, both drugs appear to carry a small risk of nephrotoxicity with regular use (defined in this study as use at least twice a week for 2 months). Is it possible that all of us baby boomers who take aspirin regularly are sacrificing our renal function to improve our cardiac function?

The results of the study by Catella-Lawson et al (Abstract 16–6) are straightforward. They show that administration of ibuprofen before aspirin inhibits the antiplatelet effects of aspirin and may thus abrogate the cardioprotective (ie, anticoagulant) properties of the drug.

B. H. Thiers, MD

Non-Steroidal Anti-Inflammatory Drugs and Risk of Serious Coronary Heart Disease: An Observational Cohort Study

Ray WA, Stein CM, Hall K, et al (Vanderbilt Univ, Nashville, Tenn; Nashville Veteran's Affairs Med Ctr, Nashville, Tenn)
Lancet 359:118-123, 2002   16–7

Background.—It is unclear whether the risk of myocardial infarction (MI) and other serious coronary heart disease is decreased or increased by the use of non-aspirin nonsteroidal antiinflammatory drugs (NANSAIDs). An observational comparison of the risk of MI and fatal coronary heart disease was made among new users of widely prescribed NANSAIDs.

Methods.—Data obtained from the Tennessee Medicaid program between 1987 and 1998 identified 181,441 new users of NANSAIDs aged from 50 to 84 years and an age- and gender-matched cohort associated with the date on which their use of NANSAIDs began. None were residents in a nursing home, nor did they have life-threatening diseases. The data for each of the users terminated with admission to a hospital for an acute MI or death of the participant from coronary heart disease.

Results.—A total of 532,634 person-years of follow-up were analyzed. Serious coronary heart disease cases numbered 6362, equivalent to a rate of 11.9 per 1000 person-years. The multivariate-adjusted rate ratio for current NANSAID use was 1.05; that for former use was 1.02. The rate ratio for naproxen was 0.95, the ratio for ibuprofen was 1.15, and that for other NANSAIDs was 1.03. Among long-term NANSAID users whose use was uninterrupted, no protective effect against coronary heart disease was found. The rate ratio for current users whose use extended for more than 60 days was 1.05. A comparison of naproxen with ibuprofen directly showed a rate ratio of 0.83 for current users.

Conclusions.—In a high-risk population of persons who were at least aged 50 years, NANSAIDs offered no protection against coronary heart disease, nor did they promote the development of serious heart problems. Thus, since nonselective NANSAIDs offer no protective effect against coronary heart disease, they should not be used for cardioprotection.

► Low-dose aspirin has been shown to prevent nonfatal MIs, a finding that suggests that other NSAIDs could have the same effect. However, non-aspirin NSAIDs have complex properties that could either prevent or even promote coronary artery disease. For example, high doses of NSAIDs inhibit synthesis of prostacyclin, a potent endogenous platelet inhibitor, which could raise the risk of coronary heart disease, as could other dose-related effects, such as hypertension, of these drugs. Indeed, a large trial of the new cyclooxygenase-2-selective drug, rofecoxib, demonstrated a higher incidence of MI in the rofecoxib group (0.4%) than in the naproxen group (0.1%).[1] Whether this reflected a protective effect of naproxen or a harmful effect of rofecoxib is unknown. The current study demonstrates the absence of a protective effect of naproxen or other non-aspirin NSAIDs on the risk of coronary heart disease and suggests that these drugs should not be used for cardioprotection.

B. H. Thiers, MD

Reference

1. Bombardier C, Laine L, Reicin A, et al: Comparison of upper gastrointestinal toxicity of rofecoxib and naproxen in patients with rheumatoid arthritis. *N Engl J Med* 343:1520-1528, 2000.

Risk of Cardiovascular Events Associated With Selective COX-2 Inhibitors
Mukherjee D, Nissen SE, Topol EJ (Cleveland Clinic Found, Ohio)
JAMA 286:954-959, 2001   16–8

Background.—Atherosclerosis is a process that involves inflammatory features, and selective cyclooxygenase 2 (COX-2) inhibitors may have antiatherogenic effects because of their ability to inhibit inflammation. However, the use of COX-2 antagonists may result in increased prothrombic activity because they decrease vasodilatory and antiaggregatory prostacyclin production. A literature search was conducted to define the cardiovascular effects of COX-2 inhibitors when used in the treatment of arthritis and musculoskeletal pain in patients without coronary artery disease.

Methods.—A MEDLINE search was conducted to identify all English-language articles on the use of COX-2 inhibitors published from 1998 through February 2001. Relevant submissions to the US Food and Drug Administration by pharmaceutical companies were included in the review.

Results.—Two major randomized trials were identified: the Vioxx Gastrointestinal Outcomes Research Study (VIGOR) with 8076 patients, and the Celecoxib Long-term Arthritis Safety Study (CLASS) with 8059 patients. Two small trials, each with approximately 1000 patients, also were identified. The VIGOR trial demonstrated that the relative risk of developing a confirmed, adjudicated thrombotic cardiovascular event with rofecoxib treatment compared with naproxen was 2.38. In the CLASS trial, no significant difference in the incidence of cardiovascular events was noted between celecoxib and other nonsteroidal anti-inflammatory agents. In both the VIGOR and the CLASS trials, the annualized myocardial infarction rates for COX-2 inhibitors were significantly higher than in the placebo group of a recent meta-analysis of 23,407 patients in primary prevention trials.

Conclusions.—The data available from these studies have indicated the need for caution regarding the risk of cardiovascular events in patients treated with COX-2 inhibitors. Further evaluation in prospective trials may provide data to aid in determining the magnitude of this risk.

▶ This study from a respected group of cardiology researchers at the Cleveland Clinic Foundation found a small increase in cardiovascular events in patients taking COX-2 inhibitors. Although prospective confirmatory trials are needed, the widespread prescription of these drugs suggests caution in their use. All nonsteroidal anti-inflammatory drugs have a specific risk:benefit profile, and each patient must be judged individually as to which drug is most appropriate. A comprehensive review of the COX-2 class of drugs appeared in another journal the same month this study was published.[1]

B. H. Thiers, MD

Reference

1. Fitzgerald GA, Patrono C: The coxibs, selective inhibitors of cyclooxygenase-2. *N Engl J Med* 345:433-442, 2001.

17 New and Unusual Therapies and Adverse Drug Reactions

Evaluation of the Efficacy and Tolerability of Oral Terbinafine (Daskil) in Patients With Seborrhoeic Dermatitis: A Multicentre, Randomized, Investigator-blinded, Placebo-controlled Trial

Scaparro E, Quadri G, Virno G, et al (Dermatologic Outpatient Dept of Genoa, Italy; Dermatologic Outpatient Dept of Savona, Italy; Dermatologic Outpatient Dept of Ventimiglia, Italy; et al)

Br J Dermatol 144:854-857, 2001

17–1

Introduction.—Seborrheic dermatitis is a common chronic inflammatory disease of the skin with no definitive cure. In previous open noncontrolled trials, topical and systemic terbinafine, an allylamine antimycotic agent, has proved effective in the treatment of seborrheic dermatitis. The clinical efficacy of oral terbinafine was evaluated in a multicenter, randomized, placebo-controlled trial.

Methods.—Sixty patients, 32 men and 28 women, were enrolled in the 12-week trial. All patients had moderate to severe seborrheic dermatitis with involvement of at least 2 body sites. A 2-week run-in period was followed by a 4-week treatment period and 8 weeks of follow-up. Study treatments were oral terbinafine tablets (250 mg once daily) and a placebo moisturizing cream (applied twice daily). Investigators who evaluated treatment efficacy were unaware of the patient's treatment. Erythema, scaling, and itching were scored on a 0-3 scale and a global clinical score was calculated.

Results.—The terbinafine and placebo groups were balanced in demographic and clinical data. The mean baseline global clinical scores were 7.4 in the placebo group and 7.7 in the terbinafine group. At 4 and 12 weeks, the mean global clinical scores were 5.9 and 6.3, respectively, in the placebo group, reductions that were not significant compared with baseline. With terbinafine treatment, both individual and global scores were significantly reduced compared with baseline values and with the placebo group. The mean global clinical scores in the terbinafine group were 1.0 at

315

week 4 and 1.2 at week 12. No serious side effects occurred in either group.

Conclusion.—Oral terbinafine is an effective treatment for seborrheic dermatitis. The clinical improvements seen at 4 weeks in this trial were maintained for 8 weeks after completion of treatment. A previous study showed that terbinafine has an anti-inflammatory action in addition to its fungicidal activity.

▶ This was a single-blind study comparing oral terbinafine with a placebo moisturizing cream in the treatment of moderate to severe seborrheic dermatitis. The results were quite impressive, with the clinical improvement from the oral terbinafine maintained 8 weeks after treatment was discontinued. Nevertheless, oral terbinafine is not an innocuous drug, and a more practical study might have been one that compared terbinafine cream with its vehicle. Several published studies have suggested the utility of topical antifungal agents in the treatment of seborrheic dermatitis.[1]

B. H. Thiers, MD

Reference

1. Dupuy P, Maurette C, Amoric J, et al: Randomized, placebo-controlled, double-blind study on clinical efficacy of ciclopiroxolamine 1% cream in facial seborrhoeic dermatitis. *Br J Dermatol* 144:1033-1037, 2001.

Potent Corticosteroid Cream (Mometasone Furoate) Significantly Reduces Acute Radiation Dermatitis: Results From a Double-blind, Randomized Study
Boström A, Lindman H, Swartling C, et al (Univ Hosp, Uppsala, Sweden; Karolinska Inst, Stockholm, Sweden)
Radiother Oncol 59:257-265, 2001   17–2

Background.—A common side effect of radiation therapy, sometimes requiring the temporary discontinuation of therapy, is radiation-induced dermatitis, an inflammatory skin reaction usually treated with topical corticosteroids. This study evaluated whether erythema intensity caused by acute radiation dermatitis could be reduced using mometasone furoate (MMF) prophylactically and therapeutically. An additional goal was the delineation of various symptoms, including pigmentation, itching, burning, and pain.

Methods.—Fifty women participated, all of whom were undergoing breast-conserving surgery for primary breast adenocarcinoma without lymph node metastasis. They were receiving tangential 5-MV photon beam radiation therapy to the breast parenchyma. The women were randomly given tubes of either MMF or an emollient cream (placebo) to be applied to the irradiated area twice a week until the 12th fraction (24 Gy) and then once a day until 3 weeks after completing radiation therapy. All women also applied an emollient cream over the irradiated area once a day from the first day of radiation therapy until 3 weeks after its completion.

Punch biopsy specimens from the treated area were obtained before and after treatment, with clinical evaluation of the skin at 24, 34, 44, and 54 Gy as well as 3 weeks after therapy was complete.

Results.—Forty-nine women completed the study. A higher patient erythema-index mean was found in the group using the emollient than in the MMF group at all of the radiation dosages. A statistically significant lowered total patient erythema index was found in the MMF group when compared to the emollient group. During follow-up, the patient melanin-index mean was higher in the emollient group, but the difference did not reach statistical significance. The maximal skin erythema reaction was statistically significantly less pronounced in the MMF group than in those using the emollient cream. Subjective severe symptoms with moist desquamation required further topical treatment for 6 patients who were using the emollient. Most patients had only mild or no symptoms during the study. Less itching and burning was reported among those using MMF than in those using the emollient cream, but this did not reach statistical significance.

Conclusions.—A significant benefit was found to accompany the use of MMF for the treatment of acute radiation dermatitis among this population of women. When used with an emollient cream, MMF was associated with less erythema, itching, and burning than the use of an emollient cream alone. The period of recommended use should begin with the first day of irradiation and continue until 3 weeks after radiation therapy is completed.

▶ The role of topical corticosteroids in the treatment of acute radiation dermatitis is controversial. This article caught the reviewer's eye because of its description of mometasone furoate (Elocon in the United States) as a potent corticosteroid cream. Mometasone furoate is often marketed as a safe topical steroid, with little risk of atrophy. It has been promoted for use in children, and its use in facial and intertriginous areas is not uncommon. My opinion is that it is perhaps the only topical corticosteroid that is actually much stronger than its manufacturer claims. I have seen numerous cases of facial telangiectasia and steroid-induced rosacea associated with long-term use of mometasone furoate.

B. H. Thiers, MD

Treatment of Prurigo Nodularis With Topical Capsaicin
Ständer S, Luger T, Metze D (Univ of Muenster, Germany)
J Am Acad Dermatol 44:471-478, 2001   17–3

Background.—Prurigo nodularis (PN) is characterized by intensely pruritic, lichenified, or excoriated papules and nodules and is assumed to be a manifestation of a cutaneous reaction pattern to repeated rubbing or scratching caused by pruritus of various origins. PN is a common occurrence in patients with atopic dermatitis and other itchy dermatoses, such as scabies, xerosis cutis, and bullous pemphigoid, and can be a signal of other systemic diseases, such as iron deficiency, hepatic or thyroid dysfunction, obstructive biliary disease, diabetes mellitus, chronic renal failure, lymphoma, leukemia, and other malignant tumors. Some studies have indicated that emotional stress or profound psychiatric illness may be another cause of PN. Topical capsaicin would appear to be a promising treatment for PN because this alkaloid interferes with the perception of pruritus and pain by depletion of neuropeptides in small sensory cutaneous nerves. The efficacy, safety, and practicability of capsaicin in the topical treatment of PN was evaluated in a large series of patients.

Methods.—A group of 33 patients with PN of various origins received topical capsaicin (0.025% to 0.3%) 4 to 6 times daily for periods ranging from 2 weeks to 10 months, with a consecutive follow-up period of up to 6 months. Skin biopsy specimens were taken from 7 patients before, during, and after therapy for histologic, immunohistochemical, and ultrastructural analysis.

Results.—After the symptoms of neurogenic inflammation subsided, all of the patients experienced complete elimination of pruritus within 12 days. Topical capsaicin also contributed to the gradual healing of the skin lesions. Pruritus returned in 16 of 33 patients within 2 months of discontinuance of therapy. Ultrastructural analysis demonstrated no degenerative changes of cutaneous nerves during or after capsaicin therapy. The depletion of substance P was demonstrated by confocal laser scanning, a finding that provided confirmation of the specific effect of capsaicin in vivo.

Conclusions.—Topical capsaicin was found to be an effective and safe treatment modality that resulted in clearing of the skin lesions.

▶ The 100% response rate is certainly striking! Unfortunately, a blinded controlled study would be difficult to perform because of the characteristic burning sensation experienced with application of capsaicin.

B. H. Thiers, MD

Clobetasol Propionate in the Treatment of Premenarchal Vulvar Lichen Sclerosus

Smith YR, Quint EH (Univ of Michigan, Ann Arbor)
Obstet Gynecol 98:588-591, 2001   17–4

Background.—Prepubertal children and postmenopausal women are the typical patients who have vulvar lichen sclerosus, with 5% to 15% of the cases occurring in children. Treatment has involved improved hygiene, hormone-containing ointments, and low-potency and high-potency topical steroids. The effectiveness, side effects, and long-term results of treating vulvar lichen sclerosus with clobetasol propionate 0.05% ointment in a group of premenarchal girls were assessed.

Methods.—The study population consisted of all premenarchal girls (15 patients) seen at the University of Michigan Pediatric and Adolescent Gynecology Clinic between January 1995 and July 2000 for treatment of vulvar lichen sclerosus. All received topical clobetasol propionate 0.05% ointment for 2 to 4 weeks, then were tapered to a lower potency steroid. Factors assessed included age at onset, symptoms, results of vulvar examination, prior management efforts, effectiveness of the treatment, follow-up information, and adverse effects. A follow-up telephone survey was conducted with parents of the girls.

Results.—The average patient age at the start of symptoms was 5.7 years. A biopsy confirmed the diagnosis in 4 cases, while visual diagnosis was sufficient in 11. Within 4 to 7 weeks after beginning treatment, 14 girls had a good response. A yeast superinfection occurred in 1 girl and transient erythema in another. Follow-up extended for 2 months to 6 years. Telephone interviews were conducted for 11 girls at least 1 year after treatment. Two showed further vulvar symptoms, 5 had 1 or 2 total flares, 3 had between 3 and 8 flares per year, and 1 girl remained unresponsive to treatment. Recurrences were successfully managed if steroid treatment was resumed as soon as the vulvar symptoms developed.

Conclusions.—Clobetasol propionate was safe and effective for these girls with premenarchal vulvar lichen sclerosus, but recurrences were noted in 82% of the cases. Most girls responded to treatment. Nearly half of those treated had occasional relapses, 36% had frequent relapses, and 18% had none. Thus, clobetasol propionate treatment was associated with good results overall.

▶ This study is compromised by a lack of histologic confirmation of the diagnosis in a majority of the patients and the absence of a control group. However, the therapeutic benefit of a brief course of superpotent topical steroids has previously been reported in female adults and children.[1,2] Still unknown are the longer term effects of such therapy on this inherently atrophogenic disease and whether such therapy might decrease (or even increase) the chance of its evolution into squamous cell carcinoma.

B. H. Thiers, MD

References

1. Lorenz B, Kaufman RH, Kutzner SK: Lichen sclerosis: Therapy with clobetasol propionate. *J Reprod Med* 43: 790-794, 1998.
2. Garzon MC, Paller AS: Ultrapotent topical corticosteroid treatment of childhood genital lichen sclerosis. *Arch Dermatol* 135: 525-528, 1999.

Tacrolimus Ointment in the Treatment of Chronic Cutaneous Graft-vs-Host Disease: A Case Series of 18 Patients

Choi CJ, Ngheim P (Harvard Med School, Boston; Harvard Univ, Cambridge, Mass)

Arch Dermatol 137:1202-1206, 2001   17–5

Introduction.—Chronic graft-versus-host disease (GVHD), which affects 50% of patients with long-term transplant survival, frequently results in cutaneous disorders. The immunosuppressive drug tacrolimus is effective in the topical treatment of patients with atopic dermatitis and is also effective when used systemically in the treatment of patients with psoriasis and GVHD. The efficacy of tacrolimus applied topically was assessed for 18 patients with refractory chronic cutaneous GVHD.

Methods.—The study included 18 patients who had undergone allogeneic bone marrow transplantation and were receiving at least 1 systemic immunosuppressive drug for control of GVHD. None was concurrently using topical corticosteroids or systemic tacrolimus. Patients applied the 0.1% tacrolimus ointment 2 to 3 times daily to affected areas. Efficacy was measured by patient reports and physician examinations.

Results.—Of the 18 patients, 13 (72%) responded to topical tacrolimus treatment with relief of erythema and/or pruritus. Response was rapid, occurring within hours or days. Side-by-side comparisons of tacrolimus ointment versus a control group of 6 patients confirmed the efficacy of tacrolimus. Even with entire-body application of the ointment, serum tacrolimus levels were low or undetectable. All patients subsequently went on to more aggressive therapies, however, because of GVHD progression or loss of drug efficacy (in 2 patients). Further treatments included increases in steroid dosage, psoralen-UV-A therapy, and extracorporeal photopheresis.

Conclusion.—In this small series of patients with steroid-refractory chronic cutaneous GVHD, 2- to 3-times daily application of tacrolimus ointment was effective in reducing erythema and pruritus. The ointment did not appear to have adverse systemic effects.

▶ Choi et al show that tacrolimus ointment may provide an alternative to topical steroid therapy for the local treatment of cutaneous GVHD. However, as noted by the authors, GVHD is a systemic disease and, for many patients, local treatment is only palliative. For patients with more aggressive GVHD, systemic immunosuppression, photochemotherapy, or extracorporeal photopheresis may be necessary.

B. H. Thiers, MD

The Use of Tetracyclines for the Treatment of Sarcoidosis
Bachelez H, Senet P, Cadranel J, et al (Hôpital Saint-Louis, Paris; Hôpital Tenon, Paris)
Arch Dermatol 137:69-73, 2001   17–6

Background.—Therapeutic difficulties in the treatment of sarcoidosis are related to the chronic course of the disease and the lack of spontaneous regression of lesions. The chronic nature of sarcoidosis has raised the balance between the benefit and the long-term tolerance of therapy. Thus, oral corticosteroids, which have been recognized as the most effective therapy for sarcoidosis, are indicated as the first-line treatment only for patients who present with severe visceral involvement. Oral steroids are not indicated for patients who present with less severe involvement, because their long-term use has been associated with many adverse effects and because relapses are a common occurrence during reduction of daily dosage. The toxicity of steroids has prompted interest recently in the efficacy of corticosteroid-sparing agents in patients with sarcoidosis. The safety and efficacy of minocycline was evaluated in the treatment of sarcoidosis.

Methods.—In a nonrandomized open study, 12 patients with cutaneous sarcoidosis were treated with minocycline, 200 mg/d, for a median duration of 12 months. Extracutaneous lesions were present in 3 patients during the study. The median length of follow-up was 26 months.

Results.—A clinical response was demonstrated by 10 patients, with 8 patients demonstrating complete responses and 2 patients demonstrating partial responses. In 1 patient, a progression of skin lesions was observed, whereas the lesions remained stable in another patient. There were minimal adverse effects with the exception of 1 patient, in whom a hypersensitivity syndrome developed. In 2 patients, slight hyperpigmentation occurred; this disappeared completely after minocycline was discontinued. In 3 patients, there was a relapse of skin symptoms after minocycline was withdrawn. These patients later received doxycycline, 200 mg/day, which allowed complete remission of the lesions.

Conclusions.—These findings support minocycline and doxycycline as beneficial for the treatment of cutaneous sarcoidosis. It would appear that randomized controlled studies are warranted for the evaluation of the true efficacy of tetracyclines in patients with cutaneous sarcoidosis.

▶ This is yet another in a series of articles claiming antibiotic responsiveness of conditions presumed to be of a noninfectious origin.[1-3] Interestingly, each of these articles comes from abroad. Is it possible that phenotypically similar diseases may have different causes in different regions?

B. H. Thiers, MD

References

1. Sharma PK, Yadav TP, Gautam RK, et al: Erythromycin in pityriasis rosea: A double-blind, placebo-controlled clinical trial. *J Am Acad Dermatol* 42 (2 Pt 1):241-244, 2000.
2. Buyuk AK, Kavala M: Oral metronidazole treatment of lichen planus. *J Am Acad Dermatol* 43 (2 Pt 1):260-262, 2000.
3. Rudnicka L, Szymanska E, Walecka I, et al: Long-term cefuroxime axetil in subacute cutaneous lupus erythematosus: A report of three cases. *Dermatology* 200:129-131, 2000.

Parathyroidectomy Promotes Wound Healing and Prolongs Survival in Patients With Calciphylaxis From Secondary Hyperparathyroidism

Girotto JA, Harmon JW, Ratner LE, et al (Johns Hopkins Med Institutions, Baltimore, Md; Univ of Wisconsin, Madison)
Surgery 130:645-651, 2001   17-7

Background.—Calciphylaxis is a rare but life-threatening condition occasionally affecting patients with secondary hyperparathyroidism. Parathyroidectomy has been advocated as the only potentially curative intervention.

Methods.—Between January 1989 and May 2000, 13 patients with pathologic/clinical criteria of calciphylaxis were treated at the study institution. Of these 13 patients, 7 were managed with medical therapy alone, and 6 were referred for parathyroidectomy. The medical records were reviewed, and patients/relatives were interviewed.

Results.—All patients had cutaneous wounds requiring local debridement predominantly located on the lower extremities or abdominal wall. Six patients underwent subtotal (3.5 gland) parathyroidectomy without morbidity. All 6 had significant reductions in parathyroid hormone levels after surgery (mean decrease, 94% ± 0%), and all reported resolution of pain and healing of cutaneous wounds. Of the remaining 7 patients who had medical management alone, 5 eventually died of complications related to calciphylaxis. In comparing the 2 groups, patients who underwent parathyroidectomy had a significantly longer median survival than those who did not have surgery (36 vs 3 months, $P = .021$) (Fig 2).

Conclusions.—Calciphylaxis frequently causes gangrene, sepsis, and eventual death. Parathyroidectomy can be performed with minimal morbidity and is associated with resolution of pain, wound healing, and a

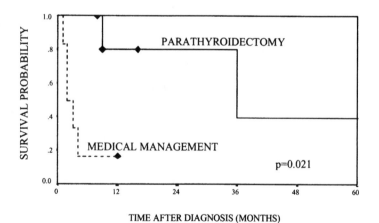

TIME AFTER DIAGNOSIS (MONTHS)

FIGURE 2.—Actuarial survival comparison of patients with secondary hyperparathyroidism and calciphylaxis treated by parathyroidectomy versus medical management alone. (Courtesy of Girotto JA, Harmon JY, Ratner LE, et al: Parathyroidectomy promotes wound healing and prolongs survival in patients with calciphylaxis from secondary hyperparathyroidism. *Surgery* 130:645-651, 2001.)

significantly longer median survival. Therefore, patients with secondary hyperparathyroidism and signs/symptoms of calciphylaxis should be referred promptly for consideration of parathyroidectomy.

▶ This article adds to the growing body of evidence demonstrating the importance of early surgical intervention for patients with calciphylaxis, although some authorities reserve the procedure only for patients with severe hyperparathyroidism.[1] Traditional surgical approaches have favored subtotal hyperparathyroidectomy because of the 5% risk of permanent hypoparathyroidism associated with total parathyroidectomy and autotransplantation. More recently, total parathyroidectomy has gained favor. This more effectively eliminates parathyroid hormone secretion (which is thought to play a key pathogenetic role in calciphylaxis), and the resulting permanent hypoparathyroidism can easily be treated.

Most patients in the current study had peripherally located lesions. Many clinicians believe such patients have a better prognosis than those with centrally located lesions. This could have influenced the results in the current study, as the 3 patients who had centrally located lesions and were treated medically all died.

B. H. Thiers, MD

Reference

1. Kang AS, McCarthy JT, Rowland C, et al: Is calciphylaxis best treated surgically or medically? *Surgery* 128:967-972, 2000.

Treatment of Perforating Collagenosis of Diabetes and Renal Failure With Allopurinol
Munch M, Balslev E, Jemec GBE (Roskilde Hosp, Denmark)
Clin Exp Dermatol 25:615-616, 2000   17–8

Introduction.—There is no uniformly successful treatment for patients with reactive perforating collagenosis associated with diabetes and renal failure. In a previous report, 2 elderly women with hyperuricemia remained in complete remission during 6 months of treatment with allopurinol. In the case described below, allopurinol led to the resolution of skin lesions and itching that developed during hemodialysis necessitated by diabetic nephropathy.

> *Case Report.*—Woman, 63, was referred for diagnosis and treatment of severely itching, ulcerated skin lesions localized to the right lower leg. Antihistamines and topical treatment with emollients had offered no relief. The patient's lesions regressed within a few days of starting treatment with allopurinol (100 mg once a day) and disappeared after 2 weeks. Remission was complete after 6 months of on-treatment follow-up.

Discussion.—The etiology of reactive perforating collagenosis of diabetes and renal failure is not known, but the disease mechanism may involve reactive changes after superficial cutaneous trauma from scratching and pruritus. Because reactive perforating dermatosis may be initiated by increased oxidative stress and glycosylated end products caused by diabetes mellitus, the antioxidant properties of allopurinol may contribute to its clinical effectiveness. Other antioxidant drugs might also be useful.

▶ The use of allopurinol in the treatment of reactive perforating collagenosis has previously been reported.[1] This condition typically affects patients with diabetes and associated renal failure. Unfortunately, it is just this group of patients that appears to be most susceptible to allopurinol-induced toxic epidermal necrolysis.

B. H. Thiers, MD

Reference

1. Krüger K, Tebbe B, Krengel S, et al: Erworbene reaktiv perforierende dermatose. *Hautartz* 50:115-120, 1999.

Efficacy and Safety of Desensitization to Allopurinol Following Cutaneous Reactions
Fam AG, Dunne SM, Iazzetta J, et al (Univ of Toronto; Toronto East Gen Hosp)
Arthritis Rheum 44:231-238, 2001   17–9

Introduction.—In about 2% of patients receiving allopurinol for the treatment of hyperuricemia and gout, a pruritic maculopapular rash will develop. To overcome this treatment-limiting complication, desensitization procedures may be used. Experience with a slow oral desensitization protocol for patients with hyperuricemia with cutaneous reactions to allopurinol was reported.

Patients.—The retrospective study included 32 patients (21 men, 11 women; mean age, 63 years). The diagnosis was gout in 30 patients and chronic lymphocytic leukemia in 2. Each had a pruritic cutaneous reaction to allopurinol that precluded continuation of needed therapy. The patients' mean serum urate level was 618 µmol/L, and mean serum creatinine 249 µmol/L. The patients followed a standard oral allopurinol desensitization procedure, with the daily dose increasing gradually from 50 µg to 100 mg over a target of 28 days; a modified protocol was used for patients at high-risk. Short-term and long-term outcomes were assessed; a successful short-term outcome was defined as the ability to tolerate an allopurinol dose of 50 to 100 mg/day.

Outcomes.—The rash recurred in 4 patients, resulting in failure of desensitization. The remaining 28 patients reached the target allopurinol dose without deviating from the protocol over a mean of 30.5 days. Seven patients developed a recurrent rash within a mean of 54 days, requiring dosage adjustment. Late cutaneous reactions occurred in 7 patients 1 to 20 months after they completed the protocol. Of these, 4 responded to dosage modification, and 3 had to stop allopurinol treatment. At a mean follow-up time of 33 months, 78% of the patients were able to continue allopurinol treatment. Their mean serum urate level after desensitization was 318 µmol/L.

Conclusions.—The slow desensitization protocol is safe and effective for patients with hyperuricemia with allopurinol-induced maculopapular eruptions. The rash may recur during or after desensitization, but most such reactions can be controlled with dosage reduction or temporary cessation of allopurinol treatment. Successful desensitization requires careful planning, discussion with the patient, and follow-up.

▶ A series of articles approximately 20 years ago documented an association between toxic epidermal necrolysis and allopurinol use in patients with chronic renal failure who also were receiving diuretic agents. It should be stressed that none of the individuals in the series reported by Fam et al had experienced such a severe allopurinol hypersensitivity reaction. Nevertheless, the desensitization protocol described should only be undertaken with caution and with appropriate monitoring. The authors stress that desensitization is not recommended for patients with previous Stevens-Johnson syndrome, toxic epidermal necrolysis, or other life-threatening reactions to the drug. A slower incremental dosing regimen, with dosage changes every 5 to 10 days or longer, increases the likelihood of successful desensitization and is recommended for patients at high risk, including the frail or elderly and those who have had widespread allopurinol-induced eruptions, especially associated with systemic symptoms or eosinophilia.

B. H. Thiers, MD

Cutaneous Adverse Reactions to Hydroxyurea in Patients With Sickle Cell Disease
Chaine B, Neonato M-G, Girot R, et al (Hôpital Tenon, Paris)
Arch Dermatol 137:467-470, 2001   17–10

Introduction.—The administration of hydroxyurea results in a lower rate of sickle polymer formation and a significant improvement in sickle cell disease (SCD). Treated patients have fewer vaso-occlusive crises, shorter hospital stays, and a decreased need for blood transfusions. Some patients, however, may experience severe adverse cutaneous reactions to hydroxyurea. A group of patients with SCD who were undergoing hydroxyurea treatment were examined by a dermatologist for cutaneous lesions.

Methods.—The patients were 17 adults (8 men and 9 women) who ranged in age from 19 to 51 years (12 were in their 20s). Sixteen were homozygous for SCD, and 1 was compound heterozygous for sickle cell–β-thalassemia. All patients had been treated with hydroxyurea for pain, acute chest syndrome, or both. The mean duration of treatment was 3.04 years, and the mean daily dose was 20.23 mg/kg.

Results.—Leg ulcers were present in 5 patients (29%). Clinical and US examinations excluded arterial or venous disorders in 4 of these patients. The fifth patient had experienced a previous episode of lower leg venous thrombosis, but her ulcers were bilateral without venous insufficiency on the opposite leg. All ulcers were cured or greatly improved when hydroxyurea was withdrawn or the dose decreased. Patients with hydroxyurea-induced ulcers were older than those without the ulcers (mean age, 35.8 vs 23.5 years) and had a higher prevalence of previous SCD ulcers.

Conclusion.—The risk of leg ulcers among hydroxyurea-treated patients with SCD was unexpectedly high (29%). Older patients had a greater risk, particularly if they had a history of SCD ulcers. Because hydroxyurea is a lifelong treatment for SCD, patients should be carefully monitored for skin changes.

▶ Leg ulcers secondary to hydroxyurea therapy have previously been described.[1,2] In the early 1990s, the efficacy of hydroxyurea in treating sickle cell disease was recognized. The drug appears to stimulate the production of fetal hemoglobin in red blood cells, which correlates with a lower rate of sickle polymer formation and significant clinical improvement. Unfortunately, the incidence of leg ulcers in sickle cell patients receiving hydroxyurea appears to be quite high.

B. H. Thiers, MD

References

1. Sirieux ME, Debure C, Baudot N, et al: Leg ulcers and hydroxyurea: Forty-one cases. *Arch Dermatol* 135: 818-820, 1999.
2. Best PJ, Daoud MS, Pittelkow MR, et al: Hydroxyurea-induced leg ulceration in 14 patients. *Ann Intern Med* 128: 29-32, 1998.

The Teratogenicity of Anticonvulsant Drugs
Holmes LB, Harvey EA, Coull BA, et al (Massachusetts Gen Hosp, Boston; Harvard Med School, Boston; Brigham and Women's Hosp, Boston)
N Engl J Med 344:1132-1138, 2001   17–11

Background.—Infants exposed to anticonvulsant drugs in utero have an increased frequency of major malformations, growth retardation, and hypoplasia of the midface and fingers. This clinical picture is known as anticonvulsant embryopathy. However, it is unclear whether the abnormalities result from the maternal epilepsy itself or from exposure to the treatment.

Methods.—Data obtained by screening 128,049 pregnant women at delivery were analyzed. Three groups of infants were identified: those exposed to anticonvulsant agents, those unexposed to such drugs but

TABLE 5.—Major Malformation Identified in Singleton Infants Enrolled and Examined by Study Physicians

ANTICONVULSANT-DRUG EXPOSURE	MALFORMATIONS*
Phenytoin	Ventricular septal defect and inguinal hernia
	Penile hypospadias
	Calcaneovalgus deformity of the foot
Phenobarbital	Tetralogy of Fallot
	Unilateral cleft lip
	Hypoplasia of the mitral valve
Carbamazepine	Tetralogy of Fallot, esophageal atresia, vertebral anomalies, and multiple terminal transverse limb defects
	Multiple ventricular septal defects
	Large cavernous hemangioma on leg (5 cm by 4 cm)
Phenytoin and Phenobarbital	Imperforate anus
	Postaxial polydactyly, postminimi (type B)
Phenytoin and mysoline	Severe hypoplasia of fingernails and toenails, with decreased flexion of interphalangeal joints
Phenytoin and carbamazepine	Ventricular septal defect
Phenytoin and valproic acid	Coarctation of the aorta
Carbamazepine, phenytoin, and valproic acid	Membranous ventricular septal defect
Carbamazepine, valproic acid	Lumbosacral spina bifida
Phenytoin, phenobarbital, carbamazepine	Aortic-valve stenosis
None	Congenital dysplasia of the hip
	Cleft palate
	Membranous ventricular septal defect
	Penile hypospadias
	Undescended testicle on right side (in two infants)
	Postaxial polydactyly, postminimi (type B), left hand
	Talipes equinovarus

*Unless otherwise noted, each set of 1 or more malformations occurred in 1 infant.
(Reprinted by permission of *The New England Journal of Medicine* from Holmes LB, Harvey EA, Coull BA, et al: The teratogenicity of anticonvuolsant drugs. *N Engl J Med* 344:1132-1138. Copyright 2001, Massachusetts Medical Society. All rights reserved.)

whose mothers had a history of seizures, and those unexposed to anticonvulsant drugs whose mothers had no history of seizures.

Findings.—Infants exposed to 1 anticonvulsant drug had a higher combined frequency of anticonvulsant embryopathy than unexposed infants whose mothers had no history of seizures, at 20.6% and 8.5%, respectively (Table 5). Among infants exposed to 2 or more drugs, the frequency was 28%. The frequency of these abnormalities in infants whose mothers had a history of epilepsy but took no anticonvulsant agents during pregnancy was similar to the control group.

Conclusions.—Exposure to anticonvulsant drugs in utero is associated with a distinctive pattern of physical abnormalities. Anticonvulsant embryopathy appears to be associated with exposure to anticonvulsant treatment rather than to the epilepsy itself.

▶ The authors show that the pattern of physical abnormalities in infants of mothers with epilepsy is associated with the use of anticonvulsant drugs during pregnancy rather than with the seizure disorder itself. Recognition of the pattern of abnormalities associated with the various anticonvulsant drugs is of particular importance to pediatric dermatologists who may see such patients in clinics for children with genetic diseases.

B. H. Thiers, MD

18 Miscellaneous Topics

Seasonal Variations in Hospital Admission for Deep Vein Thrombosis and Pulmonary Embolism: Analysis of Discharge Data
Boulay F, Berthier F, Schoukroun G, et al (Nice Teaching Hosp, France)
BMJ 323:601-602, 2001   18–1

Background.—The occurrence of fatal pulmonary embolism has been shown to vary according to season. However, seasonal variation in occurrence has not been established for deep vein thrombosis. Whether a relationship between deep vein thrombosis and the seasons exists was determined by analyzing French hospital admission data from the national hospital discharge register.

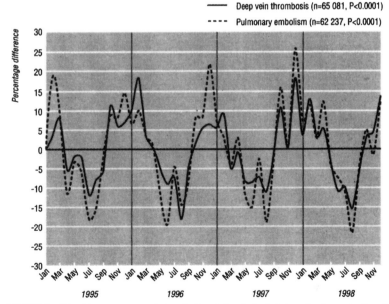

FIGURE 1.—Monthly percentage variations in French hospital admissions for deep vein thrombosis and pulmonary embolism (0 represents the sum of monthly variations). (Courtesy of Boulay F, Berthier F, Schoukroun G, et al: Seasonal variations in hospital admission for deep vein thrombosis and pulmonary embolism: Analysis of discharge data. *BMJ* 323:601-602, 2001. Reprinted with permission from the BMJ Publishing Group.)

Methods.—Cases occurring between 1995 and 1998 with a discharge diagnosis of pulmonary embolism or deep vein thrombosis were included for analysis. Monthly percentage variations in admission data were compared with the sum of monthly variations (set at zero) for pulmonary embolism (n = 62,237; median age, 68 years; 57% women) and deep vein thrombosis (n = 65,081; median age, 69 years, 58% women) (Fig 1).

Results.—The number of admissions per month for both deep vein thrombosis and pulmonary embolism was higher in the winter than in the summer (Roger's test: $P < .0001$). For deep vein thrombosis, the mean monthly admissions ranged from 18% below average (August 1996) to 18% above average (February 1996 and December 1997). For pulmonary embolism, the mean monthly admissions ranged from 22% below average (August 1998) to 26% above average (December 1997).

Conclusion.—Admissions to hospitals for pulmonary embolism and deep vein thrombosis clearly increase during the winter months, showing a seasonal variation.

▶ The authors show a striking increase in hospital admissions for vein thrombosis and pulmonary embolism during the winter months. This suggests that thrombogenic factors may have a seasonal component. Reduced physical activity and vasoconstriction induced by cold are associated with reduced blood flow in the lower limbs and may play a role as well.

B. H. Thiers, MD

Frequency and Prevention of Symptomless Deep-Vein Thrombosis in Long-Haul Flights: A Randomised Trial

Scurr JH, Machin SJ, Bailey-King S, et al (Royal Free and Univ College Med School, London; Stamford Hosp, London)
Lancet 357:1485-1489, 2001   18–2

Introduction.—Several retrospective reports suggest that as many as 20% of patients with thromboembolism have recently traveled by air. The true frequency of air travel-related deep-vein thrombosis (DVT) is unknown, however. The overall frequency of DVT in long-haul airline passengers was assessed in a randomized controlled trial. Also evaluated was the efficacy of wearing class I below-knee elastic compression stockings (20-30 mm Hg) during the flight.

Methods.—Volunteers recruited for the study were 89 men and 142 women, all of whom were older than 50 years and had no history of thromboembolic problems. The study participants were planning to travel economy class with 2 sectors of at least 8 hours' duration within 6 weeks. Excluded were individuals with cardiorespiratory problems or other serious illness and those who regularly wore compression stockings. Stockings were used by 115 participants during their flights; 116 participants did not wear stockings. The deep veins were assessed by duplex US before and after travel. Blood samples were analyzed for 2 gene mutations which predispose to venous thromboembolism: factor V Leiden (FVL) and prothrombin G20210A (PGM).

Results.—Symptomless DVT in the calf developed in 12 (10%) passengers who were not wearing elastic compression stockings; none of the passengers wearing the stockings had DVT. Two of the passengers with DVT were heterozygous for FVL. Superficial thrombophlebitis developed in 4 passengers with varicose veins who wore stockings. Once of the passengers was heterozygous for both FVL and PGM.

Conclusion.—A surprisingly large number (10%) of air passengers who were not wearing elastic compression stockings were found to have symptomless DVT after lengthy trips (median duration, 24 hours). No cases of symptomless DVT were detected in the group randomly assigned to stocking use. For individuals older than 50 years, wearing compression stockings during long-haul air travel may reduce the rate of symptomless DVT.

▶ The authors document a surprisingly high incidence of symptomless DVT in airline passengers on extended flights and suggest the use of elastic compression stockings. All passengers were more than 50 years of age, and the 10% incidence of DVT reported in this study is likely higher than would be found in the general population. Pulmonary embolism occurs in about 10% of patients seeking medical care who have an isolated calf vein thrombosis. However, such patients are generally symptomatic, with easily identifiable predisposing factors. Quite likely, for most long-haul air travelers like those reported here, spontaneous resolution of the calf vein thomboses occurs without recognizable complications.

B. H. Thiers, MD

Severe Pulmonary Embolism Associated With Air Travel
Lapostolle F, Surget V, Borron SW, et al (Université Paris XIII; George Washington Univ, Washington, DC)
N Engl J Med 345:779-783, 2001   18–3

Background.—Air travel is considered a risk factor for pulmoanry embolism. However, no one has documented the association between pulmonary embolism and distance flown. Whether air travel duration is associated with the risk of pulmonary embolism was investigated.

Methods and Findings.—All cases of pulmonary embolism necessitating medical attention on arrival at the Charles de Gaulle Airport, the busiest airport in France, between 1993 and 2000 were reviewed. Data on 56 passengers with confirmed pulmonary embolism were analyzed. Passengers traveling more than 3100 miles had a much greater incidence of pulmonary embolism than those traveling a shorter distance. These incidences were 1.5 and 0.01 cases per million, respectively. Those traveling more than 6200 miles had an incidence of 4.8 cases per million.

Conclusions.—These data strongly suggest an association between air travel duration and the risk of pulmonary embolism. A greater distance traveled significantly contributes to pulmonary embolism risk.

▶ The findings are not surprising and are consistent with those reported by Scurr et al (Abstract 18–2). The authors recommend simple behavioral and mechanical prophylactic measures for patients embarking on air travel of long duration. These measures include adequate consumption of fluids, avoidance of alcohol, smoking, and constrictive clothing, the use of elastic support stockings, avoidance of leg crossing, frequent changes in position while seated, and minor physical activity, including walking and moving the legs. In an accompanying editorial, Ansell[1] advises that until such nonpharmacologic approaches have been fully promoted, it may be premature and even dangerous to recommend aspirin or other anticoagulant drugs, even to persons considered to be at high risk. In addition, he argues that although the use of compression stockings may be helpful in preventing deep venous thrombosis, they may induce superficial venous thrombosis.[2]

B. H. Thiers, MD

References

1. Ansell JE: Air travel and venous thromboembolism, is the evidence in? *N Engl J Med* 345:828-829, 2001.
2. Machin SJ, Mackie IJ, McDonald S, et al: Airline travel: Incidence and prevention of venous thrombosis. *Thromb Haemost* 86:Suppl, 2001.

Toe Ulceration Associated With Compression Bandaging: Observational Study
Chan CLH, Meyer FJ, Hay RJ, et al (Guy's and St Thomas's NHS Trust, London)
BMJ 323:1099, 2001   18–4

Background.—This report described ulceration of the toe and cleft developing in patients treated with a compression bandage for venous ulcers.

Findings.—From 1990 to 2000, 194 new patients were referred for management of venous leg ulcers. The patients were managed with standard 3- or 4-layer compression treatment. In 12 of these patients, aged 32 to 72 years, ulceration developed after several months of 4-layer compression bandaging. This ulceration was superficial, without a distinct shape, and was either unilateral or bilateral. Ulceration predominantly occurred on the dorsum of the medial 3 toes and interdigital clefts (Figure; see color plate XV). Hematologic investigations, microbiological cultures, and viral and fungal antibody titers were all normal. Ulcer biopsy specimens revealed nonspecific inflammatory cells without malignancy or acid-fast bacilli. There was no evidence of ischemia, diabetes, peripheral neuropathy, osteomyelitis, edema, or obesity. The ulcers were resistant to healing. Amputation was successfully performed in 1 patient.

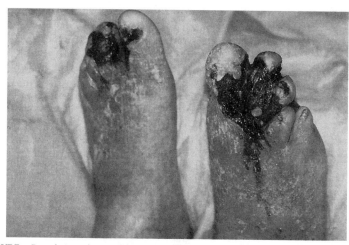

FIGURE.—Dorsal view of toe and interdigital cleft ulceration on the dorsum of the first and second toes of the left foot and toe, and interdigital cleft ulceration affecting the first, second, and third toes of the right foot. (Courtesy of Chan CLH, Meyer FJ, Hay RJ, et al: Toe ulceration associated with compression bandaging: Observational study *BMJ* 323:1099, 2001. With permission from the BMJ Publishing Group.)

Conclusion.—Toe and cleft ulcers developed in patients treated with 4-layer compression bandaging for venous leg ulceration. The ulcers were refractory to conventional healing methods.

▶ The mechanisms underlying the ulcerations observed by Chan et al are unknown. Possible contributing factors include increased local hypoxia, edema of the toes, and the development of venous hypertension. It is interesting that all 12 patients reported with these unusual ulcers had been treated with the 4-layer bandage. This bandage may be associated with increased compression pressure compared with the 3-layer bandage and may alter the biomechanics of gait, increase friction, and compress the toes.

B. H. Thiers, MD

Bone Marrow Involvement in Cutaneous Mastocytosis

Fearfield LA, Francis N, Henry K, et al (Chelsea and Westminster Hosp, London; Imperial College of Medicine, London)
Br J Dermatol 144:561-566, 2001   18–5

Introduction.—Cutaneous expressions of mastocytosis are usually benign and indolent, yet hematologic cancer is a recognized complication of mast cell disease. It has been reported that up to 60% of adult patients with cutaneous mastocytosis may experience occult bone involvement. The bone marrow was examined in adult patients with cutaneous mastocytosis to assess cytogenetic changes in bone marrow cells.

Methods.—Thirteen adult patients seen between 1993 and 1998 with clinical features of cutaneous mastocytosis were evaluated. No patients had systemic symptoms, and all had normal physical examination findings. All patients underwent bone marrow aspirate and trephine biopsies.

Results.—Twelve of the 13 patients had evidence of bone marrow involvement. Bone marrow cytogenetic abnormalities have been detected in patients with cutaneous mastocytosis, but all 6 patients in this series for whom cytogenetic analysis of the bone marrow cells was performed had a normal karyotype.

Conclusion.—The striking finding that 12 of 13 patients had increased numbers of mast cells indicates that most adult patients with cutaneous mastocytosis have underlying systemic involvement, despite being free of symptoms. The significance of this finding has yet to be determined.

▶ Fearfield et al show a surprisingly high incidence of bone marrow involvement in adults with cutaneous mastocytosis. This does not necessarily imply cancer, inasmuch as bone marrow mast cell infiltration could result from a reactive process in response to the cutaneous mast cell disease. Notably, all 6 patients in whom cytogenetic analysis of bone marrow cells was performed had a normal karyotype.

B. H. Thiers, MD

Kaposi's Sarcoma Associated With Previous Human Herpesvirus 8 Infection in Kidney Transplant Recipients

Cattani P, Capuano M, Graffeo R, et al (Università Cattolica del Sacro Cuore, Rome)
J Clin Microbiol 39:506-508, 2001   18–6

Introduction.—Human herpesvirus 8 (HHV-8) has been detected in virtually all patients with Kaposi sarcoma (KS), but the infection is not restricted to patients with KS. An above-average seroprevalence of HHV-8 has been reported in central and southern Italy, and an association between HHV-8 and KS has been demonstrated in organ transplant recipients. The seroprevalence of HHV-8 was compared between a control group and a group of patients awaiting kidney transplants. Transplant recipients were followed to evaluate the risk of HHV-8 transmission via kidney transplantation and the correlation between HHV-8 infection and the subsequent development of KS.

Methods.—The transplant group consisted of 175 patients; the 215 control subjects were patients seen at a clinic for other reasons. All study participants were from central or southern Italy. Those in the transplant group were monitored every 3 months during the first year, then every 6 months. Serum samples were collected for antibody detection.

Results.—The seroprevalence of HHV-8 was similar in patients awaiting a kidney transplant (14.8%) and control subjects (14.9%). Rates of seroprevalence were similar for men and women in the 2 groups. Among control subjects, seroprevalence tended to increase with age. One hundred of the transplant recipients were tested for anti-HHV-8 antibodies during the follow-up period. These patients showed an increase in seroprevalence, from 12% on the date of transplantation to 26%. During a follow-up period ranging from 3 months to 10 years, 7 transplant patients (4.0%) were diagnosed with KS. Six of them had been seropositive for HHV-8 before transplantation. Overall, KS developed in only 0.7% of transplant recipients who had been seronegative before the procedure.

Discussion.—The most important risk factor for development of KS after kidney transplantation is the presence of HHV-8 infection before transplantation. Antibody detection could identify patients at high risk for KS, especially in areas with a high seroprevalence.

▶ The findings suggest that reactivation of latent HHV-8 infection by immunosuppressive treatment might play an important role in the development of iatrogenic KS. Because the authors did not have access to donor data, they could not exclude the possibility that in some cases, seropositive organ recipients were reinfected with HHV-8 from donors. Nevertheless, the data indicate that pretransplant HHV-8 seropositivity is a more important risk factor for KS than infection via transplantation.

B. H. Thiers, MD

Skin Infections in Renal Transplant Recipients
Hogewoning AA, Goettsch W, van Loveren H, et al (Leiden Univ, The Netherlands)
Clin Transplant 15:32-38, 2001   18–7

Background.—Renal transplant recipients often experience skin infections. Data on the period-specific incidence of renal recipients' most common skin infections, with the exclusion of human papillomavirus infections, were evaluated in a long-term retrospective study. In addition, potential risk factors such as gender, age, and diabetes were assessed.

Methods.—The 137 participants had received their first transplant between July 20, 1967, and December 22, 1980, and were living with a functional graft as of August 1, 1989. Follow-up lasted until July 1, 1996. Skin infections were counted for each patient over different time periods, then expressed as a percentage of the infections in the entire patient group. This yielded the incidence of skin infections for the various posttransplant time periods.

Results.—Three charts from the transplant source were unavailable, leaving a total of 134 participants. Data were also pulled from 114 charts from the dermatology service. One hundred five patients had 340 skin infections. Those occurring most often in the first posttransplant year were candidal infection, herpes simplex infection, and impetigo; few new patients were affected with these infections beyond the first year. The infections most frequently seen after the first posttransplant year were dermatomycoses, herpes zoster, and folliculitis; these affected a significant number of new patients during this time period.

Conclusions.—Skin infections among renal transplant patients appear to be quite common, with differences related to the length of time after transplantation.

▶ The interesting aspect of this study was the finding that the spectrum of skin infections observed in transplant patients varies and depends to some degree on the time interval since transplantation. This implies that short-term versus long-term immunosuppression may favor the emergence of different infectious diseases. There are several limitations to the study, not the least of which is its retrospective nature. Moreover, a significant number of minor infections might not have been reported. This may explain why herpes zoster was reported more often than herpes simplex, whereas one would expect minor herpes simplex infections to occur more frequently than herpes zoster. A prospective study is needed to confirm the validity of the findings.

B. H. Thiers, MD

Skin Diseases in Children With Organ Transplants

Euvrard S, Kanitakis J, Cochat P, et al (Hôpital Edouard Herriot, Lyon, France; Hôpital Nord, Saint-Etienne, France)

J Am Acad Dermatol 44:932-939, 2001   18–8

Background.—Skin diseases are frequent in organ transplant recipients, but studies concerning children are sparse.

Objective.—We assessed skin diseases in children who had received organ transplants.

Methods.—A total of 145 children referred to our dermatologic consultation were studied.

Results.—Steroid-induced striae distensae and acne occurred only in adolescents; severe cyclosporine-related side effects were more frequent in younger children. The most common findings were warts (53.8%), tinea versicolor (14.5%), herpes simplex/zoster (9.6%), molluscum contagiosum (6.9%), and impetigo contagiosum and folliculitis (6.2%). Other notable disorders included a diffuse hyperpigmentation with a "dirty" appearance of the skin, pyogenic granulomas, melanocytic nevi proliferation, and skin tags. Two of 20 further adult patients who received transplants during childhood had squamous cell carcinomas.

Conclusion.—Children who have received organ transplants frequently present side effects of immunosuppressive drugs and infectious diseases. Most disorders are related to the age of the patients rather than to the length of immunosuppression, whereas others are favored by the reinforcement of immunosuppression. Skin cancers were not encountered, but the risk of carcinomas in early adulthood should be considered.

▶ Children with organ transplants experience various cutaneous complications, including common infectious disorders and side effects of immunosuppressive drugs. Cutaneous complications are observed more frequently in children who are receiving either systemic corticosteroids or cyclosporine; they appear to be related more to the patient's age rather than the duration of immunosuppression. In this study, no cutaneous carcinomas were noted in children. However, skin cancer (including 1 patient with metastatic squamous cell carcinoma) developed at age 32 in 2 of 20 adults who had received their transplants as children. Thus, photoprotection is mandatory in this patient population.

S. Raimer, MD

Recent Skin Injuries in Normal Children

Labbé J, Caouette G (Centre Hospitalier de l'Université Laval, Canada; Québec Dept of Public Health)
Pediatrics 108:271-276, 2001   18–9

Background.—Skin injuries are the most common and most easily recognizable signs of abuse in children, with up to 90% of victims of physical abuse being seen with skin injuries. Severe physical abuse is very likely to be identified, but minor physical abuse is less easy to distinguish from accidental injury. The most difficult situation for the physician occurs when a recent skin injury is observed in a child who is not presenting because of trauma. Are these injuries signs of physical abuse or the result of normal physical activity? The physician can contribute to the prevention of physical abuse by reporting the situation, but the reporting of innocent parents can have significant and regrettable adverse outcomes for innocent parents. Few studies have addressed skin injuries in "normal" children. Data on the totality of recent skin injuries in normal children and adolescents were collected and the relationship among the number of injuries, the age of the child, and the time of year in a temperate climate was determined.

Methods.—Study participants were children and adolescents seen consecutively over 1 year for a reason other than trauma. The total body surface, with the exception of the anal-genital area, was systematically examined, and the characteristics and location of all recent bruises, abrasions, scratches, cuts, and burns were recorded. The examiner ignored scars from old injuries. Fisher's exact test was used to analyze the data.

Results.—A total of 2040 examinations were performed in 1467 children and adolescents up to 17 years of age. Most (76.6%) had at least 1 recent skin injury, and there was no difference between the sexes. At least 5 injuries were noted in 17% of the children, whereas 4% had 10 or more injuries, fewer than 1% had 15 or more injuries, and 0.2% had 20 or more injuries. The lower limbs were the sites most often involved, with fewer than 2% of the children having injuries to the thorax, abdomen, pelvis, or buttocks and fewer than 1% having injuries to the chin, ears, or neck (Table 3). Most injuries were bruises. More injuries were seen in the summer, and more of these were bruises. Children in the 0- to 8-month age

TABLE 3.—Percentage of Children With Injuries by Site

Site	% of Children With Injuries*
Legs	50.1
Knees	32.9
Forearms	13.8
Thighs (upper legs)	12.2
Elbows	5.2
Head (other than the forehead, chin, cheeks, or ears)	4.6
Feet	4.3
Forehead	3.8
Hands	3.5
Arms	3.0
Cheeks	3.0
Back (lumbar region)	2.6
Posterior thorax	1.7
Abdomen and pelvis	1.7
Buttocks	1.6
Anterior thorax	1.0
Chin	0.7
Ears	0.3
Neck	0.2
Anal-genital region	Not evaluated

*Total exceeds 100% because many children had more than 1 site of injury.
(Reproduced by permission of *Pediatrics* from Labbé J, Caouette G: Recent skin injuries in normal children. *Pediatrics* 108:271-276, 2001.)

group rarely had any skin injuries; the injuries seen in this group were mostly scratches on the head and face.

Conclusions.—Most normal children after the age of 9 months had 1 or more recent skin injury. These injuries were mainly bruises; they were more prevalent in the summer in a region with a temperate climate and were usually observed on the limbs, although any part of the body could be involved. Physicians should be particularly attentive to children with injuries with unusual characteristics, such as an uncommon location; 15 or more injuries; bruises in a child under 9 months of age; numerous injuries other than on the lower limbs; and numerous injuries other than bruises, abrasions, or scratches. Injuries in these children could be signs of physical abuse or a bleeding disorder.

▶ Labbé and Caouette examined the skin of normal children for the presence of recent injuries. They found that injuries most commonly occur over bony prominences, such as the shins, knees, and elbows, and that 5- to 9-year-olds tend to have the most injuries. The authors concluded that bruises or other injuries to the ears, neck, trunk, or buttocks or injuries in children 0 to 8 months of age should alert the physician to the possibility of abuse.

S. Raimer, MD

Dramaturgical Study of Meetings Between General Practitioners and Representatives of Pharmaceutical Companies

Somerset M, Weiss M, Fahey T (Univ of Bristol, England)
BMJ 323:1481-1484, 2001   18–10

Background.—Commercial sources of information have great influence on general practitioners and their prescribing patterns. The pharmaceutical companies invest significant resources in promotional activities. This study explored the general practitioner–pharmaceutical representative encounter using Goffman's dramaturgical model.

Study Design.—One general practitioner met with 13 pharmaceutical representatives who requested to meet with him between January to June 2000. With the consent of the representatives, these meetings were recorded and full transcripts were prepared. The transcripts were analyzed by the dramaturgical model of Goffman, who proposed that the context of any interaction is a stage, individuals involved are actors, and the interaction is a performance.

Findings.—The encounters typically lasted for 10 to 25 minutes and could be depicted as consisting of 6 scenes. In scene 1, the pharmaceutical representative initiated the encounter and flattered the general practitioner by making him feel the more important player. Scene 2 was an opportunity for the representative to assess the practitioner's knowledge of the product. Scene 3 was used to propose clinical and cost benefits associated with the product. During scene 4, the practitioner took center stage and questioned this information. Scene 5 involved a recovery strategy on the part of the representative. In the final scene, the representative sought to ensure future purchases.

Conclusion.—Encounters between general practitioners and pharmaceutical representatives follow a consistent format. Physicians may perceive these meetings as benign and informative, but the industry views them as a cost-effective method to influence prescribing patterns. General practitioners might benefit from an alternative, unbiased, and accessible source of information.

▶ The findings concur with a recent guide published in *Pharmaceutical Marketing* that acknowledges the role of medical education as "a potent weapon to be used by the marketer in supporting promotional activities."[1] Roughead et al have described other techniques used by the pharmaceutical industry.[2] These include "reciprocity," in which someone who is given a gift will feel bound to make repayment. Clearly, the intention is for this obligation to be repaid through prescribing the company's product. Somerset et al confirmed that this marketing technique is a fundamental tactic in meetings between general practitioners and pharmaceutical representatives.

B. H. Thiers, MD

References

1. Cook J: Effective medical education. *Pharm Marketing* 12:14-22, 2001.
2. Roughead EE, Harvey KJ, Gilbert AL: Commercial detailing techniques used by pharmaceutical representatives to influence prescribing. *Aust NZ J Med* 28:306-310, 1998.

CUTANEOUS ONCOLOGY AND DERMATOLOGIC SURGERY

19 Dermatologic Surgery, Including Laser and Cosmetic Surgery

Botulinum Toxin Injection Is an Effective Treatment for Axillary Hyperhidrosis
Whatling PJ, Collin J (John Radcliffe Hosp, Oxford, England)
Br J Surg 88:814-815, 2001   19–1

Introduction.—Patients with excessive axillary sweating may seek surgical treatment after other options prove ineffective. Thoracoscopic sympathetic denervation of the axillary skin requires ablation of at least the T2 and T3 ganglia, and the incidence of compensatory hyperhidrosis is high. The patients in this study were successfully treated with intradermal injections of botulinum A toxin.

Methods.—The 16 patients, 8 men and 8 women, all had predominantly axillary hyperhidrosis. Using a 25G needle, each axilla was injected at 12 equally spaced points with botulinum A toxin (Dysport). Axillary sweating was quantitatively assessed in 10 patients before and several months after the injections. Ten patients underwent repeat injections after 1 year.

Results.—No complications were associated with the treatment. Within 3 days, all patients reported complete dryness of each axillae (40% experienced relief within 24 hours). The mean duration of action of the toxin was 9 months; sweating gradually returned in all but 1 patient. Three patients experienced a single episode of sudden breakthrough sweating, 2 at 3 months and 1 at 8 months. Those patients who had repeat injections reported good results.

Conclusion.—Intradermal injection of botulinum A toxin disrupts vesicular release in the cholinergic nerve terminals and is a highly effective and well tolerated treatment for isolated axillary hyperhidrosis. The authors do not recommend this technique for palmar hyperhidrosis because of the adverse effect of muscle weakness.

Botulinum Toxin A for Axillary Hyperhidrosis (Excessive Sweating)

Heckmann M, for the Hyperhidrosis Study Group (Ludwig-Maximilians-Universität, Munich; Technische Universität München, Munich)
N Engl J Med 344:488-493, 2001
19–2

Background.—Primary hyperhidrosis (excessive uncontrolled sweating without known cause) can be severe enough to cause substantial discomfort. It can also cause skin maceration and secondary microbial infections. Patients often suffer social stigmatization. The use of botulinum toxin A as a therapeutic agent to treat primary hyperhidrosis was examined. Botulinum A blocks acetylcholine release, which mediates sympathetic neurotransmission in sweat glands.

Methods.—The 145 patients in this multicenter trial (January 1999 to March 2000) had primary axillary hyperhidrosis for more than 1 year that was unresponsive to aluminum chloride treatment. In addition, they exhibited sweat production greater than 50 mg per minute. Each patient received, in randomized, double-blind fashion, injections of placebo or botulinum toxin A (200 U) in each axilla in 10 separate aliquots. (*Note:* The botulinum A preparation used in this study differed from other preparations reported in the literature.) After 2 weeks the treatments were revealed, and 100 U of botulinum was injected into the placebo axilla, again in 10 separate aliquots. Gravimetry was used to measure changes in the rate of sweat production.

Results.—The mean ($\pm$SD) sweat production at baseline was 192 ± 136 mg per minute. At 2 weeks, the axilla that had received therapy had mean sweat production of 24 ± 27 mg per minute ($P < .001$) compared with 144 ± 113 in the placebo axilla (also significant at $P = .004$). At 2 weeks, after injection of 100 U of botulinum toxin A into the placebo axilla, the mean rate of sweat production was reduced to 32 ± 39 mg per minute ($P < .001$). Sweat production rates (in 136 patients) still remained lower than baseline 24 weeks after treatment with 100 U. The mean rates were 67 ± 66 in the 200-U axilla and 65 ± 64 in the 100-U axilla. When the 2 doses were given in the 145 patients, 3 (2.1 %) experienced equal reduction of sweating in each axilla. Sixty-four patients (44.1 %) experienced greater reduction in sweating in the 100-U axilla. Seventy-eight patients showed greater reduction in sweating in the 200-U axilla. Ninety-eight percent of the patients said that they would recommend this well-tolerated treatment to others.

Conclusions.—Botulinum toxin A appears to be a safe and effective treatment for severe axillary hyperhidrosis.

▶ In my experience, this is a very effective therapy for axillary hyperhidrosis and is associated with high patient satisfaction. It should be noted that the potency of Botox is 2.5- to 4-fold greater than that of the Dysport used in these studies (Abstracts 19–1 and 19–2). Health care insurers will often approve the procedure after conventional therapies have failed. It is interesting to note that the reduction in sweating is significantly prolonged compared with pharmacologic denervation for rhytids.

J. Cook, MD

Type A Botulinum Toxin for the Treatment of Hypertrophy of the Masseter and Temporal Muscles: An Alternative Treatment

von Lindern JJ, Niederhagen B, Appel T, et al (Univ of Bonn, Germany)
Plast Reconstr Surg 107:327-332, 2001   19–3

Objective.—Hypertrophy of the masseter and temporal muscles can lead to symmetric or occasionally asymmetric enlargement of the affected muscle. Treatment up to now has involved the use of occlusal splints, the systemic administration of muscle relaxants, or surgical muscle reduction plus partial ostectomy of the masseteric tuberosity of mandible. The potential use of botulinum toxin to treat masseter and temporal muscle hypertrophy was tested in this study.

Methods.—Type A botulinum toxin was administered to 7 patients with unilateral and bilateral hypertrophy of the masseter and temporal muscles. Three were treated with an extraoral, transcutaneous approach, 3 with an intraoral approach, and 1 with a combined approach. In two patients, hyperactive areas of the muscles were identified electromyographically and targeted injections of botulinum delivered. Progress was recorded every 3 months, and patients were monitored for as long as 25 months. Additional doses of botulinum toxin were administered as needed.

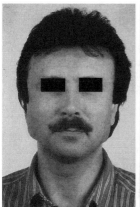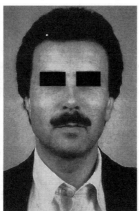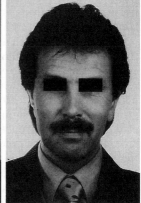

FIGURE 1.—*Left*, Patient with hypertrophy of the masseter and temporalis muscles before treatment with botulinum toxin. The same patient 3 months (*center*) and 25 months (*right*) after local injection of botulinum toxin in the masseter and temporal muscles. In this extreme case, a third injection was necessary because of a recurrence of muscle hypertrophy. The second injection was administered after 3 months, and the third injection was administered after 12 months. (Courtesy of von Lindern JJ, Niederhagen B, Appel T, et al: Type A botulinum toxin for the treatment of hypertrophy of the masseter and temporal muscles: An alternative treatment. *Plast Reconstr Surg* 107:327-332, 2001.)

Results.—Injections resulted in marked atrophy of the affected muscles between 3 and 8 weeks after injection. Three patients required a second injection, and 1 needed 3 injections (Fig 1). Patients showed no tendency to relapse over an observation period of up to 25 months.

Conclusion.—Botulinum toxin can be used to successfully treat hypertrophy of the masseter and temporal muscles.

▶ This is another interesting application of botulinum toxin with impressive results.

J. Cook, MD

Quantitative and Qualitative Effects of Chemical Peeling on Photo-Aged Skin: An Experimental Study
Butler PEM, Gonzalez S, Randolph MA, et al (Harvard Med School, Boston)
Plast Reconstr Surg 107:222-228, 2001   19–4

Objective.—Chemical peeling can improve the appearance of photo-aged skin, possibly by increasing glycosaminoglycan content and increasing the quality of collagen. The qualitative and quantitative changes that occur after a chemical peel were studied in a photo-aged animal model.

Methods.—The study included 100 hairless mice who were exposed to UVB radiation 3 times weekly for 14 weeks. The mice were divided into 5 groups of 20 mice each, comprising a a control group and 4 groups that were treated on their dorsal sides with either 50% glycolic acid, 30% trichloroacetic acid, 50% trichloroacetic acid, or phenol (Bokea-Gordon formula). Punch biopsy specimens were taken at 3, 7, 14, 28, and 60 days for histologic analysis and to assess collagen content. Glycosaminoglycan content was measured at 14, 28, and 60 days.

Results.—The dermal thickness at day 60 was increased in animals treated with 50% trichloroacetic acid (171 μm) and phenol peels (192 μm) compared with those treated with glycolic acid (83 μm) and 30% trichloroacetic acid (72 μm) and the (70 μm). The difference was significant between the 50% trichloroacetic acid and phenol groups and the control group, whereas no significant difference was noted between the glycolic acid or 30% trichloroacetic acid and the control group. Increased collagen reorganization was apparent in the upper reticular dermis at day 28 and in the papillary dermis at day 60. Treatment groups lost elastotic masses in the papillary and reticular dermis compared with the control group. The amount of collagen increased at day 3 in all treatment groups, peaked on day 28, and returned to prepeel levels by day 60. Collagen elevations were significant in the 30% and 50% trichloroacetic acid groups and the phenol group on days 3 and 28. In the 50% trichloroacetic acid and phenol groups, glycosaminoglycan levels increased and remained elevated through day 28 but declined to normal levels by day 60.

Conclusion.—Chemical peels result in qualitative and quantitative skin changes, with deeper peels increasing dermal volume and reorganizing dermal structural elements, including collagen and elastin.

▶ This animal study addresses the effect of chemical peels on photoaged skin, and attempts to identify the histologic changes that correlate with an improved clinical appearance. In this study, the investigators focused on the dermis. After deep peels with 50% trichloroacetic acid, there was a significant increase in dermal thickness. After both superficial and deep peels, there was evidence of collagen reorganization, and the amorphous clumps of elastic fibers were replaced with fine wavy elastic fibers arranged parallel to the surface. These changes were more marked with deep peels. Studies like this allow more insight into the microscopic changes associated with photoaging and how various resurfacing modalities work. Animal models such as this should also allow clinicians to make modifications in these resurfacing modalities in an effort to improve their safety and effectiveness.

P. G. Lang, Jr, MD

A Clinical and Histologic Comparison of Electrosurgical and Carbon Dioxide Laser Peels

Acland KM, Calonje E, Seed PT, et al (St Thomas' Hosp, London; GKT School of Medicine, London)
J Am Acad Dermatol 44:492-496, 2001   19–5

Background.—A radiofrequency-controlled electrosurgical device (ESD) has been adapted for skin peeling. A high-voltage, low-amperage current converts an irrigant into an ionized vapor, causing molecular dissociation and superficial damage in adjacent tissue.

Objective.—We compared the clinical and histologic effects of a scanning carbon dioxide (CO_2) laser (ESC/Sharplan 40C) and the ESD (Visage Cosmetic Surgery System, Arthrocare).

Methods.—This study was a matched clinical trial involving 9 subjects. Two strips (2×1 cm) of skin on the temple were alternately assigned to receive 2 passes with either the CO_2 laser (Silktouch mode, 260 handpiece, fluence 15 J/cm^2, 10 mm^2) or the ESD (125 V = setting 4, 5 mm handpiece). Strips were wiped with moist gauze after the first pass, and 4-mm punch biopsy specimens were taken immediately and after 3 months. Clinical assessment of re-epithelialization, erythema, and hyperpigmentation was made at 1, 2, 4, and 12 weeks.

Results.—Median erythema scores were significantly greater in skin treated with the CO_2 laser. Histologic examination showed greater epidermal loss and a significantly thicker zone of underlying thermal damage (average difference, 63 μm; 95% confidence interval, 40-87; $P = .0002$) in skin treated with the CO_2 laser compared with skin treated with the ESD. After 3 months, a band of superficial dermal fibrosis was thicker in skin treated with the CO_2 laser (average difference, 170 µm; 95% confidence interval, 69-271; $P = .0075$).

Conclusion.—Two passes with the ESD elicited a more superficial skin peel than the CO_2 laser. Despite minimal thermal damage, superficial dermal fibrosis was seen at 3 months in skin treated with the ESD.

▶ In this study comparing cold ablation (coblation) and CO_2 laser resurfacing, immediate posttreatment biopsy findings revealed a greater depth of tissue injury with the CO_2 laser. Therefore it is not surprising that at 3 months the amount and depth of dermal fibrosis was greater with the laser treatment. Although skin treated with coblation tended to reepithelialize more quickly and had less erythema, it may be that less tissue damage may also mean less improvement in wrinkles and scars.

P. G. Lang, Jr, MD

Wiping Away Debris Between Passes During Laser Surgery: Is it Really Efficient or Causing Complications?
Yuksel F, Karacaoglu E, Guler MM (GATA Haydarpasa Egitim Hastanesi, Istanbul, Turkey)
Aesthetic Plast Surg 25:184-186, 2001   19–6

Introduction.—Laser resurfacing of facial rhytids and pigmented lesions achieves better results than dermabrasion or topical caustic agents. But laser surgery can also have undesirable effects, such as scar formation or a cobblestone-like appearance on patients' faces. An experimental study was designed to determine the effects of wiping away the debris between sessions.

Methods.—The experiment was performed with the use of Sprague-Dawley rats. Laser beams were applied to the backs of the animals in 2 sessions. Half of the rats had charred skin debris removed with a saline soaked gauze, then the second pass was performed in the same manner. In the second group, the debris was not wiped and laser beams were applied directly onto the previous treatment site. All sites were excised for histologic evaluation.

Results.—The wiped group had a statistically higher ablation rate, but its surface irregularity was significantly greater when compared to the unwiped group. The difference in the values of tissue heights between wiped and unwiped groups was significant, with a more regular surface in the unwiped group.

Discussion.—Repeated passes during laser resurfacing will dehydrate and coagulate dermal collagen, limiting the penetration of laser energy. When the debris is wiped, the remaining surface is somewhat irregular, and subsequent passes may increase the irregularity. Vaporized tissue may act as a barrier, producing a more even result. Wiping vaporized debris every 2 passes is the recommended method for laser surgery.

▶ Clinicians continue to attempt to refine carbon dioxide laser resurfacing in an effort to minimize side effects such as scarring, delayed hypopigmentation, and persistent redness. Such refinements have included not wiping away the vaporized tissue after the last pass or going over the area with the erbium-YAG laser after the final pass has been made. There are several reasons to wipe away vaporized tissue between passes. One is that such tissue may interfere with deeper penetration of the laser, thus decreasing the benefit of the procedure. Another is that it may act as a heat sink, leading to unwanted thermal damage. In this study, Yuksel and associates showed that by not wiping away the vaporized tissue they achieved a smoother surface; however, at the same time less tissue was ablated. They theorize that by not wiping, areas that were missed by the previous pass absorb more energy, whereas the vaporized layer protects the previously vaporized tissue. Thus, the vaporized tissue acts as a barrier, yielding a more even result. The authors suggest wiping after every 2 passes. This would not only allow for more uniform vaporization, but would also permit sufficiently deep vaporization, which would facilitate a good cosmetic outcome. Unfortunately, this study was done in animals and we have no way of knowing what effect this protocol would have when resurfacing the skin of patients. Additionally, their modification is based on the assumption that significant areas are missed when each pass is made. With computerized pattern generators and a little attention to technique, this would not seem likely and one must wonder if their assumption is more theoretical than real.

P. G. Lang, Jr, MD

The Epidermal and Dermal Changes Associated With Microdermabrasion
Freedman BM, Rueda-Pedraza E, Waddell SP (Plastic Surgery Associates of Northern Virginia, McLean; Reston Hosp Ctr, Reston, Va)
Dermatol Surg 27:1031-1034, 2001   19–7

Introduction.—Microdermabrasion is a technique for skin rejuvenation in which a stream of fine sand particles is directed over the skin by a compressed air delivery system. Through repetitive intraepidermal injury, fibroblast activity and new collagen deposition in the dermis may be stimulated. The onset and extent of dermatologic changes associated with the treatment were analyzed in a group of volunteers who underwent facial microdermabrasion.

Methods.—Participants were 10 white individuals ranging in age from 31 to 62 years. All had 6 facial aluminum oxide microdermabrasion treatments performed at 6- to 10-day intervals. The average treatment duration was 15 minutes, and the treatment end point was clinical erythema. Photographs were taken and skin biopsy specimens obtained pretreatment, 1 week after the third treatment, and 1 week after the sixth treatment. Sections of the biopsy specimens were prepared for light microscopy and the slides were reviewed in a blinded fashion.

Results.—After 3 microdermabrasion treatments, the mean epidermal thickness increased from 45 μm to 62 μm. The mean thickness after 6 treatments was 65 μm. Papillary dermal thickness increased from a mean of 81 μm pretreatment to 114 μm after 6 treatments. Compared with control areas, treated sites also exhibited flattening of the rete pegs, vascular ectasia, perivascular inflammation, and hyalinization of the papillary dermis with newly deposited collagen and elastic fibers.

Discussion.—The inflammatory response elicited by microdermabrasion resembles a reparative process in the dermis and epidermis. Histologic changes produced by microdermabrasion could be observed after 3 treatments and became more evident after 6 treatments. Initial clinical changes appear to result from stimulation of the basal layer, with epidermal thickening, flattening of the rete pegs, and normalization of the stratum corneum.

The Evaluation of Aluminum Oxide Crystal Microdermabrasion for Photodamage

Tan M-H, Spencer JM, Pires LM, et al (New York Univ; Johnson and Johnson Consumer Products, Skillman, NJ)
Dermatol Surg 27:943-949, 2001   19–8

Introduction.—Aluminum oxide crystal microdermabrasion is a popular technique for rejuvenation of facial skin. Patients report an improvement in skin appearance and texture, but the clinical efficacy of the treatment on photodamaged skin has not been established. Ten volunteers who underwent 5 or 6 microdermabrasion treatments of facial skin were evaluated by photographs, skin thermography, sebum analysis, and histologic analysis.

Methods.—Participants had Fitzpatrick skin types I to III and photodamage. Photographs taken pretreatment and posttreatment were graded by 2 physicians on a 4-point scale (from no improvement to marked improvement [75% to 100% change]). Thermographic changes were documented before and after microdermabrasion, and sebum content was measured with an automated sebumeter. Also assessed were skin topography, elasticity, stiffness, compliance, and histology.

Results.—Analysis of clinical photography by physicians indicated mild improvement in most patients. Seven of the 10 patients reported mild improvement in the appearance of treated skin. Immediately after microdermabrasion sessions, skin temperature increased (consistent with increased blood flow), sebum content decreased, and a temporary increase in skin roughness and mild flattening of some wrinkles occurred. Dynamic skin analysis revealed a statistically significant decrease in skin stiffness and an increase in skin compliance. Histologic studies in 2 participants before and 1 week after the final treatment showed a number of changes: slight orthokeratosis and flattening of rete ridges, slight edema, and vascular ectasia. Collagen and elastin content were not significantly changed.

Conclusion.—Microdermabrasion is a simple, noninvasive, and painless procedure that yields mild improvement in the appearance of photodamaged skin. Objective biochemical analysis confirmed a decrease in skin stiffness and an increase in skin compliance consistent with persistent edema. Histologic analysis revealed marked vascular changes in the reticular dermis below the level of direct abrasion.

▶ The popularity of microdermabrasion continues to expand. This minimally invasive technique is generally met with a moderate to high degree of patient satisfaction. Both of these well-written articles (Abstracts 19–7 and 19–8) demonstrate variable results after microdermabrasion. It would appear that not all units are created equal, and operator technique is important to achieve the desired outcome. With increasing aggressiveness of both the powered suction and the crystal delivery, results may improve. However, the consequence of this may be longer periods of postprocedure erythema, which many patients, in my experience, may not be willing to accept.

J. Cook, MD

Combined Laser Therapy for Difficult Dermal Pigmentation: Resurfacing and Selective Photothermolysis
Park SH, Koo SH, Choi EO (Korea Univ, Seoul)
Ann Plast Surg 47:31-36, 2001   19–9

Introduction.—The removal of deep pigmented lesions is difficult, and complications such as scar formation or depigmentation can occur. A combined laser therapy with resurfacing lasers followed by the application of selective photothermolytic lasers was used successfully for 47 patients with nevus of Ota and 15 with congenital nevi.

Methods.—Between 1992 and 1995, 57 patients with nevus of Ota were treated with the Q-Switched Ruby Laser (QSRL) (Dermalase, Lumonics Inc, England) alone. The combined therapy, using the Tru-Pulse CO_2 laser (Tissue Technologies, Albuquerque, NM) and the QSRL, has been used at the study institution since 1995. Most patients were young adults with facial lesions. In cases of nevus of Ota, the combined treatment included 2 to 3 passes at 300 mJ of the CO_2 laser and 6 to 7 J/cm^2 of the QSRL concomitantly, followed by QSRL at 4- to 6-week intervals. For congenital nevi, initial treatment included 3 passes at 500 mJ using the CO_2 laser and 6 to 7 mJ/cm^2 using the QSRL concomitantly, followed by the QSRL at 4- to 6-week intervals. Sunblock was used daily after wound healing, and 4% hydroquinone was applied as a bleaching cream nightly. Outcome was classified as excellent, good, fair, poor, or no change.

Results.—The mean duration of combined treatment for nevus of Ota was 6 months and the mean number of treatments was 5. Excellent results were achieved in 98% of patients. Twelve patients (80%) with congenital nevi had good-to-excellent results; 20% had only fair results. With QSRL alone, 95% of patients with nevus of Ota had excellent results. Congenital nevi could not be treated with the QSRL alone. The combined treatment reduced the number of treatments and the total treatment period for patients with nevus of Ota.

Conclusion.—Resurfacing followed by selective laser treatment enhances the removal of deep dermal pigmentation. The Er:YAG laser should be studied as well because it causes less thermal damage during resurfacing and promotes faster wound healing than the CO_2 laser.

▶ These investigators focused on 2 lesions characterized by the presence of pigment deep in the dermis: nevus of Ota and congenital nevi. They hypothesized that by initially performing CO_2 laser resurfacing, they could remove the superficial pigment, thus allowing the QSRL to more effectively reach and remove the deep pigment. Although the results with nevus of Ota were impressive, it should be noted that the treatment course, on average, was only shortened by several treatments and several months. Although no long-term complications were observed, one must ask whether it is worth the added risk of scarring to minimally shorten the treatment course, especially when there was no difference in outcome when the QSRL was used alone. This dual laser technique, however, might be useful for patients with recalcitrant lesions. Also, as a comparison, it might be worthwhile to perform the same study using the Er:YAG laser instead of the CO_2 laser. Finally, as other studies have demonstrated, the response of congenital nevi to laser surgery was less predictable and the results achieved were less favorable.

P. G. Lang, Jr, MD

Long-Pulsed Nd:YAG Laser-Assisted Hair Removal in Pigmented Skin: A Clinical and Histological Evaluation
Alster TS, Bryan H, Williams CM (Washington Inst of Dermatologic Laser Surgery, DC)
Arch Dermatol 137:885-889, 2001   19–10

Background.—Most laser hair removal systems emit energy with wavelengths from 630 to 1100 nm, which can penetrate 2 to 5 mm into the dermis and thus irradiate the entire length of an anagen hair follicle. Laser hair removal in darker-skinned patients is challenging because the increased concentration of epidermal melanin absorbs the laser energy, thereby reducing follicular irradiation. The efficacy and safety of a 1064-nm Nd:YAG laser (which can penetrate from 5-7 mm into the dermis) was investigated for hair reduction in patients with darker skin.

Methods.—The subjects were 20 women 21 to 39 years old with skin phototypes IV-VI who had dark brown-to-black terminal hair on the face, axillae, or legs. Involved areas were treated by a long-pulsed (50-msec) emission from a 1064-nm Nd:YAG laser delivered once a month for 3 consecutive months. In brief, before each treatment hairs greater than 1 mm long were shaved, and the patient's skin was protected during laser irradiation by a contact cooling device. The mean fluences were 50 J/cm² for facial hair (n = 8), 45 J/cm^2 for hair on the legs (n = 4), and 40 J/cm^2 for axillary hair (n = 8). All treatment sites were photographed under identical conditions before each of the 3 treatments and 1, 3, 6, and 12 months after the last treatment. Two independent raters reviewed these photographs to evaluate hair loss and the extent of hair regrowth, as follows: less than 25% = 0, 25% to 50% = 1, 51% to 75% = 2, 76% to 90% = 3, and greater than 90% = 4. Patients also reported any adverse effects at each visit. Additionally, at baseline, immediately after the first treatment, and at 1 and 6 months after the final treatment, 3 patients provided 3-mm skin punch biopsy specimens from each of the different treatment areas. These specimens were examined by a dermatopathologist to determine histologic changes.

Results.—For all 3 body locations, after each of the 3 treatments there was a marked reduction in hair regrowth that persisted for 12 months after the final treatment. For facial hair, clinical hair reduction scores after 1, 2, and 3 treatments and at 12 months after the last treatment were 1.8, 2.3, 2.9, and 2.3, respectively. Leg hair was slightly more responsive, with corresponding clinical hair reduction scores of 2.0, 3.2, 3.5, and 2.9. Axillary hair was the most responsive to treatment, with corresponding clinical hair reduction scores of 2.8, 3.6, 4.0, and 3.5. Thus, sun-protected areas and thinner axillary skin had a greater clinical response than sun-exposed facial and leg skin. Adverse effects included mild-to-moderate pain at the treatment site (90% of sites), transient pigmentary alteration (5%), and vesiculation (1.5%); the latter 2 adverse effects occurred only in sun-exposed areas. Adverse effects were less common in sun-protected areas and thinner axillary skin than in sun-exposed facial and leg skin. Histologic examination of biopsy specimens obtained 6 months after the last treatment showed selective follicular injury but no epidermal disruption. Large terminal hair follicles had been destroyed with minimal inflammation and hair shafts were reduced in number, while pilosebaceous glands were preserved.

Conclusions.—The long-pulsed 1064-nm Nd:YAG laser can safely and effectively provide long-term hair reduction in patients with darker skin. Adverse effects were transient and generally mild. The greatest clinical response, with the fewest adverse effects, was noted for sun-protected skin and thinner axillary skin, although sun-exposed facial and leg skin also had a substantial response to 3 treatment sessions. This suggests that skin thickness influences the clinical outcome to a greater degree than does the hair growth cycle.

▶ This study supports the contention of laser manufacturers that the long-pulsed Nd:YAG 1064-nm laser is effective and safe for hair removal in patients with dark skin. Interestingly, hair-bearing areas with thinner skin were more responsive to treatment.

P. G. Lang, Jr, MD

Clinical and Pathophysiologic Correlates of 1064-nm Nd:YAG Laser Treatment of Reticular Veins and Venulectasias

Sadick NS, Prieto VG, Shea CR, et al (Cornell Univ, New York; Univ of Texas, Houston; Duke Univ, Durham, NC; et al)

Arch Dermatol 137:613-617, 2001   19–11

Introduction.—The long-pulsed Nd:YAG (1064-nm) laser has recently been used with success in the treatment of disfiguring leg veins and the removal of unwanted body hair. In a study of 13 patients with reticular veins and venulectasias, the histologic and clinical effects of a 1064-nm Nd:YAG laser system were evaluated.

Methods.—Patients were 13 women with a mean age of 38.5 years and with skin types II through V. All veins were located on the inner or outer thighs. Included in the treated vessels were blue venulectasia, 0.5 to 1.5 mm in diameter (class 2; 72%), and reticular veins, 1.5 to 4.0 mm in diameter (class 3; 28%). A single treatment was performed using the following parameters: wavelength, 1064 nm (multiple synchronized pulsing); spot size, 6 mm; pulse duration, 14 msec (single pulse); and fluence, 130 J/cm^2. Double-masked observers judged outcome according to 5 categories, with grade 0 indicating worsening and grade 4 indicating 75% to 100% improvement. Biopsy specimens were obtained for histologic examination and immunohistochemical analysis.

Results.—Eight patients (62%) had excellent results, with 75% to 100% clearing of the treated vessel surface area. In all cases, immediate intravascular pigment darkening and perivascular erythema were manifested as end points of therapy. Hyperpigmentation, observed in 3 (23%) patients, resolved within 6 weeks. One patient had telangiectatic matting. Histologically, the treated areas exhibited perivascular hemorrhage, thrombi, fragmentation and homogenization of elastic fibers, and eosinophilia of vessel walls. The treated vessels also exhibited increased expression of the heat shock protein hsp70 and transforming growth factor β.

Conclusion.—The long-pulsed 1064-nm Nd:YAG laser was able to achieve closure and long-term clearance of blue venulectasia and reticular veins up to 4 mm in diameter, probably by heat-induced vessel damage and subsequent fibrosis. Clearance remained during 6 months of posttreatment evaluation, although the finding of recanalized thrombi in some biopsy specimens suggests the possibility of long-term vessel reappearance.

▶ The long-pulsed 1064 Nd:YAG laser is fast becoming the laser of choice for treating large leg veins (less than 4 mm) and for hair removal in dark-skinned individuals. This study verifies the efficacy of this laser for treating leg veins, even in skin type V patients. However, patients should be forewarned that transient hyperpigmentation is common after treatment and that telangiectatic matting may occur.

P. G. Lang, Jr, MD

Both the Flashlamp-Pumped Dye Laser and the Long-Pulsed Tunable Dye Laser Can Improve Results in Port-Wine Stain Therapy

Scherer K, Lorenz S, Wimmershoff M, et al (Univ of Regensburg, Germany)
Br J Dermatol 145:79-84, 2001   19–12

Background.—The accepted treatment of port-wine stains (PWS) involves a flashlamp-pumped dye laser (FPDL) at 450 μs pulse duration, but an alternative, a long-pulsed tunable dye laser (LPTDL) used at 1.5 ms pulse duration originally developed for leg veins, may also prove useful. The efficacy and adverse effects accompanying each modality were compared.

Methods.—The study included 62 healthy individuals aged from 2 to 65 years with skin types ranging from Fitzpatrick I to V whose PWS were untreated previously. They were evaluated using both the FPDL and the LPTDL. The FPDL was used at 585 nm, for a 450 μs pulse duration on a 7-mm spot at a fluence of 5.75 to 7.0 J/cm². Each patient received several pulses with the laser. The LPTDL was used at 4 wavelengths, 585, 590, 595, and 600 nm, for a 1.5 ms pulse duration on a 5-mm spot up to a fluence of 20 J/cm². Several pulses were delivered to each patient with LPTDL at all 4 wavelengths. The epidermis was cooled by a dynamic cooling device. Exposure was 30 ms, with a 20 ms delay before the next exposure. The test spots chosen were representative of the color and surface structure of the PWS. Evaluations were performed 6 weeks after treatment and results graded as excellent, good, moderate, or poor in comparison with untreated areas.

Results.—Of the 62 patients, 12 (19%) had the best results with FPDL, and 30 (48%) had the best results with LPTDL. With respect to wavelength, the number of patients showing the best fading was as follows: 585 nm, 13 patients; 590 nm, 3 patients; 595 nm, 8 patients; and 600 nm, 6 patients. No differences between the FPDL and the LPTDL results were apparent in 20 patients, and 7 patients did not respond to either laser treatment. Neither the age of the patient nor the location of the PWS affected results. Twenty-eight patients who had the best result with LPTDL continued that treatment, with 22 having only LPTDL and 6 also receiving FPDL. LPTDL did not increase the incidence of adverse effects. The adverse effects reported were minor, with hyperpigmentation and/or atrophy reported by 14 patients undergoing FPDL and 13 patients after LPTDL.

Conclusions.—The LPTDL permits treatment of a wider range of vessels than FPDL. Nearly 50% achieved better fading with LPTDL, and only 19% had better fading with FPDL. For larger PWS vessels, LPTDL may be more effective than FPDL.

▶ Laser technology continues to evolve. The latest advance in lasers to treat vascular lesions has been the ability to adjust not only the wavelength but also the pulse duration. In this study, the authors compared the flashlamp-pumped pulsed dye laser (450 μs pulse) and long pulse tunable dye laser (1.5 ms pulse) for their ability to treat PWS. A side-by-side comparison was performed based primarily on test spot results rather than dividing the PWS into segments and comparing the lasers in their ability to treat a portion of the lesion. Anyone doing test spots with these lasers will often observe complete clearing within the test spot, but when the actual treatment is done, multiple treatments are often necessary to achieve good (as opposed to complete) clearing. Thus, comparing test spots may not be the best way to assess the merits of different laser systems. Also, because of power limitations, it was only possible to use a 5-mm spot size with the tunable dye laser, which could have influenced the outcome. Finally, the maximum power used with the flashlamp-pumped dye laser was only 7 J/cm^2. Although somewhat flawed in its design, this investigation does attempt to compare the 2 laser systems and most importantly points out the heterogeneity of the vessels comprising a PWS. This is important because vessels of different size require different pulse durations and energies to bring about their ablation.

P. G. Lang, Jr, MD

Myofibroblasts and Apoptosis in Human Hypertrophic Scars: The Effect of Interferon-α2b
Nedelec B, Shankowsky H, Scott PG, et al (Univ of Alberta, Edmonton, Canada)
Surgery 130:798-808, 2001   19–13

Background.—Hypertrophic scars (HSc) are a dermal fibroproliferative phenomenon that leads to considerable morbidity. Preliminary evidence suggests that interferon (IFN) may improve the clinical appearance of HSc. The aims of this study were to compare the cell density in HSc and in wounds that heal without development of HSc (normotrophic scars); to examine the presence of myofibroblasts and apoptosis in HSc and normotrophic scars over time; and to determine whether systemic administration of IFN-α2b can induce apoptosis.

Methods.—Two groups of patients underwent serial tissue biopsies. Six burn patients were studied prospectively by obtaining biopsy specimens from wound granulation tissue, normal skin, post-burn HSc, and normotrophic scars (healed donor sites). A second patient group with HSc was treated with systemic IFN-α2b, and biopsy material was taken before, during, and after IFN therapy. The tissue was analyzed by immunohistochemical staining for α-smooth muscle actin (α-SMA) and by in situ DNA fragmentation terminal deoxynucleotidyl transferase-mediated deoxyuridine triphosphate (dUTP)–biotin nick end labeling (TUNEL) assay for apoptosis.

Results.—The total numbers of fibroblasts in HSc were found to be similar to granulation tissue and twice that of normal skin and normotrophic scars. Over time the numbers of cells in HSc tissue decreased toward normal skin levels. A significantly higher percentage of fibroblasts stained for α-SMA in HSc, as compared with normotrophic scars or normal skin obtained from the same patient ($P > .05$). Serial biopsy specimens of resolving HSc tissue obtained from patients who received systemic IFN-α2b showed a general reduction in the total number of fibroblasts and myofibroblasts, which was associated with a significant increase in the percentage of apoptotic cells compared with normal dermis from the same patient.

Conclusions.—HSc tissues have greater numbers of fibroblasts and myofibroblasts than do normal skin and normotrophic scars. As HSc remodel, the numbers of fibroblasts and myofibroblasts decrease, possibly by induction of apoptosis. Systemic IFN-α2b may contribute to the resolution of HSc in part by the enhanced induction of apoptosis.

▶ Interferon has been administered systemically and intralesionally in the treatment of keloidal scarring, and anecdotal reports point to the possible effectiveness of topical application of the interferon inducer, imiquimod. Whatever the mode of administration, enhanced induction of apoptosis may be the underlying mechanism of action. Certainly, local administration of IFN or IFN induction would seem to represent a safer and more cost-effective approach than systemic injection.

B. H. Thiers, MD

Ear-Lobe Keloids: Treatment by a Protocol of Surgical Excision and Immediate Postoperative Adjuvant Radiotherapy
Ragoowansi R, Cornes PGS, Glees JP, et al (St George's Hosp, London; Royal Marsden Hosp, Sutton, England)
Br J Plast Surg 54:504-508, 2001   19–14

Background.—In a previous study, the estimated incidence of earlobe keloids after ear piercing was 2.5%; it is probable that with multiple piercings the number of keloids will increase. Keloids are distinct from hypertrophic scars in that the scars soften and flatten spontaneously, whereas the keloids remain thick and raised for extended periods, even years. Most treatments for keloids have limited success and variable results. Patients not responding to massage with topical silicone may receive monthly intralesional steroid injections over a 4-month period. If no response is then observed, excision is needed. However, a 50% recurrence rate after excision has been reported. The use of a combination of extralesional excision plus immediate postoperative adjuvant radiotherapy was assessed for its effectiveness.

Methods.—The study included 35 patients (age, 16-44 years; average, 24 years) who had not responded to intralesional steroid treatment, excision, or both. In an extralesional full-thickness excision, the entire ear-piercing track was removed from anterior to posterior. The resulting wound defects were closed with interrupted 5/0 monofilament prolene sutures and the scar covered with topical 2% lignocaine-0.25% chlorhexidine in sterile lubricant gel; the site was then covered with a transparent self-adhesive polyurethane dressing so the area could be observed without disturbing the wound or increasing the risk of sepsis. Radiotherapy was given within 24 hours of surgery at a dose of 10 Gy at the skin surface in 1 fraction. Photon irradiation of 100 kV was applied at 25 cm SSD, using a 4-mm A1 filter, which resulted in a high-voltage therapy of 4 mm A1. Non-target areas were shielded, and radiotherapy beams were angled to avoid adjacent tissues. Follow-up assessments were performed 4 weeks, 3 months, and 6 months after the procedure, then annually until relapse or 5 years postoperatively. If additional treatment was required, the case was treated as a treatment failure, and the patient was considered to have relapsed.

Results.—After 5 years' follow-up, 34 patients were still being monitored, one having been lost at 1 year. All keloids were controlled at 4 weeks, but relapse occurred in 3 patients at 1 year and in 4 additional patients at 5 years. The cumulative probability of control was 79.4%. No serious radiation toxicity occurred, and the only side effects were transient mild erythema and postradiation hyperpigmentation, generally in non-white patients and lasting for several months or years. Because of the risk of recurrence, all patients were cautioned not to have ear piercing after treatment.

Conclusions.—Adjuvant radiotherapy after extralesional excision was successful in preventing the recurrence of keloids in the majority of these high-risk patients. During the 5-year follow-up period, 79.4% of cases exhibited control of the keloids.

▶ Keloids are difficult to treat, and controlled studies are difficult to perform. In this study, keloids of the ear were surgically excised, and the patients received a single 10-Gy dose of postoperative radiation. With this protocol, the authors report a quite acceptable 5-year control rate of 79.4%. However, this reviewer would offer some criticism of the study design and conclusions. The authors contend that keloids located on the ear have the highest recurrence rate of any anatomical location. If anything, the opposite may be true. Keloids of the chest, shoulder, and jawline have a much higher recurrence rate. Indeed, in this reviewer's experience, keloids of the chest, treated with a combination of surgical excision, intralesional steroids, and postoperative radiation, still show nearly a 100% recurrence rate. Thus, to truly evaluate the proposed treatment protocol, the authors should have included keloids located on other anatomical sites.

P. G. Lang, Jr, MD

Investigation of Recurrence Rates Among Earlobe Keloids Utilizing Various Postoperative Therapeutic Modalities

Jackson IT, Bhageshpur R, DiNick V, et al (Inst for Craniofacial and Reconstructive Surgery, Southfield, Mich)

Eur J Plast Surg 24:88-95, 2001

19–15

Background.—Many treatments have been used to treat keloids of the external ear. Experience with keloids of the earlobe was reviewed to assess patient characteristics and the efficacy of various treatment modalities in preventing recurrences.

Methods.—The medical records of 24 patients (10 males and 14 females) 7 to 64 years old (mean age, 25 years) with earlobe keloids due to earlobe piercing (n = 19 patients) or trauma (n = 3) or as a complication of rhytidectomy (n = 2) were reviewed. Eighteen patients were African American, 4 were white, 1 was Hispanic, and 1 was Arabian. All patients underwent total surgical excision of the keloid and intralesional corticosteroid injection immediately after the defect was sutured. This core regimen was the only treatment received by 10 patients. The other patients also underwent the following treatments, alone or in combination: radiation (1200 cGy in 3 equal fractions at 4-day intervals beginning on postoperative day 4), interferon (3 doses of 0.1 mL α-interferon injected locally at 1-week intervals beginning 1 week postoperatively), postoperative steroid injections (once a week for 3 weeks), and pressure earrings (worn beginning 2 weeks postoperatively and continuing for 6 months). Patients were observed for 12 months to 10 years (mean, 5.6 years) to determine recurrences (ie, nodulation or raised surfaces at the excision site >0.5 cm in diameter).

Results.—Nine patients (38%) had a positive family history of keloids. Twelve patients (50%) had a history of keloids on the earlobe (n = 9) or the abdomen and extremities (n = 3). Eight of these 12 patients had been treated by surgical excision or steroid injection. Patients presented between 15 days and 24 months after the onset of new keloids or the appearance of recurrent lesions. Nine of the 24 patients (37%) had bilateral ear involvement, 10 (42%) had keloids only on the left ear, and 5 (20%) had keloids only on the right ear. Keloids ranged in size from 0.5 to 6.0 cm (mean, 2.6 cm), and all were predominantly sessile. During follow-up, 7 patients (29%) experienced a recurrence. These 7 patients included 3 males and 4 females 7 to 43 years old; 5 were African American, 1 was white, and 1 was Arabian. Time to recurrence ranged from 5 to 24 months (mean, 11.7 months). Five of these 7 patients (71%) had a history of keloids, 3 of whom had previously received intralesional steroid therapy. Recurrent lesions tended to be smaller than the original keloids (0.5-2 cm for recurrences, compared with 1-6 cm for the original lesions). Of the 10 patients who underwent the core regimen only, 8 (80%) have experienced no recurrence at a mean follow-up of 31 months. In contrast, of the 5 patients who used pressure earrings in addition to the core regimen, 3 (60%) experienced recurrence. The other 2 recurrences occurred in 1 of 4 patients (25%) who received the core regimen plus local postoperative steroid injections plus pressure earrings, and in the 1 patient (100%) who received the core regimen plus interferon. No recurrence develped in the 4 patients who received radiation (in combination with interferon or local postoperative steroid injection).

Conclusions.—Based on these findings and a review of the literature, the following guidelines for managing keloids of the earlobes are recommended. First, patients with small solitary lesions and a family history of keloids should try conservative management before proceeding to surgical excision, because the early treatment of scars may prevent hypertrophy. Minimizing trauma to the wound bed may also reduce recurrence rates; this includes the use of noncrushing instrumentation and the closing of skin edges under minimal tension with nonabsorbable sutures. Local excision, immediate intralesional corticosteroid injection, and radiation may confer the best protection against recurrence. Pressure earrings appear to be of little benefit.

▶ The title of this article suggests that the reader will be enlightened regarding the management of keloids; unfortunately, it falls short of its goal. Although the patients were stratified according to treatment modality, many of the groups contained only a few patients. Thus, definitive conclusions regarding the various approaches cannot be drawn.

P. G. Lang, Jr, MD

Treatment of Keloids by High-Dose-Rate Brachytherapy: A Seven-Year Study

Guix B, Henírquez I, Andrés A, et al (Universitat de Barcelona; Policlínica Balmes, Barcelona)
Int J Radiat Oncol Biol Phys 50:167-172, 2001   19–16

Background.—Keloid scars are notorious for their propensity to recur after treatment. Even the most effective treatment—surgical excision followed by radiation therapy—carries a recurrence rate of about 20%. Because delivery of the radiation dose can be better targeted with brachytherapy than with external beam irradiation, it was hypothesized that high-dose-rate (HDR) brachytherapy might be an effective and safe means of treating keloids. This hypothesis was tested prospectively, and results were reported after 7 years of follow-up.

Methods.—The subjects were 169 patients (35 males and 134 females) 16 to 72 years old (mean age, 42 years) with keloid scars of the face (n = 77), thorax (n = 42), abdomen (n = 31), legs (n = 12), or arms (n = 7). All but 1 patient were white. Keloids were 2 to 22 cm (mean, 4.2 cm) long and 1.0 to 2.8 cm (mean, 1.8 cm) wide. Most patients (147, or 87%) underwent surgical excision of the keloid, during which a flexible 6F plastic catheter was inserted through the center of the wound before closure. HDR brachytherapy was administered at a total dose of 1200 cGy, delivered in 4 equal fractions over the first 24 hours after surgery. The tube was withdrawn immediately after the last brachytherapy fraction was delivered, and the wound was covered with a gauze pad for 2 hours. However, 22 patients (13%) refused surgery and received HDR brachytherapy alone (total of 1800 cGy in 6 equal fractions delivered over 36 hours) via plastic tubes placed through the skin to cover the entire scar. Patients were monitored at regular intervals for at least 1 year (median, 37.3 months) to determine recurrences, late skin effects, and cosmetic results.

Results.—During follow-up, recurrence developed in 8 patients (4.7%). This included 5 of 147 patients (3.4%) who underwent surgical excision followed by HDR brachytherapy, and 3 of 22 patients (13.6%) who had been treated with HDR brachytherapy alone. Cosmetic results were excellent or good in 88.4% of patients treated with excision plus HDR brachytherapy and in 77.3% of patients treated with HDR brachytherapy alone. Clinical signs and symptoms improved over time after treatment. For example, more than 75% of the patients reported a burning sensation, redness, or pruritus before treatment, whereas less than 5% reported 1 of these signs at the 2-year follow-up visit. Skin pigmentation changes developed in 10 patients (5.9%), and limited areas of telangiectasia developed in 26 patients (15.4%). There were no cases of skin atrophy or skin fibrosis.

Conclusions.—All patients responded to HDR brachytherapy with a reduction in pruritus, redness, or burning. Additionally, all patients tolerated HDR brachytherapy well, with no reports of pain; the greatest inconvenience was that patients had to return to the radiation therapy department so often during the first 24 to 36 hours after beginning therapy. Cosmetic results were good or excellent in the vast majority of patients. Other authors have reported keloid recurrence rates of 21% to 27% after surgical excision and radiation therapy (with or without intralesional corticosteroid injection). The recurrence rate in this series was much better, 3.5% if the keloid was excised before HDR brachytherapy and 13.6% if HDR brachytherapy was used alone. Thus, HDR brachytherapy, especially when combined with surgical excision, safely and effectively treats keloid scars and prevents their recurrence. Another advantage of this approach is that it allows very accurate dosimetry and geometric treatment optimization. In fact, of the total of 720 fractions given, new dosimetry was required in 554 fractions (76.9%), and was accomplished quickly and easily. HDR brachytherapy is also economical, and its costs compare favorably with those of external beam radiation therapy for keloids. Thus, the authors recommend HDR brachytherapy as the treatment of choice for keloid scars.

▶ The quest continues for an efficacious and simple method to reduce the recurrence rate after keloid treatment. It has been reported that postoperative radiation therapy may reduce the risk of keloid recurrence after surgical excision. Most studies show that even with a combination of surgical removal and radiation treatment, recurrence rates are approximately 20% to

25%. In this study, the authors ingeniously implanted a small catheter in the base of the wound after surgical extirpation of the keloid and administered localized brachytherapy with excellent results. Although their method includes 4 to 6 visits for administration of the radiation in the first 24 to 36 postoperative hours, minimal side effects were seen. If this protocol could be designed to be cost effective, it may well prove to be an excellent method for treating difficult keloids.

J. Cook, MD

Ganglion of the Distal Interphalangeal Joint (Myxoid Cyst): Therapy by Identification and Repair of the Leak of Joint Fluid
de Berker D, Lawrence C (Bristol Royal Infirmary, England; Royal Victoria Infirmary, Newcastle upon Tyne, England)
Arch Dermatol 137:607-610, 2001   19–17

Introduction.—The authors believe that digital myxoid cysts (DMCs) result from leakage of joint fluid from a degenerative distal interphalangeal joint (DIPJ), and that sealing the point of leakage can be curative. They tested this theory by using a minimally traumatic surgical procedure after communication between the DMC and the DIPJ was confirmed with methylene blue dye injection.

Methods.—The open nonrandomized trial enrolled 54 adults (34 women, 20 men; mean age, 60.4 years). All surgery was performed with the patient under local anesthetic ring block of digital nerves at the base of the digit. After methylene blue dye was injected into the DIPJ, a skin flap was designed around the cyst and raised to identify the dye-filled communication between joint and cyst. The cyst contents were evacuated without skin excision, and the cyst roof was left intact.

Results.—Methylene blue dye injection confirmed communication between cyst and joint in 48 patients (89%). In 3 of the other 6 patients, dye was still found in adjacent tissues. Dye failed to enter the joint in the remaining 3 patients. With 8 months of follow-up, 48 patients remained cured with no visible scarring. Five of 6 relapses occurred within 4 months of treatment. Two patients experienced pain for 4 months, and another reported limited joint mobility for 2 months.

Conclusion.—A conservative surgical method that does not require tissue excision was used successfully to treat DMCs. The authors believe that the DMC is a ganglion, and they have shown that a connection between the DMC and the DIPJ is present in almost 90% of cases. Cure rates were higher on fingers (94%) than on toes (57%) because in the toe the weight of standing and walking increases the pressure of fluid escaping from the joint.

▶ This novel method involves intra-articular methylene blue injection to clearly identify the connection between the cyst and the joint space, followed by disruption of the communication. This technique involves no tissue resection, with significantly quicker healing and less operative risks. The success rate seems to be much higher in fingers than in toes, perhaps a consequence of the significant difference in hydrostatic pressures at these anatomic sites.

J. Cook, MD

Assessment of Ropivacaine as a Local Anesthetic for Skin Infiltration in Skin Surgery

Moffitt DL, de Berker DAR, Kennedy CTK, et al (Bristol Royal Hosps, England)
Dermatol Surg 27:437-440, 2001   19–18

Introduction.—Ropivacaine, a new amide local anesthetic, has a longer duration of action than lidocaine and reduced cardiac toxicity compared with equivalent doses of bupivacaine. The use of local infiltration of ropivacaine for skin surgery was assessed in 18 healthy volunteers.

Methods.—This double-blind placebo-controlled study sought to establish the concentration of ropivacaine with an optimum balance among prolonged anesthesia, maximum rate of onset, and least pain of infiltration. Four concentrations of ropivacaine (1, 2, 5, and 7.5 mg/mL) were injected intradermally for purposes of comparison, with normal saline used as a control. A sixth injection of lidocaine 2% and epinephrine 1:80,000 was compared with ropivacaine for pain on injection. Volunteers were asked to score the pain of infiltration for each injection. The onset and duration of anesthesia were assessed by pinprick testing.

Results.—Pain of infiltration varied widely among the volunteers, but there was a trend for increasing pain with higher concentrations of ropivacaine. The pain of lidocaine and epinephrine infiltration was significantly greater than both control and 7.5 mg/mL ropivacaine. Full anesthesia, with an absence of sensation to pinprick, was reached at a mean of 161 seconds with 2 mg/mL ropivacaine, a mean of 74 seconds with 5 mg/mL, and a mean of 51 seconds with 7.5 mg/mL. Estimated mean times to regain full sensation were more than 692 minutes for 5 mg/mL and more than 773 minutes for 7.5 mg/mL ropivacaine. A vasoconstrictor effect occurred in the ropivacaine infiltration sites, especially at higher concentrations.

Conclusion.—Ropivacaine has a rapid onset and long duration of anesthesia and is significantly less painful to inject than lidocaine plus epinephrine. The cost of ropivacaine is substantially greater, however, than that of lidocaine, a factor that may limit the use of ropivacaine in dermatologic surgery.

▶ Ropivacaine may represent a useful local anesthetic because of its rapid onset and long duration of action in comparison with that of lidocaine. However, the inherent vasoconstrictive properties of ropivacaine, as well as its high cost, leave me skeptical that it will replace lidocaine for cutaneous anesthesia. With proper technique, including buffering of lidocaine before injection, use of room temperature or warmer solutions, injection with small-gauge needles, and a slow rate of infiltration, local anesthesia with lidocaine can be safe, effective, and minimally painful.

J. Cook, MD

A Prospective Comparison of Octyl Cyanoacrylate Tissue Adhesive (Dermabond) and Suture for the Closure of Excisional Wounds in Children and Adolescents

Bernard L, Doyle J, Friedlander SF, et al (Univ of California, San Diego)
Arch Dermatol 137:1177-1180, 2001   19–19

Background.—2-Octyl cyanoacrylate is a tissue adhesive that has recently been approved by the Food and Drug Administration. Large trials, most of which have taken place in the emergency department, have shown that octyl cyanoacrylate is a good alternative to suturing in the repair of selected lacerations and incisions in both children and adults. This small prospective trial performed in a pediatric dermatology clinic compared the cosmetic results and complications with the use of this adhesive to close cutaneous excisional biopsy wounds with results obtained after closure with conventional monofilament sutures.

Methods.—The subjects were 42 children and adolescents undergoing excisional dermatologic procedures yielding 52 wounds on the head and neck (35%), trunk (35%), or extremities (31%). All excisions were performed in a similar manner, and deep subcutaneous sutures were used to close all wounds. At the patient's choice, 28 wounds (mean patient age, 7.7 years; 65% female, 42% nonwhite) were closed with monofilament sutures, and 24 wounds (mean patient age, 7.0 years; 45% female, 32% nonwhite) were closed with tissue adhesive. Two months after surgery, wound cosmesis was evaluated by a dermatologist using the Hollander Wound Evaluation Scale (HWES). In addition, photographs of the sites were taken and scored independently by 2 dermatologists who were blinded to the method of skin closure, based on a 100-mm visual analog scale (VAS).

Results.—Only 29 of the 42 patients (69%) returned for the 2-month evaluation. Thus, only 73% of the patients in the tissue-adhesive group and 73% of patients in the suture group were evaluable. VAS scores were available for 38 of 52 wounds (73%). No patient in either group experienced early complications. HWES scores were higher in the suture group than in the tissue-adhesive group (6 vs 5), but the difference was not statistically significant. However, VAS scores were significantly higher in the suture group (mean, 63.3 mm vs 47.8 mm). Neither HWES nor VAS scores differed significantly on the basis of the site of operative incision. Hypertrophic scars were more common in the tissue-adhesive group (5 vs 3), but the difference was not statistically significant.

Conclusions.—Wounds closed by tissue adhesive had significantly worse cosmesis than wounds closed by standard suture, and there tended to be more hypertrophic scarring in these wounds as well. Octyl cyanoacrylate is being marketed as a replacement for sutures less than 5-0 in diameter. Thus, wounds that would require 3-0 or 4-0 sutures, which typically are under higher tension, would not be candidates for this tissue adhesive. The current findings, however, must be interpreted in light of the fact that patients were not randomized; they chose their method of skin closure. Furthermore, results might not be the same in a study that examined only facial wounds under low tension. In addition, approximately 25% of patients did not return for the 2-month follow-up visit, and 2 months might not be long enough to identify the ultimate cosmetic outcome. Nonetheless, until large randomized trials can be performed, it would seem prudent to restrict the use of octyl cyanoacrylate tissue adhesive in excisional procedures and high-tension wounds.

▶ Tissue adhesives have been marketed as an alternative to suturing for cuticular closure. The speed of application may represent an advantage over suturing. However, larger prospective trials demonstrating their equivalent cosmetic end results are lacking. In this small study, suturing provided a better cosmetic outcome than did tissue adhesives. The high cost of tissue adhesives when compared with that of sutures (approximately 400% more expensive) must also be considered.

J. Cook, MD

20 Nonmelanoma Skin Cancer

Reliability of Counting Actinic Keratoses Before and After Brief Consensus Discussion: The VA Topical Tretinoin Chemoprevention (VATTC) Trial

Weinstock MA, Bingham SF, Cole GW, et al (Brown Univ, Providence, RI; VA Cooperative Studies Program Coordinating Ctr, Perry Point, Md; VA Med Ctr Long Beach, Calif; et al)

Arch Dermatol 137:1055-1058, 2001   20–1

Introduction.—Actinic keratoses (AKs) are important indicators of risk for sun-related skin cancers and markers of UV exposure in sun-sensitive skin. Large-scale investigations involving AK typically use the number of AKs as their primary measure, but counts vary widely even when performed by experienced dermatologists. The reliability of AK counts was evaluated in the context of the high-risk population enrolled in the Department of Veterans Affairs Topical Tretinoin Chemoprevention (VATTC) Trial.

Methods.—A volunteer sample of 9 patients from the ongoing VATTC Trial participated in the study. Those eligible for the trial had had 2 or more keratinocyte carcinomas (either basal or squamous cell) in the 5 years before enrollment. All patients were receiving 0.1% tretinoin cream or a vehicle cream, typically applied once daily. Seven dermatologists independently counted AKs on the patients' face and ears before (in the morning) and after (in the afternoon) a brief joint discussion of discrepancies.

Results.—The mean of all counts of AKs on the face and ears of participants was 12.7, but dermatologists varied substantially in their AK counts. The standard deviation of the parameter estimates for the dermatologists decreased from 0.45 to 0.24 after a brief joint discussion, a 47% decrease of borderline statistical significance. Although the variability in counts was reduced in the afternoon session, it remained substantial.

Conclusion.—Experienced dermatologists can vary considerably in their counts of AKs. Part of the problem is that there is a continuous spectrum of lesions ranging from sun-damaged skin to squamous-cell carcinoma in situ. A discussion of discrepancies may improve the reliability of AK counts.

▶ Consistency of evaluation methods is the Achilles heel of studies involving more than 1 investigator, especially studies conducted at different locations. Many years ago, I joined our residents in performing a study assessing the benefits of a novel electric razor for patients with pseudofolliculitis barbae. The regular evaluations included a "razor bump" count. There was tremendous variation from investigator to investigator. Weinstock et al show that this can occur with AKs as well. Although a joint discussion of the discrepancies enhanced the reliability of the counts, substantial variation remained. To quote the authors, "Counting of AKs is an imprecise business, even when performed by experts."

B. H. Thiers, MD

Topical 3.0% Diclofenac in 2.5% Hyaluronan Gel in the Treatment of Actinic Keratoses
Wolf JE Jr, Taylor JR, Tschen E, et al (Baylor College of Medicine, Houston; Univ of Miami, Fla; Academic Dermatology Associates, Albuquerque, NM; et al)
Int J Dermatol 40:709-713, 2001   20–2

Background.—Actinic keratoses (AKs) result from excessive exposure to ultraviolet irradiation. They have epidemiologic and histologic features resembling those of invasive squamous cell carcinoma. AKs show potential to develop into squamous cell carcinoma; a high incidence of p53 mutations occurs in both disorders. Most AKs are successfully treated with liquid nitrogen cryotherapy, curettage, electrocautery, dermabrasion, laser, and chemical peels, but these all have significant potential side effects, including scarring. Topical 5-fluorouracil (5-FU) is also used but requires an extended treatment period, is not completely effective, and creates painful, unattractive erosions. Topical diclofenac in a hyaluronan gel vehicle was tested for efficacy in the treatment of patients with AKs.

Methods.—Ninety-six of the 120 patients enrolled completed the study. Patients underwent a screening visit, then were randomly assigned to receive either 3% diclofenac in 2.5% hyaluronan gel or placebo (the vehicle only) in a dose of 0.5 g applied twice a day to each 5-cm^2 treatment area for 90 days. Patients were instructed to avoid excessive sun exposure and to use sunscreen. The efficacy of the treatment was determined at each visit through 2 quantitative (Target Lesion Number Score [TLNS] and Cumulative Lesion Number Score [CLNS]) and 2 qualitative (investigators' and patients' perception of the change in lesions assessed with the Investigator Global Improvement Index [IGII] and Patient Global Improvement Index [PGII]) measures.

Results.—The TLNS of 50% of the patients receiving diclofenac was zero, indicating complete resolution of all target lesions in the designated

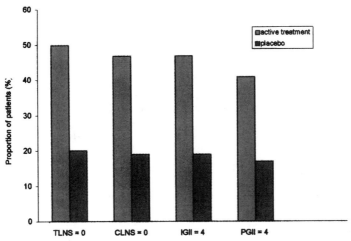

FIGURE 1.—Comparison of the results obtained for the 4 primary outcome variables for both treatment groups at follow-up (30 days after end of treatment). All comparisons are statistically significant ($P < .05$). *Abbreviations: TLNS,* Target Lesion Number Score; *CLNS,* Cumulative Lesion Number Score; *IGII,* Investigator Global Improvement Index; *PGII,* Patient Global Improvement Index. (Courtesy of Wolf JE Jr, Taylor JR, Tschen E, et al: Topical 3.0% diclofenac in 2.5% hyaluronan gel in the treatment of actinic keratoses, *Int J Dermatol* 40:709-713, 2001. Reprinted by permission of Blackwell Science, Inc.)

area. Only 20% of those receiving placebo achieved this score. Forty-seven percent of the diclofenac group also had a score of zero on the CLNS, whereas only 19% of the placebo group reached this score (Fig 1). Complete improvement was reported with the IGII in 47% of those treated with diclofenac, but in only 19% of the placebo group. The PGII score showed complete improvement in 41% of those treated with diclofenac and in only 17% of those receiving placebo. Adverse events generally involved only the skin, and no deaths or serious adverse reactions occurred.

Conclusion.—AKs were effectively treated with 3% diclofenac in 2.5% hyaluronan gel. Patients tolerated the treatment well and nearly half of all treated patients had complete resolution.

▶ The theory behind the use of diclofenac in the treatment of premaligant lesions is based on the apparent antineoplastic effects of nonsteroidal anti-inflammatory agents.[1] Inhibition of the enzymes, cyclooxygenase-1 (COX-1) and COX-2, by these drugs would impair arachidonic acid metabolism and hence decrease production of its metabolites, which may play a permissive role in a variety of tumorigenic processes including the conversion of pro-carcinogens to carcinogens, inhibition of immune surveillance, inhibition of apoptosis, stimulation of angiogenesis, and increasing tumor cell invasiveness.

B. H. Thiers, MD

Reference

1. Scioscia KA, Snyderman CH, D'Amico F, et al: Effects of arachidonic acid metabolites in a murine model of squamous cell carcinoma. *Head Neck* 22:149-155, 2000.

Topical Treatment of Actinic Keratoses With 3.0% Diclofenac in 2.5% Hyaluronan Gel

Rivers JK, Arlette J, Shear N, et al (Univ of British Columbia, Vancouver, Canada; The Dermatology Ctr, Calgary, AB, Canada; Sunnybrook & Women's Health Sciences Ctr, Toronto; et al)
Br J Dermatol 146:1-7, 2002   20–3

Background.—Treatment for actinic keratoses (AKs) is necessary to keep these premalignant skin lesions from evolving into squamous cell carcinoma. However, current treatments for AK, such as cryosurgery and 5-fluorouracil, can cause serious adverse events. The efficacy of 3% diclofenac in 2.5% hyaluronan gel in treating AK has been shown in open-label trials. This randomized, double-blind, placebo-controlled trial was undertaken to explore further the efficacy and safety of this approach.

Methods.—The subjects were 195 white patients (142 men and 53 women; average age, approximately 67 years) with at least 5 AKs in up to three 5-cim^2 treatment blocks on the forehead, central face, scalp, or the dorsum of hands. None of the patients was currently taking any drug that could affect response to the study medications. All patients were screened 6 days before beginning treatment, and the target lesion number score (TLNS) within each treatment block was recorded. At the second visit, patients were randomized into 4 equal groups to receive either placebo (topical 2.5% hyaluronan gel) for 30 (V30) or 60 (V60) days or active drug (3.0% diclofenac in 2.5% hyaluronan gel) for 30 (A30) or 60 (A60) days. Study drug dosages were 0.5 g of gel per treatment block, twice a day, with 6 hours or more between applications. During treatment, a cumulative lesion number score (CLNS; sum of remaining target lesions and new lesions) was measured within each treatment block, and the thickness of lesions was evaluated by a 4-point total thickness score (TTS; 0, lesion visible but not palpable; 3, lesion hyperkeratotic and >1-mm-thick). In addition, both patients and investigators used a 7-point scale (−2, significantly worse; 4, completely improved) to assess global improvement (PGII and IGII, respectively). Patients were assessed 30 days after the end of treatment to determine the proportions of patients with TLNS, CLNS, and TTS = 0 and IGII and PGII = 4.

Results.—At follow-up, the A60 group had significant improvements in all efficacy variables measured compared with the placebo group, whereas values for the A30 group were improved, but not significantly so, compared with those in the placebo group. Specifically, compared with placebo, the A60 group had significantly more patients with a TLNS = 0

(33% vs 10%); this corresponded to 64% improvement in the A60 group and 34% improvement in the placebo group. The A60 group also had significantly more patients with a CLNS = 0 (31% vs 8%, corresponding to improvements of 54% vs 23%), and significantly more patients with a TTS = 0 (25% vs 6%, corresponding to improvements of 59% vs 31%). Similarly, significantly more patients in the A60 group had an IGII = 4 (31% vs 10%) and a PGII = 4 (29% vs 10%). Treatments were generally well tolerated, with the most common adverse events being pruritus, rash, dry skin, and a reaction at the application site. Eleven patients withdrew from the study, 8 because of an adverse event; of these 8 patients, 4 were in the A60 group, 2 in the A30 group, and one each in the P30 and P60 groups.

Conclusions.—Twice-daily treatment with topical 3.0% diclofenac in 2.5% hyaluronan gel for 60 days effectively reduced the number and thickness of AK lesions. All treated lesions cleared in about one third of patients, and the number of lesions decreased by 50% to 65%. Treatment was generally well tolerated, and the most common adverse events were skin-related. Thus, topical 3% diclofenac in 2.5% hyaluronan gel holds promise as a noninvasive, easy-to-use, safe and effective treatment for AK.

▶ Although the reported numbers might not seem impressive, the investigators were held to quite difficult primary end points involving varying measurements of total lesion resolution (ie, complete clearance). Any evidence of residual lesions within the treatment area meant the patient had to be classified as a treatment failure. When looked at from the more liberal parameter of improvement, the percentage of positively responding patients in each objective assessment category approximately doubled.

The message to be learned from this study and the data of Wolf et al (Abstract 20–2) is that with the diclofenac preparation (marketed as Solaraze), 90 days' treatment is better than 60 days' treatment, which in turn is better than 30 days'. Although the duration of treatment is longer than with topical 5-fluorouracil, the significant irritation from the latter often turns the standard 2 to 3 week course of treatment into a much longer period of hand-holding and topical steroid therapy. Other alternatives to topical 5-fluorouracil (eg, topical imiquimod) are currently under investigation (see Abstracts 20–4 to 20–6).

B. H. Thiers, MD

Successful Treatment of Actinic Keratosis With Imiquimod Cream 5%: A Report of Six Cases
Stockfleth E, Meyer T, Benninghoff B, et al (Univ of Kiel, Germany; IPM-Hamburg, Germany; 3M-Medica, Borken, Germany)
Br J Dermatol 144:1050-1053, 2001   20–4

Introduction.—Actinic keratoses (AK) are premalignant lesions typically treated with destructive procedures, including cryotherapy, elec-

FIGURE 1

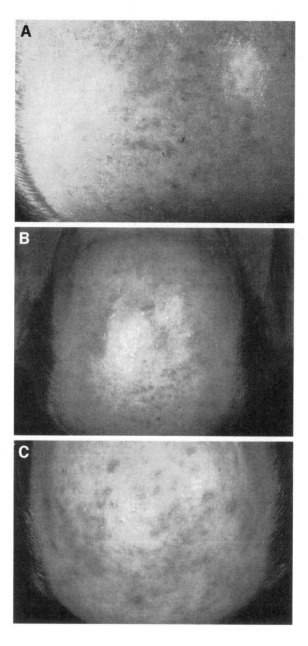

(Continued)

FIGURE 1 (cont.)

FIGURE 1.—A typical response of actinic keratosis lesions to treatment with imiquimod (patient 5). A, Beginning of treatment; B, after 2 to 5 weeks; C, after 4 to 5 weeks; and D, after 8 weeks. (Courtesy of Stockfleth E, Meyer T, Benninghoff B, et al: Successful treatment of actinic keratosis with imiquimod cream 5%: A report of six cases. *Br J Dermatol* 144:1050-1053, 2001. Reprinted by permission of Blackwell Science, Inc.)

trodessication, or topical 5-fluorouracil. Reported are 6 patients with resistant/recurrent AK of the head who were treated with imiquimod cream.

Methods.—All patients had been treated for recurrent AK for 5 to 16 years. All patients had up to 10 AK and at least 1 lesion that had a diameter of 0.5 cm or more. All lesions had responded temporarily after being treated with surgical excision, cryotherapy, or 5-fluorouracil. Histologic examination via 0.4-cm diameter punch biopsy was performed on the same lesion before and after treatment. Patients applied 5% imiquimod cream to AK 3 times weekly for 6 to 8 weeks or until the AK were resolved. Treatment was modified to 2 times weekly for the remainder of the treatment period when patients experienced local skin reactions. Before treatment, patients were instructed to protect their skin from exposure to the sun.

Results.—The AK cleared completely in all patients. After a follow-up period ranging from 2 to 12 months, there were no recurrences (Fig 1; see color plates XVI and XVII). All patients experienced mild erythema, and 3 patients experienced itching. No treatment was required for adverse events.

Conclusion.—Topical application of 5% imiquimod cream is safe and effective in the treatment of recurrent AK. There was no histologic evidence of persisting AK.

Imiquimod 5% Cream in the Treatment of Bowen's Disease

Mackenzie-Wood A, Kossard S, de Launey J, et al (Skin and Cancer Found, Darlinghurst, Australia; 3M Pharmaceuticals, St Paul, Minn)
J Am Acad Dermatol 44:462-470, 2001   20–5

Introduction.—Large diameter lesions of Bowen's disease may be challenging to treat surgically at some sites, including the shins, and may need alternate treatment modalities. The effectiveness of topical 5% imiquimod cream, a topical immune response modifier that stimulates the production of interferon alfa and other cytokines, was examined in 16 patients with Bowen's disease in a phase II open-label trial.

Methods.—All patients had a single biopsy-proven plaque of Bowen's disease that was 1 cm or greater in diameter. Lesions were treated once-daily with self-application of 5% imiquimod cream for 16 weeks. Patients were evaluated weekly for 2 weeks, then at biweekly intervals. A biopsy was performed on the treated area 6 weeks after completion of treatment. Lymphocyte CD4/CD8 rations were examined in pretreatment and post-treatment biopsy specimens by immunophenotyping of the lymphocytic infiltrate.

Results.—The mean age of the 10 women and 6 men was 75 years (range, 57-95 years). Lseion sizes ranged from 1 to 5.4 cm in diamter (0.7-21.6 cm^2 in area). Fifteen lesions were located on the legs, and 1 was located on the shoulder. Fourteen patients (93%) had no residual tumor present in their 6-week posttreatment biopsy specimens (Fig 1; see color plate XVIII). One patient died of unrelated intercurrent illness before a biopsy specimen could be obtained. The median CD4/CD8 lymphocyte ratio in pretreatment biopsy specimens was 2:1 and was 1:2.2 in post-treatment specimens. Ten patients completed 16 weeks of treatment, and 6 ceased treatment between 4 and 8 weeks because of local skin reactions.

Conclusion.—These preliminary findings indicate that topical imiquimod is effective in treating Bowen's disease, especially on the lower limbs. The dosing schedule and length of treatment for Bowen's disease requires further investigation.

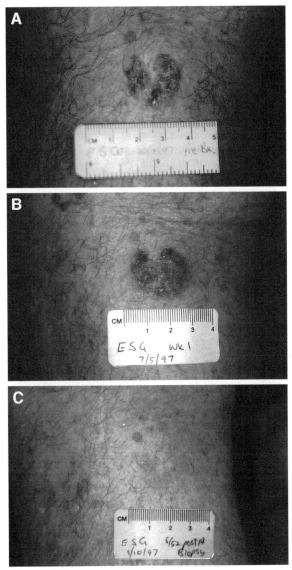

FIGURE 1.—Patient 12. **A**, Bowen's disease on left lateral calf. **B**, After 1 week of treatment with 5% imiquimod cream. **C**, Treated area 6 weeks after completing 16-week course. (Courtesy of Mackenzie-Wood A, Kossard S, de Launey J, et al: Imiquimod 5% cream in the treatment of Bowen's disease. *J Am Acad Dermatol* 44:462-470, 2001.)

Imiquimod 5% Cream in the Treatment of Superficial Basal Cell Carcinoma: Results of a Multicenter 6-Week Dose-Response Trial

Marks R, and the Australasian Multicentre Trial Group (St Vincent's Hosp, Melbourne, Victoria, Australia; Fremantle Hosp, Wash; St George Hosp, Sydney, New South Wales, Australia; et al)

J Am Acad Dermatol 44:807-813, 2001   20–6

Introduction.—Superficial basal cell carcinoma (sBCC) is becoming increasingly common in fair-skinned populations throughout the world. The efficacy and safety of various dose regimens of 5% imiquimod cream in the treatment of sBCC was examined in 99 patients with sBCC in a multicenter, randomized, open-label, dose–response trial.

Methods.—Patients were randomly assigned to treatment with imiquimod cream: twice daily, once daily, twice daily 3 times per week, or once daily 3 times per week. The treatment site was excised and evaluated histologically 6 weeks after completion of the imiquimod treatment. Because of frequent reports from another trial of severe local skin reactions in the twice daily treatment group, recruitment in this arm was ceased after 3 patients were enrolled.

Results.—Intention-to-treat analysis showed 100% histologic clearance (3/3) with the twice daily regimen, 87.9% clearance (29/33) with the once daily regimen, 73.3% clearance (22/30) with the twice daily 3 times per week regimen, and 69.7% clearance (23/33) with the once daily 3 times per week regimen (Table 2). Dose-related inflammatory skin reactions at the application site were commonly observed. Most treatment regimens were well-tolerated. Local skin reactions, especially erythema, were observed with all 4 dose regimens. One patient withdrew as a result of a medication-related skin reaction.

Conclusion.—These findings support earlier data suggesting that 5% imiquimod cream is valuable in the treatment of sBCC. Nearly 90% histologic clearance was observed when the cream was applied to tumors daily for 6 weeks. Local skin reactions were common and were well-tolerated by most patients.

▶ These are exciting findings (Abstracts 20–4 to 20–6) that suggest the possibility of topical imiquimod (Aldara) treatment of superficial skin cancers. Some tweaking of the treatment regimen may be necessary to determine the dosing frequency that provides the maximum benefit with minimal local irritation. Moreover, the cure of skin cancer is measured in years rather than

---

TABLE 2.—Complete Response Rate by Treatment Group

	Twice Daily	Daily	Twice Daily 3/wk	Daily 3/wk
Intention-to-treat data set	3/3 (100%)	29/33 (87.9%)	22/30 (73.3%)	23/33 (69.7%)
Per-protocol data set	1/1 (100%)	26/29 (89.7%)	21/28 (75%)	22/31 (71%)

(Courtesy of Marks R, and the Australasian Multicentre Trial Group: Imiquimod 5% cream in the treatment of superficial basal cell carcinoma: Results of a multicenter 6-week dose-response trial. *J Am Acad Dermatol* 44:807-813, 2001.)

in weeks or months. Long-term follow-up data are necessary to determine the durability of the treatment response.

B. H. Thiers, MD

Photodynamic Therapy of Actinic Keratoses With Topical Aminolevulinic Acid Hydrochloride and Fluorescent Blue Light
Jeffes EW, McCullough JL, Weinstein GD, et al (Univ of California, Irvine; Veterans Affairs Med Ctr, Long Beach, Calif; Veterans Affairs Med Ctr, Miami, Fla; et al)
J Am Acad Dermatol 45:96-104, 2001   20–7

Background.—Topical 20% aminolevulinic acid (ALA) HCl photoactivated with red laser light can be an effective treatment for actinic keratoses (AKs). This study investigated the efficacy of ALA photodynamic therapy with a nonlaser fluorescent blue light.

Methods.—Thirty-six patients with at least 4 AKs on the face or scalp were enrolled in this multicenter, investigator-blinded, randomized, vehicle-controlled study. The 6 women and 30 men ranged in age from 38 to 100 years, with a median age of 69 years. Two AKs on each patient were treated with vehicle and two with 20% ALA solution. All four AKs on each patient were irradiated with the same dose of nonlaser blue light at the same time 14 to 18 hours after application of ALA. Clinical response was defined as the percentage reduction of pretreatment lesion area and was rated as *complete response* (completely cleared with no evidence of adherent scale on the surface of the treated skin when palpated); *partial response,* ≥50% reduction in lesion size); or *no response* (<50% reduction in lesion size). Retreatment was permitted at 8 weeks.

Results.—Thirty-four of 36 patients completed the 16-week study. Two patients were lost to follow-up after week 8. There was a significant difference in the clearing of AKs treated with ALA versus vehicle after a single photodynamic treatment. Overall, 66% of the AKs treated with ALA were completely cleared at 8 weeks; in contrast, only 17% of AKs treated with vehicle were completely cleared. Better results (88% clearance) were seen with the optimal light dose of 10J/cm². Most patients (51%) reported a moderate burning sensation during treatment, and 18% of patients reported severe burning or stinging symptoms. However, most patients reported no burning or stinging by 24 hours after treatment, and all of the patients were able to complete treatment regardless of the burning or stinging symptoms.

Conclusions.—Photodynamic therapy with topical ALA and a nonlaser blue light source appears to be an effective treatment for patients with multiple actinic keratoses.

▶ A number of modalities are available to manage the patient with multiple AKs. The mainstay of treatment has been topical 5-fluorouracil (5FU). However, this treatment may not always be feasible, may be associated with prolonged discomfort, and often is not tolerated by patients with severe photodamage.

Dermabrasion, laser resurfacing, and chemical peeling can are alternatives to topical 5FU but are more labor-intensive, may not be covered by insurance, and are more risky (ie, they are associated with a higher incidence of scarring and pigmentary alteration). More recently, topical imiquimod has been proposed as a treatment for AKs; however, it also may be associated with considerable irritation. We now have available yet another modality to manage patients with multiple AKs: topical photodynamic therapy (PDT). Not surprisingly, most patients experience moderate burning, stinging, and pain, and some even experience significant pain. However, these symptoms usually subside within 24 hours. Erythema, edema, and varying degrees of vesiculation are also observed but appear to dissipate within a week. Thin lesions responded best. Although encouraging, if topical PDT is going to have broader application, the current protocol will have be modified to ensure effective treatment of thicker AKs.

P. G. Lang, Jr, MD

Impact of the Basic Skin Cancer Triage Curriculum on Providers' Skin Cancer Control Practices
Mikkilineni R, Weinstock MA, Goldstein MG, et al (VA Med Ctr, Providence, RI; Brown Univ, Providence, RI; Univ of Rhode Island, Kingston)
J Gen Intern Med 16:302-307, 2001   20–8

Introduction.—Current efforts aimed at the early detection of skin cancer are scattered and not uniform. Because primary care providers (PCPs) are in a unique position to provide preventive services, their ability to detect skin cancer in its early stages could reduce morbidity and mortality from these malignancies. Researchers assessed the effect of the Basic Skin Cancer Triage (BSCT) curriculum on the practice patterns of PCPs.

Methods.—The BSCT curriculum was designed to assist PCPs in the accurate and confident triage of skin lesions and to help counsel patients on skin cancer issues. Providers received 2 hours of instruction and were given a triage algorithm, skin cancer information pamphlets, and review articles. Before and 1 month after their participation, the physicians, nurses, and physician assistants were evaluated on their practice of skin cancer control measures.

Results.—Twenty-two of 28 PCPs completed both the preintervention and postintervention surveys. After participation in the BSCT curriculum, PCPs showed significant improvements in their attitudes toward and provision of the total body skin examination. Skin cancer control measures increased during initial patient visits and routine visits with patients at high risk for skin cancer. There were nonsignificant improvements in PCP attitudes toward skin cancer prevention counseling. These changes in practice patterns were confirmed by patient exit interviews.

Discussion.—The BSCT curriculum, a brief multicomponent intervention, led to improvements in the skin cancer prevention practices of PCPs. The long-term impact of the BSCT curriculum is not known, but such interventions may enhance efforts to reduce skin cancer morbidity and mortality.

Skin Cancer Screening and Prevention in the Primary Care Setting: National Ambulatory Medical Care Survey 1997
Oliveria SA, Christos PJ, Marghoob AA, et al (Mem Sloan-Kettering Cancer Ctr, New York)
J Gen Intern Med 16:297-301, 2001   20–9

Introduction.—Skin cancer screening may be the best way to reduce the rising incidence of skin cancer in the United States. Primary care physicians are in an optimal position to educate patients about primary prevention efforts and to detect early precancerous or thin lesions. Data from the 1997 National Ambulatory Medical Care Survey (NAMCS) were analyzed to determine the extent of skin cancer screening and prevention practices in the primary care setting.

Methods.—Using the NAMCS master file, researchers initially identified visits to family practitioners and internists. Because skin cancer rarely occurs in nonwhite individuals, the study sample was limited to visits where the patient was identified as being white and of non-Hispanic origin. The final study sample included information on 784 nonillness-related patient visits to 109 family practitioners and 61 internists.

Results.—The mean age of patients in the study sample was 43.4 years; 56.6% of the visits were by women. In more than 94% of visits, a physician was the health provider seen. Skin examination was reported at only 15.8% of all of the nonillness visits, and education and counseling on skin cancer prevention at only 2.3% of visits. Compared with internists, family practitioners were significantly more likely to perform pelvic and rectal examinations and the Papanicolaou test and to provide breast self-examination counseling. Skin cancer screening and prevention services, however, did not differ significantly between family practitioners and internists.

Discussion.—Family practitioners and internists are less likely to offer skin cancer screening than other forms of cancer screening at patient visits. Yet skin examination during routine care has been proposed as the optimal strategy to reduce the morbidity and mortality associated with skin cancer.

▶ In the United States, there continues to be an alarming increase in the incidence and prevalence of melanoma and non-melanoma skin cancers. Escalating health care expenditures have generated many attempts to control health care delivery (managed care). Particular emphasis has been placed on restricting a patient's ability to directly access specialists. In the United States, most patients with a primary cutaneous complaint do not see a dermatologist. This area of cost containment and continuing managed care has placed significant pressures on primary care physicians to diagnose and treat skin diseases without referral to a dermatologist.[1] These 2 articles (Abstracts 20–8 and 20–9) demonstrate that skin cancer screening and preventative counseling are not commonly done in the primary care setting.

Previous research has shown that patients are generally most satisfied with unrestricted access to specialist care.[2] Despite the relative ease of skin examination and the high prevalence of skin cancer, there are barriers that may prevent effective skin monitoring in the primary care setting. The increasing pressure to see greater numbers of patients on a daily basis, attention to other medical concerns, a lack of reimbursement for screening examinations, and a documented lack of diagnostic and procedural expertise may significantly lessen the chance for early diagnosis of cutaneous cancers by primary care physicians. Previous research has suggested that physicians recommend and perform examinations and procedures with which they are comfortable and show some degree of technical competence.[3,4] A 1995 survey of medical schools in the United States revealed that most medical students receive minimal training in dermatology and that the few contact hours they receive are frequently within the first 2 years of medical school, before the acquisition of clinical skills. Soloman and associates found that 97% to 99% of family practitioners had 1 month or less of dermatology training in medical school or residency before beginning practice.[5] Gerbert and colleagues observed that primary care residents failed to correctly identify skin cancers 50% of the time.[6] One third of the time, they failed to recommend a biopsy for a cancerous lesion. This lack of exposure and training may significantly impact the diagnosis and treatment of a patient with a cutaneous complaint seen in the primary care setting.

Primary care physicians play a critical role in the health care of our patients and the coordination of specialist and subspecialist care. Hopefully, we in the dermatology community can emphasize the importance of the skin examination to our primary care colleagues. The ease of examination of the skin and the potential for early diagnosis and management of melanoma and nonmelanoma skin cancer underscore the importance of improving the practitioner's skill and willingness to attend to cutaneous complaints. Still, the best treatment may prove to be an appropriate referral.

J. Cook, MD

References

1. Cook J: Issues in the delivery of dermatologic surgery for skin cancer. *Dermatol Clin* 18:251-259, 2000.
2. Owens SA, Maeyens E, Weary PE: Patients' opinions regarding direct access to dermatologic specialty care. *J Am Acad Dermatol* 32:250-256, 1997.
3. Lewis CE: Disease prevention and health promotion practices of primary care physicians in the United States. *Am J Prev Med* 4(suppl 4):9-16, 1998.
4. Wender RC: Cancer screening and prevention in primary care. *Cancer* 72(suppl): 1093-1099, 1993.
5. Soloman BA, Collins R, Silverberg NB, et al: Quality of care. *J Am Acad Dermatol* 34:601-607, 1996.

6. Gerbert B, Maurer T, Berger T, et al: Primary care physicians as gatekeepers in managed care. *Arch Dermatol* 132:1030-1038, 1996.

Skin Cancer Surveillance in Renal Transplant Recipients: Questionnaire Survey of Current UK Practice

Harden PN, Reece SM, Fryer AA, et al (Staffordshire Hosp, Stoke on Trent, England)
BMJ 323:600-601, 2001   20–10

Introduction.—Patients who receive an organ transplant are at increased risk for the development of nonmelanoma skin cancer. Because of the high incidence, rapid growth, and increased metastatic potential of these cancers in transplant recipients, surveillance programs are essential. A survey of centers in the United Kingdom was designed to establish current practice in skin cancer surveillance for renal transplant recipients.

Methods and Results.—A questionnaire sent to 65 centers asked whether skin cancer surveillance was performed, which staff did the surveillance, and what education was provided for patients. Twenty-six surgical and 35 nephrology centers that managed a total of 16,264 renal transplant recipients responded to the survey. Annual surveillance for skin cancer was practiced at only 13 centers, 12 of which used a full skin examination. Patients were educated about skin cancer risk before transplantation in 36 centers and after transplantation in 51. A higher proportion of surgical centers provided education for transplant recipients. There was no difference in the proportion of surgical or nephrology centers that provided skin cancer surveillance, full skin examination, or specific training for clinicians providing surveillance.

Conclusion.—All transplant recipients should receive ongoing education about the risk of skin cancer associated with long-term immunosuppression, and all clinicians caring for these patients must have adequate training to perform full skin surveillance.

▶ Often forgotten in the presurgical evaluation of transplant patients is the skin examination. Patients should be evaluated for malignant and premalignant skin lesions before transplantation and concomitant immunosuppression, and treated accordingly. As emphasized by Harden et al, more needs to be done to ensure that these patients are adequately monitored for the development of skin cancer after their transplant procedure.

B. H. Thiers, MD

Annual Incidence and Predicted Risk of Nonmelanoma Skin Cancer in Renal Transplant Recipients

Harden PN, Fryer AA, Reece S, et al (Keele Univ, Stoke-on-Trent, England)
Transplant Proc 33:1302-1304, 2001   20–11

Introduction.—Patients who have undergone solid organ transplantation are known to have an increased risk for nonmelanoma skin cancer (NMSC). In contrast to the general population, the ratio of squamous cell carcinoma (SCC) to basal cell carcinoma (BCC) is greater in the transplant population (1:4 vs 3.8:1). And NMSC appears at an earlier age, spreads more rapidly, and often occurs as multiple lesions in transplant recipients. A group of renal transplant recipients was monitored to establish the annual incidence of skin cancer in such a population and to identify clinical factors associated with NMSC risk.

Methods.—The 193 white renal transplant patients in the longitudinal study were recruited at a hospital in the United Kingdom between May 1997 and July 2000. A structured questionnaire was used to gather demographic information and calculate cumulative sun exposure. Unclothed patients were examined and any suspicious lesion biopsied. Information on the cause of renal failure and details of the pretransplantation and posttransplantation courses were obtained from patient records. At a first review, performed at a mean of 1.28 years later, 164 patients underwent skin surveillance; 107 of these patients completed a second review 24 months after initial recruitment.

Results.—The mean patient age at transplantation was 38.7 years and the mean duration of follow-up was 9.3 years. Among patients in whom tumors developed, the mean time from transplantation to appearance of the first NMSC was 8.9 years. Both older age at transplantation and male gender were significantly associated with increased risk for SCC and BCC. Compared with transplant recipients with brown eyes, those with green eyes had a significantly increased risk for SCC. A predictive index based upon age at transplantation, eye color, and gender was developed; among individuals with a total score of 8.25 or greater, the odds ratio for development of NMSC within 10 years was 12.2. The annual NMSC incidence rate was between 7.1% and 10.6% but increased with the duration of immuosuppression. Skin cancer risk was not associated with the immunosuppressant regimen, number of acute rejection episodes, or treatment for rejection.

Conclusion.—NMSC is an important issue for renal allograft recipients. Posttransplant surveillance should be performed regularly and patients at greatest risk for skin cancer identified.

▶ It is well recognized that transplant patients are at increased risk for NMSC, especially SCC. In this study from the United Kingdom, an increased risk for NMSC was seen in transplant patients who were male, older at the time of transplantation, and had green eyes. The annual incidence of NMSC increased significantly in patients having had their transplant more than 10 years earlier (18%).

P. G. Lang, Jr, MD

Non-melanoma Skin Cancers and Glucocorticoid Therapy
Karagas MR, Cushing GL Jr, Greenberg ER, et al (Dartmouth Med School, Lebanon, New Hampshire; Mount Auburn Hosp, Cambridge, Mass)
Br J Cancer 85:683-686, 2001   20–12

Background.—Organ transplant recipients who receive immunosuppressive drugs such as glucocorticoids are at significantly increased risk of developing squamous cell carcinoma (SCC) and basal cell carcinoma (BCC). Systemic glucocorticoids are also prescribed for other conditions. The association between glucocorticoid use in nontransplant recipients and the risk of nonmelanoma skin cancer (SCC, BCC) was investigated in a population-based case-control study of residents of New Hampshire.

Study Design.—The study included 603 patients with BCC, 293 patients with SCC, and 540 age- and gender-matched control subjects. All participants were aged 25 to 74 years, had no history of organ transplantation, and were New Hampshire residents. Participants were interviewed, and sociodemographic data were obtained, in addition to data regarding skin sensitivity to light, radiation treatment, tobacco use, time spent outdoors, and corticosteroid prescription. If patients had received corticosteroids for at least 1 month, they were further queried as to age at treatment, condition for which steroids were prescribed, name of drug, dosage, and treatment duration. The odds ratio of the association of BCC and SCC with use of glucocorticoids was computed using unconditional logistic regression analysis.

Findings.—The risk of SCC was significantly increased and the risk of BCC moderately increased among patients who had used oral glucocorticoids. The use of inhaled steroids had no detectable impact on the risk of developing either BCC or SCC.

Conclusions.—Use of oral glucocorticoids increases the risk of both squamous and basal cell carcinoma among nontransplant recipients. The immunosuppression induced by oral glucocorticoids may permit these cancers to escape immunosurveillance.

▶ It is well recognized that immunosuppressed transplant patients are at increased risk of developing nonmelanoma skin cancer. In this study of patients with no history of organ transplantation receiving glucocorticoids for a variety of reasons, the authors found a twofold increase in the incidence of squamous cell carcinoma and a modest increase in the incidence of basal cell carcinoma with systemic but not inhaled steroids. Although interesting, these results should be considered preliminary. First, one has to question how well matched were the controls. Second, the duration of therapy was in general quite short (<6 months). Finally, the patients apparently were not screened for the use of other immunosuppressive agents.

P. G. Lang Jr, MD

Predictors for Cutaneous Basal- and Squamous-Cell Carcinoma Among Actinically Damaged Adults
Foote JA, Harris RB, Giuliano AR, et al (Univ of Arizona, Tucson)
Int J Cancer 95:7-11, 2001   20–13

Introduction.—Actinic keratoses (AKs) indicate photodamage of the skin and are highly associated with an increased risk of both basal cell carcinoma (BCC) and squamous cell carcinoma (SCC). Individuals with multiple AKs randomly assigned to the placebo arm of a phase III vitamin A chemoprevention trial were studied to identify factors associated with the development of a first BCC or SCC.

Methods.—The double-blind 5-year chemoprevention trial conducted between 1985 and 1992 randomly allocated participants to oral vitamin A (25,000 IU daily) or placebo. All trial members were classified as "moderately sun-damaged," with 10 or more AKs on the forearm. The analysis was limited to 918 individuals who had been randomly assigned to the placebo group. They had no history of a skin cancer and none occurring within the first 3 months of the trial. Participants were followed for a mean of 57 months for the development of nonmelanoma skin cancers.

Results.—All members of the study group lived in Arizona; 69% were men and most were married and well educated. A total of 164 first BCCs and 129 first SCCs were diagnosed during the follow-up period. Incidence rates of BCC and SCC were 4106 and 3198 per 100,000 person-years, respectively. The incidence of BCC increased with age in men and women, whereas the SCC incidence increased with age only in men. Independent predictors for SCC occurrence were older age, male gender, natural red hair color, and adult residence in Arizona for at least 10 years.

Conclusion.—The incidence rates for both BCC and SCC were high among these sun-damaged adults. Sun-exposure in adulthood can significantly affect skin cancer occurrence.

► This study demonstrates that patients with significant photodamage (those with more than 10 AKs) are at significant risk for development of BCC or SCC. This risk is particularly increased for older individuals. Older age, male gender, red hair, and residence in Arizona for more than 10 years as an adult were independently predictive of SCC, whereas only increased age predicted BCC. These observations are consistent with the hypothesis that the development of SCC correlates better with the degree of photodamage than does BCC.

P. G. Lang, Jr, MD

Melanocortin-1 Receptor Gene Variants Determine the Risk of Non-melanoma Skin Cancer Independently of Fair Skin and Red Hair

Bastiaens MT, ter Huurne JAC, Kielich C, et al (Leiden Univ, The Netherlands)
Am J Hum Genet 68:884-894, 2001
20–14

Introduction.—Ultraviolet radiation is the main environmental risk factor for nonmelanoma skin cancer; fair skin and red hair may be the major genetically determined risk factors. Melanocortin-1 receptor (MC1R) gene variants are linked to fair skin and red hair. The MC1R is a G-protein coupled receptor that is expressed in several cell types, including melanocytes and perhaps keratinocytes. Common polymorphisms have been observed in the MC1R gene.

Methods.—Persons with nonmelanoma skin cancer and controls with no skin cancer history were evaluated to determine the association of MC1R gene variation with fair skin and red hair. Persons with any MC1R variant alleles were evaluated to determine whether they were at increased risk of developing cutaneous squamous cell carcinoma (SCC), nodular basal cell carcinoma, or multifocal basal cell carcinoma. The coding sequence of the human MC1R gene was examined via single-stranded confirmation polymorphism analysis, followed by sequencing of unknown variants. Persons with MC1R variant alleles were evaluated to determine whether they were at increased risk of developing nonmelanoma skin cancer, and if so, whether the increased risk was mediated by fair skin and red hair.

Findings.—Of 853 research subjects, 453 had nonmelanoma skin cancer and 385 had no skin cancer. Twenty-seven MC1R gene variants were detected. There were 379 (45.2%), 208 (24.8%), and 7 (0.9%), respectively, carriers of 1, 2, and 3 MC1R gene variants. There was a strong correlation between MC1R variants and fair skin and red hair, particularly the variants Arg151Cys and Arg160Trp ($P < .0001$). The carriers of 2 variant alleles were at increased risk for developing cutaneous SCC (odds ratio [OR], 3.77; 91% confidence interval [CI], 2.11-6.78), nodular basal cell carcinoma (OR, 2.26; 95% CI, 1.45-3.52), and superficial multifocal basal cell carcinoma (OR, 3.43; 95% CI, 1.92-6.15) compared with carriers of 2 wild-type alleles. The risk was diminished by one half in carriers of 1 variant allele. The highest relative risks of nonmelanoma skin cancer were observed in carriers of the Asp84Glu, His260Pro, and Asp294His variant alleles. The risk was slightly lower for carriers of the Val60Leu, Val92Met, Arg142His, Arg161Cys, and Arg160Trp variant alleles.

Conclusion.—When stratified by skin type and hair color, these factors did not change the relative risks. The MC1R gene variants are important independent risk factors for nonmelanoma skin cancer.

▶ The MC1R gene is highly polymorphic, with numerous possible single nucleotide change variants. Certain MC1R variant alleles have been previously associated with fair skin and red hair, and with malignant melanoma.

In the study abstracted here, MC1R genotypes were determined in a large number of individuals with nonmelanoma skin cancer and in control subjects. The data obtained convincingly indicate that certain genotypes are significantly associated with squamous cell carcinoma, nodular basal cell carcinoma, and superficial multifocal basal cell carcinoma, and that these gene variants constitute risk factors independent of the possession of fair skin and red hair. The mechanisms whereby these receptor variants predispose to skin cancer remain to be elucidated.

G. M. P. Galbraith, MD

Regulation of Cutaneous Malignancy by γδ T Cells
Girardi M, Oppenheim DE, Steele CR, et al (Yale Univ, New Haven, Conn; King's College, London)
Science 294:605-609, 2001   20–15

Background.—Many T cells are constitutively resident within the epithelium. These intraepithelial lymphocytes (IELs) have limited T-cell receptor (TCR) diversity and are commonly enriched in γδ cells. Some evidence suggests that TCRγδ+ IELs recognize autologous proteins expressed on epithelial cells after infection or malignant transformation. For example, in human bowel carcinoma, the expression of 2 molecules related to major histocompatibility complex (MHC) class I (MICA and MICB) is up-regulated. MICA and MICB are lysed by γδ+ IELs that express NKG2d, which is a receptor for MICA and MICB. With the use of a murine model, these authors investigated the ability of γδ+ IELs to down-regulate cutaneous malignancy.

Methods.—Studies were performed in mice lacking the γδ TCR. In brief, mice were inoculated with carcinoma cells or had carcinogens applied to their skin to determine their susceptibility to cutaneous malignancy. After cancer induction, their skin cells were examined to identify the expression of Rae-1 or H60; these murine MHC-related molecules are structurally similar to human MICA. Experiments were also performed to examine whether murine NKG2d could bond with RAE-1 and whether the addition of NKG2d affected the subsequent proportion of cancerous cells.

Results.—After cancer induction, the γδ−γδ− mice had significantly reduced resistance to cutaneous malignancy. The cancerous cells highly expressed Rae-1 and H60, and Rae-1ε specifically interacted with NKG2d. In vitro, TCRγδ+ IELs were able to kill squamous carcinoma cells expressing Rae-1.

Conclusions.—IELs may use evolutionarily conserved proteins to down-regulate cutaneous carcinoma.

▶ In this murine model, carcinogens cause skin cells to express antigens that are recognized by certain intraepithelial lymphocytes; mice lacking these lymphocytes are highly susceptible to skin cancer. Proof of a similar phenomenon in human skin would further our understanding of the mechanisms of cutaneous carcinogenesis and perhaps lead to new ways to prevent and treat skin cancer.

B. H. Thiers, MD

Progressive Decreases in Nuclear Retinoid Receptors During Skin Squamous Carcinogenesis
Xu X-C, Wong WYL, Goldberg L, et al (Univ of Texas, Houston; Baylor College of Medicine, Houston; Austin, Tex; et al)
Cancer Res 61:4306-4310, 2001   20–16

Background.—Squamous cell carcinoma (SCC) is clinically more aggressive than basal cell carcinoma and accounts for most nonmelanoma skin cancer deaths. Because rates of SCC continue to increase, new strategies to prevent skin cancer are being developed. One method, retinoid chemoprevention, has established clinical activity in several sites of epithelial carcinogenesis, including the skin. Retinoid effects are mediated mainly by retinoic acid receptors (RARs) and retinoid X receptors (RXRs), nuclear proteins that act as transcription factors to alter gene expression. Retinoid receptor status was analyzed in premalignant and malignant skin lesions to determine whether the levels of these receptors are related to cancer development and progression.

Methods.—Specimens were obtained from sun-exposed areas of the skin of white adult patients. Areas of actinic keratosis (AK), SCC, and adjacent normal skin were included. An in situ hybridization method was used to analyze the expression of RARs and RXRs.

Results.—In normal skin, RAR-α and -γ and RXR-α, -β, and -γ expression ranged from moderate to very strong, and expression was generally higher in the spinous and granular layers than in the basal layer. Expression of the retinoid receptors was suppressed in both AK and SCC, compared with adjacent normal skin. Expression of RAR-β ranged from weak to absent in both normal skin and lesional samples. Analysis of the degree of suppression of RXR-α and RAR-γ, the 2 predominant retinoid receptors in skin, suggests that RXR-α suppression may be an earlier event and RAR-γ suppression a later event during multistep skin squamous carcinogenesis.

Conclusions.—Suppressed expression of retinoid receptors occurs early (in AK) and appears to be associated with progression of squamous skin carcinogenesis to SCC. Pharmacologic retinoic acid (RA) levels may restore the ability of skin SCC cells to use RA, thus upregulating the skin RARs.

▶ The authors suggest that the loss of receptor expression may result in a diminished ability of epidermal cells to respond to physiologic levels of RA. This may play a role in the pathogenesis of SCC. As a corollary, they argue that pharmacologic levels of RA may restore the ability of SCC cells to use

RA by saturating the remaining signaling machinery and upregulating cutaneous RARs.

B. H. Thiers, MD

Vitamin C-Induced Decomposition of Lipid Hydroperoxides to Endogenous Genotoxins
Lee SH, Oe T, Blair IA (Univ of Pennsylvania, Philadelphia)
Science 292:2083-2086, 2001   20–17

Background.—Protection against cancer may be a role of antioxidants in the diet. Thus, supplementing the diet with antioxidants may contribute to the prevention of some diseases. However, vitamin C supplementation has not proved effective in studies of chemoprevention for cancer. In addition, concern exists regarding the potential disadvantages of transition metal ion-mediated pro-oxidant effects.

Methods.—Whether vitamin C induces the decomposition of lipid hydroperoxides into endogenous genotoxins was examined experimentally.

Results.—Lipid hydroperoxide decomposition was induced by vitamin C, producing the DNA-reactive bifunctional electrophiles 4-oxo-2-nonenal, 4,5-epoxy-2 *(E)*-decenal, and 4-hydroxy-2-nonenal. The compound 4,5-epoxy-2*(E)*-decenal is a precursor of etheno-2'-deoxyadenosine, a significant mutagenic lesion found in human DNA.

Conclusions.—Genotoxins were formed from lipid hydroperoxides through the mediation of vitamin C and in the absence of transition metal ions. Such action may underlie the lack of efficacy in cancer chemoprevention noted with vitamin C despite its antioxidant properties.

▶ Topical and oral vitamin C products and supplements have been touted as important tools to fight skin aging. This study from the University of Pennsylvania suggests that vitamin C can promote DNA damage by mediating the production of harmful genotoxins. Although vitamin C is a proven antioxidant, its ability to promote DNA damage may be a significant negative and may help explain why megadoses of the vitamin have failed to show efficacy as a cancer chemopreventive strategy.

B. H. Thiers, MD

Ultraviolet Exposure as the Main Initiator of p53 Mutations in Basal Cell Carcinomas From Psoralen and Ultraviolet A-Treated Patients With Psoriasis
Seidl H, Kreimer-Erlacher H, Bäck B, et al (Karl-Franzens Univ, Graz, Austria)
J Invest Dermatol 117:365-370, 2001   20–18

Background.—Among the risk factors for basal cell carcinoma (BCC) is chronic exposure to sunlight. Patients who have psoriasis and are treated with psoralen and ultraviolet A (PUVA) have a greater frequency of BCC.

The reasons behind this increased frequency are unclear because PUVA's carcinogenic properties are difficult to separate from its immunosuppressive activities and the frequent presence of other carcinogenic risk factors. Studies have shown that PUVA exposure may initiate the development of skin cancer by producing mutations of the *p53* gene. Genetic samples of 13 BCCs from 5 patients with psoriasis treated with PUVA were analyzed to detect mutations of the *p53* tumor suppressor gene.

Methods.—The DNA was extracted, submitted to polymerase chain reaction–single-strand confirmation polymorphism (PCR-SSCP) analysis, and underwent nucleotide sequencing.

Results.—Of the 13 BCCs examined, 7 had abnormalities on DNA sequencing, including 11 mis-sense, 2 non-sense, and 4 silent mutations. Ninety-two percent of the combined mis-sense and non-sense mutations occurred at dipyrimidine sites, and 69% were of the ultraviolet fingerprint type, reflecting the findings among the general population. Fewer mutations were found at 5'-TpA sites, which is a potential psoralen-binding site and a target for PUVA mutagenesis.

Conclusions.—The main cause of the mutations at *p53* and a principal contributor to the development of BCC may be exposure to ultraviolet B light either in the environment or through therapeutic means, but PUVA may also directly produce some of the mutations. Only half of the BCC samples had *p53* mutations, suggesting that other tumor suppressor genes or oncogenes may be damaged by PUVA and lead to BCC tumorigenesis.

▶ Two previous studies have included analysis of the molecular sequence of the *p53* tumor suppressor gene in PUVA-associated squamous cell carcinoma (SCC); both showed a large portion of the detected *p53* mutations were at dypyrimidine sites and were of the UV fingerprint type, suggesting that DNA damage caused by UVB exposure may be a significant factor in the formation of SCC in PUVA-treated patients.[1,2] In one of the studies, approximately half of the mutations were detected at locations considered to be possible psoralen-binding sites and targets for PUVA mutagenesis.[1] This indicates that PUVA exposure may directly initiate a substantial portion of skin cancers by causing *p53* mutations at psoralen-binding sites. In the current study, the majority of *p53* mutations in BCC from PUVA-treated patients occurred at sites similar to those found in the general population, with a small percentage being found at psoralen-binding sites. This suggests that even though the major cause of *p53* mutations (and possibly BCC tumorigenesis) appears to be environmental or therapeutic UVB exposure, PUVA may itself directly cause some *p53* mutations as well. As the number of patients studied was small, it is impossible to state with certainty whether PUVA-related mutations are detected more frequently in SCC or BCC. This is a finding that would be of interest in that SCC is more consistently related to PUVA exposure. Moreover, *p53* mutations may not be the only story, as only half the BCC in the current study harbored *p53* mutations. Other tumor suppressor genes and/or oncogenes may also be targets of PUVA-associated damage.

B. H. Thiers, MD

References

1. Nataraj AJ, Wolf P, Cerroni L, et al: *p53* mutations in squamous cell carcinomas from psoriasis patients treated with psoralen + UVA (PUVA). *J Invest Dermatol* 109:238-243, 1997.
2. Wang XM, McNiff JM, Klump V, et al: An unexpected spectrum of *p53* mutations from squamous cell carcinomas in psoriasis patients treated with PUVA. *Photochem Photobiol* 66:294-299, 1997.

A Correlation of Alpha-Smooth Muscle Actin and Invasion in Micronodular Basal Cell Carcinoma

Christian MM, Moy RL, Wagner RF, et al (Univ of Texas, Dallas; Univ of California, Los Angeles; VA-West Los Angeles Med Ctr, California; et al)
Dermatol Surg 27:441-445, 2001   20–19

Introduction.—Microfilaments composed primarily of actin are largely responsible for cell motility. Normal epithelial cells contain little actin, and the altered expression of actin may influence the invasive potential of some cancers. Nine micronodular basal cell carcinomas (BCC) were examined to determine whether the presence of alpha-smooth muscle actin (α-SMA) correlated with aggressive invasion. Compared with nodular BCC, micronodular BCC require more surgical stages, wider tissue margins, and deeper defects during Mohs micrographic surgery (MMS).

Methods.—Seven primary and 2 recurrent micronodular BCC were removed by MMS or excision. The tumors were evaluated for neural invasion and depth of tissue invasion and with α-SMA antibodies. Neural invasion was strictly defined as tumor within the nerve or perineural sheath. Immunoperoxidase staining was used to identify α-SMA antibodies; findings were positive if either the tumor cells or stroma stained. The BCC were compared with 13 morpheaform and 12 nodular BCC.

Results.—Six (67%) micronodular and 8 (62%) morpheaform BCC stained positive for α-SMA; all nodular BCC stained negative. Three of the 6 micronodular BCC that stained positive for α-SMA invaded the fascia or muscle and 3 exhibited neural invasion. None of the 3 micronodular BCC that stained negative for α-SMA invaded the fascia or muscle and only 1 showed neural invasion. All α-SMA–positive micronodular tumors displayed a purely micronodular pattern. Two of the 3 α-SMA–negative tumors, however, had a mixed nodular-micronodular pattern.

Conclusion.—Actin was identified in 66% of micronodular, 62% of morpheaform, and 0% of nodular BCC. The micronodular BCC that stained positive for α-SMA exhibited a higher incidence of neural or deep invasion, or both, than the micronodular BCC that stained negative. Actin within tumor cells may increase cell motility, leading to increased invasion.

▶ As tumors progress from in situ to invasive lesions, critical elements include disruption of the basement membrane and the ability to migrate into surrounding stroma. Previous studies have shown the poor transplantability of basal cell carcinoma. This tumor is critically dependent on stromal inter-actions for continued growth. Here the authors demonstrate that the more aggressive types of basal cell carcinoma are characterized by increased staining for α-SMA, which probably represents a marker for myofibroblasts and their associated stromelysin-3. This enzyme degrades the stromal ma-trix surrounding the tumor, potentially facilitating tumor invasion.

J. Cook, MD

The Specialty of the Treating Physician Affects the Likelihood of Tumor-Free Resection Margins for Basal Cell Carcinoma: Results From a Multi-Institutional Retrospective Study

Fleischer AB, Feldman SR, Barlow JO, et al (Wake Forest Univ, Winston-Salem; Indiana Univ, Indianapolis; Univ of Colorado, Denver; et al)
J Am Acad Dermatol 44:224-230, 2001   20–20

Background.—Basal cell carcinoma (BCC) is the most common cutane-ous malignancy. Surgical experience and physician specialty may affect the outcome quality of surgical excision of BCC.

Methods.—We performed a multicenter retrospective study of BCC excisions submitted to the respective Departments of Pathology at 4 major university medical centers. Our outcome measure was presence of histo-logic evidence of tumor present in surgical margins of excision specimens (incomplete excision). Clinician experience was defined as the number of excisions that a clinician performed during the study interval. The analytic sample pool included 1459 tumors that met all inclusion and exclusion criteria. Analyses included univariate and multivariate techniques involv-ing the entire sample and separate subsample analyses that excluded 2 outlying dermatologists.

Results.—Tumor was present at the surgical margins in 243 (16.6%) of 1459 specimens. A patient's sex, age, and tumor size were not significantly related to the presence of tumor in the surgical margin. Physician experi-ence did not demonstrate a significant difference either in the entire sample ($P < .09$) or in the subsample analysis ($P > .30$). Tumors of the head and neck were more likely to be incompletely excised than truncal tumors in all the analyses ($P < .03$). Compared with dermatologists, otolaryngologists ($P < .02$) and plastic surgeons ($P < .008$) were more likely to incompletely excise tumors; however, subsample analysis for plastic surgeons found only a trend toward significance ($P < .10$). Dermatologists and general surgeons did not differ in the likelihood of performing an incomplete excision ($P > .4$).

Conclusion.—The physician specialty may affect the quality of care in the surgical management of BCC.

▶ This multicenter study addresses the likelihood that physician specialty might influence the completeness of resection of BCCs. Fleischer et al found that otolaryngologists and plastic surgeons typically had higher rates of incomplete tumor excision than dermatologists or general surgeons. This may be explained to some extent by the high likelihood of tumors occurring on the head and neck in these 2 surgical disciplines. A retrospective study cannot completely assess all the variables evaluated by these authors. Although the consequences of too-narrow surgical margins were well demonstrated, the contrary of too-wide surgical margins could not be examined.

Many previously reported studies have clearly shown that dermatologists are indeed the skin cancer experts who can accurately determine the appropriate method of treatment for BCCs, including destructive modalities, excisional surgery, radiation therapy, and Mohs' micrographic surgery. Nevertheless, further studies supporting the expertise of dermatologists in treating nonmelanoma skin cancer are always welcome.

J. Cook, MD

Dense Inflammation Does Not Mask Residual Primary Basal Cell Carcinoma During Mohs Micrographic Surgery
Katz KH, Helm KF, Billingsley EM, et al (Pennsylvania State Univ, Hershey; Univ of Massachusetts Med Ctr, Worcester)
J Am Acad Dermatol 45:231-238, 2001   20–21

Background.—Primary basal cell carcinoma is a contiguous, unifocal tumor. Theoretically, the cure rate should be 100% when primary basal cell carcinoma is treated with Mohs' micrographic surgery. The actual cure rate is estimated to be 99%. Recurrences can be attributed to misinterpretation of the histologic sections, either because of faulty processing of the tissue or the misinterpretation of "hidden tumor." The concern that dense lymphocytic inflammation could mask residual tumor had led surgeons performing the Mohs' micrographic procedure to remove additional layers of tissue to maintain a high cure rate at the expense of tissue conservation. The concept that inflammation can hide residual tumor has never been convincingly demonstrated. This study sought to determine whether inflammation masks tumor during Mohs' surgery for primary basal cell carcinoma.

Methods.—Twenty-five consecutive patients who underwent Mohs' micrographic surgery for primary basal cell carcinoma were studied. In these patients, areas of dense inflammation were encountered during surgery. The areas of dense inflammation were sectioned and stained with hematoxylin and eosin and Ber-EP4, a sensitive although relatively nonspecific stain for detecting basal cell carcinoma.

Results.—In 12 of 25 patients, the area of dense inflammation did not correspond to basal cell carcinoma in the immediate vicinity. In the remaining 13 patients, basal cell carcinoma was discovered in the immediate area of the dense inflammation. In all of the patients in whom basal cell carcinoma was present, the carcinoma was progressively easier to identify as sections were taken deeper into the block. In none of the patients did the dense inflammation mask residual tumor.

Conclusions.—Areas of dense inflammation do not mask primary basal cell carcinoma during Mohs' surgery. These areas should be carefully evaluated before additional surgery is performed.

▶ The authors argue that Mohs' surgeons routinely take extra layer(s) of tissue if dense inflammation is present when tracing out a basal cell carcinoma. Is this true? It is well recognized that tumor cells can be concealed by dense inflammation. For this study, deeper sectioning revealed basal cell carcinoma in 52% of cases, especially if the tumor was of the infiltrating type. This investigation reveals that it is not necessary to arbitrarily take an extra layer of tissue when inflammation is present—simply cut deeper into the block!

P. G. Lang, Jr, MD

Risk of Synchronous and Metachronous Second Nonmelanoma Skin Cancer When Referred for Mohs Micrographic Surgery
Schinstine M, Goldman GD (Univ of Vermont, Burlington)
J Am Acad Dermatol 44:497-499, 2001   20–22

Background.—Patients with basal cell carcinoma and cutaneous squamous cell carcinoma are at substantial risk for the onset of a second nonmelanoma skin cancer (NMSC).

Objective.—Our purpose was to determine the incidence of multiple (synchronous) NMSC at presentation to an academic Mohs micrographic surgery referral center and to note the incidence of second lesions occurring in a metachronous fashion.

Methods.—A retrospective study was conducted of 456 consecutive patients who presented for Mohs surgery over a 2-year period. Patients were assessed at initial visits for the presence of multiple NMSCs and were subsequently examined over 2 years for the onset of new NMSCs.

Results.—More than 39% of patients initially referred for Mohs surgery with a basal cell or squamous cell carcinoma either presented with multiple primary lesions or experienced a subsequent NMSC within 2 years. These tumors were divided almost equally between multiple primary NMSC at presentation and subsequent (metachronous) tumors.

Conclusion.—Patients referred for Mohs surgery in an academic setting are a select group at extremely high risk of additional NMSCs at or shortly after presentation for the index lesion.

▶ Nearly one half of patients referred to these investigators' academic Mohs' surgery practice had an additional NMSC at presentation or one that developed within 2 years. Although some selection bias is possible because of the authors' practice profile, this article underscores the importance of both careful follow-up and patient education in the early postoperative period so that any additional NMSCs can be appropriately managed.

J. Cook, MD

Perineural Spread of Cutaneous Squamous and Basal Cell Carcinoma: CT and MR Detection and Its Impact on Patient Management and Prognosis

Williams LS, Mancuso AA, Mendenhall WM (Univ of Florida, Gainesville)
Int J Radiat Oncol Biol Phys 49:1061-1069, 2001   20–23

Background.—The spread of head and neck cancers along cranial nerves is not uncommon, but its detection can be challenging. The diagnostic and prognostic utility of CT and MRI was investigated retrospectively in patients with perineural spread of basal or squamous cell carcinoma of the face and scalp.

Methods.—The subjects were 35 patients (26 men and 9 women; median age, 66 years) with basal or squamous cell carcinoma of the face or scalp. All patients had clinical or pathologic evidence of perineural spread along the divisions of the trigeminal or facial nerves. All patients underwent CT and MRI before receiving radiation therapy with curative intent. Two radiologists independently estimated the volume of perineural disease on CT and MRI scans as minimal (abnormal enhancement without obvious enlargement of the nerves), moderate (nerve enlargement to 2-3 times normal diameter, with or without abnormal enhancement), or gross (nerve enlargement to >5 times normal diameter or an obvious mass, with or without abnormal enhancement). Perineural extension on CT and MRI was divided into 3 zones of involvement: zone 1 (peripheral), zone 2 (central/skull base), and zone 3 (cisternal). Patients were followed up for 2 years or more (median, 4.3 years) to compare clinical characteristics and disease-free survival between patients with and without CT or MRI evidence of perineural spread.

Results.—Eighteen patients had positive CT or MRI findings for perineural spread, while 17 patients had clinical or pathologic evidence of perineural spread but negative imaging findings (n = 17). Sixteen of 24 patients (66.7%) with symptoms of perineural spread at diagnosis had positive imaging findings, and 6 of these patients experienced disease progression. Conversely, 9 of 11 patients (81.8%) who were asymptomatic at diagnosis had negative imaging findings, and only 1 had disease progression. Symptoms of perineural spread did not correlate significantly with outcomes, however. Absolute survival rates at 2 years were similar in the imaging-positive and imaging-negative groups (83% and 94%, respectively). However, absolute 5-year survival was significantly worse in the patients with positive imaging findings (50% vs 86%). Among the imaging-positive patients, there was a trend (*P* = .054) for those with a greater degree and extent of perineural spread to have an increased likelihood of disease progression.

Conclusions.—CT and MRI were useful in identifying patients with advanced perineural spread of cutaneous basal and squamous cell carcinoma of the head or scalp. Patients with clinical symptoms at diagnosis were significantly more likely to have positive imaging findings, and positive imaging findings were associated with significantly poorer 5-year survival. Outcomes were also worse in patients with greater perineural tumor volume and more central disease. Thus, CT and MRI in this population have prognostic value as well.

▶ Patients with documented perineural involvement by cutaneous squamous cell and basal cell carcinomas should undergo imaging to determine the extent of spread and whether cure is possible. It is generally agreed that MRI is superior to CT in the detection of perineural disease. In this study, only approximately 50% of patients had positive scan results, but many of the patients underwent CT rather than MRI. Unfortunately, the authors did not subdivide the patients on the basis of the type of scan they had, and it cannot be determined how sensitive MRI is in this setting. Regardless, patients with positive scan results usually fared worse. Although this study did not demonstrate a worse prognosis for symptomatic patients, larger studies have.[1] This has been my experience as well.

P. G. Lang, Jr, MD

Reference

1. McCord MW: Perineural invasion by skin cancer of the head and neck. Presented at the 27th Annual Radiation Oncology Clinical Research Seminar, Gainesville, Fla, Feb 2-8, 1997.

Photofrin-Mediated Photodynamic Therapy for Treatment of Aggressive Head and Neck Nonmelanomatous Skin Tumors in Elderly Patients
Schweitzer VG (Henry Ford Health System, Detroit)
Laryngoscope 111:1091-1098, 2001   20–24

Introduction.—Hematoporphyrin-derivative photodynamic therapy (PDT), a modality using light-activated drugs and low-power nonthermal light, has proved effective in treating a variety of malignancies that fail to respond to conventional methods. In dermatologic oncology, PDT has been used for primary and recurrent nonmelanoma skin cancer, Kaposi sarcoma, mycosis fungoides, and palliation of tumors that have metastasized to the skin. The patients reviewed in this study were referred specifically for PDT for aggressive, recurrent nonmelanomatous tumors of the head and neck.

Methods.—Patients were 8 men and 4 women with an age range of 60 to 92 years. Many had comorbidities. A variety of causes of cutaneous head and neck cancer and of previous treatment modalities were represented by the group. Therapy consisted of injection with 1.0 mg/kg Photofrin (dihematoporphyrin derivative) followed 60 hours later by intraoperative laser light activation. Light was delivered through microlens fiber using an argon dye laser. For 4 weeks after treatment, patients had to follow detailed precautions to minimize drug-related sensitivity, wear proper clothing and modify their travel and daily activities.

Results.—Five patients received intraoperative PDT combined with surgical resection (including radical mastoidectomy and lateral temporal bone resection) and 7 were treated with PDT alone. At follow-up periods ranging from 6 months to 5 years, 10 patients achieved complete responses with excellent wound healing and cosmetic outcome. The mean survival time for these 10 patients was 35 months. One patient experienced a partial response and required 3 additional treatments for local recurrences over a 6-year period. The remaining patient died of renal failure 3 months after PDT.

Conclusion.—Photofrin-mediated PDT was found to be an effective locoregional oncologic modality for patients with aggressive primary or recurrent basal cell carcinoma and squamous cell carcinoma of the head and neck. The treatments were well tolerated in these elderly patients who had progressive disease despite previous surgical and radiation therapy.

▶ PDT utilizing systemic, topical, and intralesional photosensitizers is an evolving technology that holds great promise, and new photosensitizers are being developed. The greatest experience has been with IV dihematoporphyrin (Photofrin). PDT represents an alternative to extensive surgery and reconstruction or multiple surgeries in debilitated or elderly patients with extensive or recurrent cancers, or in patients prone to the development of multiple skin cancers (eg, patients with basal cell nevus syndrome, xeroderma pigmentosum, or transplants). By lowering the dose of the photosensitizer but giving high energies of light, better selectivity of the photoreaction can be achieved. Moreover, the persistent photosensitivity can be taken advantage of, by allowing multiple treatments to be given over a 2-week period. PDT also can be combined with surgery when necessary. In this report, the author demonstrates the usefulness of PDT and summarizes her experience with 12 patients.

P. G. Lang, Jr, MD

Human Papillomavirus Infection as a Risk Factor for Squamous-Cell Carcinoma of the Head and Neck
Mork J, Lie AK, Glattre E, et al (Cancer Registry of Norway, Oslo; Natl Hosp, Oslo, Norway; Norwegian Radium Hosp, Oslo, Norway; et al)
N Engl J Med 344:1125-1131, 2001   20–25

Background.—A number of studies indicate that oncogenic human papillomaviruses (HPVs) are associated with various cancers, but the results of case series and case-control studies are inconsistent. To evaluate causality, studies must be based on samples from healthy persons in whom the disease develops later. Reliable markers of either previous or present HPV infection are antibodies to HPV capsid antigens; when assessed by seroepidemiologic methods, HPV-16 infection has been associated with cervical and anogenital cancers. The possibility that HPV infection may be a risk factor for the development of head and neck squamous cell carcinoma was assessed.

Methods.—Serum samples were obtained from serum banks to which 900,000 residents of Norway, Finland, and Sweden had donated. Serum bank files were used to link donated samples with persons who were given a diagnosis at least a month later of head or neck cancer. Three hundred one invasive squamous cell carcinomas and 8 carcinomas (not otherwise specified) of the head and neck were found, of which 292 proved useable. Control subjects were alive and free of head and neck cancer at the time the corresponding patient's condition was diagnosed; they were matched for age, sex, and length of serum storage. The standard enzyme-linked immunosorbent assay was used to detect antibodies against HPV. Serum cotinine, which indicates exposure to tobacco smoke, was also assessed, and tissues were evaluated for HPV DNA by means of polymerase chain reaction assay.

Results.—Patients with head and neck cancer had a prevalence of seropositivity for HPV-16 more than twice as high as that of controls. The seroprevalance for HPV-18, HPV-33, and HPV-73 was similar between patients and controls. A significant association between HPV-16 seropositivity and risk of squamous cell carcinoma was found after adjusting for cotinine levels, but none was found for the other HVP types. Of 228 tumor specimens, DNA extraction was successful in 160. Of these, 9% were positive for HPV-16 DNA; they were generally specimens from oropharyngeal tumors. Thus, individuals positive for HPV-16 had a significant risk of having a head and neck cancer containing HPV-16 DNA (odds ratio, 37.5) compared with those without this viral genome (odds ratio, 2.1).

Conclusion.—Infection with HPV-16 may be a risk factor for the development of squamous cell carcinoma of the head and neck.

▶ The data suggest that HPV-16 infection may be a risk factor not only for cervical and anogenital cancers, but also for squamous cell carcinoma of the head and neck. The findings, however, do not clearly prove a cause-and-effect relationship between the infection and these head and neck tumors.

B. H. Thiers, MD

DNA Content as a Prognostic Marker in Patients With Oral Leukoplakia

Sudbø J, Kildal W, Risberg B, et al (Univ of Oslo, Norway)
N Engl J Med 344:1270-1278, 2001   20–26

Background.—Squamous cell carcinoma, which has a poor prognosis, may develop in patients with oral leukoplakia. Risk factors for oral carcinoma have been identified, but there have been no reliable predictors of the outcome of oral carcinoma in individual patients with oral leukoplakia.

Methods.—One hundred fifty patients with oral leukoplakia classified as epithelial dysplasia were identified. The nuclear DNA content (ploidy)

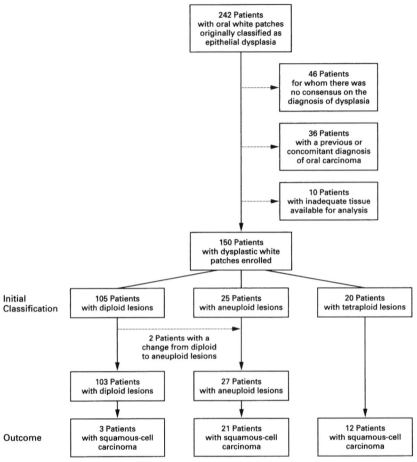

FIGURE 1.—Selection, classification, and outcome of patients with oral leukoplakia according to the analysis of the DNA content of the lesions. There were no changes in ploidy from aneuploid to either tetraploid or diploid or from tetraploid to either diploid or aneuploid. Carcinoma did not develop during follow-up in either of the patients with lesions that changed from diploid to aneuploid during follow up. (Reprinted by permission of *The New England Journal of Medicine*, from Sudbø J, Kildal W, Risberg B, et al: DNA content as a prognostic marker in patients with oral leukoplakia. *N Engl J Med* 344:1270-1278. Copyright 2001, Massachusetts Medical Society. All rights reserved.)

of these lesions was measured to determine whether DNA ploidy could be used to accurately predict clinical outcome. Biopsy specimens were obtained at annual follow-up and graded histologically. The specimens were also classified with respect to DNA content in a blinded fashion. Disease-free survival was assessed in relation to DNA ploidy and histologic grade. The mean duration of follow-up was 103 months.

Results.—Among the 150 patients, carcinoma developed in 36 (24%). Of the total group, 105 patients (70%) had diploid (normal) lesions, 20 (13%) had tetraploid (intermediate) lesions, and 25 (17%) had aneuploid (abnormal) lesions at initial diagnosis (Fig 1). Carcinoma developed in 3

(3%) of the 105 patients with diploid lesions, compared with 21 (84%) of 25 patients with aneuploid lesions. This translated to a negative predictive value of 97% for the diploid lesions and a positive predictive value of 84% for aneuploid lesions. Of the 20 patients with tetraploid lesions, carcinoma developed in 12 (60%). The mean time from initial assessment of the DNA content to the development of a carcinoma was 35 months in the aneuploid group and 49 months in the tetraploid group. Cumulative disease-free survival was 97% for patients with diploid lesions, 40% for patients with tetraploid lesions, and 16% for patients with aneuploid lesions.

Conclusions.—Assessment of the DNA content of cells in patients with oral leukoplakia can be used to predict risk for oral carcinoma.

▶ Sudbø et al demonstrate that oral leukoplakia lesions with aneuploid DNA content clearly have a worse prognosis than those with diploid DNA content. The obvious conclusion is that more aggressive treatment of aneuploid lesions may be warranted. Tetraploid lesions appear to represent an intermediate group with an uncertain clinical outcome. An editorial in the same journal discussed the implications of this study for the management of patients with leukoplakia.[1]

B. H. Thiers, MD

Reference

1. Lippmann SW, Hong WK: Molecular markers of the risk of oral cancer. *N Engl J Med* 344:1323-1326, 2001.

High Incidence of Lichen Sclerosus in Patients With Squamous Cell Carcinoma of the Penis

Powell J, Robson A, Cranston D, et al (The Churchill, Oxford, England; Oxford Radcliffe Hosps, England)
Br J Dermatol 145:85-89, 2001   20–27

Background.—Lichen sclerosis (LS) has been clearly associated with vulval carcinoma in women. Until recently, however, only anecdotal reports of penile squamous cell carcinoma (SCC) in men with LS have appeared. The incidence of penile carcinoma in men with LS was investigated.

Methods and Findings.—A review of 20 patients with penile SCC in a center's 4-year pathology database was done. Evidence of LS was detected in the excised specimen in 8 (40%) patients. Seven of these men had well-differentiated SCC. Of the 12 patients with no evidence of LS, only 3 (25%) had well-differentiated SCC. A case note review indicated that 7 patients had a history of LS, sometimes preceding the SCC by 10 years. All of these patients had well-differentiated SCC. Ten patients had died, 7 from metastatic disease. The deaths included 4 patients in the well-differentiated group.

Conclusions.—Penile SCC and LS appear to be associated. Clinical presentation of LS or a need for circumcision may precede the SCC by many years. Counseling at the time of diagnosis is very important. Clinicians must be aware of the association of LS and penile SCC to reduce the subsequent risk from SCC.

▶ The authors advocate that all adult circumcision samples should be sent for histologic examination to establish the diagnosis of LS. If the diagnosis is established, patients and their physicians should be given full information about the disease and the possible future risk of penile cancer, and about its signs and symptoms upon presentation.

B. H. Thiers MD

Sentinel Lymph Node Dissection for Merkel Cell Carcinoma

Vandeweyer E, Sales F, Bourgeois P (Brussels, Belgium; Jules Bordet Cancer Inst, Brussels, Belgium)
Eur J Plast Surg 24:147-149, 2001   20–28

Introduction.—Merkel cell carcinoma, an aggressive cutaneous neuroendocrine tumor, exhibits some of the same features as malignant melanoma. Lesions generally appear as a pink, red, or blue nodule ranging in size from a few millimeters to several centimeters. The role of lymph node dissection in the treatment of Merkel cell carcinoma is controversial, and sentinel lymph node dissection for disease staging is under evaluation. The patient presented had a sentinel lymph node isolated and biopsied for tumor involvement.

> *Case Report.*—Man, 50, was seen for a rapidly growing asymptomatic lesion on the lateral aspect of the left arm. The subcutaneous nodule had been present for at least 6 weeks. An incisional biopsy specimen revealed a Merkel cell carcinoma. Histologic examination of the tumor removed during wide radical excision confirmed the diagnosis. The patient's lymph nodes were not palpable, and imaging studies showed no distant metastases. Preoperative lymphoscintigraphy indicated a single sentinel lymph node in the axillary region. The sentinel lymph node was free of tumor involvement, and the patient recovered with no additional treatment.

Discussion.—Because lymph node metastases in Merkel cell carcinoma are associated with a poor prognosis, elective lymph node dissection is often recommended. With the use of sentinel lymph node biopsy, some patients may be able to avoid the morbidity associated with unnecessary lymph node dissection.

▶ Although the follow-up period was short, this case report suggests that sentinel lymph node biopsy may have a role in the management of Merkel cell carcinoma.

P. G. Lang, Jr, MD

Early Experience With Sentinel Lymph Node Mapping for Merkel Cell Carcinoma
Rodrigues LKE, Leong SPL, Kashani-Sabet M, et al (Univ of California, San Francisco; Univ of Hawaii, Honolulu)
J Am Acad Dermatol 45:303-308, 2001   20–29

Merkel cell or cutaneous neuroendocrine carcinoma is a malignant tumor with a propensity toward local and systemic recurrence. A new surgical technique, intraoperative lymphatic mapping and selective sentinel lymph node dissection (SSLND), has been demonstrated to have a high predictive value for the detection of metastatic disease in the regional lymphatic basin in cutaneous melanoma. The use of this technology may be particularly useful to accurately stage patients with Merkel cell carcinoma (MCC) because this tumor has a frequent propensity toward regional nodal metastases. Intraoperative lymphatic mapping and SSLND were performed on 6 patients with biopsy-proven MCC. Three patients with MCC had positive disease in the sentinel lymph node(s). SSLND is a feasible technique with minimal procedural morbidity to detect clinically occult disease in patients with MCC.

▶ From the standpoint of sentinel lymph node biopsy (SLNB), the tumor other than melanoma and breast cancer that probably has been investigated most is Merkel cell carcinoma. This study represents yet another small series of patients examined to assess the usefulness of SLNB in managing Merkel cell carcinoma. SLNB can be successfully used to identify metastatic nodal disease in patients with Merkel cell carcinoma. This study does not answer whether early identification of metastatic disease and appropriate treatment alters prognosis.

P. G. Lang, Jr, MD

Prognostic and Therapeutic Implications of Sentinel Lymphonodectomy and S-Staging in Merkel Cell Carcinoma
Düker I, Starz H, Bachter D, et al (Klinikum Augsburg, Germany)
Dermatology 202:225-229, 2001   20–30

Introduction.—Merkel cell carcinoma (MCC) is a rare cutaneous malignancy with a poor prognosis. Among node-positive patients, mortality is 67%. Because MCC usually affects the elderly, elective lymph node dissection is not routinely performed. The prognostic and therapeutic relevance of sentinel lymph node excision (SLNE) was examined in a study of 5 patients with MCC of the skin.

Methods.—Four of the 5 patients were aged 73 years or older. Sites of MCC were the head and neck region, the upper extremities, the lower extremities, and the trunk. All patients received wide local excision. Gamma-probe–guided SLNE assisted by lymphatic mapping was performed, and paraffin sections from each sentinel lymph node (SLN) were examined for the presence of micrometastases. Four S stages could be distinguished by documenting the number of metastatically involved slices of the SLN and the depth of invasion.

Results.—All SLNs were successfully identified and excised, with no procedure-related complications. Four patients had a positive SLN. Radical lymph node dissection was performed in 3 patients with S_2 disease. The patient with S_3 disease refused the procedure and died within 1 year with widespread metastasis.

Conclusion.—The use of SLNE in patients with MCC allows identification of those who do not require a complete regional SLNE. In this series, the patient with negative findings was alive at 21 months and free of recurrent disease. For patients with nodal disease, an aggressive treatment strategy can be followed.

▶ This is yet another small series of cases that addresses the reliability and prognostic implications of SLNE in the management of MCC. These authors have previously utilized the S staging system in melanoma patients to help further refine the prognostic significance of SLNE and to attempt to define which patients with a positive SLNE specimen require a complete node dissection. This study applies this S staging system to patients with MCC. Although the results are preliminary, it would appear that patients with a negative SLNE fare much better, and that patients in whom there is limited penetration (less than 1 mm) of the tumor into the depths of the node are less likely to have involvement of nonsentinel nodes. These latter patients may not require a complete dissection of the nodal basin and may have a better prognosis than patients with non–sentinel node metastases.

P. G. Lang, Jr, MD

Merkel Cell Carcinoma of the Head and Neck: Effect of Surgical Excision and Radiation on Recurrence and Survival
Gillenwater AM, Hessel AC, Morrison WH, et al (Univ of Texas, Houston)
Arch Otolaryngol Head Neck Surg 127:149-154, 2001   20–31

Introduction.—Merkel cell carcinoma (MCC) is a rare malignant neoplasm of the skin that usually arises in the head and neck region. In spite of the innocuous appearance of the primary lesion, MCC often has an aggressive clinical course with frequent locoregional recurrences and distant metastases. A retrospective analysis was performed to ascertain whether excision of the primary lesion with wider surgical margins affected the rate of locoregional control. The effect of postoperative radiation therapy (XRT) on locoregional recurrence and survival rates was also examined.

Methods.—A database was used to identify patients with either MCC or a neuroendocrine carcinoma of the skin who were seen in the years from 1945 to 1995. Sixty-six patients with MCC were identified. Medical records were examined for demographic information; tumor size and location; type of initial therapy; number, site, and time to onset of recurrence; and final outcome. Survival curves were constructed for 3 groups of patients: those who did not receive postoperative XRT, those who received postoperative XRT, and those who received XRT as their definitive therapy.

Results.—The mean age of the 55 men and 11 women was 68.4 years (range, 41-91 years). The 18 patients with adequate data were grouped according to the width of their surgical margins: smaller than 1 cm, 1 to 2 cm, and larger than 2 cm. The groups were similar in rates of locoregional control and survival because of the small patient population. Among patients who did and did not receive postoperative XRT (26 and 34 patients, respectively), there was a significant difference in local recurrence rates (3 [12%] and 15 [44%], respectively; $P < .01$) and regional recurrence rates (7 [27%] and 29 [85%], respectively; $P < .01$). These groups did not differ significantly in disease-specific survival ($P = .30$). Regardless of type of therapy, distant disease developed in 36% of all patients.

Conclusion.—No effect of the width of surgical margins on outcome could be determined in this small patient population. Postoperative XRT was correlated with a significant improvement in locoregional control. There were no significant associations between type of initial therapy and rates of distant metastases or survival.

▶ Controversy exists over whether postoperative radiation after the resection of a MCC offers any benefit. The usual recommended margins of excision have been 2 to 3 cm. In this study, the authors attempted to look at the role of margins, postoperative radiation, and neck dissection in the management of MCC of the head and neck. Unfortunately, the data available for analysis were somewhat limited, making it difficult to draw definitive conclusions. In the small number of cases studied, it did not appear that margins of 2 to 3 cm offered any advantage over 1-cm margins. Postoperative radiation to the area of excision, regional nodes, and intervening lymphatics appeared to decrease the local and regional recurrence rate in patients without clinical node involvement but had no impact on the incidence of distant metastases or overall survival. This latter observation suggests the need for effective adjuvant (systemic) therapy. There were too few cases to assess the role of elective neck dissection either with or without postoperative radiation, in the management of MCC of the head and neck. Radiation as a primary treatment appeared to be associated with a significant incidence of recurrence. The authors also cite the encouraging preliminary results observed with sentinel lymph node biopsy in these patients but admit that their follow-up time was too short and their experience too limited to draw any definitive conclusions.

P. G. Lang, Jr, MD

Multimodality Treatment of Merkel Cell Carcinoma: Case Series and Literature Review of 1024 Cases
Medina-Franco H, Urist MM, Fiveash J, et al (Univ of Alabama, Birmingham)
Ann Surg Oncol 8:204-208, 2001   20–32

Background.—The most effective treatment of Merkel cell carcinoma (MCC), an unusual and potentially aggressive form of skin cancer, is currently undetermined, with roles for surgery, chemotherapy, and radiotherapy. These therapeutic options were analyzed retrospectively with respect to the cancer's natural history, patient factors, tumor characteristics, and treatment variables. The English-language literature on MCC was also reviewed.

Methods.—A search of the Tumor Registry and Radiation Oncology records from the University of Alabama at Birmingham (UAB) from 1986 through June 2000 identified 16 patients who had localized primary MCC. Demographics, tumor characteristics, treatment, and outcome were documented, and tumors were staged according to the presence or absence of metastases to regional lymph nodes. A χ^2 test or Fisher's exact test was done as appropriate. The literature review covered January 1990 to June 2000 and included patient age, gender, medical history, state at presentation, treatment, and outcome.

Results.—The patients comprised 12 white men and 4 white women and were aged from 37 to 94 years (median age, 67 years). Three patients were taking immunosuppressant agents for kidney or heart transplant, and 5 had a history of squamous cell carcinoma (SCC). The primary MCC size ranged from 0.7 to 7.3 cm (mean, 2.73 cm), and sites included the head and neck, trunk, and extremities (Table 1). Wide local excision was used

---

TABLE 1.—Clinicopathological Characteristics of Merkel Cell Carcinoma

Characteristic	UAB Experience (n = 16) No. (%)	Literature Review (n = 1024) No. (1%)
Location		
Head and neck	10 (62.5%)	416 (40.6%)
Trunk	0	236 (23.0%)
Extremities	6 (37.5%)	338 (33.0%)
Unknown	0	34 (3.4%)
Stage at presentation		
I	10 (62.5%)	751 (73.4%)
II	6 (37.5%)	231 (22.6%)
III	0	41 (4.0%)

Abbreviation: UAB, University of Alabama at Birmingham.
(Courtesy of Medina-Franco H, Urist MM, Fiveash J, et al: Multimodality treatment of Merkel cell carcinoma: Case series and literature review of 1024 cases. *Ann Surg Oncol* 8:204-208, 2001.)

in all cases, with 3 having modified radical neck dissection and 2 having axillary sentinel lymph node biopsy for forearm lesions; both had metastasis at presentation. None of the stage I patients had elective lymph node dissection. Adjuvant radiotherapy was used for 7 patients, 4 with stage II disease, 1 with a positive surgical margin, 1 with a 7-cm MCC of the scalp, and 1 with a lip tumor. Adjuvant chemotherapy was used for 2 patients with stage II disease; 1 died 4 months later and the other has no evidence of disease after 20 months. Recurrences were found in 7 patients at a mean of 6.9 months (range, 2 to 11 months): 3 tumors recurred in regional lymph nodes only, 3 at distant sites, and 1 at both local and distant sites.

The median survival overall was 32 months; actuarial 2-year survival rate was 59%, and 3-year survival rate was 31%. Prognostic significance attended finding of positive nodes at presentation. Stage I patients had a median survival of 97 months, whereas stage II patients' median survival was only 15 months. The literature revealed 58% of patients were men, 42% women, and mean patient age was 69 years (range, 18 to 98 years); more than 98% of patients were white. The incidence of SCC of the skin was reported as 13.5%. Immunosuppression was found in 14.5% of patients. The head and neck area was the most common primary site; 3% of cases involved metastatic disease of unknown primary, usually in lymph nodes. Localized disease was the presenting stage in 75% of patients. Excluding patients with distant metastases at presentation, 55.5% had lymph node metastases at presentation or during follow-up. Distant metastases usually affected the lymph nodes, distant skin, lung, CNS, or bone. Local recurrence was found in 30.1% of stage I and II patients during follow-up. An average disease-free interval of 7.4 months was noted. With adjuvant radiotherapy, the local recurrence rate was 10.5%; without it, the recurrence rate was 52.6%. Survival rates in the various studies ranged from 75% at 5 years to 35% at 3 years, with the most consistent prognostic factor being tumor stage at presentation. Two series reported male sex as an adverse prognostic factor. The incidence of MCC was increased, and the prognosis was poorer, when immunosuppressive therapy was a factor.

Conclusions.—MCC represents an aggressive disorder that recurs both locally and distantly at a high rate. It may be useful to perform sentinel lymph node biopsy to identify patients who can benefit from elective node dissection to control the disease regionally. Radiotherapy was a positive influence in several cases.

▶ This article presents a comprehensive review of the prognosis and management of Merkel cell carcinoma (MCC). A number of key points are presented: (1) ultraviolet light probably plays a role in the pathogenesis of MCC, as the majority of these tumors occur in white individuals and on sun-exposed skin. Moreover, a significant number of affected patients have a history of nonmelanoma skin cancer; (2) immunosuppression may be associated with the development of MCC, just as it is with nonmelanoma skin cancer. In some studies, immunosuppression has been also shown to have an adverse effect on prognosis; (3) MCC is an aggressive tumor. In the series of Medina-Franco et al, the 3-year survival was 31%; (4) the most important prognostic factor is the stage of disease at the time of diagnosis. Patients with localized disease do much better than those with nodal metastases (median survival, 97 vs 15 months); (5) although the findings have varied from study to study, postoperative radiation appears to improve locoregional control; and (6) although many patients with systemic disease respond to chemotherapy, it does not appear to prolong life, and it can be quite toxic.

P. G. Lang, Jr, MD

Second Neoplasms in Patients With Merkel Cell Carcinoma
Brenner B, Sulkes A, Rakowsky E, et al (Rabin Med Ctr, Petah Tiqva, Israel; Kaplan Med Ctr, Rehovot, Israel; Tel Aviv Univ, Israel; et al)
Cancer 91:1358-1362, 2001   20–33

Background.—Data on the epidemiologic and clinical features of Merkel cell carcinoma (MCC) are incomplete, yet some studies have detailed a relationship between MCC and other skin tumors as well as with hematologic malignancies. Data from the Israel Cancer Registry were analyzed to see if an association indeed exists between MCC and second neoplasms and to determine the effect on patients' survival.

Methods.—Sixty-seven patients were diagnosed with MCC from August 1983 to December 1999. For each patient, age, gender, ethnic origin, date of MCC diagnosis, date of diagnosis for other neoplasms, and date and cause of death were recorded, as applicable. A group of age- and ethnic-matched patients (comprised of 5751 with malignant melanoma) served as control subjects against whom the MCC group was measured for the incidence of second neoplasms.

Results.—Most MCC patients were elderly Ashkenazi Jews (age range, 19 to 90 years; median age, 73 years). Among the 17 patients with a second neoplasm, the median age was 72 years. The control group had a significantly lower incidence of second neoplasms than did the MCC group (5.8% vs 25%). The calculated standardized incidence ratio of 2.8 was significantly higher in the MCC group. Twelve of the MCC patients had a history of a previous neoplasm, diagnosed a median of 4 years before the MCC diagnosis. Four patients had a second neoplasm develop within a median of 3 years after their MCC diagnosis. One patient had a synchronous tumor at the periphery of the MCC specimen, and 2 had a third primary tumor. Thus, 19 second tumors were found in 17 patients with MCC. Nearly half of these second tumors were squamous cell carcinomas, with the remainder being hematologic malignancies, breast or ovarian adenocarcinomas, and 1 anaplastic meningioma. Patients with a second neoplasm at any point in their history had a significantly higher mortality from MCC, with 65% of these patients dying of generalized metastatic MCC and only 40% of the remaining patients doing so. The estimated actuarial risk of a second primary tumor was 2.1% for each year of observation among patients who developed a second neoplasm during the follow-up period.

Conclusions.—Patients with MCC have a high risk of having a second neoplasm develop, including noncutaneous solid tumors. In addition, patients in whom these second tumors develop have a greater MCC-specific mortality.

▶ This study attempts to address the incidence of second cancers in patients with MCC. Unfortunately, the presence of immunosuppression was not detailed in either the patients or the control group. It is well known that the incidence of MCC is increased in patients who are immunosuppressed (eg, from hematologic malignancies, chronic disease, or transplantation). The association with hematologic malignancies may be partially explained by the frequent use of corticosteroids in managing these conditions. The failure to detail the level of immune competence in the patients and control subjects seriously flaws the reported data. Additionally, the nature of the procedures used in the evaluation and search for second malignancies was not detailed. One would assume that patients with MCC would likely have undergone staging workups more exhaustive than a routine history, physical exam, and chart review.

Like other studies that attempt to ascertain the risk of a second malignancy in patients with nonmelanoma skin cancer, this article fails to clearly establish a linkage. Nevertheless, the treating physician should be aware of published reports of an increased incidence of second malignancies when evaluating and managing these patients.

J. Cook, MD

Mohs Micrographic Surgery for the Treatment of Spindle Cell Tumors of the Skin

Huether MJ, Zitelli JA, Brodland DG (Northwest Med Ctr, Tucson, Az; Univ of Pittsburgh, Pa)
J Am Acad Dermatol 44:656-659, 2001   20–34

Background.—Because of the uncommon nature of dermal spindle cell tumors, the effectiveness of various treatment modalities is difficult to assess.

Objective.—Our purpose was to measure the effectiveness of treating dermatofibrosarcoma protuberans, atypical fibroxanthoma, malignant fibrous histiocytoma, and leiomyosarcoma by means of Mohs micrographic surgery (MMS). In addition, we attempted to determine whether MMS is useful in treating dermal spindle cell tumors when no definitive histopathologic diagnosis can be rendered.

Methods.—In a retrospective chart review, demographic data, tumor data, treatment characteristics, recurrence, and follow-up data were tabulated.

Results.—The recurrence rate for dermatofibrosarcoma protuberans treated by MMS was 3.0%, for atypical fibroxanthoma was 6.9%, for malignant fibrous histiocytoma was 43%, and for leiomyosarcoma was 14%. The recurrence rate for spindle cell tumors not otherwise specified was 0%.

Conclusion.—These data establish the effectiveness of MMS in the treatment of dermal spindle cell tumors, including those for which no definitive histopathologic diagnosis can be rendered.

▶ This article reflects the experience of 2 highly respected Mohs surgeons in the management of malignant spindle cell tumors of the skin. On the basis of a literature review, Mohs micrographic surgery appears to yield cure rates that equal or exceed those of routine wide excision. Somewhat disappointing was the high recurrence rate seen with tumors such as malignant fibrous histiocytoma (43%) and leiomyosarcoma (14%). However, the total number of these tumors treated was small, and with leiomyosarcoma it was unclear if the tumors arose superficially or deep. Although it is presumed that these recurrences represented true local recurrences and not satellite lesions, this is not specifically stated. Finally, would the outcome have been different if permanent sections and not frozen sections had been used?

P. G. Lang, Jr, MD

21 Nevi and Melonoma

Giant Congenital Melanocytic Nevi: The Significance of Neurocutaneous Melanosis in Neurologically Asymptomatic Children
Foster RD, Williams ML, Barkovich AJ, et al (Univ of California, San Francisco)
Plast Reconstr Surg 107:933-941, 2001   21–1

Introduction.—Neurocutaneous melanosis, a rare syndrome characterized by the development of benign or malignant melanocytic tumors of the CNS, is associated with pigmented nevi on the head and neck or dorsal spine area. Previously, the authors reported distinct MR findings of T1 shortening, strongly suggestive of neurocutaneous melanosis, in 6 of 20 neurologically asymptomatic children with giant congenital melanocytic nevi. The incidence and long-term clinical significance of neurocutaneous melanosis were examined in similarly high-risk patients.

Methods.—Forty-nine children (27 boys and 22 girls) with giant congenital melanocytic nevi involving the head and neck or overlying dorsal spine were referred between March 1990 and April 1997. The average age at referral was 5 months. All children had MRI of the brain consisting of standard T1- and T2-weighted spin echo images. Spinal MR scanning was also performed when the giant nevus overlay the lumbosacral spine. Gadolinium-enhanced scans were obtained when abnormalities were identified on nonenhanced scans. Patients were then referred for surgical excision of the nevi.

Results.—MR scans of 42 children were available for review; 11 of these patients also had MR scans of the spinal cord. Fourteen MR studies revealed abnormalities and 10 had T1 shortening, indicative of melanocytic rests within the brain or meninges. There were no associated masses or cases of leptomeningeal thickening. In the 10 patients with T1 shortening, the most common areas of involvement were the amygdala, cerebellum, and pons. One patient who underwent spinal imaging was found to have a tethered spinal cord. Neither the location nor size of the nevus appears to correlate completely with the presence or absence of abnormalities revealed by MRI. During an average follow-up period of 5 years, only 1 patient showed neurologic symptoms (developmental delay, hypotonia, and questionable seizures). This child had no other signs, however, of neurocutaneous melanosis. In addition, there have been no cases of cutaneous or CNS melanoma in the entire patient group.

Conclusion.—In these neurologically asymptomatic children with giant congenital melanocytic nevi, CNS melanocytosis was present in almost 25%. Symptomatic disease has developed in only 1 patient, however. Asymptomatic children with giant congenital melanocytic nevi may have an increased lifetime risk of CNS melanoma, but they do not have the poor prognosis of children with symptomatic disease.

Central Nervous System Imaging and Congenital Melanocytic Naevi
Kinsler VA, Aylett SE, Coley SC, et al (Hosp for Children NHS Trust, London)
Arch Dis Child 84:152-155, 2001   21–2

Introduction.—Before the development of noninvasive imaging techniques such as MRI, intracranial melanosis (ICM) in children with congenital melanocytic nevi (CMN) would only become apparent if neurologic symptoms occurred. The clinical notes and MRI scans of 43 children with CMN were examined to determine which patients should be imaged for CNS abnormalities and what imaging findings mean for the individual patient.

Methods.—Because symptomatic intracranial abnormalities are more often associated with CMN located on the head or over the spine, the children offered MRI had CMN with a diameter greater than 2 cm on the head or overlying the spine. The mean age at MRI was 4.35 years. In 32 patients, the CMN size was greater than 10 cm. Satellite lesions were present in 34 cases. All children underwent a neurologic examination, and findings were compared with those of MRI.

Results.—Nine children had abnormal neurologic symptoms or signs, 6 had both abnormal clinical and radiologic findings, and 7 had abnormal MRI findings. Only 3 of the 7 children with abnormal scans had ICM, but 6 of 7 showed abnormal neurologic symptoms or signs in the first 3 months of life. Structural brain abnormalities (a choroid plexus papilloma, a cerebellar astrocytoma, and a posterior fossa arachnoid cyst) were present in 3 of 4 children with abnormalities on MRI but without ICM. The only patient with an abnormal MRI scan and no clinical neurologic problems had changes suggestive of immature myelination.

Conclusion.—In this series of patients with CMN, 7 of 43 had CNS abnormalities on MRI. Three children had typical scan findings of ICM, and 4 had nonmelanocytic lesions. Six of the 7 children with MRI abnormalities had neurologic symptoms or signs. The use of early routine MRI in children with a CMN greater than 2 cm in diameter on the head or over the spine is recommended because treatable nonmelanocytic lesions may be found.

▶ In the past, ICM was diagnosed only if a patient had neurologic symptoms develop. With the advent of noninvasive imaging technology, such as MRI, it has become apparent that CMN may be associated with a variety of nonmelanocytic anomalies of the CNS, and that there are patients with CMN who have asymptomatic ICM. Foster et al (Abstract 21–1) identified abnormalities in 14 of 42 MRI studies. However, only one of these children had neurologic symptoms during the follow-up period. Twenty-three percent of patients with abnormal scans had T1 shortening, indicative of melanocytic rests within the brain or meninges. Eleven patients had spinal MRI scans; a tethered cord was demonstrated in 1. The authors note that T1 shortening is more difficult to detect after myelinization of the CNS, which begins at approximately 4 months of age; thus, melanosis is more likely to be detected if the MRI is done on very young infants. Although Foster et al recommend MRI studies for their patients with large CMN of the scalp or CMN overlying the spine, they acknowledge that cost factors, the risk of general anesthesia (which is often necessary), and the lack of effective treatment of CNS disease should it be found make such a recommendation questionable. Imaging studies definitely are recommended for infants with neurologic symptoms or for those with nevi over the lumbosacral area, which can indicate a tethered cord.

Kinsler et al (Abstract 23–2) noted abnormalities in 7 of 43 children studied with MRI. The mean age was 4.35 years. Six of these children had abnormal neurologic signs within the first 18 months of life. Because in 2 of the infants operable lesions were detected (a benign fibrotic choroid plexus lesion and a juvenile cerebellar astrocytoma), which may or may not have been related to their CMN, these authors recommend imaging of all children with large CMN over the scalp or spine.

It would seem reasonable to suggest MRI in newborns to detect CNS melanosis. The procedure can usually be done in this age group without the need for general anesthesia. The risk of a melanoma developing in lesions of CNS melanosis is approximately equivalent to that in skin lesions. Thus, these children are at increased risk for melanoma even if all CMN could be removed. Spinal imaging for those with lumbosacral lesions and a complete workup for those with neurologic signs should be recommended.

S. Raimer, MD

Automatic Differentiation of Melanoma From Melanocytic Nevi With Multispectral Digital Dermoscopy: A Feasibility Study

Elbaum M, Kopf AW, Rabinovitz HS, et al (Electro-Optical Sciences, Inc, Irvington, NY; New York Univ; Skin and Cancer Associates, Plantation, Fla; et al)
J Am Acad Dermatol 44:207-218, 2001   21–3

Background.—Cure of malignant melanoma is dependent on early identification and prompt removal. The challenges facing dermatologists are the diagnosis of melanoma in the early stages of progression and the differentiation of melanoma from benign neoplasms that resemble melanoma. The development of clinical *ABCD* (asymmetry, border, color, diameter) rules and the use of dermoscopy have led to further improvements in diagnostic accuracy. However, dermoscopic technique is predicated on the subjective interpretation of findings, for which extensive training is necessary. Thus, interest has grown in objective, computer-assisted analysis of dermoscopic images. This study describes the development of a novel multispectral digital dermascope with "expert system" software that performs the image processing sequence automatically from beginning to end. This system provides fully automated differentiation of melanoma from dysplastic and other melanocytic nevi.

Methods.—Before biopsy, images were obtained of pigmented lesions suspected of being melanoma at 4 clinical centers. A total of 10 gray-level images were taken for each lesion, with each image in a different area of the visible and near-infrared spectrum. Images of 63 melanomas (33 invasive, 30 in situ) and 183 melanocytic nevi (111 dysplastic nevi) were processed with the multispectral digital dermoscopy software to separate melanomas from nevi by using either a linear or a nonlinear classifier. Concordant diagnosis by 2 dermatopathologists was used as the gold standard control for the training and testing of the 2 classifiers.

Results.—On resubstitution, the 13-parameter linear classifier yielded a 100% sensitivity and 85% specificity, whereas the 12-parameter nonlinear classifier yielded 100% sensitivity and 73% specificity. Leave-one-out cross-validations yielded a sensitivity of 100% with a specificity of 84% for the linear classifier and a sensitivity of 95% with a specificity of 68% for the nonlinear classifier. Infrared-image features and features based on wavelet analysis were significant.

Conclusions.—Multispectral digital dermoscopy can provide accurate, automated differentiation of invasive and in situ melanomas from melanocytic nevi.

▶ Even experts are not infallible when it comes to correctly diagnosing malignant melanoma. For this reason, dermoscopy was developed as an aid to distinguish benign pigmented lesions from melanoma. Although numerous studies have demonstrated that this technique can increase diagnostic accuracy, it requires much experience and clinicopathologic correlation. To eliminate human error, and to make dermoscopy a valuable aid to the less-experienced clinician, investigators have linked dermoscopy to computers by using digital imaging. As illustrated in this article, this technology has continued to evolve. Although computer-assisted digital imaging will never replace good clinical judgment, it should help the clinician distinguish benign pigmented lesions from melanoma and decrease the number of atypical nevi that require biopsy.

P. G. Lang, Jr, MD

Is Dermoscopy (Epiluminescence Microscopy) Useful for the Diagnosis of Melanoma? Results of a Meta-analysis Using Techniques Adapted to the Evaluation of Diagnostic Tests

Bafounta M-L, Beauchet A, Aegerter P, et al (Assistance Publique-Hôpitaux de Paris)
Arch Dermatol 137:1343-1350, 2001   21–4

Background.—Dermoscopy is a method by which fluid is applied to the skin (to make the stratum corneum more translucent), and handheld microscopes or videomicroscopes are used to examine the pigmented anatomic structures of the epidermis, dermoepidermal junction, and superficial papillary dermis. Whether dermoscopy improves the accuracy of melanoma diagnosis remains a matter of controversy. The effectiveness of dermoscopy performed by experienced operators was compared with that of naked-eye clinical examination in the diagnosis of melanoma.

Methods.—Four databases (MEDLINE, EMBASE, PASCAL-BIOMED, and Bibliothèque Inter Universitaire Médicale), plus textbooks and relevant reference lists, were searched to identify articles in any language that included the following keywords: *melanoma skin neoplasm, sensitivity, specificity,* and either *dermoscopy, dermatoscopy, epiluminescence microscopy, diascopy, surface microscopy,* or *incident light microscopy.* Only studies that met the following criteria were considered for analysis: the spectrum of lesions was well described, histologic findings were provided as the standard criterion, and the sensitivity and specificity were calculated or calculable. Of the 672 studies identified, only 8 met the inclusion criteria. Data from these 8 studies were extracted by 3 independent investigators (2 dermatologists and 1 statistician). Summary receiver operating characteristics (ROC) curves were constructed to compare the sensitivity and specificity of dermoscopy performed by formally trained operators with that of naked-eye clinical examination.

Results.—The 8 studies analyzed were published between 1993 and 2000, and included 328 melanomas (most <0.76-mm-thick) and 1865 benign pigmented skin lesions (mostly melanocytic lesions). For clinical diagnosis, the sensitivity, specificity, positive predictive value, and negative predictive value for melanomas ranged from 0.50 to 0.94, 0.55 to 0.89, 1.91 to 10.66, and 0.61 to 0.08. Corresponding values for dermoscopy were 0.75 to 0.96, 0.79 to 0.98, 4.21 to 76.62, and 0.28 to 0.04. ROC analysis indicated that the discriminating power of dermoscopy was significantly higher than that of clinical examination: The estimated odds ratios for dermoscopy and clinical examination were 76 and 16, respectively, whereas the corresponding positive likelihood ratios were 9 and 3.7, and the corresponding negative likelihood ratios were 0.11 and 0.27. Furthermore, the sensitivity of dermoscopy did not vary according to the number of lesions analyzed, the percentage of melanoma lesions, or the type of dermoscope or dermoscopic criteria used in each study.

Conclusions.—When performed by experienced operators, dermoscopy improves the accuracy of melanoma diagnosis compared with naked-eye clinical examination. Further research is needed to determine whether performing dermoscopy can reduce the number of excisional biopsies performed on benign pigmented lesions without increasing the number of melanomas that are missed.

▶ Although dermoscopy has been found to be a useful diagnostic adjunct in the detection of melanoma, some question remains regarding its real value. The authors reviewed and subjected to meta-analysis 8 published series on dermoscopy. After doing so, they concluded that dermoscopy, when performed by formally trained clinicians, can increase their ability to diagnose melanoma, especially thin melanoma. Thus, if more clinicians would develop expertise in dermoscopy, the number of biopsies performed to distinguish between melanoma and benign pigmented lesions might decrease.

P. G. Lang, Jr, MD

Detection of Clinically Amelanotic Malignant Melanoma and Assessment of Its Margins by In Vivo Confocal Scanning Laser Microscopy
Busam KJ, Hester K, Charles C, et al (Mem Sloan-Kettering Cancer Ctr, New York; Harvard Med School, Boston)
Arch Dermatol 137:923-929, 2001   21–5

Introduction.—Amelanotic melanomas lack pigment and may be mistaken for other types of skin cancer or inflammatory processes. Near-infrared confocal scanning laser microscopy (CSLM) is a new imaging technique that allows in vivo microscopic examination of the epidermis and papillary dermis. Lesions from 2 patients were imaged and analyzed with CSLM to explore the feasibility of this technique for detecting and assessing clinically amelanotic cutaneous malignant melanoma.

Methods.—Images obtained with this technique have the appearance of elongate (oblique) vertical histologic sections. The biopsy specimens or excised tissue from these 2 patients were stained for melanin pigment and analyzed immunohistochemically for the expression of melanosomal markers. One biopsy specimen was also examined by electron microscopy.

Results.—Both patients were white women in their sixties. One had a history of basal and squamous cell carcinoma and multiple actinic keratoses and had recently been found to have a malignant melanoma. Areas examined with CSLM were on the lower part of the left leg and appeared as various areas of erythema and ill-defined hypopigmentation with normal-appearing intervening skin. The other patient, with a history of biopsy-proven and narrowly excised in situ melanoma on her left cheek, was examined for facial erythema near the scar. No apparent pigmentation was seen in or around the scar on visual examination. In both patients, images obtained by CSLM revealed an abnormal intraepidermal melanocytic proliferation that differed markedly from normal skin. After excision, clinically amelanotic melanoma cells containing melanosomes and rare melanin granules were demonstrated by Fontana-Masson stains and immunohistochemical and ultrastructural studies.

Conclusion.—Amelanotic melanomas often escape early detection because of their lack of distinct pigmentation. It was not known whether CSLM would be able to visualize the cells of a clinically amelanotic tumor. But, as demonstrated in these 2 cases, reflectance CSLM offers promise as a noninvasive screening tool for these lesions in which residual melanin pigment or melanosomes provide cytoplasmic contrast.

▶ In vivo CSLM has been proposed as a means of assessing margins in skin cancer. It is limited, however, in that it only penetrates to the level of the papillary dermis. Melanin provides a bright white image in contrast to the surrounding skin that, in theory, could allow one to determine the subclinical extent of a melanoma. Amelanotic melanomas represent not only a diagnostic challenge but their margins are often indistinct, even with the aid of a Wood's lamp, making surgery difficult. In this study, 2 patients with amelanotic melanomas were examined by CSLM. Despite a clinical lack of pigment, CSLM was able to detect subclinical spread of the melanomas. This is probably because even amelanotic melanomas produce some pigment. Based on this small series of cases, one would hope that in vivo CSLM might eventually obviate the need for multiple biopsies when mapping out an amelanotic melanoma preoperatively.

P. G. Lang, Jr, MD

The Relation Between Mortality From Malignant Melanoma and Early Detection in the Cancer Research Campaign Mole Watcher Study

Melia J, Moss S, Coleman D, et al (Inst of Cancer Research, Sutton, Surrey, England; Royal Devon & Exeter Hosp, England; Leicester Royal Infirmary, England; et al)
Br J Cancer 85:803-807, 2001   21–6

Background.—The Cancer Research Campaign (CRC) conducted a health education program for 2 years aimed at early detection of cutaneous malignant melanoma in 6 health districts of England and 1 in Scotland (overall population, 3 million persons). The effects of this intervention on annual and cumulative mortality rates for melanoma were assessed, comparing rates for the intervention areas with those for comparison areas also in England and Scotland. Data collection extended for 9 years after the 2-year intervention.

Methods.—A CRC Mole Watcher leaflet was distributed, which outlined the early signs of melanoma using a 7-point checklist and encouraged reporting suspicious lesions early in their course to general practitioners. A pigmented lesion clinic was funded in each area to back up the local dermatology clinics. The mortality rate study was limited to include only those individuals aged 15 to 74 years, because melanoma rarely occurs at younger ages, and other causes of death may confound the data for older ages. Data were categorized by age, gender, and area of residence to calculate annual mortality rates. Each registry maintained its own coding system for cause of death, from which the underlying cause of death could be identified. Quality control checks were done using a random sample of death certificates in the respective areas. Outcome measures were the annual and cumulative mortality rates.

Results.—The annual mortality rate did not differ between men and women in the various areas at the beginning of the study, but melanoma mortality rates for women decreased somewhat for all areas after 1993. Regression analysis, however, revealed no significant differences in the trends between areas. Age-adjusted cumulative mortality rates also showed no significant differences between areas, with no improvement resulting from the intervention. Heterogeneity testing showed no significant differences in the melanoma mortality rates between the intervention areas and the other areas, nor was a difference noted between the rates of men and women.

Conclusions.—No significant reduction in mortality rates for melanoma occurred after the CRC early detection intervention. This applied to both cumulative and annual rates. It is possible that a longer follow-up period would be required for differences to be apparent.

▶ In the hope of reducing the mortality rate from melanoma, many countries have developed public education programs to encourage early detection. The preliminary results from some of these interventional programs seem to suggest that they do impact the death rate from melanoma. In this study, however, public education did not appear to reduce melanoma-associated mortality rates. Nevertheless, there may be several explanations for this. First, the time period studied may have not been sufficiently long. Second, the campaign lasted only 2 years. To make a significant impact on mortality rates from melanoma, an ongoing educational campaign would likely have the greatest chance of success.

P. G. Lang, Jr, MD

Outdoor Activities in Childhood: A Protective Factor for Cutaneous Melanoma? Results of a Case Control Study in 271 Matched Pairs
Kaskel P, Sander S, Kron M, et al (Univ of Ulm, Germany; Univ of Munich)
Br J Dermatol 145:602-609, 2001   21–7

Background.—A relationship between melanoma and sun exposure has been proposed, because of an increased incidence of melanoma among white people who are exposed to excessive amounts of ultraviolet (UV) radiation. Occupational and leisure behavior with respect to sun exposure and melanoma incidence were assessed by the case-control method among persons in Southern Bavaria, Germany.

Methods.—Included in the assessment for the melanoma patients were past medical, social, and family history; total body inspection, including precursor lesions for skin cancer; and phenotypic factors (skin reaction to sunlight, skin phototype, hair color, eye color). They had all been diagnosed with melanoma at least 6 months before beginning the study. Each completed a standardized questionnaire and physical examination. The results were compared with patients with healthy skin from the same geographic region. The risk factors for cutaneous melanoma were preselected using a local significance level of 5% and were identified as exposure to UV radiation, occupational exposure, and a family history of cancer, particularly melanoma. These risk factors were subjected to multiple conditional logistic regression analysis to identify the most important factors and assess their effect.

Results.—Forty percent of the melanomas were located on the trunk, 25% on the lower extremities, 11% on the head, 16% on the upper extremities, and 6% were acral. Male patients tended to have lesions on the trunk, whereas female patients tended to have them on the extremities. Five melanoma patients and 3 control subjects were immunosuppressed. UV radiation had been used for treatment purposes in 4 melanoma patients, and ionizing radiation had been used in 4 others; no control subjects had UV radiation therapy and 7 had ionizing radiation. The crude odds ratio (OR) for 56 possible risk factors showed strong associations for 20. The multiple regression analysis identified the following risk factors: melanoma in first-degree relatives; the presence of solar lentigines, actinic keratoses, and actinic cheilitis; skin phototype, with a higher risk for type I/II than for type III/IV; immediate skin reaction to short periods of sun exposure at the beginning of the outdoor season; exposure during holidays 20 years before the melanoma diagnosis; and a history of sunburn in childhood. Engaging in outdoor activities, however, (playing soccer or gardening) in childhood served a protective function.

Conclusions.—Among the preventable risk factors for melanoma were sunburn in childhood and heightened sun exposure during annual holidays. Exposure during outdoor recreational activities in childhood offered some protection against melanoma.

▶ This article represents yet another epidemiologic study that addresses risk factors for melanoma. As with previous studies, melanoma risk is increased in (1) fair skinned individuals with a history of sunburns; (2) individuals with atypical nevi; (3) individuals with evidence of chronic skin damage (eg, actinic keratoses); and (4) individuals with a family history of melanoma. Previous articles such as this have shown that melanoma correlates better with intense intermittent sun exposure rather than with chronic sun exposure. This study, however, goes one step further and suggests that regular outdoor activities, such as soccer and gardening, may actually protect against melanoma. An explanation for this observation is not clear but would include (1) hardening of the skin to the effects of UV light, or (2) more judicious exposure to the sun and a willingness to protect the skin from the sun when outdoors on a regular basis.

P. G. Lang, Jr, MD

Timing of Excessive Ultraviolet Radiation and Melanoma: Epidemiology Does Not Support the Existence of a Critical Period of High Susceptibility to Solar Ultraviolet Radiation-Induced Melanoma
Pfahlberg A, for the FEBIM Study Group (Univ of Erlangen-Nuremberg, Germany; et al)
Br J Dermatol 144:471-475, 2001   21–8

Introduction.—A history of sunburn is considered a risk factor for melanoma, and some studies suggest that the risk is greatest when exposure to excessive ultraviolet radiation occurs during childhood. In a recent case-control study, sun protection during childhood was reported to have a greater impact on reducing melanoma risk than sun protection during adulthood. The existence of a "critical period" early in life was examined in a multicenter case-control study.

Methods.—A total of 603 patients with histopathologically verified melanoma of the skin and 627 population control subjects was recruited from centers in 7 European countries. Control subjects were matched to the patients for age, sex, and ethnic origin. Participants were interviewed to determine the frequency and timing of painful sunburns during 2 periods: childhood (up to age 15) and adulthood (after age 15).

Results.—A consistent increase in melanoma risk was associated with an increased frequency of sunburn, whether the sunburns occurred in childhood or adulthood. Thus, the hazardous impact of sunburns on melanoma persists throughout life. Melanoma risk was doubled with more than 5 sunburns, whenever they occurred.

Conclusion.—The findings of this study do not support the existence of a "critical period" of high melanoma susceptibility. Sunburn increases melanoma risk whether it occurs in childhood or adulthood, and preventive programs should focus on all age groups.

▶ Although intermittent exposure to ultraviolet light throughout life is thought to predispose to the development of melanoma, much emphasis has been placed on the role of severe sunburns in childhood. In this multicenter study, the investigators found a correlation between the frequency of sunburns and the development of melanoma; however, they were not able to document that sunburns before the age of 15 years were more harmful than those after the age of 15 years.

P. G. Lang, Jr, MD

Recent Trends in Cutaneous Melanoma Incidence Among Whites in the United States
Jemal A, Devesa SS, Hartge P, et al (Natl Cancer Inst, Bethesda, Md)
J Natl Cancer Inst 93:678-683, 2001   21–9

Background.—Skin melanoma is one of the most rapidly increasing cancers among white persons in the United States. However, whether this increase in melanoma incidence is real or simply attributable to greater public awareness and improved diagnosis remains a matter of debate. To shed light on this controversy, the incidence patterns of melanoma among white US residents over the past 30 years were examined with respect to age, sex, tumor stage, and tumor thickness.

Methods.—Incidence data from the Surveillance, Epidemiology, and End Results (SEER) Program were used to determine rates of invasive melanoma in whites since 1970. Age at diagnosis was examined in 5-year cohorts (15-19 years through ≥85 years), as was year of diagnosis (1973-1977 through 1993-1997). Trends in incidence rates were also examined by comparing rates in the earlier (1973-1979) and later (1980-1997) periods. In addition, trends in tumor stage (local, regional, or distant) and tumor thickness (<1, 1 to <4, and ≥4 mm) since 1988 were examined according to broader age groups (≤40, 40-59, and >60 years old). Incidence rates were reported as the number of cases per 100,000 person-years of observation.

Results.—Between 1973 and 1997, the incidence rates of invasive melanoma more than doubled in white women (from 5.9% to 13.8%) and almost tripled in white men (from 6.7% to 19.3%). Incidence rates for both sexes rose less rapidly in the more recent period compared with the earlier period. Since 1980, incidence rates tended to stabilize in white men younger than 40 years of age but increased in older men, particularly those 60 years or older. In contrast, incidence rates since 1980 tended to remain stable in middle-aged white women but increased somewhat in white women younger than 30 years old. In the earlier period, the incidence of localized tumors was significantly higher in men and women of all ages (<40, 40-59, and ≥60 years), whereas rates of regional and distant disease were significantly higher only in men. In the more recent period, the incidence of local and regional diseased continued to increase significantly in men of all ages, but local disease rates in women increased significantly only in those 60 years or older. Within each age cohort, incidence rates for each tumor stages were higher in men than in women. From 1988 through 1997, the incidence of tumors of thin and intermediate thickness increased significantly in women of all ages, but the incidence of thick tumors remained stable. For men, the incidences of tumors of thin and intermediate thickness increased significantly after age 40 years, and the incidence of thick tumors increased significantly after age 60 years.

Conclusions.—The incidence of melanoma among white persons in the United States has continued to increase since the early 1970s. Men 60 years or older are at highest risk because rates have increased most rapidly in this group. Thick lesions and distant disease are also more common in older white men.

▶ The debate continues whether there has been a true increase in the incidence of melanoma or if this simply reflects increased public awareness and an increase in the diagnosis of early lesions. Jemal et al suggest that the increase is real and not solely a reflection of improved diagnosis. Although the rate of increase in the incidence of melanoma appears to have declined in both males and females, its incidence is still rising rapidly in the United States. A large proportion of this increase is in individuals 60 years or older, especially men. There also continues to be an increase in the incidence of thick lesions and in distant metastases in men 60 years or older, which may explain why the mortality from melanoma has stabilized or is declining in females but is still rising in males. From a public health standpoint, it would seem that men, particularly those 60 years or older, should be targeted for increased education and surveillance.

P. G. Lang, Jr, MD

Primary Cutaneous Melanoma in Hidden Sites Is Associated With Thicker Tumours: A Study of 829 Patients
Nagore E, Oliver V, Moreno-Picot S, et al (Hosp Gen Universitario, Valencia, Spain; Univ of Valencia, Spain)
Eur J Cancer 37:79-82, 2001   21–10

Introduction.—Breslow thickness is the most important pathologic prognostic feature of a primary cutaneous melanoma, and tumors that occur in more hidden areas may be thicker at the time of diagnosis. Data from 829 consecutive patients with a cutaneous malignant melanoma were analyzed for the relationship between tumor thickness and degree of visibility of the tumor's location.

Methods.—The melanomas had been diagnosed between January 1976 and July 1998. Variables collected included gender, age at diagnosis, anatomical site, tumor stage and histological type, and Breslow thickness.

Three categories of anatomical site were defined as follows: body regions visible to patients during normal activities (group 1; 493 patients), body regions visible to patients or their partners in privacy (group 2; 281 patients), and body regions hidden to patients and their partners (group 3; 55 patients).

Results.—Group 3 patients, including patients with lesions on anatomical sites, such as the plantar surface, scalp, and buttock fold, tended to have thicker melanomas, including a higher percentage of acral lentiginous melanomas, and had a higher proportion of older men. In multivariate analysis with adjustment for gender, age, and histological type, tumor site remained an independent factor affecting Breslow thickness. When groups 2 and 3 were combined and compared with group 1, there were statistically significant differences between these 2 groups in age, sex, histologic type, stage, Breslow category, and Breslow thickness.

Conclusion.—Primary cutaneous melanomas located in hidden body regions have a larger Breslow thickness and a higher rate of metastatic disease than tumors in visible regions, perhaps because of delay in diagnosis. But most patients with tumors in hidden sites were elderly men, and both increasing age and male gender are associated with a poorer prognosis. Patients need to be aware that sun-protected, hidden body areas are potential sites of melanoma.

▶ Not surprisingly, these authors found that melanomas in "hidden areas" (oral cavity, plantar surface, and intergluteal cleft) were thicker at the time of diagnosis and more likely to have metastasized than melanomas located in more readily accessible areas. This was especially true for males and for older patients. The results emphasize that it is important for the physician to examine these less accessible areas and to educate patients to examine these areas themselves.

P. G. Lang, Jr, MD

Clinical and Histologic Features of Level 2 Cutaneous Malignant Melanoma Associated With Metastasis
Taran JM, Heenan PJ (Univ of Western Australia, Nedlands)
Cancer 91:1822-1825, 2001   21–11

Background.—Metastatic melanoma is rarely reported in patients with level 2 primary cutaneous malignant melanoma (CMM) and has accrued up to 15 years after the initial diagnosis. The pathology reports from a nationwide cancer registry over a 15-year period were reviewed to determine the incidence and characteristics of metastases associated with level 2 CMM.

Methods.—Since 1981, by law, the Western Australia Cancer Registry has received copies of pathology reports for all invasive malignant melanomas in the region. This registry information was used to identify all patients with a primary CMM 1 mm thick or smaller that was diagnosed between 1982 and 1989. Patients were observed through 1996 to identify metastases. Histologic sections were reviewed under blind conditions to confirm the level and thickness of the CMM, and to identify regression (ie, an area of tumor-free epidermis and dermis that was flanked by melanoma, with fibrosis, increased vascularity, and lymphocytic infiltration in the papillary dermis deep to the tumor-free epidermis).

Results.—The registry contained reports of 2834 patients with a primary invasive CMM diagnosed from 1982 to 1989. Of these, 1716 reports (60.6%) noted a maximum tumor thickness of 1 mm or less. During follow-up through 1996, 67 of these 1716 patients (3.9%) had a confirmed metastatic melanoma. Of these 67 patients with CMM smaller than 1 mm thick who had metastases, 49 had only 1 primary CMM and 18 had multiple primary CMMs. Of the 49 patients reported to have a single primary CMM 1 mm thick or smaller and metastases, further examination revealed that all but 5 of them had a level 3 or 4 CMM from 0.3 to 1.0 mm thick. All 5 of the patients with a confirmed single primary level 2 CMM 1 mm thick or smaller and metastasis had either focal (1 case) or extensive (4 cases) areas of regression. Of the 18 patients reported to have multiple primary CMMs 1 mm thick or smaller and metastases, 17 had their first metastasis diagnosed simultaneous with a subsequent primary CMM. Nine of these 18 patients had a level 2 CMM among their primary CMMs. Eight of these 9 patients had another primary CMM of level 3-5 invasion that occurred before the metastasis had been reported.

Conclusions.—Within this large group of specimens, the only solitary level 2 CMMs to metastasize were those with established regression. Thus, metastasis from level 2 CMMs without regression must be very rare, if it occurs at all.

▶ Thin melanomas (≤1 mm thick) do not commonly metastasize. In this study of Clark level II primary melanomas 1 mm thick or smaller, only those showing regression metastasized. This suggests that before regression occurred, the lesions may have been much deeper.

P. G. Lang, Jr, MD

The Vertical Dimension in the Surgical Treatment of Cutaneous Malignant Melanoma—How Deep Is Deep?

Wolf Y, Balicer RD, Amir A, et al (Tel-Aviv Univ, Israel)
Eur J Plast Surg 24:74-77, 2001   21–12

Background.—Most authorities agree that the optimal width of the surgical margins around cutaneous malignant melanomas should be 0.5 to 3.0 cm, depending on the thickness of the tumor. But what is the optimal depth of the tumor-free surgical margin? Ten-year follow-up data were analyzed from patients who underwent surgery for primary cutaneous malignant melanoma to evaluate the influence of the thickness of the tumor-free deep margin on outcomes.

Methods.—The subjects were 48 patients (21 men and 27 women) 31 to 84 years old (mean age, 60.2 years) who underwent surgery for primary cutaneous malignant melanoma in 1987-1988. Most patients (30, or 62.5%) underwent wide resection after the primary excision. Maximum tumor thickness was measured from histologic specimens according to the Breslow classification. The thickness of the tumor-free margin under the primary resection and the depth of the wide resection were measured as well. Clinical and histologic features at surgery were analyzed in light of recurrences and survival during 10 years of follow-up.

Results.—The mean Breslow thickness was 1.6 mm; 20 lesions were less than 1 mm thick, 21 were 1 to 4 mm thick, and 4 were more than 4 mm thick. During follow-up, local (n = 5) or distant (n = 5) recurrence developed in 10 patients (21%) and 13 patients (27%) died. When patients were grouped according to tumor thickness, patients in whom recurrence developed tended to have a tumor-free margin thickness deep to the tumor that was less than that in patients in whom recurrence did not develop. For example, the only patient with a melanoma larger than 4 mm who did not experience recurrence had a tumor-free margin deep to the tumor that was 5 mm thick, whereas the other 3 patients with very thick lesions (all of whom had a recurrence) had an average 2.26-mm margin. Ten-year survival was significantly greater in patients with a tumor-free margin deep to the tumor of 3 mm or larger than in those with a thinner margin (82% vs 50%). Multivariate analyses identified 5 significant independent predictors of 10-year survival: age, gender, histologic type, Breslow thickness, and tumor-free margin deep to the tumor. The ratio of the vertical dimension of the tumor-free margin to the thickness of the tumor was calculated, and was also shown to be a significant independent predictor of outcome. Patients with a margin/tumor thickness ratio less than 1 were almost 5 times more likely to have a recurrence than patients with a higher margin/tumor thickness ratio (66% vs 14%). Ten-year survival was also related to the margin/tumor thickness ratio, with survival rates of 33% for a ratio less than 1, 62% for a ratio of 1.0 to 4.0, and 88% for a ratio more than 4.0.

Conclusions.—The tumor-free margin thickness deep to the tumor is an important factor in determining clinical outcomes among patients with cutaneous malignant melanoma. The tumor-free margin under a malignant melanoma should be 3 mm or greater. Additionally, the ratio of the resected deep tumor-free margin to tumor thickness also impacts recurrence and survival. Thus, the margin/tumor thickness ratio should be more than 1.

▶ A great deal of attention has been directed at the width of excisional margins for melanoma, but much less attention has been paid to the depth of the excision. Most of the controversy has centered around whether or not to include fascia in the excision, with most authorities recommending that it is not necessary to take fascia. This study suggests that the depth of the excision significantly impacts recurrence rate and overall survival. Based on their findings, the authors propose that for invasive melanomas, the tumor free margin, in terms of depth, should be at least 3 mm and the ratio of the depth of the deep margin to the thickness of the lesion should be greater than 1. Although this is an interesting observation and one of potential therapeutic importance, it is unclear if the depth of excision significantly impacted recurrence rates and overall survival for lesions of all thicknesses.

P. G. Lang, Jr, MD

Gender and Other Survival Predictors in Patients With Metastatic Melanoma on Southwest Oncology Group Trials
Unger JM, Flaherty LE, Liu PY, et al (Southwest Oncology Group Statistical Ctr, Seattle; Wayne State Univ, Detroit; Loyola Unit, Maywood, Ill; et al)
Cancer 91:1148-1155, 2001   21–13

Introduction.—Some studies suggest that women with metastatic melanoma have better survival rates than men, but other reports have not confirmed this finding. To better understand the effect of gender on survival, while accounting for other clinical and treatment variables, 813 patients from 15 consecutive Southwest Oncology Group trials were analyzed.

Methods.—Fourteen trials were phase II studies and 1 was a combination phase II and phase III study. All patients had stage IV malignant melanoma; were at least partially ambulatory; and had adequate hematologic, renal, and hepatic function. A variety of agents and combinations of agents were tested in the trials. The patients were registered between March 15, 1982, and August 15, 1995. Survival data included in the analysis was received through November 15, 1997. A multivariate Cox regression model was used.

Results.—Trial participants were 292 women (36%) with a median age of 53 years and 521 men (64%) with a median age of 55 years. Men had a significantly shorter disease-free interval before diagnosis of metastatic disease (median, 1.4 years vs 2.3 years for women), and a greater proportion of men had 3 or more organ sites with metastases at registration (34% vs 24% of women). Performance status was similar for men and women, and visceral involvement was present in 81% of both groups. Highly significant predictors of worse survival were poor performance status, more organ sites with metastases, liver involvement, and nonliver visceral involvement. The disease-free interval before metastasis had borderline significance. A total of 781 (96%) patients died. The median overall survival time was 6.5 months for women and 5.3 months for men, but gender was not a predictor of survival in the Cox regression model.

Conclusion.—The database of patients analyzed for this study consisted of a large cohort of consistently staged, consecutively treated patients with stage IV disease. Female gender was not an independent predictor of better survival in advanced metastatic melanoma, but women in this series had fewer metastatic sites at registration and a longer disease-free interval from initial diagnosis.

▶ Previous reports have suggested that women with disseminated melanoma may fare better than men. However, in this study, multivariate analysis did not confirm this conclusion. Although women demonstrated a slight survival advantage, this reflected their pattern of disease and was not gender-related. Performance studies and the number of organ sites involved with metastases were the best correlates with survival. The use of cisplatin-based chemotherapy or dacarbazine also correlated with survival, but the use of interferons or interleukins did not.

P. G. Lang, Jr, MD

Inactivation of Apoptosis Effector *Apaf-1* in Malignant Melanoma

Soengas MS, Capodieci P, Polsky D, et al (Cold Springs Harbor Lab, NY; Mem Sloan Kettering Cancer Ctr, New York; Johns Hopkins Univ, Baltimore, Md)
Nature 409:207-211, 2001   21–14

Introduction.—Metastatic melanoma is a deadly cancer that fails to respond to conventional chemotherapy. It is poorly understood at the molecular level. Mutations in p53 frequently occur in aggressive and chemoresistant cancers. They are rarely seen in melanoma. Melanoma is extremely resistant to apoptosis-inducing agents yet retains wild-type p53. Several tumor types, including melanoma, were examined for loss-of-function mutations in the *Apaf-1* gene, whose product, Apaf-1, acts as a cell-death effector that works with cytochrome *c* and caspase-9 to mediate p53-dependent apoptosis.

Findings.—A series of metastatic melanoma samples were evaluated for their p53 and Apaf-1 status. A low rate of p53 mutation was identified in these tumors. A strikingly high rate of allelic loss was observed for polymorphic markers encompassing the Apaf-1 locus on chromosome 12q23 (>40%). This allelic loss could be recovered by treatment with the methylation inhibitor 5-aza-2'-deoxycytidine (5aza2dC). Tumors with loss of heterozygosity expressed little Apaf-1 message via in situ hybridization compared with tumors with no loss of heterozygosity. Apaf-1 expression also was examined in a series of 19 cell lines derived from metastatic melanomas. Five lines expressed Apaf-1 levels similar to those of normal melanocytes (Apaf-1 positive), 4 lines expressed intermediate Apaf-1 levels (70% to 30%), and 10 lines expressed little Apaf-1 (Apaf-1 negative).

Conclusion.—Metastatic melanomas often lose Apaf-1. Apaf-1-negative melanomas are invariably chemoresistant and are not capable of performing a typical apoptotic program in response to p53 activation. Restoring physiologic levels of Apaf-1 through gene transfer or 5aza2dC treatment markedly enhanced chemosensitivity; it rescued the apoptotic defects related to Apaf-1 loss. Thus, Apaf-1 loss may contribute to the low rate of p53 mutations seen in this highly chemoresistant tumor type. It is likely that Apaf-1 is a tumor suppressor.

▶ The authors show that Apaf-1, which functions as a tumor suppressor, is inactivated in metastatic melanomas, leading to defects in the execution of apoptotic cell death. They also demonstrate that restoring physiologic levels of Apaf-1 markedly enhances chemosensitivity and restores the apoptotic defect associated with loss of Apaf-1. If, as the authors suggest, Apaf-1 loss contributes to the aggressive nature and extreme chemoresistance of melanomas, the findings reported here offer an exciting possible new avenue of future therapy for this devastating disease.

B. H. Thiers, MD

Increased Soluble CD95 (sFas/CD95) Serum Level Correlates With Poor Prognosis in Melanoma Patients
Ugurel S, Rappl G, Tilgen W, et al (Saarland Univ, Homburg/Saar, Germany)
Clin Cancer Res 7:1282-1286, 2001   21–15

Introduction.—Recent research indicates that functional impairment of the Fas/CD95 receptor-ligand system is associated with malignant proliferation. The function and clinical significance of serum sFas/CD95 in patients with cancer, however, is a matter of debate. The correlation of sFas/CD95 serum concentration with clinical parameters and prognosis in patients with malignant melanoma was examined.

Methods.—Study subjects were 125 unselected patients with histologically confirmed malignant melanoma at different stages of disease and 30 healthy controls matched with patients for age and gender. Patients were classified as free of tumor or having detectable tumor mass and as under ongoing therapy or untreated. Serum samples from patients and controls were assessed with a commercially available ELISA kit.

Methods.—Compared with healthy controls, sFas/CD95 serum level was significantly elevated in patients with melanoma (mean, 8.6 vs 6.27 ng/mL). In univariate analysis, serum concentration of sFas/CD95 was correlated with advanced disease stage. There was a slight increase of sFas/CD95 serum concentrations in patients with detectable tumor compared with tumor-free patients. Patients treated with IFN-α alone or combined with cytostatics showed no change in serum sFas/CD95 concentration. In contrast, serum sFas/CD95 concentrations were strongly increased in those currently undergoing therapy with cytostatic agents. Both overall survival and progression-free survival were worse for patients with elevated sFas/CD95 serum levels, but only the association with progression-free survival remained significant in multivariate analysis.

Conclusion.—This is the first study to demonstrate a highly significant correlation between elevated sFas/CD95 serum level and poor prognosis in patients with melanoma. Evaluation of serum sFas/CD95 may provide information relevant to the selection of therapeutic strategies.

► Interaction between membrane-bound type I protein Fas/CD95 and its ligand, FasL, appears to play a key role in maintaining tissue homeostasis by induction of apoptosis and may be important in the control of malignant proliferations.[1,2] Apoptosis mediated by Fas/CD95 is often impaired in neoplastic cells because of the downregulation, total loss, or dysfunctional signaling of Fas/CD95, and the Fas/CD95-FasL system has been shown to suppress metastatic progression in mice. Ugurel et al have shown that increased soluble Fas/CD95 serum levels correlate with a poor prognosis in patients with melanoma. It is possible that this excess soluble Fas/CD95 inhibits the functional Fas/CD95-FasL interaction that leads to apoptosis. This might enable tumor cells to evade the immune response or impair their apoptosis induced by cytostatic drugs. Interestingly, although the stage of the disease correlated with the soluble Fas/CD95 serum concentration, the tumor burden did not. Thus, the source of the high levels of soluble Fas/CD95 remains unknown.

B. H. Thiers, MD

References

1. Nagata S: Fas and Fas ligand: A death factor and its receptor. *Adv Immunol* 57:129-144, 1994.
2. Chouaib S, Asselin-Paturel C, Mami-Chouaib F, et al: The host-tumor immune conflict: From immunosuppression to resistance and destruction. *Immunol Today* 18:493-497, 1997.

Usefulness of Preoperative Lymphoscintigraphy for the Identification of Sentinel Lymph Nodes in Melanoma
Morris T, Stevens JS, Pommier RF, et al (Oregon Health Sciences Univ, Portland)
Am J Surg 181:423-426, 2001   21–16

Introduction.—Sentinel lymph node biopsy (SLNB) is becoming the standard of care for patients with melanoma and intermediate tumor thickness and is also proposed for some patients with thin or thick lesions. The majority of patients undergo initial preoperative lymphoscintigraphy (LS) before the SLNB; however, the routine use of preoperative LS is controversial. The scans of 87 patients were reviewed to evaluate the efficacy of preoperative LS in surgical planning for patients with primary melanomas at various sites. The effect of previous wide local excision (WLE) was also investigated.

Methods.—The data analyzed included patient demographics, location and thickness of the primary lesion, findings of preoperative LS, operative findings, and findings from pathologic examinations. Lymphoscintigraphy was defined as both lymph node drainage scans (LS performed before the day of surgery) and sentinel node scans (LS performed just before surgery). The number of standard and aberrant drainage patterns by location of primary lesions were recorded.

TABLE 2.—Summary of Aberrant Drainage Patterns by Location of Primary Lesion

Anatomical Sites by Drainage Pattern	Number Aberrant Drainage/Total
Truncal	41
Standard	29 (71%)
Aberrant drainage	12 (29%)
Contralateral axilla	1
Axilla and groin	2
Cervical nodes	3
Bilateral axilla	5
Lumbar triangle	1
Head and neck	14
Standard	5 (36%)
Aberrant drainage	9 (64%)
Extremity	32
Standard	30 (94%)
Aberrant drainage	2 (6%)
Upper thigh (interval sentinel lymph node)	1
Popliteal	1

(Reprinted with permission from Morris KT, Stevens JS, Pommier RF, et al: Usefulness of preoperative lymphoscintigraphy for the identification of sentinel lymph nodes in melanoma. *Am J Surg* 181:423-426, 2001. Copyright 2001, Excerpta Medica Inc.)

Results.—Truncal lesions were present in 41 patients, head and neck lesions in 14, and extremity lesions in 32. The mean tumor thickness, from reports of 76 patients, was 2.6 mm. Thirty-eight patients had LS on the morning of their operation, and 49 had preoperative LS on a previous day. Ambiguous drainage (Table 2) was demonstrated in 9 (64%) head/neck lesions and in 12 (29%) truncal lesions, but in only 2 (6%) extremity lesions. Forty-one patients (47%) had undergone previous WLE of their primary lesion before LS. No significant difference was noted in the number of drainage basins for the WLE (average, 1.34) and non-WLE groups (average, 1.22), and at least 1 SLN was found for all WLE patients. Rates of aberrant drainage were 27% for the prior WLE group and 26% for the group without prior WLE.

Conclusion.—Preoperative LS adds little information for patients with melanoma lesions of the extremities, but the imaging technique is important in the treatment planning of SLN biopsy for head/neck and truncal lesions. The presence of a previous WLE is not a contraindication for lymph node drainage scans and subsequent SLN biopsies.

▶ Although this study includes a relatively small number of patients, it provides data that confirm results from larger studies and reports important new information. As in previous studies, the data indicate that for truncal lesions and head and neck lesions, classic anatomical teachings cannot be relied on to predict lymph node drainage. For these areas, drainage to aberrant nodes and to multiple basins is common. Thus, preoperative LS is mandatory to sample the appropriate nodal basin(s). Aberrant drainage (interval, popliteal, and epitrochlear nodes) for extremity lesions is uncommon (6% in this series), but significant enough in this reviewer's opinion to justify

LS. The new information presented in this study is that prior WLE apparently did not impact the LS findings or the ability to detect the sentinel lymph node(s). This is important because many patients are being denied sentinel node biopsy because of a prior wide excision. Although limited, the experience at our institution has been similar, not only for melanoma patients, but also for patients with high-risk squamous cell carcinomas that have been treated with Mohs surgery. We have found that prior wide excision or Mohs' surgery does not affect our ability to identify the sentinel nodes.

P. G. Lang, Jr, MD

Reproducibility of Lymphoscintigraphy in Cutaneous Melanoma: Can We Accurately Detect the Sentinel Lymph Node by Expanding the Tracer Injection Distance From the Tumor Site?
Rettenbacher L, Koller J, Kässmann H, et al (Salzburg State Hosp, Austria; Hosp Barmherzige Brüder, Salzburg, Austria)
J Nucl Med 42:424-429, 2001   21–17

Introduction.—Many patients with cutaneous melanoma undergo lymphoscintigraphy after diagnosis to determine the feasibility of sentinel lymph node (SLN) biopsy. It is not known, however, if a diagnostic excisional biopsy up to 10 mm from the primary tumor can alter the lymphatic flow, causing the original SLN associated with the primary tumor to be missed. In a group of 100 patients, the radiotracer was injected at different distances and the localization of the SLNs was compared.

Methods.—Study participants were 42 women and 58 men, 24 to 78 years old. Excluded were patients with clinically known metastases. In 81 patients, diagnostic biopsy (<1.0 cm margins) had been performed at least 1 week before lymphoscintigraphy. The melanoma was still present in 19 patients. Depth of invasion was less than 1.5 mm in 63 patients and more than 1.5 mm in 37. Lymphoscintigraphy was performed twice. Intracutaneous injection of a total of 30 MBq ^{99m}Tc nanocolloid were performed at 4 separate sites at a 2- to 5-mm distance from the melanoma or the biopsy scar; these were followed by dynamic imaging until the SLN became visible. On another day, the radiopharmaceutical agent was injected exactly 10 mm from each of the previous sites. Imaging was again performed.

Results.—The SLN identification rate was 94% with close injection and 100% with 10-mm distant injection, a statistically significant difference. With close injection, the mean number of detected lymph nodes per patient was 1.5. An additional SLN was apparent in 16 patients on lymphoscintigraphy with the 10-mm distant injection, yielding a mean of 1.7 detected lymph nodes per patient. All SLNs detected with close injection were identified with distant injection. In 6 patients, only distant injection detected a SLN. Twelve patients (11 with a Breslow thickness >1.5 mm) had a SLN that was positive for tumor.

Conclusion.—The reproducibility of lymphoscintigraphy with the use of close and distant injection distances was 84%. In the remaining 16%, distant injection identified a lymph node in addition to the original SLN. Conservative excision of the primary tumor was performed without preventing detection of the original SLN.

▶ A concern regarding the use of a 1-cm margin for a diagnostic biopsy for melanoma is that it could disrupt the lymphatics, resulting in an inability to accurately localize the SLNs. This study compared the localization of the SLNs when the colloid tracer used for lymphoscintigraphy was injected adjacent to the biopsy scar or primary lesion, or 10 mm from it. Rettenbacher and associates found that the more distant injection allowed the identification of additional SLNs, especially if an excisional biopsy had been done. The authors concluded that small excisional biopsies do not appear to interfere with the recovery of SLNs. However, it appears to this reviewer (assuming the additional nodes identified were SLNs) that this is not necessarily the case, and that in patients having undergone an excisional biopsy, the colloid may need to be injected at least 10 mm from the biopsy site.

P. G. Lang, Jr, MD

A Micromorphometry-Based Concept for Routine Classification of Sentinel Lymph Node Metastases and Its Clinical Relevance for Patients With Melanoma
Starz H, Balda B-R, Krämer K-U, et al (Klinikum Augsburg, Germany; Univ of California, Los Angeles)
Cancer 91:2110-2120, 2001   21–18

Background.—Selective sentinel lymph node (SLN) removal from patients with cutaneous melanoma may allow prognostic assessment. Patients who may benefit were identified with the use of a staging system for metastatic SLN involvement, which was studied for its prognostic significance in comparison with the pTNM system.

Methods.—Sentinel lymph nodectomy (SLNE) under γ probe guidance was used for 342 patients with 344 primary cutaneous melanomas. SLNE was done immediately or soon after primary tumor removal. Histologic criteria verified the diagnosis and the T class of the primary melanoma. Ten persons had cutaneous metastases, leading to upstaging into the next higher T classification. Fifty-three patients with T1 melanomas were included to define a lower limit for SLNE. Primary tumor thickness was 0.2 to 12 mm. No extracutaneous metastases were found. SLNs were divided into 3 consecutive paraffin sections to conserve the total profile. One section was stained routinely (hematoxylin and eosin), 1 was immunolabeled (polyclonal anti-S100 antiserum), and 1 had monoclonal antibody labeling (HMB45). The number of SLN sections where melanoma cells were detected (n) and the maximal distance of melanoma cells from the lymph node capsule interior margin (d) were the basis of the S classifica-

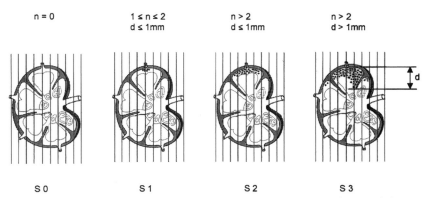

FIGURE 1.—Schematic depiction of the S-staging concept, including the definitions of the 4 S classifications based on the parameters n (the number of 1-mm-thin sentinel lymph node slices with [immuno-]histologically detectable tumor cells) and d (the maximum distance of tumor cells to the interior margin of the lymph node capsule). (Courtesy of Starz H, Balda B-R, Krämer K-U, et al: A micromorphometry-based concept for routine classification of sentinel lymph node metastases and its clinical relevance for patients with melanoma. *Cancer* 91:2110-2120, 2001. Copyright 2001 American Cancer Society. Reprinted by permission of Wiley-Liss, Inc, a subsidiary of John Wiley & Sons, Inc.)

tion (Fig 1). Melanoma-positive SLNs were found in 62 patients, who were further divided into 42 who received regional complete lymph node dissection (RCLND) and 20 who did not. Distribution of T and S categories was similar between the 2 groups. A few patients received adjuvant chemotherapy or immunotherapy with monitoring at a special melanoma

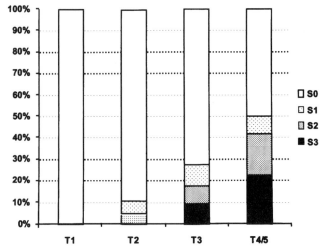

FIGURE 4.—The frequency of the different S categories in relation to the T categories of 344 melanomas (342 patients). In patients with sentinel lymph nodes in 2 or more different lymph node regions, the highest S classification was used for this evaluation. (Courtesy of Starz H, Balda B-R, Krämer K-U, et al: A micromorphometry-based concept for routine classification of sentinel lymph node metastases and its clinical relevance for patients with melanoma. *Cancer* 91:2110-2120, 2001. Copyright 2001 American Cancer Society. Reprinted by permission of Wiley-Liss, Inc, a subsidiary of John Wiley & Sons, Inc.)

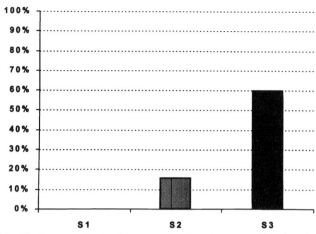

FIGURE 5.—The frequency of regional metastases in at least 1 nonsentinel lymph node in relation to the S categories. These data are based on the exact histologic and immunohistochemical evaluation of 40 lymph node regions in 39 patients who underwent regional completion lymph node dissection(s) because of melanoma positive sentinel lymph nodes. (Courtesy of Starz H, Balda B-R, Krämer K-U, et al: A micromorphometry-based concept for routine classification of sentinel lymph node metastases and its clinical relevance for patients with melanoma. *Cancer* 91:2110-2120, 2001. Copyright 2001 American Cancer Society. Reprinted by permission of Wiley-Liss, Inc, a subsidiary of John Wiley & Sons, Inc.)

clinic. Correlations between T and S categories and their relation to the presence or absence of non-SLN metastases after RCLND were assessed.

Results.—Twenty-three patients with melanoma-positive SLNS were in category S1. In 22 others, metastases occurred only in subcapsular sinuses and adjacent areas, but these were multifocal or more cohesive and affected more than 2 SLN sections, earning an S2 classification. Seventeen patients were placed into class S3. S categories correlated with T categories (Fig 4). No melanoma-positive SLNs came from patients with T1 melanomas; thus, these were classified as S0. S3 patients all had high-risk T category lesions. An average of 29 non-SLNs per RCLND were obtained from 39 patients who had 40 RCLNDs, and 11 patients had at least 1 positive non-SLN (9 S3 and 2 S2). A significant correlation existed between S classification and non-SLN metastases (Fig 5). The follow-up period ranged from 2 to 66 months (median, 31.5 months); 19 patients had distant metastases, primarily in lungs, pleura, and brain. Time from SLNE to distant metastases ranged from 5 to 50 months (median, 19 months). Risk for the development of distant metastases was highly significantly related to T classification and S category. Multivariate analysis showed tumor thickness, category S3, and trunk location were independent significant risk factors for distant metastases and survival. The 36 S3 patients showed a significantly higher risk for distant metastases than those in the S0, S1, or S2 categories. Adding T and S categories yielded a score of 1 to 8 and defined a staging scheme to predict distant metastases.

Conclusions.—Several components predicted the development of distant metastatic disease, but the S staging concept could decisively determine whether RCLND was advisable. A combined T and S staging system may also stratify melanoma patients in a prognostically relevant way.

▶ The sentinel lymph node biopsy (SLNB) provides critical staging and prognostic information in patients with melanoma. Currently, if a patient is found to have a positive SLNB they are usually subjected to a complete lymph node dissection and prognostically grouped with other patients having a positive SLNB. In this study, the authors attempt to subdivide patients with a positive SLNB into different prognostic categories based upon the extent of involvement of the SLN, the so-called S classification. Preliminary results of this microstaging suggest that the S classification may be useful in predicting which patients require a complete node dissection and which patients are at significant risk for developing distant metastases. When the S classification is combined with the T (thickness) classification, one has an even more powerful tool for predicting distant metastases. As more effective adjuvant therapies become available, assigning a score based on the S and T classifications to a patient with a positive SLNB may allow the physician to better select those patients who would benefit the most from such therapy.

P. G. Lang, Jr, MD

Sentinel Lymph Node Biopsy in the Management of Patients With Primary Cutaneous Melanoma: Review of a Large Single-Institutional Experience With an Emphasis on Recurrence

Clary BM, Brady MS, Lewis JJ, et al (Mem Sloan-Kettering Cancer Ctr, New York)
Ann Surg 233:250-258, 2001   21–19

Background.—The optimal surgical management for patients with primary cutaneous melanoma has not been established. Elective lymph node dissection (ELND) is associated with improved survival rates for these patients, but sentinel lymph node mapping and biopsy (SLNB) is also effective in staging nodal basins at risk of regional metastases. SLNB was performed and recurrence patterns were described in a prospective study

TABLE 2.—SLN Identification in 387 Mapped Basins in 357 Patients

Basin	Total Number	SLN Identified	%
Axillary	211	199	94
Inguinal	127	121	95
Cervical	45	36	80
Popliteal/brachial	4	4	100
Total	387	360	93

Abbreviation: SLN, Sentinel lymph node.
(Courtesy of Clary BM, Brady MS, Lewis JJ, et al: Sentinel lymph node biopsy in the management of patients with primary cutaneous melanoma: Review of a large single-institutional experience with an emphasis on recurrence. *Ann Surg* 233:250-258, 2001.)

TABLE 4.—Incidence of SLN Metastases According to Tumor Thickness

Tumor Thickness (mm)	Number of Patients (Total)	Number of Patients With Positive Nodes	%	P Value*
≤1.0	27	1	4	
>1.0-2.0	132	14	11	.24
>2.0-3.0	79	20	25	.01
>3.0-4.0	42	8	19	.06
>4.0	50	12	24	.02
Unknown	2	1		
Total	332	56	17	

*Versus ≤1.0 mm.
Abbreviation: SLN, Sentinel lymph node.
(Courtesy of Clary BM, Brady MS, Lewis JJ, et al: Sentinel lymph node biopsy in the management of patients with primary cutaneous melanoma: Review of a large single-institutional experience with an emphasis on recurrence. *Ann Surg* 233:250-258, 2001.)

of a large, consecutive, single-institution patient group with primary cutaneous melanoma.

Study Design.—From May 1991 to December 1998, 357 patients with primary cutaneous melanoma had SLNB at Memorial Sloan-Kettering Cancer Center. Postoperative follow-up examinations occurred every 3 to 4 months for the first year, every 3 to 6 months for the second year and every 6 to 12 months afterward. Follow-up studies included the taking of chest radiographs, measurements of serum lactate dehydrogenase levels, and complete blood counts.

Findings.—The median primary tumor thickness was 2.1 mm. A Clark IV or V depth of invasion was detected in 81%, and ulceration was present in 29% of primary lesions. Of the 357 patients, SLNB was successfully performed in 332 (93%). A total of 387 nodal basins were mapped and 360 SLN were identified (Table 2). SLN metastases were detected in 17% of patients. Of these, 13 were not identified by hematoxylin and eosin staining and required either step-sectioning or immunohistochemical (IHC) analysis. SLN metastases were significantly associated with primary tumor thickness (Table 4). No significant difference was noted in age,

TABLE 5.—Factors Associated With SLN Positivity

Prognostic Factor	SLN Negative	SLN Positive	P Value
Age, mean (yr)	55	52	.22
Male (%)	56	57	1.00
Axial location (%)	51	43	.31
Clark level >III (%)	80	89	.17
Thickness, mean (mm)	2.5	3.4	.01
Ulceration (%)	28	38	.19

Abbreviation: SLN, Sentinel lymph node.
(Courtesy of Clary BM, Brady MS, Lewis JJ, et al: Sentinel lymph node biopsy in the management of patients with primary cutaneous melanoma: Review of a large single-institutional experience with an emphasis on recurrence. *Ann Surg* 233:250-258, 2001.)

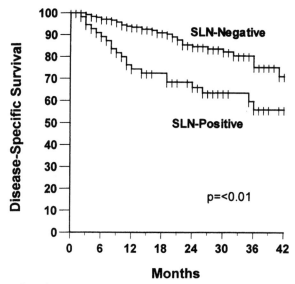

FIGURE 1.—Relapse-free survival according to sentinel lymph node (SLN) status. (Courtesy of Clary BM, Brady MS, Lewis JJ, et al: Sentinel lymph node biopsy in the management of patients with primary cutaneous melanoma: Review of a large single-institutional experience with an emphasis on recurrence. *Ann Surg* 233:250-258, 2001.)

gender (Table 5), Clark depth of invasion, tumor location or ulceration between patients with SLN metastases and those without. The median recurrence interval was 13 months. For those patients with SLN metastases, the recurrence rate was 40%, and for those without SLN metastases, it was only 14%. The 3-year relapse-free survival rate was 58% for those patients with SLN metastases and 75% for those without (Fig 1). A univariate analysis (Table 6) indicated that SLN status was the most important predictor of disease-free survival. A multivariate analysis indi-

TABLE 6.—Prognostic Factors Influencing Relapse-Free Survival

Prognostic Factor	Univariate P Value	Disease-Free Survival		P Value
		HR	Multiple Covariate 95% Confidence Interval	
Male gender	.25	1.09	0.35-1.46	.43
Age (increasing)	.01	1.03	1.01-1.05	<.01
Axial primary	.89	NT	NT	NT
Ulceration	.13	1.02	0.78-1.36	.89
Clark level IV-V	.10	1.05	0.69-1.74	.80
Tumor thickness	<.01	1.26	1.10-1.40	<.01
SLN positive	<.01	1.50	1.11-2.01	<.01

Note: Age and tumor thickness treated as continuous variables. Node-negative patients undergoing confirmatory elective lymph node dissection (n = 24) were excluded from analyses.

Abbreviation: NT, Not tested.

(Courtesy of Clary BM, Brady MS, Lewis JJ, et al: Sentinel lymph node biopsy in the management of patients with primary cutaneous melanoma: Review of a large single-institutional experience with an emphasis on recurrence. *Ann Surg* 233:250-258, 2001.)

TABLE 8.—Incidence and Pattern of First-Site Recurrences

Site	All Patients (n = 308)			SLN-Negative (n = 252)			SLN-Positive (n = 56)		
	Incidence (%)	Recurrences (n)	% of All Recurrences	Incidence (%)	Recurrences (n)	% of All Recurrences	Incidence (%)	Recurrences (n)	% of All Recurrences
Local	2.9	9	15	2.8	7	18	3.6	2	9
Nodal	4.6	14	23	4.4	11	28	5.4	3	14
In-transit	4.6	14	23	2.8	7	18	12.5	7	32
Systemic	7.8	24	39	5.6	14	36	17.9	10	45
Total	19	61	NA	14	39	NA	39	22	NA
Locoregional		37	61		25	64		12	55

Note: Node-negative patients undergoing confirmatory elective lymph node dissection (n = 24) were excluded from analyses.
Abbreviation: SLN, Sentinel lymph node.
(Courtesy of Clary BM, Brady MS, Lewis JJ, et al: Sentinel lymph node biopsy in the management of patients with primary cutaneous melanoma: Review of a large single-institutional experience with an emphasis on recurrence. Ann Surg 233:250-258, 2001.)

TABLE 11.—Pattern of Recurrence After Sentinel Lymphadenectomy and ELND

Author	Year	Patients (n)	Follow-Up (Median)	Recurred	Site of First Recurrence			
					Nodal	In-transit	Local	Systemic
SLN								
Gershenwald (SLN Neg)	1998	243	35 mo	27 (11%)	10 (32%)	8 (26%)	4 (13%)	9 (29%)
Gadd (SLN-Neg)	1999	89	23 mo	11 (12%)	7 (64%)	2 (18%)	NR	2 (18%)
Essner (SLN-Neg)	1999	225	45 mo	26 (12%)	11 (42%)	6 (23%)	NR	9 (34%)
Essner (SLN-Pos)	1999	42	45 mo	16 (38%)	5 (31%)	4 (25%)	NR	7 (44%)
Present series (SLN-Neg)	2000	252	23 mo	35 (14%)	11 (28%)	7 (18%)	7 (18%)	14 (36%)
Present series (SLN-Pos)	2000	56	27 mo	22 (39%)	3 (14%)	7 (32%)	2 (9%)	10 (45%)
ELND								
McCarthy	1988	636	9.8 yr	204 (32%)	10 (5%)	24 (12%)	44 (21%)	116 (55%)
Essner	1999	267	14 yr	54 (20%)	9 (17%)	11 (20%)	NR	34 (63%)

Abbreviations: SLN, Sentinel lymph node; *NR,* not reported; *ELND,* elective lymph node dissection.
(Courtesy of Clary BM, Brady MS, Lewis JJ, et al: Sentinel lymph node biopsy in the management of patients with primary cutaneous melanoma: Review of a large single-institutional experience with an emphasis on recurrence. *Ann Surg* 233:250-258, 2001.)

cated that SLN status, primary tumor thickness, and age were the only significant independent predictors of disease-free survival. Locoregional recurrences accounted for 61% of all first recurrences (Table 8).

Conclusions.—Sentinel lymph node mapping and biopsy is an accurate method for staging the nodal basins of patients with primary cutaneous melanoma. SLN status is the most important prognostic factor for determining the risk of recurrence (Table 11), especially if performed with step-sectioning and IHC analysis. First recurrences are usually locoregional, emphasizing the need for careful follow-up of these patients.

▶ This study from Memorial Sloan-Kettering Cancer Center may not add new data but reaffirms the data from previous studies and provides a good review of prior investigations on sentinel lymph node biopsy (SLNB). Of 6 variables studied, only tumor thickness appeared to influence SLN positivity. This is interesting in light of the new proposed staging classification for melanoma[1] and some of the current proposed guidelines for SLNB. In the new proposed classification system, Clark's level of invasion does not assume a high degree of importance. The results of this study seem to confirm the decision to de-emphasize the role of Clark's level, yet current recommendations for SLNB in patients with thin lesions (<1 mm) suggest that this procedure may be advisable for Clark's level IV lesions. In the new proposed classification system, ulceration is given considerable weight as a prognostic indicator, but in this study, ulceration apparently did not influence the incidence of positive SLNB. Finally, this study, as others, demonstrates that the result of the SLNB is the most important variable in determining prognosis for patients without clinical evidence of metastases. This finding alone, in this reviewer's opinion, justifies the performance of the procedure. Prior studies have shown the importance of the physical exam in the follow-up of melanoma patients. This is driven home in this article by the fact that 61% of recurrences were locoregional.

P. G. Lang, Jr, MD

Reference

1. Balch CM, for the AJCC Melanoma Staging Committee: A new American Joint Committee on Cancer staging system for cutaneous melanoma. *Cancer* 88:1484-1491, 2000.

Melanoma Thickness and Histology Predict Sentinel Lymph Node Status
Nguyen CL, McClay EF, Cole DJ, et al (Med Univ of South Carolina, Charleston)
Am J Surg 181:8-11, 2001   21–20

Introduction.—For patients with a primary melanoma and clinically negative nodes, elective lymph node dissection increases morbidity and may offer no survival benefit. An alternative, minimally invasive procedure—intraoperative lymphatic mapping with blue dye or radioactive tracer and sentinel lymphadenectomy—may be useful in some cases. Primary melanoma histologic features were assessed in a group of patients who underwent sentinel node biopsy for the ability of these features to predict sentinel lymph node status.

Methods.—The mean age of the 112 patients was 51 years; 49% were male. Most tumors were located on the extremities (46%) or trunk (41%). ^{99m}Tc-sulfur colloid and isosulfan blue dye were injected at the site of the primary melanoma, and lymph node specimens were stained with routine hematoxylin-eosin. Histologic variables were analyzed by univariate and multivariate analysis.

Results.—The sentinel lymph node was located successfully in 105 (94%) patients, 21 (20%) of whom had nodes that were positive for metastatic disease. Subsequent lymph node dissections performed in 18 of these patients found additional positive nodes in 3 (17%). Two patients with initially negative sentinel nodes returned with lymphadenopathy at 7 and 18 months and underwent formal lymph node dissections. In multivariate analyses, predictors of the presence of micrometastases were tumor thickness greater than 1.5 mm, ulceration, and lymphovascular invasion. None of the other histologic or clinical features examined were significantly associated with occult micrometastases.

Conclusion.—Patients with primary melanoma whose lesions are greater than 1.0 mm in thickness and have unfavorable histologic characteristics such as ulceration and lymphovascular invasion can benefit from sentinel lymphadenectomy. Patients with thinner lesions may not require the procedure. The false-negative rate for sentinel lymphadenectomy in this series was 2.4%.

▶ This is yet another study that correlates sentinel lymph node (SLN) positivity with a variety of histologic variables in the primary lesion. A thickness greater than 1.5 mm, ulceration, and lymphovascular invasion correlated with SLN positivity, whereas mitotic rate, regression, gender, and location did not. No patient with a melanoma less than 1 mm thick had a positive SLN biopsy specimen, and only 17% of patients with a positive SLN biopsy specimen had involvement of nonsentinel nodes.

P. G. Lang, Jr, MD

The Sentinel Lymph Node Status Is an Important Factor for Predicting Clinical Outcome in Patients With Stage I or II Cutaneous Melanoma
Muller MGS, van Leeuwen PAM, de Lange-de Klerk ESM, et al (Vrije Univ, Amsterdam)
Cancer 91:2401-2408, 2001   21–21

Introduction.—Because it has not been proved that early removal of lymph node micrometastases has a favorable impact on overall survival of patients with malignant melanoma, the value of assessing sentinel lymph node (SLN) status is uncertain. A cohort of patients with clinical stage I or

TABLE 4.—Multivariate Predictive Value of Several Factors for at Least 3-Year Disease Free Survival

Prognostic Factor	Odds Ratio	95% CI	P Value
Negative SLN status	5.2	2.0-13.7	0.0007*
Breslow thickness			
0.5-1.0	5.8	0.7-46.9	0.1
1.01-2.0	21.9	2.6-183.3	0.004*
2.01-4.0	9.7	0.8-112.4	0.07
Ulceration absent	2.5	1.0-6.5	0.05*
Lymphatic invasion absent	5.7	1.4-22.1	0.01*
Age (yrs)			
18-30	3.2	0.5-22.2	0.24
30-40	3.7	0.5-25.6	0.18
40-50	10.9	1.8-66.8	0.01*
50-60	5.9	0.9-39.3	0.08
60-70	6.2	0.8-46.2	0.07

*Significant.
Abbreviations: CI, Confidence interval; *SLN,* sentinel lymph node.
(Courtesy of Muller MGS, van Leeuwen PAM, de Lange-de Klerk ESM, et al: The sentinel lymph node status is an important factor for predicting clinical outcome in patients with Stage I or II cutaneous melanoma. *Cancer* 91:2401-2408, 2001. Reprinted by permission of Wiley-Liss, Inc, a subsidiary of John Wiley & Sons, Inc.)

II cutaneous melanoma was monitored to determine whether SLN status can predict the probability of remaining disease free for at least 3 years.

Methods.—An SLN biopsy was performed on 263 consecutive adult patients between August 1993 and December 1997. All patients had Breslow thickness, Clark invasion level, the presence of ulceration, and lymphatic invasion recorded, and all were subjected to the same treatment protocol. The triple technique SLN procedure was used: preoperative visualization of the lymph channels from the initial site of the melanoma toward the SLN by (dynamic) lymphoscintigraphy, intraoperative visualization of those lymph channels and lymph nodes with blue dye, and a gamma probe to measure accumulated radioactivity in the radiolabeled lymph nodes.

Results.—The median follow-up time was 48 months. The SLN was tumor positive in 52 (20%) patients, 49 of whom underwent a completion lymphadenectomy. Four of the 207 patients with a negative SLN had a clinically evident positive lymph node develop in the same regional basin during follow-up. Thus the false-negative rate of the procedure was 7% and the failure rate 1.5%. The 5-year disease-free survival rate was 91% for SLN-negative patients and 49% for SLN-positive patients. Five variables exhibited a strong and statistically significant independent prognostic association with outcome: SLN status, thickness of the primary melanoma, ulceration, lymphatic invasion of the primary melanoma, and age (Table 4).

Conclusion.—Patients with stage I or II malignant melanoma have a poorer prognosis if the SLN proves tumor positive rather than tumor negative. Status of the SLN, along with the variables of Breslow thickness, lymphatic invasion, ulceration, and age, is predictive of 3-year survival.

▶ It is still unknown if the removal of microscopic nodal disease alters the prognosis of patients with melanoma. Thus, controversy exists regarding the value of sentinel lymph node biopsy (SNLB). Although this study did not address whether SLNB alters prognosis, it did demonstrate that it provides important prognostic information, as does Breslow thickness, the presence or absence of ulceration, the presence or absence of lymphatic invasion, and the age of the patient. In this study, patients with a negative SLNB were 5 times more likely to remain disease free for 3 years compared to patients with a positive SLNB. This study thus demonstrates that SLNB provides important staging information and helps select patients who might benefit from adjuvant therapy.

P. G. Lang, Jr, MD

Sentinel Lymph Node Micrometastasis and Other Histologic Factors That Predict Outcome in Patients With Thicker Melanomas
Cherpelis BS, Haddad F, Messina J, et al (Univ of South Florida, Tampa)
J Am Acad Dermatol 44:762-766, 2001   21–22

Background.—In patients with melanoma, lymph node staging information is obtainable by the surgical techniques of lymphatic mapping and sentinel lymph node (SLN) biopsy. Although no survival benefit has been proven for the procedure, the staging information is useful in identifying patients who may benefit from further surgery or adjuvant therapy. Currently, however, it is not being recommended for patients with thick melanomas (>3-4 mm). The risk of hematogenous dissemination is considered too great in these patients. Recent studies indicate, however, that a surprising number of patients with thick melanomas become long-term survivors, and the lymph node status may be predictive. None of the conventional microscopic features used to gauge prognosis in patients with melanoma have proven helpful in distinguishing the survivors with thick melanoma from those who will die of their disease.

Objective.—Our purpose was to evaluate the influence of SLN histology and other microscopic parameters on survival of patients with thick melanomas.

Methods.—A computerized patient database at the Cutaneous Oncology Clinic at H. Lee Moffitt Cancer Center was accessed to obtain records on patients with melanomas thicker than 3.0 mm (AJCC T3b). A retrospective analysis was conducted with attention paid to histologic variables, sentinel node status, and survival. Survival curves were constructed with the Kaplan-Meier method, and a Cox-Mantel rank testing was used to establish statistical significance.

Results.—Between 1991 and 1999, 201 patients were diagnosed with melanoma thicker than 3.0 mm, and 180 were alive at an average follow-up of 51 months. Of these, 166 were alive without disease. The mean overall and disease-free survival rates were 78% and 66%, respectively. There was a statistically significant difference in disease-free survival (3-

TABLE 2.—Disease-Free Survival (DFS) and Overall Survival in Patients
With Positive and Negative Sentinel Lymph Nodes (SLN)

Node Status	3-y DFS (SE)	3-y Survival (SE)
SLN+	0.37 (0.14)	0.70 (0.30)
SLN−	0.73 (0.06)	0.82 (0.06)
P value	.02	.08

Abbreviation: SE, Standard error.
(Courtesy of Cherpelis BS, Haddad F, Messina J, et al: Sentinel lymph node micrometastasis and other histologic factors that predict outcome in patients with thicker melanomas. *J Am Acad Dermatol* 44:762-766, 2001.)

year) between SLN-positive and SLN-negative patients (37% vs 73%, respectively; $P = .02$). The overall survival (3-year) for the SLN-positive patients was less than the node-negative patients (70% vs 82%), but it was not statistically significant ($P = .08$) (Table 2). The disease-free survival for patients with ulcerated lesions was less than for nonulcerated lesions (77% vs 93%, $P = .05$) (Table 3). None of the other histologic parameters studied, including Breslow thickness, Clark level, mitotic rate, or regression, had an influence on the overall or disease-free survival in this group of patients with thick tumors.

Conclusions.—The results indicate that the SLN node status is predictive of disease-free survival for patients with thick melanomas. A surprising number of patients in the study were free of disease after prolonged follow-up. None of the histologic features of the primary tumor were helpful in predicting outcome, except for ulceration. SLN biopsy appears to be justified for prognostic purposes in patients with thick melanomas.

▶ Many clinicians do not believe that sentinel lymph node biopsy (SLNB) is indicated in patients with a melanoma greater than 4 mm thick because of the likelihood of preexisting for systemic spread, which would preclude any potential therapeutic benefit. As in a previous study,[1] performing SLNB, even in patients with thick lesions, provided important prognostic information. In patients with thick lesions but negative SLNB findings, 3-year disease-free survival was significantly longer. However, overall survival was not different from that in patients with positive SLNB results. The only feature of the primary lesion that affected survival was the presence or absence of ulcer-

TABLE 3.—Disease-Free Survival (DFS) and Overall Survival in Patients
With Ulcerated and Nonulcerated Tumors

Ulceration	3-y DFS (SE)	3-y Survival (SE)
Yes	0.77 (0.07)	0.61 (0.08)
No	0.93 (0.05)	0.77 (0.08)
P value	.05	.13

Abbreviation: SE, Standard error.
(Courtesy of Cherpelis BS, Haddad F, Messina J, et al: Sentinel lymph node micrometastasis and other histologic factors that predict outcome in patients with thicker melanomas. *J Am Acad Dermatol* 44:762-766, 2001.)

ation. However, like the SLNB, ulceration affected only disease-free survival and not overall survival.

P. G. Lang, Jr, MD

Reference

1. Schacter J, Laish A, Mikhmandarov S, et al: Standard and nonstandard applications of sentinel node-guided melanoma surgery. *World J Surg* 247:491-494, 2000.

Evaluation of Sentinel Lymph Node Status in Spindle Cell Melanomas
Thelmo MC, Sagebiel RW, Treseler PA, et al (Univ of California, San Francisco)
J Am Acad Dermatol 44:451-455, 2001   21–23

Background.—The propensity for spindle cell melanoma to metastasize to the lymph node is relatively low despite its relative thick depth. To date, there are no published reports on the sentinel lymph node (SLN) status in patients diagnosed with spindle cell melanoma and desmoplastic malignant melanoma (DMM).

Objective.—Our purpose was to report our experience on the SLN status in spindle cell melanoma and DMM.

Methods.—We undertook a retrospective database and medical record review from Oct 21, 1993 to Sept 29, 1999. At the University of California at San Francisco Melanoma Center, patients with tumor thickness greater than 1 mm or less than 1 mm with high-risk features are managed with preoperative lymphoscintigraphy, selective SLN dissection, and wide excision.

Results.—Of 29 patients diagnosed with spindle cell melanoma and DMM, 28 had negative SLNs and are free of disease except for one patient who experienced splenic, bony, and brain metastases. The mean follow-up in this population was 16.5 and 11 months, respectively.

Conclusion.—Our preliminary findings show that SLNs from patients diagnosed with spindle cell melanoma and DMM only rarely harbor micrometastasis despite their relative thickness. A larger number of cases from multicenter databases may further define the true biology of SLNs in this melanoma variant.

▶ Previous studies have suggested that for melanomas of comparable thickness, desmoplastic melanomas may have a lower incidence of regional nodal metastasis than other melanomas. In keeping with this finding, this study demonstrates a low incidence of positivity of SLN biopsy specimens even though these lesions were deeply invasive. Should these observations be confirmed, this subset of patients with spindle cell and desmoplastic melanomas, with and without perineural involvement, should be studied separately with respect to survival, tumor biologic behavior and response to therapy. Although preliminary evidence suggests that these patients do better, this conclusion should be tempered with caution because the follow-up period was relatively short (11 to 16.5 months) and spindle cell melanomas may bypass the regional nodes when metastasizing.

P. G. Lang, Jr, MD

Evaluation of Micrometastases in Sentinel Lymph Nodes of Cutaneous Melanoma: Higher Diagnostic Accuracy With Melan-A and MART-1 Compared With S-100 Protein and HMB-45

Shidham VB, Qi DY, Acker S, et al (Med College of Wisconsin, Milwaukee)
Am J Surg Pathol 25:1039-1046, 2001   21–24

Introduction.—To evaluate micrometastases in sentinel lymph nodes of patients with cutaneous melanoma, S-100 protein (S-100) and HMB-45 are the traditionally used immunohistochemical markers. The interpretation of micrometastases by these markers is difficult, however. S-100 demonstrates immunoreactivity for other nonmelanoma cells and obscures nuclear details, and HMB-45 may not detect some melanoma cells. The new melanoma markers, Melan-A (clone A103) and MART-1 (clone M2-7C10), were compared with S-100 and HMB-45 for diagnostic accuracy.

Methods.—The various markers were used to examine 77 formalin-fixed paraffin-embedded sections of sentinel lymph nodes from 13 patients with primary cutaneous melanoma (stages I and II). Also studied were CD68 (PG-M1) and hematoxylin-eosin (HE)–stained sections. In a double-blind manner, 4 pathologists interpreted all immunostained slides independently for micrometastases. Findings were classified as definitely negative for metastasis, probably negative, indeterminate, probably positive, and definitely positive.

Results.—One section had inadequate material, leaving 76 sections in the analysis. Microscopic foci of metastatic melanoma, observed in 23 sections, were subtle and difficult to detect on the HE-stained sections alone. All 23 micrometastases were immunoreactive for Melan-A and MART-1, and all 4 pathologists interpreted them independently and correctly with these markers. Fifteen (65%) micrometastases were immunoreactive for HMB-45. In 13 micrometastases, interpretation was difficult with S-100, and findings were characterized variously as negative, probably negative, indeterminate, or probably positive. The ancillary use of CD68 (PG-M1) increased the diagnostic accuracy of S-100 and HMB-45 but not that of Melan-A and MART-1.

Conclusion.—Micrometastases of melanoma are difficult to detect with routine HE sections alone, and diagnostic accuracy is not high when S-100 and HMB-45 are used. Melan-A and MART-1 are superior in detecting micrometastases and are recommended as a routine alternative to the traditionally used immunomarkers.

▶ Previous studies have demonstrated that the use of immunostains, such as S-100 and HMB-45, enhances the detection of melanoma cells in sentinel lymph node biopsy specimens. Although S-100 is quite sensitive, it also stains macrophages, Langerhans cells, and dendritic cells, which can make its interpretation difficult. HMB-45 is less sensitive and may not detect some melanoma cells. It also can sometimes stain mononuclear cells, which can be a source of confusion.

In this study, the authors compared the immunostains Melan-A and MART-1 with S-100 and HMB-45 for their ability to detect melanoma cells in sentinel lymph node biopsy specimens. Melanoma cells were present in 23/76 histologic sections. These were easily identified in all 23 sections with Melan-A and MART-1 stains. S-100 staining proved to be less sensitive and more difficult to interpret, and HMB-45 staining results were positive in only 15/23 sections. Melan-A and MART-1 stains were also more specific for melanocytes. In ambiguous cases (especially those staining positively with S-100 and HMB-45), the simultaneous use of an immunostain (CD68) for macrophages helped to distinguish between staining for melanocytes and macrophages.

In general, when compared with Melan-A, MART-1 demonstrated stronger immunoreactivity and stained more melanoma cells. The authors concluded that MART-1 and Melan-A are better immunostains for detecting melanoma cells in sentinel lymph node biopsy specimens, and if immunostain S-100 is used, simultaneous staining with CD68 enhances the diagnostic accuracy of the stain.

P. G. Lang, Jr, MD

Detection of Melanoma Cells in Sentinel Lymph Nodes, Bone Marrow and Peripheral Blood by a Reverse Transcription–Polymerase Chain Reaction Assay in Patients With Primary Cutaneous Melanoma: Association With Breslow's Tumour Thickness

Blaheta H-J, Paul T, Sotlar K, et al (Eberhard-Karls-Univ, Tübingen, Germany)
Br J Dermatol 145:195-202, 2001   21–25

Background.—The 2 primary tumor characteristics on which primary cutaneous melanoma is classified are Breslow's tumor thickness and Clark's level of invasion. The use of tyrosinase reverse transcription-polymerase chain reaction (RT-PCR) has allowed the detection of tumor cells in melanoma patients. It was hypothesized that minimal residual disease could be detected with greater accuracy by analyzing sentinel lymph nodes (SLNs), bone marrow (BM), and peripheral blood (PB) with RT-PCR and that the rate of detection would be associated with Breslow's tumor thickness.

Methods.—The study included 26 consecutive patients with primary cutaneous melanoma who were staged using results of the SLN biopsy, BM, and PB examinations. Breslow's tumor thickness was at least 0.75 mm and/or Clark's level of invasion was at least level III. No metastatic disease was detected in any patient. SLN biopsy was performed; half of each SLN was used for histopathologic testing and half reserved for RT-PCR.

Results.—Thirty-five SLNs were obtained. RT-PCR detected melanoma cells in 13 (50%) of the patients, with 7 (27%) patients having positive SLN results, 2 (8%) having positive BM results, and 6 (23%) having positive PB results. The ability to detect tumor cells in SLNs using RT-PCR did not correlate with either the presence of cells in BM or in PB. When SLN RT-PCR results were positive, patients' median tumor thickness was significantly greater than when RT-PCR results were negative. The 2 patients who had RT-PCR positivity in BM had thick tumors (2 and 4.5 mm). With respect to PB findings, no significant difference in tumor thickness was found between RT-PCR-positive and RT-PCR-negative patients.

Conclusions.—When SLNs were found to be positive on RT-PCR analysis, tumors tended to be thicker, which indicates a predictive value for SLN positivity. BM results may improve the prognostic information obtained in early stages of melanoma, but PB findings did not correlate with increased tumor thickness. The use of RT-PCR findings in PB may not provide clinically relevant information.

▶ Investigators continue to look for more sensitive ways to detect subclinical disease for patients with high-risk melanoma. One of the more common assays employed has been RT-PCR. The results from study to study have varied, and the correlation with prognosis has not always been consistent. In this study, the authors used the RT-PCR assay to detect tyrosinase and Melan-A in the SLN, BM, and PB of patients with primary melanoma. The authors found that the presence of melanoma cells in the SLN and BM correlated with tumor thickness, but this was not true for patients with melanoma cells in their PB. Unfortunately, long-term follow-up was not available, and thus the significance of the detection of melanoma cells in the BM and PB is not clear, especially in that there was no correlation with SLN positivity. With respect to the BM, breast cancer may serve as a model in that node-negative breast cancer patients with occult tumor cells in the BM (detected by immunoassay) have a worse prognosis. With regard to the PB, patients with primary melanoma may periodically shed cells into the circulation that often do not survive; this may explain the inconsistent results of PB positivity and its effect on prognosis.

P. G. Lang, Jr, MD

Reverse Transcriptase-Polymerase Chain Reaction (RT-PCR) Analysis of Nonsentinel Nodes Following Completion Lymphadenectomy for Melanoma
Wrightson WR, Wong SL, Edwards MJ, et al (Univ of Louisville, Ky; Natl Genetics Inst, Los Angeles)
J Surg Res 98:47-51, 2001   21–26

Introduction.—Most melanoma patients with sentinel lymph nodes (SLN) that are histologically positive for metastasis have no additional positive lymph nodes found upon completion lymph node dissection (CLND). Therefore, it has been suggested that CLND may not be required for all patients with positive SLN. This study was undertaken to determine the frequency with which nonsentinel nodes contain melanoma cells detected by RT-PCR.

Methods.—Negative control lymph nodes were obtained from patients with breast and colon cancer. Positive control lymph nodes contained histologic evidence of melanoma. Nonsentinel nodes were harvested from melanoma patients undergoing CLND for a positive SLN. RT-PCR analysis for melanoma markers tyrosinase, gp100, MART-1, and MAGE-3 was performed, with Southern blot detection. The RT-PCR test was considered positive for the presence of melanoma cells if tyrosinase and at least one other marker were detected above background levels.

Results.—RT-PCR analysis detected the presence of melanoma cells in 0/100 (0%) of negative control lymph nodes and 28/29 (97%) of positive control lymph nodes. A total of 117 histologically negative nonsentinel nodes from 13 patients who underwent CLND for positive SLN were evaluated. RT-PCR analysis was positive in 18/117 histologically negative nonsentinel nodes (15%) from 7/13 patients (54%).

Conclusion.—RT-PCR analysis suggests that when the SLN contains histologic evidence of melanoma, the remaining nodes in that basin are at risk for metastatic disease, despite the fact that these nonsentinel nodes are infrequently histologically positive.

▶ When patients with positive SLN biopsy findings undergo CLND, the remaining nodes often are found to be free of disease. This raises the question of whether CLND should be performed in all patients with positive findings. Only well-controlled long-term studies will resolve this controversy, which prompts other relevant questions. For example, if the nonsentinel nodes (NSN) are not removed, will the body be able to destroy any residual microscopic disease, or will interferon treatment alone be adequate to eliminate any remaining microscopic disease? This study does not address these issues. However, one concern it does address is how often disease in the NSN might be missed because of sampling error. To assess this, the authors used RT-PCR to examine a series of NSN from patients with positive SLN findings. These nodes were negative with routine histopathologic examination. Fifteen percent of the nodes were positive with RT-PCR analysis, suggesting that involvement of NSN in patients with a positive SLN may be higher than previously assumed. Whether the disease was missed because of sampling error or because the disease was submicroscopic could not be determined. Based on their observations, the authors conclude that until more data are collected CLND should be performed in patients with positive SLN biopsy results.

P. G. Lang, Jr, MD

Early Recurrence After Lymphatic Mapping and Sentinel Node Biopsy in Patients With Primary Extremity Melanoma: A Comparison With Elective Lymph Node Dissection
Clary BM, Mann B, Brady MS, et al (Mem Sloan-Kettering Cancer Ctr, New York; Royal Melbourne Hosp, Australia)
Ann Surg Oncol 8:328-337, 2001   21–27

Background.—Results of prospective randomized trials assessing the efficacy of elective lymph node dissection (ELND) in the treatment of primary cutaneous melanoma of the extremities have been mixed. Thus, many surgeons have embraced sentinel lymph node mapping and biopsy with selective lymph node dissection (SLND) as the preferred method for staging disease in these patients. But are these 2 approaches therapeutically equivalent? These authors reviewed 25 years of experience at their institution to compare outcomes after ELND and SLND in patients with primary cutaneous melanoma of the extremities.

Methods.—Medical records since 1974 were examined to identify all 418 patients with primary cutaneous melanoma of the extremities who underwent either ELND (1974-1994) or SLND (1991-1998). Clinical characteristics and outcomes were compared between the 2 groups.

Results.—The ELND group consisted of 329 patients (43% men, median age 51 years) who were followed for a mean of 80 months. The SLND group consisted of 152 patients (44% men; median age, 55 years) who were followed for a mean of 26 months. A significantly greater proportion of the patients in the SLND group were older than 50 years (65% vs 55%). Tumor thickness did not differ significantly between the groups; median tumor thickness (n = 383) was 2.1 mm. Significantly more patients in the SLND group had a Clark level IV/V melanoma (78% vs 46%). The mean numbers of lymph nodes harvested in the SLND and ELND groups were 2.2 and 1.7, respectively. Nodal metastases were significantly more common among the patients in the SLND group (20% vs 13%). The only significant predictor of nodal metastases was tumor thickness (Table 2). The ELND and SLND groups did not differ significantly in disease-free survival at 3 years (91% overall), nor in relapse-free survival at 3 years (80% and 71%, respectively). However, among node-negative patients at increased risk of recurrence, 3-year relapse-free survival rates were significantly lower in the SLND group: for patients older than 50 years old, rates were 80% for the ELND group and 65% for the SLND group, whereas for patients with a tumor thickness larger than 3.0 mm, rates were 73% for

TABLE 2.—Nodal Metastases According to Tumor Thickness

Tumor Thickness (mm)	Number of Patients (Total)	Number of Patients (Node Positive)	%	P-Value (vs. >1.0-2.0 mm)
≤1.0	33	2	6	.75
>1.0-2.0	156	12	8	N/A
>2.0-3.0	88	18	20	<.01
>3.0-4.0	46	8	17	.05
>4.0	60	21	35	<.01
Unknown	2	1		
Total	385	61	16	

(Courtesy of Clary BM, Mann B, Brady MS, et al: Early recurrence after lymphatic mapping and sentinel node biopsy in patients with primary extremity melanoma: A comparison with elective lymph node dissection. *Ann Surg Oncol* 8: 328-337, 2001.)

the ELND group and 51% for the SLND group. The pattern of early first site recurrence differed significantly between the 2 groups, with systemic sites more common in the ELND group (61% vs 28% in the SLND group) and locoregional sites more common in the SLND group (72% vs 39% in the ELND group). Seven node-negative patients in the SLND group experienced a nodal recurrence. On subsequent reexamination, 5 of these 7 patients had evidence of metastases within the sentinel node.

Conclusions.—Overall disease-free and relapse-free survival was similar for patients with primary cutaneous melanoma of the extremity undergoing either ELND or SLND. However, among node-negative patients at increased risk of recurrence (older patients, thicker tumor), the rate of relapse was significantly higher after SLND. Thus, ELND and SLND should not be considered equally effective approaches until more follow-up data become available.

▶ This retrospective study represents a comparison of the efficacy of elective lymph node dissection (ELND) and sentinel lymph node biopsy (SLNB) in patients with primary melanoma of the extremities. Unfortunately, the study is flawed by several factors. In a significant number of patients undergoing ELND, the thickness of the lesion was unknown. In other patients who underwent SLNB and subsequently experienced regional node relapse, retrospective analysis revealed missed tumor. Overall, there was no difference in disease-free and overall survival between the 2 groups. However, when patients who were older than 50 years or who had lesions larger than 3.0 mm thick and were node-negative were considered separately, those who had undergone ELND fared better. However, this may have been, in part, a consequence of the subset of patients in the SLNB group who had false-negative biopsy specimens. Likewise, false-negative SLNB specimens also may have accounted, in part, for the fact that these patients were more likely to relapse regionally (eg, nodal and in transit metastases) in comparison to node-negative ELND patients, who were more likely to relapse at distant sites (eg, lungs).

P. G. Lang, Jr, MD

Risk Factors for Nodal Recurrence After Lymphadenectomy for Melanoma

Pidhorecky I, Lee RJ, Proulx G, et al (State Univ of New York, Buffalo)
Ann Surg Oncol 8:109-115, 2001   21–28

Introduction.—The ability of lymphadenectomy to control regional disease in patients with melanoma and microscopic lymph node involvement is not well defined. Risk factors for nodal recurrence after elective lymph node dissection and therapeutic lymph node dissection (ELND/TLND) were examined in a retrospective study of 338 patients with pathologically involved lymph nodes.

Methods.—The tumor registry at the Roswell Park Cancer Institute was searched for patients treated for cutaneous malignant melanoma from 1970 through 1996. Of the 2455 patients identified, 338 (13.8%) had pathologically involved regional lymph nodes and underwent ELND or TLND; none received adjuvant radiotherapy. Details of the disease, treatment, and outcome were entered into analysis.

Results.—The median age of the 338 patients was 50 years and the median follow-up time was 29 months. Regional recurrence was reported in 12 patients (14%) treated with ELND and in 72 (28%) of those treated with TLND. Risk factors associated with nodal recurrence were advanced age, a primary lesion in the head and neck, depth of the primary lesion, number of involved lymph nodes, and extracapsular extension. Patients in the ELND group had a lower incidence of recurrence than those in the TLND group. Patients who underwent TLND had larger lymph nodes, a greater number of involved nodes, and a higher incidence of extracapsular extension.

The 10-year disease-specific survival was greater in the ELND group (51% vs 30% for TLND). Nodal basin failure was predicted by distant metastasis, which occurred in 87% of patients with and 54% of patients without nodal recurrence. More relapses occurred in patients with palpable disease (28%) than in those with microscopic disease (14%). Five of 6 patients who underwent a second dissection of the regional lymph node basin after isolated nodal recurrence have had a median disease-free interval of 79 months; the remaining patient died of metastatic disease.

Conclusion.—Because nodal basin failure is associated with a poor prognosis, the prevention of initial failure is crucial. The risk factors for nodal recurrence identified here can be used to stratify patients into low- and high-risk categories. Adjuvant radiotherapy can then be considered for the high-risk group.

▶ In this study, the authors examined the regional nodal recurrence rate in patients undergoing either ELND or TLND for metastatic melanoma. None of the patients had received postoperative radiation therapy and all patients who had undergone ELND had evidence of microscopic disease. The overall recurrence rate was 25%. The 10-year disease-specific survival rate for those who experienced a recurrence was less than for those who did not

(10% vs 45%). Older patients, patients with head and neck lesions, patients with deeper tumors, patients with extracapsular extension, and those with matted nodes and with multiple involved nodes were more likely to relapse. Nodal recurrence was strongly predictive of distant metastases; in 87% of patients with recurrent nodal disease, distant metastases developed, compared with 54% of patients without nodal recurrence. Patients without evidence of distant metastases who underwent a second node dissection often experienced prolonged disease-free survival. Patients undergoing ELND were less likely to suffer nodal recurrence, probably because they usually had fewer and smaller nodes that were less likely to have extracapsular extension. Because they were less likely to suffer a recurrence, patients undergoing ELND had a significantly greater disease-free and overall survival rate.

Based on these observations, the authors propose that (1) the results in their patients undergoing ELND for microscopic disease can be extrapolated to patients with a positive sentinel lymph node biopsy specimen who subsequently undergo node dissection (ie, there may be an impact on disease-free survival and possibly even overall survival) and (2) postoperative radiation therapy should be considered for patients at high risk for nodal recurrence, especially those with head and neck lesions. This would include patients with matted nodes, those with more than 4 nodes involved, and those with extracapsular extension.

P. G. Lang, Jr, MD

Do Nodal Metastases From Cutaneous Melanoma of the Head and Neck Follow a Clinically Predictable Pattern?
Pathak I, O'Brien CJ, Petersen-Schaeffer K, et al (RPAH Med Centre, Newtown, Australia; Royal Prince Alfred Hosp, Camperdown, Australia)
Head Neck 23:785-790, 2001   21–29

Introduction.—The lymphatic drainage patterns from cutaneous melanomas of the head and neck have been described as highly variable, but investigators at the Sydney (Australia) Melanoma Unit (SMU) reported that the site of metastases can be predicted accurately in the majority of cases. Their aim in this study of 169 patients was to correlate the anatomical sites of primary cutaneous melanomas of the head and neck with sites of pathologically proven nodal metastases and to determine the extent to which these metastatic patterns conform to clinical predictions.

Methods.—Patients were treated at the SMU between 1987 and 1997. Clinical and pathologic findings were obtained from the SMU database, and the patients' clinical charts and pathologic and operative records were reviewed. The skin of the head and neck was divided into 12 subsites, with each primary melanoma assigned to 1 of these areas. It was predicted that melanomas of the anterior scalp, forehead, and face could metastasize to the parotid and neck lymph node levels I to III; the coronal scalp, ear, and neck to the parotid and levels I to V; the posterior scalp to occipital nodes and levels II to V; and the lower neck to levels III to V. Patients were followed for episodes of recurrence of metastatic disease after lymphadenectomy. The median follow-up period was 3 years for all patients and 4.5 years for those currently alive.

Results.—Therapeutic lymphadenectomies were performed in 141 patients, including 97 with comprehensive and 44 with selective dissections. The remaining 28 patients underwent elective lymphadenectomies. There were 112 parotidectomies (44 therapeutic and 68 elective). Pathologically positive nodes involved clinically predicted nodal groups in 156 (92.3%) cases. Postauricular node involvement occurred in only 3 (1.5%) cases. No patient was initially seen with contralateral metastatic disease, but 5 (2.9%) patients failed in the contralateral neck after therapeutic dissection. Metastatic disease involved the nearest nodal group in 68% of patients.

Conclusion.—In these cases of cutaneous melanoma of the head and neck, the distribution of involved nodes conformed to a clinically predictable pattern in 92% of cases. Variations indicate that unusual events occasionally occur, but not that the metastatic process is haphazard and unpredictable.

▶ Recent studies have suggested that lymphatic drainage of the head and neck is quite unpredictable and that lymphoscintigraphy is essential when planning a sentinel lymph node biopsy. In this article from the SMU, the authors claim that in 92% of melanomas of the head and neck, the site(s) of metastases can accurately be predicted. Furthermore, they state that lymphoscintigraphy may yield conflicting results in up to one third of patients. Although these authors are quite experienced in the surgical management of melanoma, their findings conflict with those of well-designed studies. Furthermore, it should be noted that of 169 node dissections, only 28 were elective, ie, 141 patients had clinical evidence of metastatic disease. Moreover, it is not clear what percentage of those patients undergoing elective node dissection had pathologic evidence of disease, and the average thickness of the primary lesions was not stated.

P. G. Lang, Jr, MD

The Use of Lymphoscintigraphy and PET in the Management of Head and Neck Melanoma

Kokoska MS, Olson G, Kelemen PR, et al (Saint Louis Univ Health Sciences Ctr; Mayo Clinic Found, Rochester, Minn; Pennsylvania State Univ, Hershey)
Otolaryngol Head Neck Surg 125:213-220, 2001   21–30

Introduction.—New methods of searching for lymph node metastasis of malignant melanoma have emerged in recent years. Two such techniques are 18 fluoro-2-deoxyglucose positron emission tomography (PET) and lymphoscintigraphy, with the use of technetium-99 radiolabeled sulfur colloid, followed by sentinel node dissection.

Study Design and Setting.—From July 1, 1998, through December 30, 2000, 18 patients diagnosed with head and neck melanomas underwent PET scans as well as lymphoscintigraphy and sentinel node dissection. All patients had tumors of Breslow depth greater than 1.0 mm and clinically negative regional nodes.

Results.—Sentinel nodes were located in 17 of 18 patients (94.4%); 15 of 18 patients (27.8%) had metastases. There were 3 patients with negative PET scans who had positive sentinel node biopsy specimens. The overall sensitivity of PET for detecting regional metastases was 40%.

Conclusion.—PET scans and lymphoscintigraphy with sentinel node dissection offer complementary methods for detecting metastatic melanoma.

▶ In general, PET has not been shown to be worthwhile for staging patients with primary melanoma localized to the skin. For high-risk lesions, the sentinel lymph node biopsy is preferable for such patients. In this study, only 40% of patients with positive sentinel lymph node biopsy specimens were diagnosed preoperatively by PET, reaffirming the limited ability of this scan to detect occult microscopic disease. Even though the authors acknowledge the limited usefulness of PET in this setting, they still suggest that it might help to detect distant metastases from a tumor not initially presenting with regional nodal metastases (which occurs in 10% of patients with head and neck melanoma) or to serve as a baseline if metastases develop later.

P. G. Lang, Jr, MD

Efficacy of Ultrasound B-Scan Compared With Physical Examination in Follow-up of Melanoma Patients
Voit C, Mayer T, Kron M, et al (Humboldt Univ, Berlin; Armed Forces Hosp Ulm, Germany; Univ of Ulm, Germany; et al)
Cancer 91:2409-2416, 2001   21–31

Background.—Ultrasound B-scans (UBS) are not done routinely in the postoperative follow-up of melanoma patients. A comparison of UBS with physical examination (PE) was done to assess whether the use of UBS can improve the early detection of metastases and increase the relapse-free and overall survival rates for melanoma patients.

Methods.—The study included 829 consecutive macroscopically disease-free patients, aged from 9 to 94 years (median, 56 years), who were followed prospectively, and who received 3011 UBS procedures. A 7.5-MHz linear scanner was used, and suspicious lesions were recorded, with unclear lesions rechecked within 4 to 6 weeks. Physical examinations were also done, including palpation of regional lymph node basins as required, recording size and number of suspicious nodes, and noting whether the patient had palpated a suspicious node before consulting the physician. Of the 242 recurrences, 103 (42%) were first-time regional lymph node recurrences. These were followed until the next recurrence to evaluate relapse-free survival rates and overall survival intervals. Follow-up examinations were performed yearly for the low-risk group and every 6 months or every 3 months as risk increased.

Results.—At scheduled melanoma follow-up examinations, 242 recurrences were noted. Only 25 were found by different examination procedures: 3 by CT scan; 2 by ear, nose, and throat examination of mucous membranes; and 20 by biopsy of skin metastases. PE detected 61 recurrences, equivalent to a sensitivity of 25.2%. Of these 61, physicians detected 27 and patients detected 34. False-positive results were noted in 45 PEs, of which 35 were done by physicians. The predictive value of PE was 57.5%. UBS examination after PE found 240 of the recurrences, equivalent to a sensitivity of 99.2%. Eighteen were highly suspicious, and 222 were definite melanoma metastases. False-positive results were obtained in 48 patients, equivalent to a positive predictive value of 83.3% and a negative predictive value of 99.9%. The UBS specificity was 98.3%. The 99% sensitivity of UBS and the 25.2% value for PE were comparable to the values found in other studies. Combining the sensitivity of PE of 25.2% and its specificity of 98.4% indicated that metastases were suspected only when they were definitely present. Thus, PE cannot provide both high sensitivity and high specificity. UBS, however, had both high sensitivity and high specificity, suggesting that when no lesion is found on UBS, further diagnostic procedures are unnecessary.

Prognosis was most closely related to the number of affected lymph nodes, with a 2-year overall survival rate of 77% when 1 metastatic lymph node was present, decreasing to 45% when more than 1 was found. In addition, when the largest lesion was 15 mm or less, the 4-year overall survival rate was 68%; when it was more than 15 mm, it was 35%. The corresponding relapse-free survival rates were 34% and 19%. Lead-time bias, which refers to an increased survival because metastatic lesions are found earlier using more sophisticated techniques, was not sufficient to explain the differences between the 2 methods.

Conclusions.—UBS was both highly sensitive and highly specific in testing for recurrent melanoma when compared with PE. The number and size of any melanoma metastases correlated with survival rates.

▶ There are at least 2 reasons for melanoma patients to come for follow-up examinations: (1) to detect a new primary lesion; and (2) to detect signs of a recurrence as early as possible. Physical examination is cost-effective but limited in its ability to detect recurrent disease. Several studies have now been published on the use of US to detect nodal recurrences. Compared with CT, MRI, and positron emission tomography, US scanning is relatively inexpensive. In this study, the specificities of the physical exam and US scanning were similar (98%); however, the US scan was much more sensitive in detecting metastases (99% vs 25%). The authors used US to determine the diameter of the largest metastatic node and found that prognosis was directly related to the size of the largest node and the number of nodes containing metastases. After reviewing this article, one must wonder if US scanning shouldn't be used more frequently to detect early recurrence in patients with high-risk melanoma.

P. G. Lang, Jr, MD

Developing Indications for the Use of Sentinel Lymph Node Biopsy and Adjuvant High-Dose Interferon Alfa-2b in Melanoma
Dubois W, Swetter SM, Atkins M, et al (Protocare Sciences Inc, Santa Monica, Calif; Stanford Univ, Calif; VA Palo Alto Health Care System, Calif; et al)
Arch Dermatol 137:1217-1224, 2001   21–32

Background.—The appropriate use of sentinel lymph node (SLN) biopsy and high-dose adjuvant interferon α-2b therapy in the management of patients with stage I to III malignant melanoma remains controversial. A multidisciplinary panel, including dermatologists, surgical oncologists, and medical oncologists was convened to formally review the available data and make recommendations using a well-validated, evidence-based consensus methodology.

Study Design.—The multidisciplinary panel was composed of 4 dermatologists, 4 oncologists, and 5 surgeons from geographically diverse areas. Eight of these physicians practiced in community settings, and 5 were based at academic institutions. The MEDLINE database from 1996 through June 2000 was searched, and supplementary information was contributed by cancer societies. The RAND/UCLA Appropriateness Method was used to review and assess multiple clinical scenarios for SLN biopsy and interferon therapy.

Conclusions.—The panel rated SLN biopsy for 48 real-world clinical situations. SLN biopsy was considered to be appropriate for patients with lesions thicker than 1.0 mm (T2) or less when ulceration or reticular dermal invasion (Clark level of at least 4) was present. SLN biopsy was considered inappropriate for patients with lesions of no more than 0.75 mm thick because nodal involvement was unlikely. Patients with lesions whose thickness was between 0.76 mm and 1.0 mm were rated as uncertain candidates for SLN biopsy. The panel also rated 56 clinical scenarios for the use of high-dose adjuvant interferon α-2b therapy. The use of adjuvant interferon therapy was considered appropriate for patients either with thick lesions (more than 4.0 mm [T4 N0 lesions]) or with positive lymph nodes (N1-N3). For node-negative lesions, interferon therapy was considered inappropriate for lesions of less than 2.0 mm thickness (T2 lesions) or from 2.0 to 4.0 mm without ulceration (T3a lesions). Use of interferon therapy was considered uncertain for patients with lesions between 2.0 and 4.0 mm with ulceration (T3b lesions). It is hoped that these guidelines will assist the decision-making process for clinicians and patients with melanoma.

▶ This article, which in essence represents a multidisciplinary consensus statement, provides an excellent review on the indications for sentinel lymph node biopsy (SLNB) and the use of interferon (IFN) α-2b therapy in the management of melanoma patients. The panel concluded that SLNB was indicated for patients with lesions more than 1.0 mm thick and for lesions less than 1 mm thick that were ulcerated or for Clark's level IV or deeper tumors. IFN was indicated for patients with nodal or in-transit metastases or for node-negative patients with lesions more than 4 mm thick.

P. G. Lang, Jr, MD

Effect of Long-term Adjuvant Therapy With Interferon Alpha-2a in Patients With Regional Node Metastases From Cutaneous Melanoma: A Randomized Trial
Cascinelli N, Belli F, MacKie RM, et al (Natl Cancer Inst, Milan, Italy; Univ of Glasgow, Scotland; S Paolo, Milan, Italy)
Lancet 358:866-869, 2001   21–33

Introduction.—Survival is substantially reduced in patients with melanoma that has spread to local draining lymph nodes, and various adjuvant therapies have not consistently demonstrated a survival advantage. In the World Health Organization Melanoma Programme Trial 16, the benefits and toxic effects of interferon α-2a were evaluated.

Methods.—A total of 444 patients from 23 centers entered the randomized trial. Those eligible had primary cutaneous malignant melanoma and histologic confirmation of regional node metastases. None had received any previous nonsurgical treatment for melanoma. After total removal of the involved regional lymph node basin, assignment was made to surgical treatment alone or surgical treatment followed by interferon α-2a (3 MU subcutaneously 3 times a week for 3 years). Patients were monitored for survival and quality of life.

Results.—There were 218 evaluable patients in the surgery-plus-interferon group and 208 in the surgery-alone group. The 5-year disease-free survival rate was 28% in both groups. Kaplan-Meier 5-year cumulative survival was also similar in the 2 groups (35% with interferon and 37% with surgery alone). Treatment with interferon had no adverse effect on patients' quality of life or daily activities. Overall, the outcome was better for women than for men and for patients with single-node involvement compared with patients with 4 or more positive nodes.

Conclusion.—Interferon α-2, administered as 3 MU 3 times weekly for 3 years, had no impact on the disease-free or overall survival of patients with melanoma and regional node metastases that were detectable after surgery. A pilot study designed to examine the value of administering interferon for 1 month before surgery is planned.

▶ In this study, patients with melanoma metastatic to the regional lymph nodes were randomly assigned to have either surgery alone or surgery plus low-dose interferon α-2a, 3 MU injected subcutaneously thrice weekly for 3 years. Although this dose of interferon was well tolerated, it had no effect on disease-free or overall survival. Most clinical trials have suggested that higher doses may be more effective.

P. G. Lang, Jr, MD

Paroxetine for the Prevention of Depression Induced by High-Dose Interferon Alfa

Musselman DL, Lawson DH, Gumnick JF, et al (Emory Univ, Atlanta, Ga)
N Engl J Med 344:961-966, 2001   21–34

Background.—Treatment with interferon-α is often associated with symptoms characteristic of depression, including anhedonia, fatigue, anorexia, impaired concentration, sleep disturbance, and suicidal ideation. These psychiatric side effects have been addressed in laboratory animals with the use of tricyclic antidepressants such as imipramine. The efficacy of paroxetine for patients who were undergoing high-dose interferon-α therapy for malignant melanoma was evaluated.

Methods.—Forty patients with malignant melanoma whose disease was estimated to have at least a 50% chance of recurrence were randomly assigned to receive paroxetine or placebo along with interferon-α2b (20 million U/m² of body surface area IV 5 days a week for 4 weeks, then 10 million U/m² subcutaneously 3 days a week for 8 weeks). Treatment with paroxetine or placebo began 2 weeks before interferon-α therapy was initiated and continued for the first 12 weeks of this therapy. There were 20 patients in each group. The average daily dose of paroxetine used was 31 mg. Evaluations were carried out at baseline and at regularly scheduled times over the first 12 weeks. The tests used included the Hamilton Depression Rating Scale, the Carroll Depression Scale, the Hamilton Anxiety Scale, and the Neurotoxicity Rating Scale.

Results.—Among the patients receiving interferon-α and paroxetine, the incidence of major depression was significantly reduced. Eleven percent of patients receiving paroxetine and 45% of those receiving placebo had symptoms associated with major depression, considered an indication of the substantial psychiatric adverse effects accompanying therapy with interferon-α. The severity of depressive symptoms over the course of the study was reduced by the paroxetine, especially anxiety and neurotoxicity. These symptom scores were about 50% lower in the paroxetine group than in the placebo group at the 8th and 12th week assessments. After completing the 12-week study, 15 patients chose to continue receiving paroxetine, and 9 had definite improvement in depressive symptoms. Side effects led to discontinuation in 3 patients, 1 had no change, and 2 were lost to follow-up.

Conclusion.—Overall, paroxetine was tolerated well by these patients with malignant melanoma who were receiving high doses of interferon-α. Paroxetine minimized symptoms characteristic of depression or eliminated them in a significant number of patients.

▶ The mechanism by which interferon-α causes depression and how the symptoms are relieved by paroxetine is unknown. Additionally, although the clinical benefits of paroxetine therapy were clear in this 12-week study, it is uncertain whether these salutory effects could be sustained over a longer period. Also unclear is whether paroxetine might inhibit the therapeutic effects of interferon-α.

B. H. Thiers, MD

Double-blind Trial of a Polyvalent, Shed-Antigen, Melanoma Vaccine
Bystryn J-C, Zeleniuch-Jacquotte A, Oratz R, et al (New York Univ)
Clin Cancer Res 7:1882-1887, 2001   21–35

Introduction.—Few treatments are available for melanoma that has metastasized to regional nodes, and prognosis is poor in such cases. In animal models, vaccines have proved effective in preventing melanoma. A polyvalent melanoma vaccine prepared from shed antigens was studied in a double-blind trial involving patients with resected stage III melanoma.

Methods.—Patients eligible for the trial had a particularly high risk of disease recurrence, with clinically palpable nodes or ≥2 histologically positive nodes, and had intact cellular immunity at baseline. A melanoma vaccine was prepared from material shed into culture medium by 4 lines of melanoma cells adapted to long-term growth in serum-free medium. Three

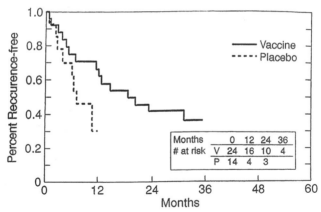

Months	0	12	24	36
# at risk V	24	16	10	4
P	14	4	3	

FIGURE 1.—Kaplan-Meier estimates of time to recurrence among patients treated with a polyvalent, shed-antigen melanoma vaccine or a placebo vaccine. The estimated median time to recurrence in the melanoma vaccine-treated group was 1.6 years compared with 0.6 years for the placebo-treated group. Data are based on an intention-to-treat analysis. (Courtesy of Bystryn J-C, Zeleniuch-Jacquotte A, Oratz R, et al: Double-blind trial of a polyvalent, shed-antigen, melanoma vaccine. *Clin Cancer Res* 7:1882-1887, 2001.)

of the lines were allogeneic, and 1 was xenogeneic. Randomization on a 2:1 ratio was to 40 µg of melanoma vaccine or placebo vaccine. Immunizations were administered intradermally, every 3 weeks for 4 cycles, monthly for 3 cycles, every 3 months for 2 cycles, then every 6 months for a total of 5 years or until disease progression.

Results.—Twenty-four patients received the melanoma vaccine and 14 the placebo vaccine. The 2 groups were similar in prognostic factors. At the time of analysis, surviving patients had been followed for a median of 39 months. The median time to disease progression (Fig 1) was significantly longer in patients treated with the melanoma vaccine (1.6 years) than in those given placebo vaccine (0.6 years); the median overall survival was 3.8 years versus 2.7 years, respectively, not a statistically significant difference. Neither group experienced systemic adverse events, and only minor reactions occurred at the injection sites.

Conclusion.—In this small series of patients, immunization with a melanoma vaccine slowed the progression of stage III melanoma. Shed antigens may be useful in developing clinically effective cancer vaccines.

▶ These are encouraging results in a subset of patients who otherwise would have an unfavorable prognosis. The recurrence-free survival was significantly prolonged although the increase in overall survival did not quite reach statistical significance. The authors' approach using shed antigens might also be useful in constructing vaccines against other cancers.

B. H. Thiers, MD

Perilesional Injection of r-GM-CSF in Patients With Cutaneous Melanoma Metastases

Hoeller C, Jansen B, Heere-Ress E, et al (Univ of Vienna)
J Invest Dermatol 117:371-374, 2001   21–36

Background.—Currently there is no effective treatment for melanoma metastases, and mean survival after diagnosis is only 6 months. The predominant cell types that infiltrate melanoma are lymphocytes and monocytes/macrophages. Some studies suggest that the injection of granulocyte-macrophage colony-stimulating factor (GM-CSF) can stimulate potent systemic antitumor activity. This study examined whether the perilesional intracutaneous injection of recombinant CM-CSF would have a therapeutic effect in patients with skin metastases of malignant melanoma.

Methods.—The subjects were 7 patients (5 men and 2 women; mean age, 76.4 years) with histologically proven cutaneous melanoma metastases. None of the patients had visceral metastases, but 3 had undergone lymphadenectomy because of lymph node metastases. All patients underwent two 5-day treatment cycles (separated by 21 days) of daily 400-µg injections of recombinant GM-CSF at 8 to 10 sites around 3 to 6 cutaneous lesions. All lesions (injected and noninjected) were studied histologically and immunohistochemically at baseline and after the last treatment to identify GM-CSF receptors, CD14+ monocytes/macrophages, and CD4+ and CD8+ lymphocytes. Patients were followed clinically at 6-month intervals for a mean of 59.7 months.

Results.—After 2 cycles of recombinant GM-CSF, the injected lesions decreased in size in 6 of 7 patients, and the total number of cutaneous metastases decreased in 5 of 7 patients. In one patient the size of the injected lesions did not decrease, but the number of metastases decreased by one third (from 91 to 62), indicating that recombinant GM-CSF had an effect beyond the injection site. White blood cell counts increased to 22,700 ± 8600 cells/mL during each 5-day treatment cycle, and eosinophil counts increased by 11.6% ± 4.4%. All patients tolerated treatment well, with the only side effects being mild drowsiness and local erythema at the site of injection. After a mean follow-up period of 5 years, 4 patients had died; 3 deaths were caused by progressive disease, but 1 died free of melanoma metastases at the age of 93 years. The remaining 3 patients were alive at the end of the follow-up period. One of the survivors was free of melanoma metastases and thus considered to be in complete remission. A second survivor had undergone excision of cutaneous metastases, and the third patient had undergone interferon-α therapy. Overall, the mean long-term survival after recombinant GM-CSF treatment was 33 months. Immunohistochemical analysis showed that treatment did not alter the expression of the GM-CSF receptor in cutaneous lesions. However, after treatment, staining for CD14-positive monocytes/macrophages and for CD4+ and CD8+ lymphocytes increased dramatically in both the injected and the noninjected lesions.

Conclusions.—For these patients with stage IV cutaneous melanoma metastases, intracutaneous treatment with recombinant GM-CSF reduced the size and number of lesions and was associated with a mean survival of 33 months. This survival is superior to that reported after surgical treatment alone (median survival, 15.7 months), and was not associated with adverse effects. Histologic and immunohistochemical changes in both the injected and the noninjected lesions, plus a dramatic increase in the white blood cell count during treatment, indicate a systemic effect of treatment. Thus, the perilesional injection of recombinant GM-CSF appears to augment host antimelanoma immunity and to provide a long-lasting reduction in melanoma metastases.

▶ Satellite lesions can be problematic from a management standpoint. If only a few lesions are present, these can be excised but this does not address the problem of subclinical lesions. Intralesional interferon or bacille Calmette-Guérin vaccination can be used, but the former is often ineffective and the latter can be accompanied by dissemination of the organism and systemic side effects. For lower-limb lesions, regional perfusion is often effective but carries with it considerable morbidity. The inflammatory cells that infiltrate melanoma include monocytes-macrophages, as well as lymphocytes. In certain models these monocytes-macrophages have been shown to possess antitumor activity. On the basis of these observations, the authors injected recombinant granulocyte-macrophage colony-stimulating factor (r-GM-CSF) perilesionally in 7 patients with cutaneous metastases from melanoma. Immunohistochemical analysis of the metastatic lesions revealed an increase in tumor-infiltrating lymphocytes and macrophages. Five of the 7 patients showed a response to treatment, not only locally, but also in lesions distant to the sites of injection; this suggests a systemic—as well as a local—effect. As postulated by Spitler et al[1], such a systemic effect may prolong survival, although only a controlled study can definitively answer this question.

P. G. Lang, Jr, MD

Reference

1. Spitler LE, Grossbard ML, Ernstoff MS, et al: Adjuvant therapy of stage III and IV malignant melanoma using granulocyte-macrophage colony stimulating factor. *J Clin Oncol* 18:1614-1621, 2000.

Intralesional Injection of Herpes Simplex Virus 1716 in Metastatic Melanoma
MacKie RM, Stewart B, Brown SM (Univ of Glasgow, Scotland; Glasgow Univ, Scotland)
Lancet 357:525-526, 2001   21–37

Introduction.—Melanocytes from which malignant melanomas are derived originate in fetal life from the neural crest; neurotropic viruses localize in melanoma cells. The a-virulent yet replication-competent mutant herpes simplex virus (HSV) 1716 causes cell death in human melanoma lines in vitro and selectively replicates in melanoma tissue in nude mice. This virus, which is deficient in the protein ICP34.5, has a median lethal dose of greater than 10^6 plaque-forming units (pfu) compared with 2 pfu for the parental wild-type strain 17. In spite of this reduced lethality, it replicates as efficiently as the wild-type virus in actively dividing cells. Reported are findings of a pilot investigation in which HSV1716 was intratumorally injected into subcutaneous metastatic nodules of 5 patients with pathologically confirmed stage 4 melanoma.

Methods.—All patients had disease that was not surgically resectable, including soft tissue nodules accessible to direct intratumoral injection at sites other than the face. In 2 patients, the injected nodules were excised 14 days after injection for pathologic and immunohistochemical examination. In 3 patients, a second 1-mL injection of 10^6 pfu HSV1716 was injected on day 14, and the nodule was excised on day 21. In addition, the last patient had a second set of 2 injections of 10^3 pfu HSV 2 weeks apart injected into a different nodule 8 weeks after the first series of injections, for a total of 4 injections. Fresh frozen sections from excised nodules were stained with use of ZIF11 antibody, which is specific for the 65-kd HSV DNA-binding protein.

Results.—The HSV1716 injections were well tolerated in all patients. All were seropositive for HSV before undergoing virus injection; their IgG and IgM titers did not substantially change during the trial. No patients experienced reactivation of endogenous latent HSV infection. No clinical changes were observed in the HSV-injected nodules in 4 patients. The 1 patient in whom 2 nodules were injected had a flattening in both injected nodules. No patients had evidence of regression of their tumor mass at any other adjacent or distant tumor site. Pathologic examination of the excised nodules revealed necrotic melanoma cells in the 3 patients who had 2 injections on days 1 and 14 and excision on day 21. Nodules in 2 of these patients showed necrosis adjacent to areas of apparently viable tumor cells yet no morphological evidence of damage to adjacent normal tissues. The nodule from the patient who had the second set of 2 injections 2 weeks apart had the most striking tumor cell necrosis; there were adjacent foci of free melanin. No cell death was observed in saline-injected nodules. Immunohistochemical examination of the excised HSV1716-injected nodules revealed evidence of viral replication within the limits of the tumor mass. In all 5 patients, the 65-kd HSV DNA-binding protein was observed in the melanoma cells from the virus-treated nodules, whereas no antigen staining was noted in the adjacent normal connective tissue.

Conclusion.—The findings indicate that HSV1716 replicates in melanoma cells, causes tumor-cell necrosis, and is not toxic. These encouraging results are sufficient to proceed with higher doses of HSV1716 in patients with metastatic melanoma.

▶ The findings are clearly preliminary and require additional confirmation. Another interesting approach involves insertion of HSV thymidine kinase into melanoma cells, followed by treatment with acyclovir or a similar drug that is activated by that enzyme. The activated triphosphate moiety would then bind to cellular DNA polymerase, which would terminate chromosomal replication and, hence, tumor cell division.

B. H. Thiers, MD

Long Term Response in a Patient With Neoplastic Meningitis Secondary to Melanoma Treated With ^{131}I-Radiolabeled Antichondroitin Proteoglycan Sulfate Mel-14 F(ab')$_2$: A Case Study
Cokgor I, Akabani G, Friedman HS, et al (Duke Univ, Durham, NC)
Cancer 91:1809-1813, 2001   21–38

Introduction.—Patients with neoplastic meningitis caused by malignant melanoma have a poor prognosis. In the case reported here, intrathecal administration of ^{131}I-labeled monoclonal antibody Mel-14 F(ab')$_2$ fragment has led to a long-term response.

> *Case Report.*—White woman, 46, was seen in March 1996 with progressive hearing loss, headaches, profound nausea, and vomiting. Resection of enlarged right axillary lymph nodes revealed malignant melanoma. A parenchymal brain mass and evidence of

leptomeningeal disease were revealed at MRI. Stereotactic biopsy did not confirm melanoma, but tumor cells consistent with melanoma were found in the CSF. The patient's condition deteriorated despite systemic chemotherapy, whole-brain radiotherapy, and intrathecal methotrexate. She became unable to walk and was completely deaf.

Cytology of the CSF revealed malignant tumor cells that were specifically reactive with Mel-14 F(ab')$_2$. In a phase I trial, the patient underwent intrathecal administration of ^{131}I-labeled monoclonal antibody Mel-14 F(ab')$_2$ fragment. The only treatment-related toxicity was a 1-minute seizure without neurologic sequelae. At 6-month follow-up, the patient was able to walk; 1 year after treatment, she had recovered and had normal neurologic examination results except for residual bilateral hearing loss. As of February 2001, the patient was radiographically and clinically free of disease.

Discussion.—Conventional interventions have yielded only minimal increases in survival time for patients with tumor spread to the leptomeninges. In cases of neoplastic meningitis caused by melanoma, the mean survival time ranges from 2 to 6 months. The use of the ^{131}I Mel-14 F(ab')$_2$ conjugate treatment produced a remarkable and sustained response in this patient.

▶ Cancer metastatic to the CNS portends a poor prognosis. In this case report, a patient with melanoma metastatic to the meninges was successfully treated using a novel approach—a radiolabeled antichondroitin proteoglycan sulfate (PGS) antibody. PGS is an antigen found in almost all melanoma cells; the F(ab')2 portion of the antibody was used to provide better tumor localization and a higher tumor:normal tissue ratio.

P. G. Lang, Jr, MD

Suppression of Melanoma Cell Proliferation by Histidine Decarboxylase Specific Antisense Oligonucleotides

Hegyesi H, Somlai B, Varga VL, et al (Semmelweis Univ, Budapest, Hungary; Univ of Buenos Aires, Argentina; Natl Academy of Sciences, Budapest, Hungary)
J Invest Dermatol 117:151-153, 2001   21–39

Background.—Melanoma cells, which tend to have a relatively high histamine content, express histidine decarboxylase (HDC). Expression of HDC in clinical samples from patients with melanoma was assessed.

Methods.—Thirty-five tissue samples were obtained during surgical excision from 28 patients. The samples included 3 dysplastic nevi, 20 melanomas, 5 metastatic melanoma lesions, and 10 samples from skin regions surrounding the primary cutaneous melanoma.

Findings.—Samples from the 25 patients with melanoma showed high HDC expression on Western blot analysis using a polyclonal HDC-specific antibody. Anti-HC antibody specificity was confirmed by HDC translation inhibition in melanoma cells by HDC-specific antisense oligonucleotide. The inhibition of HDC protein synthesis strongly affected the proliferation of melanoma cell lines in culture.

Conclusions.—The reduction in proliferation resulting from HDC antisense oligonucleotides highlights the functional relevance of histamine synthesis in melanoma growth. Specific antisense oligonucleotides for HDC may have an in situ application in the treatment of melanoma.

▶ Local application of antisense oligonucleotides has shown promise for the treatment of a variety of tumors in a number of preclinical studies. This research is ongoing as is investigation of the role of H_2 antagonists in the treatment of neoplasia.[1]

B. H. Thiers, MD

Reference

1. Bolton E, King J, Morris D: H_2 antagonists in the treatment of colon and breast cancer. *Semin Cancer Biol* 10:3-10, 2000.

Isolated Limb Infusion for Melanoma: A Simple Alternative to Isolated Limb Perfusion
Milan R, Henderson MA, Speakman D, et al (Bernard O'Brien Inst of Microsurgery, Fitzroy, Victoria, Australia: Univ of Melbourne, Fitzroy, Australia; Peter MacCallum Cancer Inst, East Melbourne, Victoria, Australia)
Can J Surg 44:189-192, 2001   21–40

Introduction.—When in-transit metastases (ITM) develop in patients with advanced melanoma, the ulcerating lesions cause considerable pain and functional impairment. Isolated limb perfusion (ILP), a complicated procedure usually reserved for extensive, large, or recurrent ITM, is associated with substantial morbidity and mortality. Patients in this prospective study were treated with isolated limb infusion (ILI), a safer alternative with results comparable to those achieved with ILP.

Methods.—Nine patients were treated with ILI from August 1997 to April 1999. All patients had extensive disease with multiple limb ITM and had previously been treated with a variety of modalities, including resection and radiation therapy. A second ILI was planned at 4 to 6 weeks after the initial treatment, and further treatments were considered for responding patients with recurrent or persistent disease. In the ILI protocol, anesthetized patients received melphalan 5 mg/L and actinomycin D 50 mg/L, added to 400 mL of normal saline, in a rapid, pressure infusion.

Results.—All 9 patients were treated for lower limb ITM. One patient received 3 ILIs, 2 received 2 ILIs, 2 had a second ILI planned, 2 had a complete response after their first ILI, and 2 died after their first ILI. One

TABLE 2.—Results of Isolated Limb Infusion (ILI) on 9 Patients Having Advanced Melanoma

Patient No.	No. of ILIs	Days F/U	Outcome	Complication	Toxicity
1	1	76	PR	None	II
2	1	113	PR	None	II
3	3	107	CR	None	II
4	1	75	PR/died	None	I
5	1	165	PR/died	None	II
6	1	534	CR	DVT, PE	III
7	2	45	PR	None	I
8	1	103	CR	None	I
9	2	540	CR	None	I

Patient 4 died of progressive systemic disease, patient 5 died of ischemic heart disease. Toxicity of limb perfusion is graded according to the Wieberdink Toxicity Scale.

Abbreviations: PR, Partial response, a reduction of at least 50% in either the number or total volume of ITMs (in-transit metastases); *CR,* complete response; *DVT,* deep vein thrombosis; *PE,* pulmonary embolism.

(Reprinted by permission of the publisher, *Canadian Journal of Surgery,* from Mian R, Henderson MA, Speakman S, et al: Isolated limb infusion for melanoma: A simple alternative to isolated limb perfusion. *Can J Surg* 44:189-192, 2001.)

patient had a procedure-related complication: 6 weeks after an uncomplicated ILI, a deep vein thrombosis and pulmonary embolism occurred. This patient was alive and well with limited ITM 18 months after the initial procedure. In most cases, toxicity was reported as mild or did not occur (Table 2).

Conclusion.—ILP can be an effective modality for ITM, but this procedure is expensive and has the potential for significant complications. In contrast, ILI is safe and inexpensive and provides response rates comparable to those of ILP. Isolated limb infusion was successful in this small series of patients, some of whom had other serious medical problems and had been treated previously with radiation therapy and/or chemotherapy.

▶ Isolated limb perfusion for in-transit metastases of melanoma is often effective but is associated with a significant morbidity. In this article, the authors present their experience with isolated limb infusion, a procedure that they claim is effective but carries lower morbidity.

P. G. Lang, Jr, MD

22 Lymphoproliferative Disorders

Are Alcohol Intake and Smoking Associated With Mycosis Fungoides?
A European Multicentre Case-Control Study
Morales Suárez-Varela MM, Olsen J, Kaerlev L, et al (Univ of Valencia, Spain; Dr Peset Hosp, Valencia, Spain; Univ of Aarhus, Denmark; et al)
Eur J Cancer 37:392-397, 2001   22–1

Background.—Mycosis fungoides (MF) is a rare cancer, a subgroup of cutaneous T-cell lymphoma that may develop in the presence of various risk factors (changes in Langerhans' cell-mediated cellular immune responses, viral infections, occupational exposures, or a family history of allergy or atopy). Wine consumption has been associated with a low incidence of cancers affecting the upper digestive tract. The role of wine consumption as a possibly protective factor against MF and smoking as another possible risk factor were evaluated.

Methods.—Conducted in 6 European countries as part of the European Rare Cancers Study, this was a multicenter case control study. The 76 cases of MF had been confirmed histologically; 2899 controls were chosen.

Results.—No significant association was found between smoking and MF, and wine consumption exerted no protective effect. A dose-response association was noted for alcohol intake after making an adjustment for smoking, and the odds ratio rose slightly for smoking after adjustment for alcohol intake. An increased risk for development of MF accompanied both a high consumption of alcohol (more than 24 g of alcohol per day) and a high intake of tobacco when adjustments were made for center, country, age, sex, and education level. Combining exposure to high levels of tobacco and high levels of alcohol produced a significantly increased risk for MF.

Conclusion.—Wine consumption held no protective benefit against MF; on the contrary, there was a positive association between MF and alcohol intake. Smoking did not increase the risk of MF or modify the effect of alcohol ingestion.

► Although alcohol intake and, to a lesser extent, tobacco use was associated with an increased risk for MF, a cause-and-effect relationship is far from proven. Alcohol consumption may be correlated with poor dietary habits, and it is possible that high alcohol concentrations may cause liver damage that might impair the metabolism of carcinogens. It is unlikely that alcohol is a risk factor that operates alone.

B. H. Thiers, MD

A Modified Staging Classification for Cutaneous T-Cell Lymphoma

Kashani-Sabet M, McMillan A, Zackheim HS (Univ of California, San Francisco)
J Am Acad Dermatol 45:700-706, 2001   22–2

Background.—Most cancer staging systems correspond to established models of tumor progression for a particular tumor, with survival worsening with advancing stage. This usually involves the use of a continuous measurement of tumor size or volume or an anatomic correlate of depth of tumor invasion. Most cancers are staged according to the TNM system, with the *T* stage denoting factors in the primary tumor, *N* denoting the nodal status, and *M* indicating the presence or absence of metastasis. The current method for staging cutaneous T-cell lymphomas stratifies patients

TABLE 1.—TNM and Staging Classification for CTCL
(Bunn and Lamberg)

T:Skin
T0: Clinically and/or histopathologically suspect lesions
T1: Limited plaques, papules, or eczematous patches covering <10% of the skin surface
T2: Generalized plaques, papules, or erythematous patches covering ≥10% of the skin surface
T3: Tumors (≥1)
T4: Generalized erythroderma
N: Lymph nodes
    N0: No clinically abnormal peripheral lymph nodes, pathology negative for CTCL
    N1: Clinically abnormal peripheral lymph nodes, pathology negative for CTCL
    N2: No clinically abnormal peripheral lymph nodes, pathology positive for CTCL
    N3: Clinically abnormal peripheral lymph nodes, pathology positive for CTCL
B: Peripheral blood
    B0: Atypical circulating cells not present (<5%)
    B1: Atypical circulating cells present (>5%)
M: Visceral organs
    M0: No visceral organ involvement
    M1: Visceral organ involvement
Staging

Staging	T	N	M
IA	T1	N0	M0
IB	T2	N0	M0
IIA	T1,2	N1	M0
IIB	T3	N0,1	M0
III	T4	N0,1	M0
IVA	T1-4	N2,3	M0
IVB	T1-4	N0-3	M1

(Courtesy of Kashani-Sabet M, McMillan A, Zackheim HS: A modified staging classification for cutaneous T-cell lymphoma. *J Am Acad Dermatol* 45:700-706, 2001.)

TABLE 2.—Modified TNM and Staging Classification for CTCL

T:Skin
T1: Patches and /or plaques covering <10% of the skin surface
T2a: Patches covering ≥10% of the skin surface
T2b: Plaques covering ≥10% of the skin surface
T3: Tumor stage
T4: Generalized erythroderma (80% or more of skin surface)
N: Lymph nodes
    N0: No clinically abnormal peripheral lymph nodes, pathology negative for CTCL
    N1: Clinically abnormal peripheral lymph nodes, pathology negative for CTCL
    N2: No clinically abnormal peripheral lymph nodes, pathology positive for CTCL
    N3: Clinically abnormal peripheral lymph nodes, pathology positive for CTCL
B: Peripheral blood
    B0: Atypical circulating cells not present (<5%)
    B1: Atypical circulating cells present (≥5%)
M: Visceral organs
    M0: No visceral organ involvement
    M1: Visceral organ involvement (confirmed by pathology)
Staging

Staging	T	N	M
IA	T1	N0	M0
IB	T2a	N0	M0
IIA	T1,2a	N1	M0
IIB	T2b	N0,1	M0
IIIA	T3	N0,1	M0
IIIB	T4	N0,1	M0
IVA	T1-4	N2,3	M0
IVB	T1-4	N0-3	M1

(Courtesy of Kashani-Sabet M, McMillan A, Zackheim HS: A modified staging classification for cutaneous T-cell lymphoma. *J Am Acad Dermatol* 45:700-706, 2001.)

on the basis of the extent of cutaneous involvement and the presence of tumors or erythroderma (Table 1). This study presents a modified staging scheme for cutaneous T-cell lymphoma and analyzes the survival of patients with mycosis fungoides and Sézary syndrome on the basis of the present classification scheme and the proposed modified staging system.

Methods.—Patients registered with the cutaneous lymphoma clinic of the University of California, San Francisco, the Veterans Administration Medical Center, San Francisco, or the private practice of one of the investigators were included in the study. The overall survival of 450 patients with mycosis fungoides and Sézary syndrome was determined by using the current classification and a modified staging classification (Table 2).

Results.—No significant differences were noted between the survival of patients with stage IB (patches and/or plaques involving more than 10% of body surface area [BSA]) and stage IIA (peripheral adenopathy) disease and those with stage IIB (tumor) and stage III (erythroderma) disease. However, a significant difference in survival was observed between patients with extensive patch versus extensive plaque stage disease. A modified classification that splits T2 into patch versus plaque stage disease and incorporates tumors and erythroderma into stage III was found to better predict overall survival than does the present classification.

Conclusions.—The proposed modification of the current staging system for cutaneous T-cell lymphoma provides subgroups that aid in the prognostic assessment of patients with cutaneous T-cell lymphoma.

▶ The proposed modification provides important prognostic information for patients with cutaneous T-cell lymphoma with varying degrees of skin involvement. As suggested by the authors, the incorporation of molecular techniques such as T-cell receptor gene rearrangement studies may someday further refine the staging classification.

B. H. Thiers, MD

Clinical Characteristics and Outcome of Patients With Extracutaneous Mycosis Fungoides
de Coninck EC, Kim YH, Varghese A, et al (Stanford Univ, Calif)
J Clin Oncol 19:779-784, 2001   22–3

Background.—The malignant lymphoproliferative T-cell disorder mycosis fungoides (MF) is generally characterized by its initial presentation in the skin. Usually the early stages of disease manifest as indolent, pruritic, scaly patches and plaques, with or without erythroderma. There may be progression to the cutaneous tumors with a mushroom-like appearance from which MF derives its name. Prognostic factors that are predictive of the outcome in patients with extracutaneous (stage IV) MF were identified, and the risk of progression to extracutaneous disease by initial extent of skin involvement was evaluated.

Methods.—The study group was composed of 112 patients with extracutaneous disease at presentation or with progression and 434 patients whose disease was initially cutaneous only. The Kaplan-Meier technique was used for the plotting of actuarial survival curves.

Results.—Documented nodal disease only was found in 78 of the 112 patients, whereas the remaining 34 patients had evidence of visceral involvement. The median length of survival for all stage IV patients from the date of first treatment for stage IV disease was 13 months. No significant effect on survival outcome was noted for sex, age, race, extent of skin involvement, and peripheral blood Sézary cell involvement. A complete response to therapy was experienced by 11 patients (10%), which resulted in a significantly improved median survival compared with patients with a partial or no response. The risk for progression to extracutaneous disease by initial extent of skin involvement at 20 years from diagnosis was 0% for limited patch/plaque, 10% for generalized patch/plaque, 35.5% for tumorous disease, and 41% for erythrodermic involvement.

Conclusions.—This was a larger-scale investigation of extracutaneous MF than has been performed previously. It was found that the prognostic factors that are important in the cutaneous stages of the disease are no longer of significance once extracutaneous disease has developed. It is possible that patients in this study who experienced a more favorable response to therapy may have had disease that was biologically less aggressive than that of other patients. The risk of development of stage IV MF was found to be highest in patients who present with tumorous or erythrodermic skin disease, whereas patients with limited skin involvement had the lowest risk of having stage IV MF develop.

▶ In this series, the risk of extracutaneous disease developing was highest in patients with tumors or erythroderma and lowest in patients with limited skin involvement. Once extracutaneous disease develops, prognostic factors important in the earlier stages of the disease (eg, the nature and extent of skin involvement) are no longer relevant to overall survival.

B. H. Thiers, MD

Phase 2 and 3 Clinical Trial of Oral Bexarotene (Targretin Capsules) for the Treatment of Refractory or Persistent Early-Stage Cutaneous T-Cell Lymphoma

Duvic M, for the Worldwide Bexarotene Study Group (M. D. Anderson Cancer Ctr, Houston; et al)

Arch Dermatol 137:581-593, 2001   22–4

Background.—A phase 1 study suggested that bexarotene (Targretin capsules; Ligand Pharmaceuticals, Inc, San Diego, Calif), a selective antagonist of retinoid X receptors (RXR), may be effective in treating cutaneous T-cell lymphoma (CTCL). A phase 2 and phase 3 clinical trial was undertaken to examine the effectiveness and safety of oral bexarotene in patients with early stage refractory or persistent CTCL, and the results were reported.

Methods.—The subjects were 58 adults (40 men and 18 women; median age, 64 years) who had biopsy-proven early (stage IA through IIA) CTCL. In each case, either patients could not tolerate prior treatments (primarily topical nitrogen mustard, topical corticosteroids, or carmustine therapy), their disease did not respond to prior therapies, or their response to 2 or more previous therapies had reached at least a 6-month plateau. Patients were randomly assigned to daily oral therapy with either 6.5 mg/m^2 bexarotene (low-dose group; n = 15), 500 to 650 mg/m^2 bexarotene (high-dose group; n = 15), or 300 mg/m^2 bexarotene (optimal-dose group, n = 28). Patients in the low-dose group could cross over to one of the higher-dose groups if their symptoms progressed after 8 weeks of therapy or if they failed to respond after 16 weeks of therapy. The primary end point was the overall response rate (ie, >50% improvement) according to the Physician's Global Assessment of Clinical Condition or the Composite Assessment of Index Lesions Severity scales. Secondary end points included body surface area (BSA) involvement and duration of response.

Results.—Responses occurred in 20% of the patients (3 of 15) in the low-dose group, 54% of the patients (15 of 28) in the optimal-dose group, and 67% of the patients (10 of 15) in the high-dose group. No influence of age, sex, or race on response was evident. Among patients who remained at the same dosage level, disease progression rates were 47% in the low-dose group, 21% in the optimal-dose group, and 13% in the high-dose group. Of the 15 patients in the low-dose group, 11 crossed over to 1 of the other 2 groups. After crossover, 8 of the 11 (73) responded. BSA involvement in all 3 groups improved over time (up to 50 weeks of therapy), decreasing from median baseline values of 20% to 40% to less than 5% in each group. The median duration of response in the higher-dose groups was 516 days. All but 1 patient experienced adverse effects (mostly mild to moderate in severity), and adverse effects increased in number and severity as the dosage of bexarotene increased. The most common adverse effects were hypertriglyceridemia (46 patients, or 79%), hypercholesterolemia (28 patients, or 48%), headache (27 patients, or 47%), central hypothyroidism (23 patients, or 40%), asthenia (21 patients, or 36%), and leukopenia (16 patients, or 28%). In addition, pancreatitis developed in 3 patients in the higher-dose groups with elevated triglyceride levels ($\geq$1300 mg/dL); all 3 recovered. There were no cases of drug-related neutropenic fever or sepsis, and no patient died of adverse effects during or within 4 weeks of discontinuing bexarotene therapy.

Conclusions.—At daily dosages of 300 mg/m^2 (the optimum-dose group), oral bexarotene was effective in treating refractory or persistent early stage CTCL in 54% of the patients. Hypertriglyceridemia and hypothyroidism were common but were reversible with drug therapy. Overall, bexarotene was effective and safe and provided a durable response in these patients.

▶ Bexarotene, the first RXR-selective rexinoid, is currently approved for the treatment of CTCL. Available retinoid A receptor (RAR)-selective retinoids are used most often to treat acne (isotretinoin) and psoriasis (acitretin), although both drugs have been used "off label" to treat CTCL as well. No data exist on the comparative efficacy and tolerability of the rexinoids and retinoids in the treatment of CTCL. Their toxicities are somewhat different, although hyperlipidemia and headache characterize both groups of drugs. RAR agonist symptoms include cheilitis, alopecia, arthritis, and myalgias. Patients treated with bexarotene may quickly develop reversible central hypothyroidism, manifested by suppressed TSH production and low thyroxine levels[1]; thyroid hormone replacement therapy was necessary in 40% of the patients reported in this study. The hypothyroidism may contribute to the hyperlipidemia seen in these patients, which may be more frequent and more severe than that noted with isotretinoin or acitretin. However, the relatively advanced age of the patients reported by Duvic et al may have predisposed them to increased lipid levels.

B. H. Thiers, MD

Reference

1. Sherman SI, Gopal J, Haugen BR, et al: Central hypothyroidism associated with retinoid X receptor-selective ligands. *N Engl J Med* 340:1075-1079, 1999.

Photodynamic Therapy With Topical 5-Aminolevulinic Acid for Mycosis Fungoides: Clinical and Histological Response

Edström DW, Porwit A, Ros A-M (Karolinska Hosp, Stockholm)
Acta Derm Venereol 81:184-188, 2001   22–5

Background.—Mycosis fungoides (MF) is the most common primary cutaneous T-cell lymphoma. No cure for MF has been reported to date. The response of single lesions to photodynamic therapy (PDT) was investigated.

Methods.—Ten plaque MF lesions and 2 tumor MF lesions in 10 patients were treated. After the topical application of 20% 5-aminolevulinic acid to the lesion and adjacent skin for 5 to 6 hours, the lesion was exposed to red light at about 630 nm. Skin biopsies were performed before treatment, after clinical improvement, and again after clinical remission.

Findings.—Of 9 plaque lesions that could be evaluated, 7 completely cleared. The tenth patient discontinued treatment because of pain. PDT, however, did not resolve either of the tumors (Fig 1; see color plate XIX). Biopsy specimens confirmed infiltrate regression after treatment. A few CD4+ and CD8+ cells were found in the sparse remaining infiltrate. Most of these cells showed normal bcl-2. In addition, fewer proliferating cells were present, as evidenced by a decline in Ki-67 and CD71 positivity.

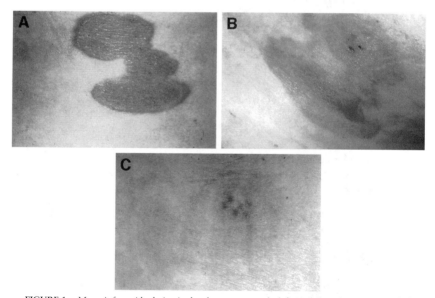

FIGURE 1.—Mycosis fungoides lesion in the plaque stage on the left trunk in patient No. 9: (**A**) before photodynamic therapy; (**B**) after 2 treatments; and (**C**) 2 weeks after completed treatment, with scars from biopsies. (Courtesy of Edstrom DW, Porwit A, Ros A-M: Photodynamic therapy with topical 5-aminolevulinic acid for mycosis fungoides: Clinical and histological response. *Acta Derm Venereol* 81:184-188, 2001.)

Conclusions.—Treatment of plaque-stage MF with PDT yields good clinical and histologic results. Most patients respond after 2 or 3 treatments.

▶ These results are encouraging but need to be confirmed by a larger, controlled study.

B. H. Thiers, MD

"High-Dose" UVA1 Therapy of Widespread Plaque-Type, Nodular, and Erythrodermic Mycosis Fungoides
Zane C, Leali C, Airò P, et al (Azienda Spedali Civili di Brescia, Italy; Univ of Brescia, Italy)
J Am Acad Dermatol 44:629-633, 2001   22–6

Background.—The clinical course of mycosis fungoides (MF) progresses slowly over years, offering ample opportunity for therapeutic interventions. Standard treatment for early stages of MF involves the use of photochemotherapy with methoxsalen along with ultraviolet A (UVA) exposure (PUVA therapy). Adverse effects may limit the effectiveness of PUVA therapy, so UVA1 (340 to 400 nm) phototherapy has been proposed as an alternative without the risks associated with the use of psoralens. The safety and efficacy of UVA1 radiation for treating widespread plaque-type, nodular, and erythrodermic MF lesions were evaluated. Changes in skin infiltrating and circulating lymphocytes induced by the UVA1 therapy were also noted.

Methods.—Six men and 7 women who had biopsy-proven MF (8 patients with stage IB, 4 with stage IIB, and 1 with stage III MF) were given 100 J/cm^2 UVA1 for 5 days each week until the lesions were in remission (complete clearing or partial improvement with no further amelioration). Four patients had lesions inaccessible to UVA1 therapy (perineocrural area, internatal cleft, and armpits), and these were considered control lesions. The UVA1 was delivered using a Dermalight UltrA1-24KW irradiation unit (Hönle GmbH, Martinsried, Germany). Before therapy began and after its completion, results were assessed by means of immunocytologic studies of skin infiltrates and circulating T-cell.

Results.—Complete response at both the clinical and the histologic level occurred in 11 patients. Partial improvement was achieved in 2 patients (1 with stage IB and 1 with stage IIB lesions). The cumulative doses of UVA1 were 2148.5 ±752.1 J/cm^2. There was no clearing of the unirradiated control lesions. Before treatment, immunocytochemical studies revealed infiltrates consistent with MF that were heavily populated by cells of the CD2+, CD3+, CD4+, CD5+, CD45RO+, CD7−, or CD8− immunophenotype. These were not found in the lesions of patients resistant to treatment. A significant reduction in the T lymphocytes of immunophenotypes CD4+/CD45RO+ and CD4+/CD95+ was found after high-dose UVA1 therapy. Follow-up extended for just over 7 months after phototherapy was discontinued, with remission maintained in 7 patients and relapse in 4, all of whom responded to a second course of UVA1.

Conclusion.—Advanced MF appears to respond well to high-dose UVA1 therapy with none of the drug intolerance or excessive erythema that often characterizes PUVA therapy. It is encouraging that patients who suffered relapses did respond to a second course of UVA1. The effects on circulating lymphocytes could not be established, since nonirradiated lesions did not respond.

▶ The excellent results of this study require confirmation in a larger group of subjects. Still unknown is the sustainability of the clinical response and the long-term side effects of this therapy.

B. H. Thiers, MD

Treatment of Stage II Cutaneous T-Cell Lymphoma With Interferon Alfa-2a and Extracorporeal Photochemotherapy: A Prospective Controlled Trial

Wollina U, Looks A, Meyer J, et al (Friedrich-Schiller Univ, Jena, Germany; Waldklinikum Gera, Germany; Heinrich-Braun-Klinikum Zwickau, Germany; et al)

J Am Acad Dermatol 44:253-260, 2001   22–7

Background.—The treatment of early stages of cutaneous T-cell lymphoma (CTCL) can be aggressive and produce a rapid response, but the long-term disease-free period is unaffected. Treatment options currently used include total electron beam radiation, topical chemotherapy, phototherapy, photochemotherapy, extracorporeal photochemotherapy (ECP), and systemic chemotherapy or chemoimmune therapy. Response rates using ECP for the Sézary syndrome are especially high (50% to 88%). This study evaluated the use of ECP along with interferon-α (IFN-α) to treat patients with stage II CTCL to assess whether combination therapy offers improved efficacy and safety.

Methods.—Three patients with histologically proven stage IIb CTCL received ECP plus IFN-α before the study began. Fourteen men (age range, 38 to 72 years) had CTCL of the mycosis fungoides type and were in stage IIa or IIb; one 72-year-old man had Ki-1 lymphoma. All received treatment with ECP (on 2 consecutive days) twice a month for 6 months combined with subcutaneous IFN-α2a (three times a week at the maximum dosage tolerated). Oral 8-methoxypsoralen was used as the photosensitizer. Skin biopsy was performed after 6 months and 12 months of therapy, and patients were checked for evidence of toxic reactions monthly. Histologic examinations were carried out at baseline, after 6 months of therapy, and again after 12 months of treatment. Staging was redone after 6 months, with further treatment individualized, based on the results.

Results.—A complete response was seen in 4 patients after 6 months. Three had a partial response, and 7 had stable disease. The time to best response for those who responded was 4.3 months. A decrease in mean skin score occurred, falling from 22.5 to 15.1; the histologic score fell from 2.57 to 1.21. A decline from 75% to 51% was noted in the percentage of CD4 cells in skin lesions. The percentage of cells positive for Ki-67 declined from 6.7% to 2.4%. The total T-cell count per microliter decreased from 1018.9 to 667.9. The ratio of CD4 to CD8 also declined from 1.88 to 1.51. No significant changes were found in the sIL-2R levels over the first 4 months of treatment. Only 25% of those who had stage IIb disease responded, whereas 60% of those with stage IIa did so. No additional therapy was needed, but the dose of interferon was decreased because of side effects. One year after discontinuation of therapy, the total response rate was 46.2%. Of the 6 patients responding, 5 (of 9) had stage IIa disease and 1 (of 4) had stage IIb disease.

Conclusion.—The combination of ECP and IFN-α2a was found to be effective for patients with stage IIa CTCL and of some value for patients with stage IIb disease. The time to best response averaged 4 months. Side effects were minimal.

▶ Unfortunately, no controlled trial has been published assessing the benefits of IFN-α as an adjunct to ECP; benefits of the combination are suggested mainly from previously published uncontrolled observations.[1,2] More data are clearly needed, including an assessment of the durability of the clinical response and the effect of this treatment regimen on prognosis.

B. H. Thiers, MD

References

1. Gottlieb SL, Wolfe JT, Fox FE, et al: Treatment of cutaneous T-cell lymphoma with extracorporeal photopheresis monotherapy and in combination with recombinant interferon alfa: A 10-year experience at a single institution. *J Am Acad Dermatol* 35:946-957, 1996.
2. Dippel E, Schrag H, Goerdt S, et al: Extracorporeal photopheresis and interferon-α in advanced T-cell lymphoma. *Lancet* 350:32-33, 1997.

Pivotal Phase III Trial of Two Dose Levels of Denileukin Diftitox for the Treatment of Cutaneous T-Cell Lymphoma
Olsen E, Duvic M, Frankel A, et al (Duke Univ, Durham, NC; Univ Texas, Houston; Univ of Texas, San Antonio; et al)
J Clin Oncol 19:376-388, 2001   22–8

Background.—Denileukin diftitox ($DAB_{389}IL-2$) is a novel recombinant fusion protein that consists of peptide sequences for the enzymatically active and membrane translocation domains of diphtheria toxin and human interleukin (IL)-2. The safety, efficacy, and pharmacokinetics of $DAB_{389}IL-2$ therapy were evaluated in patients with stage Ib to IVa cutaneous T-cell lymphoma (CTCL) who had previously received other therapeutic interventions.

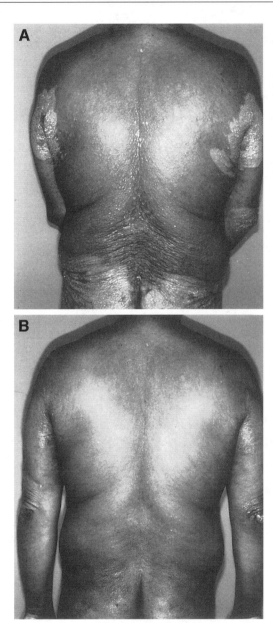

FIGURE 1.—A 44-year-old man with stage Ib cutaneous T-cell lymphoma who completed 17 courses of DAB$_{389}$IL-2. At the end of treatment, he had a partial remission but went on to a complete response off therapy and remains in remission 18 months off treatment. **A,** Baseline, pretreatment; **B,** status after 10 cycles of DAB$_{389}$IL-2. (Courtesy of Olsen E, Duvic M, Frankel A, et al: Pivotal phase III trial of two dose levels of denileukin diftitox for the treatment of cutaneous T-cell lymphoma. *J Clin Oncol* 19:376-388, 2001.)

Methods.—Patients in this phase III study had biopsy-proven CTCL that expressed the IL-2 receptor protein CD25 on 20% or more of lymphocytes. They were assigned to 1 of 2 dose levels (either 9 or 18 µg/kg/day) of $DAB_{389}IL$-2 administered for 5 consecutive days every 3 weeks for up to 8 cycles. The patients were monitored for toxicity and clinical efficacy. Clinical efficacy was assessed by measurements of changes in disease burden and quality of life. Also measured were antibody levels of antide-nileukin diftitox and anti–interleukin-2 and serum concentrations of $DAB_{389}IL$-2. A total of 71 patients were included in the trial.

Results.—Overall, 30% of the patients with CTCL treated with $DAB_{389}IL$-2 had an objective response. A complete response was experienced by 10% of the patients, and 20% of the patients had a partial response (Fig 1; see color plate XX). There was no statistically significant difference between the 2 doses in the response rate and duration of response based on the time of the first dose of study drug for all responders. Adverse effects noted were flu-like symptoms, acute infusion-related events, and a vascular leak syndrome. Transient elevations of hepatic transaminase levels occurred in 61% of the patients, with 17% experiencing grade 3 or 4 changes. Hypoalbuminemia was experienced by 79% of the patients, including 15% who experienced grade 3 or 4 changes. There was similar tolerability at 9 and 18 µg/kg/day, with no evidence of cumulative toxicity.

Conclusions.—Denileukin diftitox was shown to be a useful and important agent in the treatment of patients whose CTCL is persistent or recurrent, even after other therapeutic interventions.

▶ Despite its significant toxicities, denileukin diftitox can be remarkably effective in a small, carefully chosen group of CTCL patients recalcitrant to other therapies. It is unlikely that CD25 is an adequate screen for predicting response to the drug. Immunhistochemical findings of biopsy specimens taken from different sites are often conflicting, and the results may vary as the disease evolves. Better methods of patient selection are sorely needed.

B. H. Thiers, MD

Transmission of a T-Cell Lymphoma by Allogeneic Bone Marrow Transplantation
Berg KD, Brinster NK, Huhn KM, et al (Johns Hopkins School of Medicine, Baltimore, Md; Geisinger Med Ctr, Danville, Pa)
N Engl J Med 345:1458-1463, 2001   22–9

Background.—This case report described the transmission of a subcutaneous panniculitic lymphoma through bone marrow transplantation.

> *Case Report.*—Woman, 19, was seen in 1993 with stage IVB anaplastic large-cell lymphoma of T-cell lineage (Ki-1 lymphoma). She received chemotherapy and achieved complete remission. Lym-

phomatous meningitis developed and, after conditioning, the patient received a T-cell depleted bone marrow transplant from her HLA-identical sister and again achieved remission. Three and a half years after transplantation, the donor was seen with eczematous dermatitis on her legs, a nodule on her arm, and fever. Biopsy of the nodule revealed lobular lymphocytic panniculitis with perivascular lymphocytes. There was a dense lobular subcutaneous infiltrate of pleomorphic, atypical lymphocytes surrounding the adipocytes. The atypical cells were positive for CD3+, CD8+, granzyme B+ and TIA-1+. They were negative for CD56 and CD20. The infiltrate contained a monoclonal population of T cells with rearranged TCRγ genes. Specimens were negative for both Epstein-Barr virus and human T-cell lymphotropic virus type I. Despite treatment, the donor died 2 years after presentation.

One month before her sister's death, the recipient was seen with a 1-year history of skin lesions with persistent nodules on her legs. Histologic examination revealed a subcutaneous panniculitic T-cell lymphoma with atypical T cells. These cells had the same markers and contained the same monoclonal TCRγ rearrangement. The discovery of an identical type of tumor in these 2 sisters suggested that the lymphoma had been transmitted from the apparently healthy donor to the recipient during bone marrow transplantation. The recipient also died 7.5 years after the transplant.

Conclusion.—This case report describes the transmission of a subcutaneous panniculitic T-cell lymphoma during bone marrow transplantation. As the incidence of transplantation increases, such cases may also increase. The development of sensitive screening assays for neoplastic cells or the transplantation of purified stem cells may be necessary to avoid cases of tumor transfer during transplantation.

▶ The authors used elegant immunohistochemical and molecular techniques to document transmission of T-cell lymphoma from one sister to another during bone marrow transplantation. The recipient originally had an anaplastic large-cell lymphoma, whereas the donor had subcutaneous panniculitic T-cell lymphoma. There was no evidence for a common genetic or infectious cause for these 2 conditions, and tests of the bone marrow recipient for Epstein-Barr virus and human T-cell lymphotrophic virus type I—which have been associated with familial lymphoma syndromes—were negative. As noted by the authors, with increasing age and a corresponding increase in the frequency of occult neoplasms in older donors, the likelihood of transfer of a malignancy during transplantation may increase. To prevent such transfers may require the development of more sensitive screening assays for neoplastic cells or the transplantation of highly purified stem cells.

B. H. Thiers, MD

23 Vascular Malformations

A Unique Microvascular Phenotype Shared by Juvenile Hemangiomas and Human Placenta
North PE, Waner M, Mizeracki A, et al (Univ of Arkansas, Little Rock; Harvard Univ, Boston)
Arch Dermatol 137:559-570, 2001   23–1

Background.—Juvenile hemangiomas, ranging from small and harmless to large and deforming, are the most common tumors of childhood, affecting 10% of children. Hemangiomas develop within weeks of birth or are congenital, proliferate quickly, and involute spontaneously, although some remain disfiguring. Juvenile hemangiomas express the erythrocyte-type glucose transporter protein GLUT1 at all stages. Although it is undetectable on immunohistochemical assessment of normal skin and subcutaneous vessels, normal endothelia express GLUT1 at blood-tissue barriers, such as those of the brain, eye, nerve, and placenta. The capillaries of juvenile hemangiomas share a distinct immunophenotype with placental fetal microvessels, possibly leading to other similarities between hemangiomas and placental vessels. The existence and nature of other possible similarities was investigated in a retrospective study.

Methods.—The patients (age, 22 days to 7 years) were chosen from those who had vascular lesions excised at Arkansas Children's Hospital of Little Rock between 1997 and 1999 and for whom frozen and paraffin-embedded tissue samples were available (111 cases). Twenty-eight additional vascular lesions, including 14 angiosarcomas, were also included. Placental samples were taken within 30 minutes of delivery from the central villus parenchyma. Immunohistochemical analysis of the cryosections was performed, and immunoreactivities were scored blindly as none, weak, moderate, or intense. Electron microscopic analysis was performed.

Results.—The gender and site distributions of patients with proliferative involutive phase hemangiomas were similar to those in larger epidemiologic studies. In addition, the age range for patients with other vascular lesions (except angiosarcoma) overlapped that for patients with hemangiomas. Normal brain, placental chorionic villi, and placental trophoblasts showed specific microvascular GLUT1 immunoreaction; normal skin and subcutis, granulation tissues, and the neovasculature of nonvascular malignant tumors did not show such an immunoreaction. All juvenile hemangiomas had intensive microvascular, entirely endothelial GLUT1 immunoreactivity. None of the vascular malformations, pyogenic granulomas, tufted angiomas, or hemangioendotheliomas expressed lesional GLUT1. Five of the 14 angiosarcomas had a weak-to-moderate focal GLUT1 reactivity. Intense endothelial immunoreactivity was seen in placental intravillous fetal capillaries. All 66 juvenile hemangiomas had marked lesional endothelial immunoreactivity for FcγRII and Lewis Y antigen (LeY) that appeared in a diffuse granular cytoplasmic-membranous pattern resembling that of the placenta. Adjacent native dermal capillaries, arterioles, or arteries did not show such immunoreactivity, nor was it present in vascular malformations, pyogenic granulomas, granulation tissue, or tumor neovasculature. Only weak-to-moderate LeY immunoreactivity was shown in 2 of 7 epithelioid hemangioendotheliomas and 5 of 14 angiosarcomas; this was absent in tufted angiomas and a kaposiform hemangioendothelioma.

Conclusions.—Four functionally unrelated but shared markers of cellular specialization were noted between juvenile hemangioma and placental fetal microvessels, suggesting that these are linked. Two possible pathogenic mechanisms may account for these findings. Hemangiomas may originate from invading angioblasts that differentiate aberrantly, moving toward the phenotype of placental microvasculature in the mesenchyme of skin and subcutis, or they may originate from embolized placental cells.

▶ The authors report that 4 functionally unrelated markers of cellular specialization are expressed in both the fetal microvessels of human placenta and in juvenile hemangiomas but not in vascular lesions, such as vascular malformations, pyogenic granulomas, or granulation tissue. This suggests that hemangiomas may originate from placental chorionic villi. The pathogenic mechanism for development is uncertain. The increased incidence of hemangioma development after chorionic villus sampling suggests embolization of placental cells as a possible mechanism.

S. Raimer, MD

Congenital Nonprogressive Hemangioma: A Distinct Clinicopathologic Entity Unlike Infantile Hemangioma
North PE, Waner M, James CA, et al (Univ of Arkansas, Little Rock; Univ of California, San Francisco; Harvard Univ, Boston)
Arch Dermatol 137:1607-1620, 2001   23–2

Background.—Infantile hemangioma is a commonly occurring tumor that is characterized by perinatal presentation, rapid growth in the first year of life, and subsequent involution. This tumor is also distinctive for its expression of a unique immunophenotype that is shared by placental microvessels. The congenital nonprogressive hemangioma differs from the classic form in that it presents fully formed at birth and follows a static or rapidly involuting course. It has been assumed that this congenitally fully formed lesion is a clinical variant of the typical postnatal hemangioma; however, this assumption has not previously been tested. The histologic and immunohistochemical features of congenital nonprogressive hemangioma were compared with those of the typical postnatally proliferating hemangioma.

Methods.—All cellular vascular tumors resected from infants under age 4 months at a university-affiliated pediatric hospital over the past 20 years were characterized histologically and immunohistochemically before clinical characterization by chart review. A total of 43 lesions from 36 patients were included in the study. The hemangiomas were evaluated for histologic appearance, immunoreactivity for antigens GLUT1 and LeY, and clinical behavior.

Results.—There were differences in the histologic appearance and immunohistochemical profile of congenital nonprogressive hemangiomas in comparison with postnatally proliferating infantile hemangiomas. The congenital nonprogressive hemangiomas had lobules of capillaries within densely fibrotic stroma containing hemosiderin deposits and exhibited focal lobular thrombosis and sclerosis. There was a frequent association with multiple thin-walled vessels in the congenital nonprogressive hemangiomas, as well as an absence of "intermingling" of the neovasculature with normal tissue elements. In addition, the congenital nonprogressive hemangiomas demonstrated a lack of immunoreactivity to GLUT1 and LeY.

Conclusions.—The congenital nonprogressive hemangioma is histologically and immunophenotypically distinct from the classically presenting hemangioma of infancy and likely of different pathogenesis.

▶ The authors offer convincing evidence that the lesions described in this article and referred to as congenital nonprogressive hemangiomas represent a distinct clinical entity. As the name would suggest, these lesions are present at birth and do not appear to progress thereafter. Unfortunately, all 6 lesions described in this paper were completely excised, so it is not known whether spontaneous resolution of the lesions would have occurred. As is mentioned by the authors, there are descriptions in the literature of rare fully formed hemangiomas that are present at birth. Some of these lesions have been reported to involute at a much more rapid pace than is typical of classic infantile hemangiomas. Rogers et al[1] recently reported a series of 10 infants with what has been referred to as rapidly involuting congenital hemangiomas, which likely represents the same entity as congenital nonprogressive hemangiomas. The clinical presentation was nearly identical to that described above, and all 10 infants had very similar sonographic findings that differed from infantile hemangiomas and also enabled separation from other entities such as fibrosarcoma, malignant hemangiopericytoma, and dermatofibrosarcoma protuberans, each of which might present at birth as large, firm, purple tumors or plaques. In the series of Rogers et al, resolution began by age 8 weeks and was generally complete by age 12 months. It would therefore appear that a 2- to 3-month observation period for initiation of resolution represents appropriate management for congenital hemangiomas with clinical and sonographic features typical of rapidly involuting congenital hemangiomas.

S. Raimer, MD

Reference

1. Rogers M, Lam A, Fischer G: Sonographic findings in a series of rapidly involuting congenital hemangiomas (RICH). *Pediatr Dermatol* 19:5-11, 2002.

Oral Corticosteroid Use Is Effective for Cutaneous Hemangiomas: An Evidence-Based Evaluation

Bennett MI, Fleischer AB Jr, Chamlin SL, et al (Wake Forest Univ, Winston-Salem, NC; Univ of California-San Francisco)
Arch Dermatol 137:1208-1213, 2001   23–3

Background.—Hemangiomas are the most common of childhood tumors. They do not require treatment unless they interfere with normal functioning. The primary treatment for cutaneous hemangiomas of infancy is corticosteroid therapy, but there is significant variation to the dosage recommendations, duration of treatment, recommendations for follow up, and tapering methods. This study was performed as a meta-analysis of the efficacy of systemic corticosteroid therapy in the treatment of enlarging, problematic cutaneous hemangiomas and evaluation of the relationship of dose to response and incidence of adverse effects.

Methods.—A quantitative, systematic literature review was performed on the basis of a search of the PubMed and MEDLINE databases for articles on the combined topics of hemangiomas and corticosteroids. Studies included in this review were original case series with at least 5 patients age 2 years or under with enlarging, problematic cutaneous hemangiomas treated with systemic corticosteroids. A total of 10 case series comprising 184 patients were included in the final analysis. The mean age of patients at the initiation of systemic corticosteroid administration was 4.5 months. Patients received a mean prednisone equivalent daily dose of 2.0 mg/kg for a mean of 1.8 months. The main outcome measures were response and rebound rates and dose-response and adverse effects–response relationships in responders versus nonresponders.

Results.—The overall response rate was 84%, whereas the rebound rate was 36%. There was a significant difference between the mean dose administered to responders and the mean dose administered to nonresponders. However, there was no significant difference in the occurrence of adverse effects. Overall, adverse effects were reported in 35% of patients; however, none of the reported patients experienced catastrophic adverse effects. Serious temporary growth retardation was reported in four patients. The most commonly reported adverse effects were behavior changes and irritability, cushingoid appearance, and temporary growth retardation. On multivariate analysis, the only significant factor associated with clinical response was the prednisone equivalent dose.

Conclusions.—These findings would appear to indicate that systemic corticosteroid therapy is an effective treatment for infants with problematic cutaneous hemangiomas.

▶ Systemic corticosteroids are the treatment of choice for problematic hemangiomas of infancy. This study was a quantitative systemic review of cutaneous lesions in children younger than 2 years; it was designed to help determine the optimal dosage of corticosteroids and the duration of therapy. The analysis indicated that between 2 to 3 mg/kg per day of prednisone appeared to be the most appropriate initial dosage. Dosages less than 2 mg/kg per day were less effective and those greater than 3 mg/kg per day had a higher incidence of side effects. The mean duration of treatment in these studies was 1.8 months before the corticosteroids were tapered. Hemangiomas treated with very short treatment regimens (eg, 2-3 weeks before tapering was initiated) were more likely to rebound. The speed at which corticosteroids should be tapered has not been determined.

S. Raimer, MD

High Injection Pressure During Intralesional Injection of Corticosteroids Into Capillary Hemangiomas
Egbert JE, Paul S, Engel WK, et al (Univ of Minnesota, Minneapolis)
Arch Ophthalmol 119:677-683, 2001   23–4

Background.—Intralesional corticosteroid injection is an effective treatment for a variety of benign and malignant proliferative lesions of the head and neck. However, such treatment can result in ocular embolization with permanent vision loss. It is thought that the ocular embolization results from retrograde flow of injected drug from the target tissue into the ophthalmic artery proximal to the central retinal artery. Retrograde flow is only possible if the injection pressure of corticosteroid exceeds the systemic arterial pressure. The authors of this study have designed a custom device that facilitates the simultaneous measurement of injection pressure and volume during intralesional injection of medications. This device was used to investigate the mechanism responsible for ocular embolization during intralesional injection of corticosteroids into capillary hemangiomas.

Methods.—The participants included 3 fellowship-trained pediatric ophthalmologists and 4 patients. The patients underwent 5 separate treatment sessions of an intralesional injection of a 50/50 mixture of triamcinolone diacetate (40 mg/mL) and betamethasone sodium phosphate and betamethasone acetate (6 mg/mL) into capillary hemangiomas. The specially designed cannula was used to monitor injection pressures during the procedure. Maximum and mean pressure and volume of corticosteroid were measured for each injection.

Results.—A total of 71 injections were performed, and in 63 of these injections the maximum pressure exceeded 100 mm Hg. The total volume of corticosteroid delivered ranged from 0.9 to 2.1 mL. Each surgeon produced injection pressures that were greater than the systemic arterial pressures of each patient.

Conclusions.—Injection pressures during intralesional injection of corticosteroids into capillary hemangiomas routinely exceed the systemic arterial pressures of patients. The experienced surgeons in this report were unable to prevent this occurrence. This mechanism would account for the embolization of corticosteroid particles into the ocular circulation from retrograde arterial flow. It is recommended that the volume of corticosteroid be limited and that indirect ophthalmoscopy be performed on all patients who receive injection of long-acting corticosteroids into capillary hemangiomas.

▶ Because most physicians avoid intra-arterial injection by aspiration before injection and by limiting the volume of steroids delivered per injection, ocular embolization occurs only rarely. Nevertheless, as demonstrated by this article, high injection pressures may increase the risk of retrograde flow and possible ocular embolization. The authors recommend indirect ophthalmoscopy during or after injection into the orbit or periorbital soft tissue. This would allow the physician to immediately diagnose and treat this rare but serious complication. Because dermatologists are not trained to treat the complications of ocular embolization, intralesional steroid injections into periocular hemangiomas are probably best performed by ophthalmologists.

S. Raimer, MD

Cryogen Spray Cooling and Pulsed Dye Laser Treatment of Cutaneous Hemangiomas
Chang C-J, Kelly KM, Nelson JS (Chang Gung Univ, Taipei, Taiwan; Univ of California, Irvine)
Ann Plast Surg 46:577-583, 2001   23–5

Introduction.—Hemangiomas that fail to resolve spontaneously are treated with a variety of modalities, including carbon dioxide snow, liquid nitrogen, radiation, steroids, and surgery. Laser treatment has been successful but carries a risk of thermally induced damage to the epidermis and papillary dermis. Skin cooling, however, can minimize epidermal injury. Cryogen spray cooling plus laser treatment (CSC-LT) was compared for safety and efficacy with noncooled laser treatment (NC-LT) in a large series of patients with cutaneous hemangiomas.

Methods.—The retrospective review included 164 patients treated over an 8-year period. The average patient age at treatment was 2 years 11 months. Laser treatment was administered for a mean of 24 months. Eighty patients received NC-LT using light doses of 5.5 to 8 J/cm^2. Subsequently, the remaining 82 patients underwent CSC-LT using light doses

TABLE 2.—Number of Pulsed Dye Laser Treatments in 164 Patients With
Cutaneous Hemangiomas

Group	No. of Treatments						Total
	1	2	3	4	5	6	
NC-LT, N (%)	30 (36.59)	21 (25.61)	18 (21.95)	5 (6.10)	8 (9.76)	0 (0)	82 (100)
CSC-LT, N (%)	63 (76.83)	15 (18.29)	2 (2.44)	1 (1.22)	0 (0)	1 (1.22)	82 (100)
No. of patients	93	36	20	6	8	1	164

Note: $\chi^2 = 37.176$, $P = .001$.
Abbreviations: NC-LT, Noncooled laser treatment; CSC-LT, cryogen spray cooling and laser treatment.
(Courtesy of Chang C-J, Kelly KM, Nelson JS: Cryogen spray cooling and pulsed dye laser treatment of cutaneous hemangiomas. *Ann Plast Surg* 46(6):577-583, 2001.)

of 9 to 10 J/cm². Patients were monitored for adverse effects and followed for at least 1 year for improvements in lesional volume, texture, and color.

Results.—The majority of hemangiomas (74.3%) were located on the head and neck. Average volumes of the lesions were 14.5 cm² for the NC-LT group and 16.0 cm² for the CSC-LT group. In 16 patients, the lesions involved obstruction of orifices. Significantly more pulsed dye laser (PDL) treatments were needed in the NC-LT group (2.27 vs 1.33), indicating that improvement was greater in the CSC-LT group (Table 2). All patients achieved good or excellent improvement in volume reduction, texture, and color, but volume reduction and texture were significantly better with CSC-LT. There were no permanent adverse effects with either form of PDL therapy.

Conclusion.—The use of a cooling device with PDL treatment allows higher incident light doses to be administered to patients with cutaneous hemangiomas. With CSC-LT, fewer treatments are required than with NC-LT, and improvements in lesional volume and texture are superior.

▶ A number of studies have documented the usefulness of epidermal cooling in conjunction with PDL treatment for vascular lesions of the skin. Epidermal cooling allows the use of higher energy fluences that facilitate the clearing of recalcitrant lesions and, in theory, should reduce the number of treatments required for clearance. Based on statistical analysis, this article seems to confirm these observations, but some comments should be made. Although statistically significant, the differences in volume reduction and textural change noted between the 2 groups (ie, cooled and noncooled) were small. The cooled group required, on average, only 1 less treatment (1 treatment versus 2 treatments). Although details of the treated lesions were not given and the desired end point of treatment was not described, based on the table in this article it would appear that a good number of lesions were of significant size. Thus, it is difficult for this reviewer to fathom how such lesions could effectively be treated in only 1 or 2 sessions.

P. G. Lang, Jr, MD

Subject Index

A

Abscess
  persistent, after hair transplantation, 36
  sterile, formation after collagen
      implantation, 21
  management, 22
Abuse
  physical, and recent skin injuries in
      normal children, 337
Accutane (*see* Isotretinoin)
Acetaminophen
  renal failure and, chronic, 309
Acne, 193
  contraceptive for, low-dose, ethinyl
      estradiol and levonorgestrel in, 196
  epidemiology in general population, 194
  hyperandrogenemia and, 195
  infantile, clinical and therapeutic study,
      193
  isotretinoin for (*see* Isotretinoin)
  after laser resurfacing, 33
  photodynamic therapy with topical
      δ-aminolevulinic acid and
      incoherent light for, 205
Acquired immunodeficiency syndrome (*see*
      AIDS)
Actin
  alpha-smooth muscle, correlation with
      invasion in micronodular basal cell
      carcinoma, 390
Actinic
  keratoses (*see* Keratoses, actinic)
  prurigo, candidate gene analysis of, 227
Actinically
  damaged adults, predictors for basal
      and squamous cell carcinoma
      among, 384
Actinomycin D
  /melphalan in isolated limb infusion for
      melanoma, 464
Activin
  -receptor–like kinase 1 mutations in
      pulmonary hypertension in patients
      with hereditary hemorrhagic
      ectasia, 302
Activities
  outdoor, in childhood, as protective
      factor for melanoma, 417
Adenocarcinoma
  breast, after Merkel cell carcinoma, 406
  ovarian, after Merkel cell carcinoma,
      406

Adenoviral
  gene transfer restores lysyl hydroxylase
      activity in type VI Ehlers-Danlos
      syndrome (in rat), 292
Adhesive
  tissue, octyl cyanoacrylate, *vs.* suture,
      for closure of excisional wounds in
      children and adolescents, 364
Admission
  hospital, for deep vein thrombosis and
      pulmonary embolism, seasonal
      variations in, 329
Adolescents
  AIDS diagnosis in, survival after, 182
  prevalence of atopic dermatitis, asthma,
      allergic rhinitis, and hand and
      contact dermatitis in, 66
  wound closure in, excisional,
      Dermabond *vs.* suture for, 364
Advertising
  of prescription products, consumer,
      spending on, in U.S., 58
African American(s)
  children
    pubertal, upper lip hair prevalence in,
        218
    tinea capitis in, and hair care
        practices, 162
    patch test results with standard series
        among, 85
Age
  AIDS cases listed by, in U.S., 47
  dermatologists by, non-federal, 52
  as predicting factor of malignancy in
      dermatomyositis and polymyositis,
      240
AIDS
  (*See also* HIV)
  cases
    by age group and exposure category,
        in U.S., 47
    worldwide, 45
  diagnosis in adolescents and adults,
      survival after, 182
  incidence rates, in U.S., 49
Air
  travel
    long-haul, frequency and prevention
        of symptomless deep vein
        thrombosis in, 330
    pulmonary embolism associated with,
        severe, 331
Albendazole
  oral, for cutaneous larva migrans, 190

Alcohol
-based gel, hand cleansing with, effect on microbial colonization of artificial fingernails worn by health care workers, 139
intake and mycosis fungoides, 467
Aldara (*see* Imiquimod cream)
Alefacept
for psoriasis, chronic plaque, 97
Alendronate
for calcinosis of juvenile dermatomyositis, 250
2-year effects on bone mineral density and vertebral fractures in patients receiving glucocorticoids, 278
ALK1
mutations in pulmonary hypertension in patients with hereditary hemorrhagic ectasia, 302
Allergic
rhinitis
prevalence in adolescents, 66
seasonal, effect of omalizumab on symptoms of, 64
Allergy
development after exposure to farming in early life, 69
metal, dental, in patients with oral, cutaneous, and genital lichenoid reactions, 91
thiuram, changing frequency in healthcare workers with hand dermatitis, 88
Allopurinol
desensitization after cutaneous reactions, efficacy and safety of, 324
Alopecia
areata
extensive, topical diphenylcyclopropenone for, 214
immunotherapy with diphencyprone, predictive model for, 215
severe, high-dose pulse corticosteroid therapy for, 213
chemotherapy-induced, prevention by CDK inhibitors (in rat), 211
Alpha-smooth muscle
actin correlated with invasion in micronodular basal cell carcinoma, 390
Aluminum
oxide crystal microdermabrasion for photodamage, 350

Amelanotic
melanoma, clinically, detection and assessment of margins by in vivo confocal scanning laser microscopy, 414
American Academy of Dermatology
skin cancer screening program results, 59
American Board of Dermatology
diplomates certified by, 54
Aminolevulinic acid
topical, photodynamic therapy with fluorescent blue light and, for actinic keratoses, 377
incoherent light and, for acne, 205
for mycosis fungoides, 473
Amino-terminal
propeptide of type III procollagen in routine screening for methotrexate-induced liver fibrosis, 10-year follow-up, 112
Amoxicillin
for Lyme disease, 119
Anaplastic
meningioma after Merkel cell carcinoma, 406
Anesthetic
local, ropivacaine as, for skin infiltration in skin surgery, 363
Angiogenesis
VEGF-mediated, control of hair growth and follicle size by (in mice), 209
Angioneurotic
edema, hereditary, improvement after eradication of *Helicobacter pylori*, 65
Anthrax
lethal factor, Kif1C mediates macrophage resistance to (in mice), 137
Antibiotic(s)
-resistant *Enterococcus faecium* ingestion from chicken and pork, intestinal carriage after, 147
-resistant *Salmonella* isolated from retail ground meats, 146
therapy
appropriateness, practice guideline for penicillin skin testing improves, 143
in Lyme disease patients with persistent symptoms and history, 124
use in the European Union, variation in, 144
Antibody(ies)
desmoglein 1 and 3

blisters in human skin grafted onto
SCID mice induced by, 271
pemphigus severity related to,
cutaneous and oral, 272
formation, blocking, and Botox, 25
monoclonal
anti-CD11a, for moderate to severe
psoriasis, 99
anti-tumor necrosis factor α (*see*
Infliximab)
Anti-CD11a
monoclonal antibody for moderate to
severe psoriasis, 99
Antichondroitin
proteoglycan sulfate Mel-14 F(ab')$_2$,
I-131, long-term response in
neoplastic meningitis secondary to
melanoma, 462
Anticoagulants
bleeding problems and, postoperative, 2
Anticonvulsant
drugs, teratogenicity of, 326
Anti-epiligrin
cicatricial pemphigoid and relative risk
for cancer, 270
Antifungals
for toenail onychomycosis, long-term
efficacy of, 158
topical, for seborrheic dermatitis, 316
Antigen
shed-antigen melanoma vaccine,
polyvalent, 458
superantigen-induced T-cell proliferation
patterns, streptococcal, in guttate
vs. chronic plaque psoriasis, 93
Anti-inflammatory
drugs, nonsteroidal, 305
for arthritis of inflammatory
childhood myositis syndromes, 249
Helicobacter pylori infection and, role
in peptic ulcer disease, 307
risk of serious coronary heart disease
and, 311
steroids combined with, upper
gastrointestinal complications from,
306
treatment with, long-term, eradication
of *Helicobacter pylori* and risk of
peptic ulcers in patients starting,
308
Antimicrobial(s)
for immunobullous disease of
childhood, mixed, 277
peptide
innate, skin protection from invasive
bacterial infection by (in mice), 141
secreted by sweat glands, dermcidin
as, 142

soap, hand cleansing with, effect on
microbial colonization of artificial
fingernails worn by health care
workers, 139
Antiplatelet(s)
bleeding problems and, postoperative, 2
effects of aspirin, and cyclooxygenase
inhibitors, 309
Antiretroviral
therapy
combination, for HIV,
cost-effectiveness of, 184
combination, for HIV, herpes zoster
as immune reconstitution disease
after initiation of, 185
highly active, effect on frequency of
oral warts, 186
highly active, expenditures for care of
HIV-infected patients in era of, 183
Antisense
oligonucleotides, histidine decarboxylase
specific, suppression of melanoma
cell proliferation by, 463
Anti-tumor necrosis factor α
monoclonal antibody (*see* Infliximab)
Apaf-1
inactivation in melanoma, 425
Apoptosis
effector *Apaf-1* inactivation in
melanoma, 425
Fas-induced, of systemic sclerosis
dermal fibroblasts, decreased
susceptibility to, 234
in hypertrophic scars, effect of
interferon-α2b on, 356
Arteriolysis
radial and ulnar, with palmar
sympathectomy for ischemic pain
and Raynaud's phenomenon in
scleroderma, 239
Arteritis
giant cell, risk factors for visual loss in,
261
Arthritis
in Behçet's disease, and papulopustular
skin lesions, 255
of inflammatory childhood myositis
syndromes, 248
psoriatic, infliximab for, 101
rheumatoid
comorbidity and lifestyle,
reproductive factors, and
environmental exposures associated
with, 253
etanercept for, rapid onset of
cutaneous squamous cell carcinoma
after, 105
seropositive, early, treatment, 254

Articular
  involvement in cryoglobulinemia, 259
Aspirin
  antiplatelet effects of, and
    cyclooxygenase inhibitors, 309
  renal failure and, chronic, 309
Asthenia
  after bexarotene, oral, for cutaneous
    T-cell lymphoma, 472
Asthma
  development after exposure to farming
    in early life, 69
  prevalence in adolescents, 66
Atopic
  dermatitis (*see* Dermatitis, atopic)
  disease, probiotics in primary
    prevention of, 72
  disorders, 63
  eczema (*see* Dermatitis, atopic)
Autoimmune
  disease and cryoglobulinemia, 259
Axillary
  hyperhidrosis, botulinum toxin A for,
    343, 344
Azithromycin
  for glanders, 137

B

Bacteremia
  Staphylococcus aureus, nasal carriage as
    source of, 129
Bacteria
  periodontopathic, in Papillon-Lefèvre
    syndrome, 303
Bacterial
  infection, 117
    invasive, innate antimicrobial peptide
      protects skin from (in mice), 141
    superficial, after chemical peel, 31
    toe web, gram-negative, 134
Baldness
  male pattern, biochemical roles of
    testosterone and epitestosterone to
    5α-reductase as indicators of, 216
Bandaging
  compression, associated with toe
    ulceration, 332
Basic Skin Cancer Triage
  curriculum, impact on providers' skin
    cancer control practices, 378
Basophils
  peripheral blood, pimecrolimus inhibits
    mediator release from, 77
Behavior
  changes after oral corticosteroids for
    cutaneous hemangioma, 484

Behçet's disease
  arthritis in, and papulopustular skin
    lesions, 255
  panuveitis in, sight-threatening, effect of
    infliximab on, 257
Behçet's syndrome
  remission with tumor necrosis factor a
    blocking therapy, 256
Betamethasone
  sodium phosphate and diacetate
    injection, intralesional, high
    injection pressure during, for
    capillary hemangiomas, 485
Bexarotene
  oral, for early stage refractory or
    persistent cutaneous T-cell
    lymphoma, 471
Biochemical
  roles of testosterone and epitestosterone
    to 5α-reductase as indicators of
    male pattern baldness, 216
  study of pseudoporphyria, 288
Biopsy
  -proven inflammatory myopathy,
    malignancy incidence in, 245
  sentinel node, in melanoma
    primary, 433
    primary extremity, early recurrence
      after, 448
    use of, developing indications for, 455
  sentinel node, in Merkel cell carcinoma,
    400
    early experience with, 401
    S-staging and, prognostic and
      therapeutic implications of, 401
Bite
  tick, *Ixodes scapularis,* doxycycline for
    prevention of Lyme disease after,
    123
Black tea
  orally administered, inhibitory effects
    on skin carcinogenesis after UVB
    therapy (in mice), 282
Blacks (*see* African Americans)
Bladder
  cancer in polymyositis, 242
Bleeding
  gastrointestinal, upper, among
    corticosteroid-treated patients, risk
    of hospitalization from, 305
  problems after excisional and
    reconstructive surgery, 1
Blistering
  disorders, 265
Blisters
  in human skin grafted onto SCID mice
    induced by antibodies to
    desmogleins 1 and 3, 271

in pseudoporphyria, 288
Blood
 peripheral
  basophils, pimecrolimus inhibits
   mediator release from, 77
  melanoma cells in, detection by
   reverse transcription–polymerase
   chain reaction, 445
Blue light
 fluorescent, and topical aminolevulinic
  acid, photodynamic therapy of
  actinic keratoses with, 377
Bone
 marrow
  involvement in cutaneous
   mastocytosis, 333
  melanoma cells in, detection by
   reverse transcription–polymerase
   chain reaction, 445
  transplantation, allogeneic, HHV-6
   infection and skin rash after, 174
  transplantation, allogeneic,
   transmission of T-cell lymphoma
   by, 478
 mineral density in patients receiving
  glucocorticoids, 2-year effects of
  alendronate on, 278
Borrelia burgdorferi
 outer surface protein A vaccine in
  prevention of Lyme disease in
  children and adolescents, 125
Botox (*see* Botulinum toxin)
Botulinum toxin
 A
  for axillary hyperhidrosis, 343, 344
  for hypertrophy of masseter and
   temporal muscles, 345
 A and B
  blocking antibody formation due to,
   25
  complications of, 25
  dry mouth after, 28
  ecchymosis after, 27, 28
  headache after, 27
  hyperesthesia after, short-term, 28
  pain after, 27
  ptosis after, 26
  ptosis after, methods of minimizing,
   27
  reactions to, adverse, 26
  reactions to, idiosyncratic, 26
  reactions to, localized, 27
 B (*see* A and B *above*)
Bowen's disease
 imiquimod cream for, 374
Brachytherapy
 high-dose-rate, for keloids, 360

Breast
 adenocarcinoma after Merkel cell
  carcinoma, 406
 cancer, radiation for, acute dermatitis
  due to, mometasone furoate for,
  316
Bruising
 after lipotransfer, 38, 39
Bullous
 pemphigoid (*see* Pemphigoid, bullous)
Burkholderia mallei
 glanders due to, in military research
  microbiologist, 136

C

Caffeine
 orally administered, inhibitory effects
  on skin carcinogenesis after UVB
  therapy (in mice), 282
Calcifications
 role of phosphorus metabolism in
  development of, 251
Calcinosis
 of juvenile dermatomyositis
  new insight into, 250
  probenecid for, 251
Calciphylaxis
 from hyperparathyroidism, secondary,
  parathyroidectomy for, 322
Calcipotriol
 topical
  alone or with PUVA therapy for
   vitiligo, 222, 224
  plus low-dose UVA1 phototherapy in
   childhood morphea, 232
Calcium
 channel blockers for Raynaud's
  phenomenon in systemic sclerosis,
  236
Cancer
 (*See also* Carcinoma; Malignancy)
 breast, radiation for, acute dermatitis
  due to, mometasone furoate for,
  316
 epidermal, proneness, clues revealed by
  reconstruction of DNA
  repair-deficient xeroderma
  pigmentosum skin in vitro, 295
 hematologic, after Merkel cell
  carcinoma, 406
 incidence in U.S., 50
 prostate, and exposure to ultraviolet
  radiation, 286
 risk, relative, with anti-epiligrin
  cicatricial pemphigoid, 270

skin
Basic Skin Cancer Triage curriculum, impact on providers' skin cancer control practices, 378
nonmelanoma, 367
nonmelanoma, and glucocorticoid therapy, 383
nonmelanoma, in renal transplant recipients, annual incidence and predicted risk of, 382
nonmelanoma, risk determined by melanocortin-1 receptor gene variants, 385
nonmelanoma, synchronous and metachronous, risk when referred for Mohs micrographic surgery, 393
prevention in primary care setting, 379
regulation by γδ T cells (in mice), 386
screening, in primary care setting, 379
screening program, American Academy of Dermatology, results of, 59
surveillance in renal transplant recipients, 381
in xeroderma pigmentosum, effect of topical T4 endonuclease V in liposomes on, 296
types, specific, frequency in dermatomyositis and polymyositis, 242
Candida
albicans
hypersensitivity to, IgE-mediated, systemic ketoconazole for atopic dermatitis with, 82
osteomyelitis and diskitis after spinal surgery due to artificial nail use, 138
infection in renal transplant recipients, 335
role in diabetic foot disease, 154
Capillary
hemangioma, high injection pressure during intralesional injection of corticosteroids into, 485
Capsaicin
topical, for prurigo nodularis, 317
Carbon dioxide
laser peel *vs.* electrosurgical peel, clinical and histologic study, 347

Carcinogenesis
skin
squamous, progressive decreases in nuclear retinoid receptors during, 387
after UVB therapy, inhibitory effects of orally administered green tea, black tea, and caffeine on (in mice), 282
Carcinoma
(*See also* Cancer)
basal cell
among actinically damaged adults, predictors for, 384
glucocorticoid therapy and, 383
head and neck, aggressive, photofrin-mediated photodynamic therapy for, 396
micronodular, correlation of alpha-smooth muscle actin and invasion in, 390
perineural spread, CT and MR detection of, 394
primary, residual, dense inflammation does not mask during Mohs micrographic surgery, 392
from PUVA-treated patients with psoriasis, ultraviolet exposure as main initiator of p53 mutations in, 388
resection margins, tumor-free, specialty of treating physician affects likelihood of, 391
superficial, imiquimod cream for, 376
synchronous and metachronous, risk when referred for Mohs micrographic surgery, 393
Merkel cell
biopsy in, sentinel node (*see* Biopsy, sentinel node, in Merkel cell carcinoma)
head and neck, effect of surgical excision and radiation on recurrence and survival, 402
second neoplasms and, 406
treatment, multimodality, 404
nasopharyngeal, in dermatomyositis and polymyositis, 241
squamous cell
in adults after childhood organ transplant, 336
among actinically damaged adults, predictors for, 384
glucocorticoid therapy and, 383
head and neck, aggressive, photofrin-mediated photodynamic therapy for, 396

head and neck, papillomavirus
infection as risk factor for, 396
after Merkel cell carcinoma, 406
onset after etanercept for rheumatoid
arthritis, rapid, 105
penis, high incidence of lichen
sclerosus in men with, 399
perineural spread, CT and MR
detection of, 394
after PUVA and cyclosporine, 106
synchronous and metachronous, risk
when referred for Mohs
micrographic surgery, 393
Cardiac (*see* Heart)
Cardiovascular
events, risk with selective COX-2
inhibitors, 312
Care
health care workers (*see* Health, care
workers)
primary
providers, skin cancer control
practices of, impact of Basic Skin
Cancer Triage curriculum on, 378
setting, skin cancer screening and
prevention in, 379
Cathelicidin
protects skin from invasive bacterial
infection (in mice), 141
CD11a
monoclonal antibody against, for
moderate to severe psoriasis, 99
CD95
soluble, increased serum levels
correlates with poor prognosis in
melanoma, 426
CDK
inhibitors, prevention of
chemotherapy-induced alopecia by
(in rat), 211
Ceftriaxone
IV, for Lyme disease, 119
in patients with persistent symptoms
and history of Lyme disease, 124
Cefuroxime axetil
for Lyme disease, 119
Celecoxib
risk of cardiovascular events with, 312
Cell(s)
basal, carcinoma (*see* Carcinoma, basal
cell)
giant cell arteritis, risk factors for visual
loss in, 261
mast
dermal, pimecrolimus inhibits
mediator release from, 77
role in neutrophil recruitment in
bullous pemphigoid (in mice), 268

melanoma
detection in sentinel nodes, bone
marrow and peripheral blood by
reverse transcription–polymerase
chain reaction, 445
proliferation of, suppression by
histidine decarboxylase specific
antisense oligonucleotides, 463
Merkel cell carcinoma (*see* Carcinoma,
Merkel cell)
sickle, disease, cutaneous adverse
reactions to hydroxyurea in, 325
spindle
melanoma, sentinel node status in,
443
tumors of skin, Mohs micrographic
surgery for, 407
squamous, carcinoma (*see* Carcinoma,
squamous cell)
stem, autologous transplantation in
systemic sclerosis, 237
T (*see* T cell)
Central nervous system
imaging and congenital melanocytic
nevi, 410
Chemical
peels (*see* Peels, chemical)
Chemotherapy
-induced alopecia prevention by CDK
inhibitors (in rat), 211
Chicken
Enterococcus faecium on,
quinupristin-dalfopristin-resistant,
147
ingestion of antibiotic-resistant
Enterococcus faecium from,
intestinal carriage after, 147
Children
(*See also* Juvenile)
adolescents (*see* Adolescents)
dermatitis in, atopic
diabetes and, insulin-dependent, 76
SDZ ASM 981 for, 79
eczema in first 2 years of life,
environmental associations with, 68
exposure to farming and development
of asthma and allergy in, 69
fever and hemorrhagic rash in,
diagnostic assessment, 127
hemangioma in (*see* Hemangioma)
immunobullous disease in, mixed,
antimicrobials for, 277
infant (*see* Infant)
melanoma in, outdoor activities as
protective factor for, 417
morphea in, calcipotriol ointment plus
low-dose UVA1 phototherapy in,
232

myositis syndromes in, inflammatory, arthritis of, 248
nevi in, congenital melanocytic
giant, significance of neurocutaneous melanosis in neurologically asymptomatic children with, 409
imaging and, central nervous system, 410
normal, recent skin injuries in, 337
organ transplantation in, skin diseases after, 336
pseudomonas hot-foot syndrome in, 135
psoriasis in, 113
generalized pustular, low-dose cyclosporine for, 115
scabies diagnosis in, high-magnification videodermatoscopy in, 189
tinea capitis in (*see* Tinea, capitis)
varicella vaccine in, effectiveness in clinical practice, 171
warts in, recalcitrant, cimetidine/levamisole for, 167
wound closure in, excisional, Dermabond *vs.* suture for, 364
Cicatricial
pemphigoid, anti-epiligrin, and relative risk for cancer, 270
Cigarette
smoking (*see* Smoking)
Cimetidine
/levamisole for recalcitrant warts in children, 167
Cleansing
hand, with antimicrobial soap or alcohol-based gel, effect on microbial colonization of artificial fingernails worn by health care workers, 139
Clinics
patch test, occupation of patients evaluated in, 90
Clobetasol propionate
cream *vs.* oral prednisone for bullous pemphigoid, 267
for vulvar lichen sclerosus, premenarchal, 318
CNS
imaging, and congenital melanocytic nevi, 410
Collagen
implantation
abscesses after, sterile, management, 22
adverse events associated with, 19
ectopic, 24
filler substances in, complications of, 19

granulomatous reactions to, 21
herpes simplex reactivation after, 23
hypersensitivity reactions to, localized, 19
hypersensitivity reactions to, systemic, 21
necrosis after, local tissue, 22
necrosis after, local tissue, management, 23
vision loss after, unilateral, 24
vascular disorders, 227
Zyderm (*see* Zyderm)
Collagenosis
perforating, of diabetes and renal failure, allopurinol for, 323
Colony-stimulating factor
granulocyte-macrophage, perilesional injection for cutaneous melanoma metastases, 459
Colorectal
cancer in dermatomyositis, 242
Comorbidity
of rheumatoid arthritis, 253
Compression
bandaging associated with toe ulceration, 332
Computed tomography
of perineural spread of squamous and basal cell carcinoma, 394
Condoms
effect on reducing transmission of herpes simplex virus type 2 from men to women, 168
Condylomata (*see* Warts)
Connective tissue
growth factor production in fibroblasts and skin of scleroderma patients, iloprost suppresses, 236
Consumer
advertising of prescription products, spending on, in U.S., 58
Contact
dermatitis (*see* Dermatitis, contact)
Contraceptives
oral
low-dose, containing ethinyl estradiol and levonorgestrel, for acne, 196
myocardial infarction and, 197
third-generation, and risk of venous thrombosis, 198
Cooling
cryogen spray, and pulsed dye laser treatment of cutaneous hemangiomas, 486
Coronary
heart disease, serious, risk with NSAIDs, 311

Corticosteroid(s), 305
    bone mineral density and vertebral
        fracture in patients receiving,
        2-year effects of alendronate on,
        278
    cream *(see* topical *below)*
    gastrointestinal bleeding among patients
        on, upper, risk of hospitalization
        from, 305
    gastrointestinal complications and,
        upper, 306
    injection
        immediate, after excision of earlobe
            keloids, recurrence rates after, 359
        intra-articular, for arthritis of
            inflammatory childhood myositis
            syndromes, 249
        intralesional, high injection pressure
            during, for capillary hemangiomas,
            485
        oral, for cutaneous hemangiomas, 484
    therapy
        pulse, high-dose, for severe alopecia
            areata, 213
    skin cancers and, nonmelanoma, 383
    topical
        for dermatitis, acute radiation, 316
        for pemphigoid, bullous, 265
        vs. oral, for bullous pemphigoid, 267
Cosmetic
    surgery, 343
        collagen in *(see* Collagen,
            implantation)
        complications of, 19
        filler substances in, complications of,
            19
        silicone in, complications of, 24
Cost
    -effectiveness of combination
        antiretroviral therapy for HIV
        disease, 184
COX
    inhibitors and antiplatelet effects of
        aspirin, 309
    -2 inhibitors, selective, and risk of
        cardiovascular events, 312
Crohn disease
    pyoderma gangrenosum and psoriasis
        associated with, anti-tumor necrosis
        factor α monoclonal antibody for,
        100
Cryogen
    spray cooling and pulsed dye laser
        treatment of cutaneous
        hemangiomas, 486
Cryoglobulinemia
    etiologic factors and clinical and
        immunologic features, 258

Cryotherapy
    for acne, infantile, 193
CT
    of perineural spread of squamous and
        basal cell carcinoma, 394
Curriculum
    Basic Skin Cancer Triage, impact on
        providers' skin cancer control
        practices, 378
Cushingoid appearance
    after oral corticosteroids for cutaneous
        hemangioma, 484
Cutaneous
    (See also Skin)
    graft-*vs.*-host disease, tacrolimus
        ointment for, 319
    hemangiomas
        corticosteroids for, oral, 484
        cryogen spray cooling and pulsed dye
            laser treatment of, 486
    involvement in cryoglobulinemia, 259
    larva migrans in returning traveller,
        clinical features and management,
        190
    leukocytoclastic vasculitis in
        dermatomyositis suggests
        malignancy, 241
    lichenoid reactions, dental metal allergy
        in patients with, 91
    lupus erythematosus *(see* Lupus,
        erythematosus, cutaneous)
    lymphoma, T-cell *(see* Lymphoma,
        T-cell, cutaneous)
    mastocytosis, bone marrow involvement
        in, 333
    melanoma metastases, perilesional
        injection of GM-CSF for, 459
    pemphigus severity related to
        desmoglein 1 and 3 antibody levels,
        271, 272
    protection from ultraviolet photoinjury
        by green tea polyphenols, 281
    reactions
        adverse, to hydroxyurea in sickle cell
            disease, 325
        desensitization to allopurinol after,
            efficacy and safety of, 324
Cyclin
    -dependent kinase 2, prevention of
        chemotherapy-induced alopecia by
        (in rat), 211
Cyclooxygenase
    inhibitors and antiplatelet effects of
        aspirin, 309
    -2 inhibitors, selective, and risk of
        cardiovascular events, 312

Cyclosporine
low-dose, for generalized pustular
psoriasis, 114
PUVA and, squamous cell cancer of skin
after, 106
Cyst
inclusion, inflamed epidermal, in
posterior triangle of neck, 15
myxoid, digital, therapy by
identification and repair of leak of
joint fluid, 362
Cytokine
gene polymorphisms in psoriasis, 95

D

Dalfopristin
-quinupristin-resistant *Enterococcus
faecium* on chicken and in stool
specimens, 147
Dapsone
for mixed immunobullous disease of
childhood, 277
Daskil
for seborrheic dermatitis, 315
Death
(*See also* Mortality)
causes of, in U.S., 48
Debridement
therapy, maggot, in outpatients, 191
Debris
wiping away between passes during
laser surgery (in rat), 348
Deformity
pincushion, 7
of transposition flap, 8
Dehiscence
wound, 4
traumatic, 5
Demarcation
problems after chemical peel, 31
Denileukin
diftitox for cutaneous T-cell lymphoma,
476
Dental
metal allergy in patients with oral,
cutaneous, and genital lichenoid
reactions, 91
Depigmentation
lupus erythematosus causing, discoid,
epidermal grafting for, 229
Depression
interferon alfa causing, high-dose,
prevention with paroxetine, 457
in isotretinoin-treated patients, 201

Dermabond
vs. suture for closure of excisional
wounds in children and
adolescents, 364
Dermabrasion
microdermabrasion (*see*
Microdermabrasion)
spot, for full-thickness graft color and
contour problems, 12
Dermal
changes after microdermabrasion, 349
fibroblasts, systemic sclerosis, decreased
susceptibility to Fas-induced
apoptosis of, 234
invasion, deep, directly from epidermis
by *Trichophyton rubrum*, in
immunosuppressed patients, 151
mast cells, pimecrolimus inhibits
mediator release from, 77
pigmentation, difficult, combined laser
therapy for, 351
Dermatitis
atopic
adult, phototherapy in, narrow-band
UVB and broad-band UVA, 80
in adults, house dust mite control
measures in, 74
diabetes and, insulin-dependent, 76
with IgE-mediated hypersensitivity to
yeasts, systemic ketoconazole for,
82
mycophenolate mofetil for, 81
prevalence in adolescents, 66
risk in infancy, exposure to endotoxin
decreases, 71
SDZ ASM 981 for, 78
SDZ ASM 981 for, in children, 79
contact, 85
prevalence in adolescents, 66
statistics relating to, in Belgium, 51
hand
prevalence in adolescents, 66
thiuram allergy in healthcare workers
with, changing frequency of, 88
radiation, acute, mometasone furoate
for, 316
seborrheic
antifungal agents for, topical, 316
terbinafine for, oral, 315
Dermatofibrosarcoma
protuberans, Mohs micrographic
surgery for, 407
Dermatologic
subspecialties, physicians certified in, 55
surgery, 343
Dermatologist(s)
non-federal, by age and sex, 52
number of, 53

statistics of interest to, 43
Dermatology
American Academy of Dermatology
skin cancer screening program
results, 59
American Board of, diplomates certified
by, 54
journals, leading, 60
trainees, in U.S., 54
Dermatomycoses
in renal transplant recipients, 335
Dermatomyositis
juvenile
calcinosis of, new insight into, 250
lipodystrophy and, 246
probenecid for, 251
malignancy in
predicting factors of, 240
risk and follow-up implications, 243
risk of, 245
specific types, 242
prognostic factors and short-term and
long-term outcome, 244
Dermatophyte
infection in diabetic foot disease, 154
toenail onychomycosis, terbinafine and
itraconazole for, in elderly, 157
Dermcidin
study of, 142
Dermoscopy
in melanoma diagnosis, 413
multispectral digital, automated
differentiation of melanoma from
melanocytic nevi with, 412
Desensitization
to allopurinol after cutaneous reactions,
efficacy and safety of, 324
Desmoglein
1 and 3 antibodies
blisters in human skin grafted onto
SCID mice induced by, 271
levels, severity of cutaneous and oral
pemphigus related to, 272
Diabetes mellitus
foot infection in, fungal, 153
insulin-dependent, and atopic
dermatitis, 76
renal failure and, perforating
collagenosis of, allopurinol for, 323
Diclofenac
in hyaluronan gel for actinic keratoses,
368, 370
Didanosine
prophylaxis against HIV after sexual or
injection drug use exposure, 177

Digital
dermoscopy, multispectral, automated
differentiation of melanoma from
melanocytic nevi with, 412
myxoid cyst, therapy by identification
and repair of leak of joint fluid,
362
Diltiazem
for calcinosis in juvenile
dermatomyositis, 252
Diphencyprone
immunotherapy for alopecia areata,
predictive model for, 215
Diphenylcyclopropenone
topical, for extensive alopecia areata,
214
Diplomates
certified by American Board of
Dermatology, 54
Discoid
lupus erythematosus causing
depigmentation, epidermal grafting
for, 229
Diskitis
Candida, after spinal surgery, due to
artificial nail use, 138
DNA
content as prognostic marker in oral
leukoplakia, 397
damage, UV-induced epidermal, effect
of solar-stimulated skin adaptation
on, 284
repair-deficient xeroderma pigmentosum
skin in vitro, clues to epidermal
cancer proneness revealed by
reconstruction of, 295
Docosanol
for herpes simplex labialis, 170
Doxycycline
for glanders, 137
for Lyme disease, 119
in patients with persistent symptoms
and history, 124
for sarcoidosis, 321
single-dose, for prevention of Lyme
disease after *Ixodes scapularis* tick
bite, 123
Dramaturgical
study of meetings between general
practitioners and pharmaceutical
representatives, 339
Drug(s)
anticoagulant, and postoperative
bleeding problems, 2
anticonvulsant, teratogenicity of, 326
antifungal
for toenail onychomycosis, long-term
efficacy of, 158

topical, for seborrheic dermatitis, 316
anti-inflammatory, nonsteroidal (*see*
   Anti-inflammatory, drugs,
   nonsteroidal)
antimicrobial, for mixed
   immunobullous disease of
   childhood, 277
antiplatelet, and postoperative bleeding
   problems, 2
reactions, adverse, 315
use exposure, injection, postexposure
   prophylaxis against HIV infection
   after, 177
Dry mouth
   after Botox, 28
Dust
   mite, house, control measures, in adults
      with atopic dermatitis, 74
Dye
   hair, exposure, and rheumatoid arthritis,
      in women, 253
   laser
      flashlamp-pumped and long-pulsed
         tunable, for port-wine stains, 355
      pulsed, plus cryogen spray cooling for
         cutaneous hemangiomas, 486
Dyskeratosis
   congenita, autosomal dominant,
      mutated RNA component of
      telomerase in, 298

E

Earlobe
   keloids
      recurrence rates after various
         postoperative therapeutic
         modalities, 359
      surgical excision and immediate
         postoperative adjuvant
         radiotherapy for, 357
Ecchymosis
   after Botox, 27, 28
Ectropion
   after excisional and reconstructive
      surgery, 10
   after laser resurfacing, 34
Eczema
   atopic (*see* Dermatitis, atopic)
   in early life, environmental associations
      with, 68
Edema
   angioneurotic, hereditary, improvement
      after eradication of *Helicobacter
      pylori*, 65
   prolonged, after lipotransfer, 38

Ehlers-Danlos syndrome
   absence of inferior labial and lingual
      frenula in, 291
   recessive form, due to tenascin-X
      deficiency, 293
   type VI, adenoviral gene transfer
      restores lysyl hydroxylase activity
      in (in rat), 292
Elderly
   collagenosis of diabetes and renal
      failure in, perforating, allopurinol
      for, 323
   fasciitis of head and neck in,
      necrotizing, 130
   Merkel cell carcinoma in (*see*
      Carcinoma, Merkel cell)
   onychomycosis of toenail in,
      dermatophyte, terbinafine and
      itraconazole for, 157
   pemphigoid in, bullous, clobetasol
      propionate cream *vs.* oral
      prednisone for, 267
   skin tumors in, aggressive head and
      neck nonmelanomatous,
      photofrin-mediated photodynamic
      therapy for, 395
Electrosurgical
   vs. carbon dioxide laser peels, clinical
      and histologic study, 347
Elidel (*see* SDZ ASM 981)
Embolism
   pulmonary (*see* Pulmonary, embolism)
Endonuclease V
   T4, topical, in liposomes, effect on skin
      cancer in xeroderma pigmentosum,
      296
Endothelial
   growth factor, vascular, as mediator of
      angiogenesis, control of hair
      growth and follicle size by (in
      mice), 209
Endotoxin
   exposure decreases risk of atopic
      eczema in infancy, 71
Enterococcus faecium
   antibiotic-resistant, ingestion from
      chicken and pork, intestinal
      carriage after, 147
   quinupristin-dalfoprostin-resistant, on
      chicken and in stool specimens,
      147
Environmental
   associations with eczema in early life,
      68
   exposures and rheumatoid arthritis, 253

Epidermis
  cancer proneness, clues revealed by reconstruction of DNA repair-deficient xeroderma pigmentosum skin in vitro, 295
  changes after microdermabrasion, 349
  DNA damage, UV-induced, effect of solar-stimulated skin adaptation on, 284
  grafting for depigmentation due to discoid lupus erythematosus, 229
  inclusion cyst, inflamed, in posterior triangle of neck, 15
  necrolysis, toxic, high-dose IV immunoglobulins for, 275
  Trichophyton rubrum showing deep dermal invasion directly from, in immunosuppressed patients, 151
Epiluminescence
  microscopy in melanoma diagnosis, 413
Epitestosterone
  biochemical role as indicator of male pattern baldness, 216
Eruption
  polymorphic light, candidate gene analysis of, 227
Erythema
  after laser resurfacing, 32
  persistent, after chemical peel, 30
  prolonged, after chemical peel, 31
  after Zyderm I implant, 20
Erythrodermic
  mycosis fungoides, high-dose UVA1 therapy of, 474
Erythromycin
  for acne, infantile, 193
  for mixed immunobullous disease of childhood, 277
ESD
  vs. carbon dioxide laser peel, clinical and histologic study, 347
Estradiol
  ethinyl, and levonorgestrel in low-dose contraceptive for acne, 196
Etanercept
  for arthritis, rheumatoid, rapid onset of squamous cell carcinoma after, 105
  for psoriasis
    malignancy risk associated with, 109
    plaque, 104
Ethinyl estradiol
  /levonorgestrel in low-dose contraceptive for acne, 196
Etidronate
  for calcinosis of juvenile dermatomyositis, 251

Examination
  physical, *vs.* ultrasound B-scan in follow-up of melanoma, 453
Excisional
  surgery
    complications of, 1
    complications of, acute, 1
    facial nerve in, 13
    wound closure, octyl cyanoacrylate tissue adhesive *vs.* suture for, in children and adolescents, 364
Expenditures
  for care of HIV-infected patients in era of highly active antiretroviral therapy, 183
  on consumer advertising of prescription products, in U.S., 58
  health, national, 1970 *vs.* 2000, 58
Extracorporeal
  photochemotherapy and interferon-α2a for stage II cutaneous T-cell lymphoma, 475
Extracutaneous
  mycosis fungoides, clinical characteristics and outcome, 470
Extremity
  melanoma, primary, early recurrence after lymphatic mapping and sentinel node biopsy in, 448
Eyebrow
  elevation, asymmetric lateral, secondary to surgical repair, 9

F

$F(ab')_2$
  I-131 Mel-14, long-term response in neoplastic meningitis secondary to melanoma, 462
Fabry's disease
  cardiac variant, galactose infusion therapy for, 300
  α-galactosidase A replacement therapy in, recombinant, safety and efficacy of, 299
Face
  carcinoma, basal or squamous cell, perineural spread, CT and MR detection of, 394
  danger zones in excisional and reconstructive surgery, 13
Facial
  nerve in excisional and reconstructive surgery, 13
Famciclovir
  for herpes simplex reactivation
    after chemical peel, 31
    after collagen implantation, 24

Family
income, nonelderly population with
selected sources of health insurance
by, 56
Farming
exposure in early life to, and
development of asthma and allergy,
69
Fas
/CD95, soluble, increased serum level
correlates with poor prognosis in
melanoma, 426
-induced apoptosis of systemic sclerosis
dermal fibroblasts, decreased
susceptibility to, 234
Fasciitis
necrotizing, of head and neck, 130
Fat
tissue, decreased after oral
administration of green tea, black
tea, and caffeine after UVB therapy,
and skin carcinogenesis (in mice),
282
Fever
hemorrhagic rash and, diagnostic
assessment, 127
Fibroblasts
dermal, systemic sclerosis, decreased
susceptibility to Fas-induced
apoptosis of, 234
of scleroderma patients, iloprost
suppresses connective tissue growth
factor production in, 236
Fibrosis
liver, methotrexate-induced,
amino-terminal propeptide of type
III procollagen in routine screening
for, 10-year follow-up, 112
Fibrous
histiocytoma, malignant, Mohs
micrographic surgery for, 407
Fibroxanthoma
atypical, Mohs micrographic surgery
for, 407
Filler
substances in cosmetic surgery,
complications of, 19
Fingernails
artificial, worn by health care workers
Candida osteomyelitis and diskitis
after spinal surgery due to, 138
microbial colonization of, effect of
hand cleansing with antimicrobial
soap or alcohol-based gel on, 139
Flap
design complications, 4

distal, full- and partial-thickness
necrosis in, 6
margins, free, complications of, 7
transposition
hematoma under, 3
pincushion deformity of, 8
Flights
long-haul, frequency and prevention of
symptomless deep vein thrombosis
in, 330
pulmonary embolism associated with,
severe, 331
Fluconazole
for onychomycosis of toes,
Scopulariopsis brevicaulis, 156
vs. griseofulvin for *Trichophyton* tinea
capitis, 164
for yeast infection after chemical peel,
31
Fluorescent
blue light and topical aminolevulinic
acid, photodynamic therapy of
actinic keratoses with, 377
Fluoroquinolones
for yeast infection after chemical peel,
31
Follicle
hair (in mice)
regression, p53 involvement in
control of, 210
size, control by VEGF-mediated
angiogenesis, 209
Folliculitis
in organ transplant recipients, pediatric,
336
in renal transplant recipients, 335
Foot
diabetic, fungal infection of, 153
pseudomonas hot-foot syndrome, 135
Fracture
vertebral, in patients receiving
glucocorticoids, 2-year effects of
alendronate on, 278
Fragrances
patch testing for, false-positive findings,
87
Frenula
inferior labial and lingual, absence in
Ehlers-Danlos syndrome, 291
Functional
ability related to skin score in systemic
sclerosis, 234
Fungal
infections, 151
of diabetic foot, 153

G

Gadolinium
-enhanced MRI for neurocutaneous
melanosis in neurologically
asymptomatic children with giant
congenital melanocytic nevi, 409
Galactose
infusion therapy in cardiac variant of
Fabry's disease, 300
α-Galactosidase A
replacement therapy, recombinant,
safety and efficacy in Fabry's
disease, 299
Ganglion
of distal interphalangeal joint, therapy
by identification and repair of leak
of joint fluid, 362
Gangrene
peripheral, during infancy, 230
Gastrointestinal
bleeding, upper, among
corticosteroid-treated patients, risk
of hospitalization from, 305
complications, upper, risk with steroids,
306
GB virus C
coinfection, effect on survival among
HIV-infected patients, 178, 179
Gel
alcohol-based, hand cleansing with,
effect on microbial colonization of
artificial fingernails worn by health
care workers, 139
Gender
dermatologists by, non-federal, 52
differences
for dermatitis, allergic contact, in
adolescents, 67
for hand eczema in adolescents, 67
as predicting factor of malignancy in
dermatomyositis and polymyositis,
240
as predictor of survival from metastatic
melanoma, 424
Gene(s)
candidate, of 3 related photosensitivity
disorders, analysis of, 227
cytokine, polymorphisms, in psoriasis,
95
hairless, mutation in congenital hair loss
disorders encodes novel nuclear
receptor corepressor, 212
melanocortin-1 receptor, variants
determine risk of nonmelanoma
skin cancer, 385

p53, mutations in basal cell carcinomas
from PUVA-treated patients with
psoriasis, ultraviolet exposure as
main indicator of, 388
TGM1, mutations in autosomal
recessive lamellar ichthyosis, 297
transfer, adenoviral, lysyl hydroxylase
activity in type VI Ehlers-Danlos
syndrome restored by (in rat), 292
General practitioners
meetings between pharmaceutical
representatives and, dramaturgical
study of, 339
Genetic
features, molecular, of pulmonary
hypertension in patients with
hereditary hemorrhagic
telangiectasia, 301
Genital
herpes, recurrent, effect of resiquimod
gel on recurrence rate of, 169
lichenoid reactions, dental metal allergy
in patients with, 91
Genodermatoses, 291
Genotoxins
endogenous, vitamin C-induced
decomposition of lipid
hydroperoxides to, 388
Giant cell arteritis
visual loss in, risk factors for, 261
Glabellar
area ulceration after Zyderm II
implantation, 22
Glanders
in military research microbiologist, 136
Glucocorticoids (*see* Corticosteroids)
Glycolic acid
peel for photoaged skin, quantitative
and qualitative effects of (in mice),
346
GM-CSF
injection, perilesional, for cutaneous
melanoma metastases, 459
Graft
epidermal, for depigmentation due to
discoid lupus erythematosus, 229
skin
full-thickness, complications of, 10
full-thickness, necrosis of, 11
full-thickness, poor color and texture
match of, 12
human, on SCID mice, antibodies to
desmogleins 1 and 3 induce blisters
in, 271
-*vs.*-host disease, cutaneous, tacrolimus
ointment for, 319

Granulocyte
-macrophage colony-stimulating factor injection, perilesional, for cutaneous melanoma metastases, 459
Granuloma
formation, nodular, after silicone implantation, 25
Granulomatous
reactions to collagen implantation, 21
Green tea
orally administered, inhibitory effects on skin carcinogenesis after UVB therapy (in mice), 282
polyphenols, cutaneous photoprotection from ultraviolet injury by, 281
Griseofulvin
for onychomycosis of toes, *Scopulariopsis brevicaulis*, 156
vs. terbinafine for tinea capitis, 163
vs. terbinafine, itraconazole, or fluconazole for *Trichophyton* tinea capitis, 164
Ground meats
retail, isolation of antibiotic-resistant *Salmonella* from, 146
Growth
factor
connective tissue, production in fibroblasts and skin of scleroderma patients, iloprost suppresses, 236
vascular endothelial, as mediator of angiogenesis, control of hair growth and follicle size by (in mice), 209
retardation, temporary, after oral corticosteroids for cutaneous hemangiomas, 484
Guideline
practice, for penicillin testing, appropriateness of antibiotic therapy improved by, 143

H

Hair
care practices and tinea capitis, 162
disorders, 209
dye exposure and rheumatoid arthritis, in women, 253
follicle (in mice)
regression, p53 involvement in control of, 210
size control by VEGF-mediated angiogenesis, 209
growth control by VEGF-mediated angiogenesis (in mice), 209
lip, upper, prevalence in black and white girls during puberty, 218
loss disorders, congenital, *hairless* gene mutation encodes novel nuclear receptor corepressor in, 212
removal, long-pulsed Nd:YAG laser-assisted, in pigmented skin, 352
transplantation, complications of, 34
Hairless
gene mutation in congenital hair loss disorders encodes novel nuclear receptor corepressor, 212
Hand
cleansing with antimicrobial soap or alcohol-based gel, effect on microbial colonization of artificial fingernails worn by health care workers, 139
dermatitis
prevalence in adolescents, 66
thiuram allergy in healthcare workers with, changing frequency of, 88
Head and neck
carcinoma, squamous cell, papillomavirus infection as risk factor for, 396
fasciitis of, necrotizing, 130
melanoma
lymphoscintigraphy and PET in management of, 452
metastases from, nodal, clinically predictable pattern of, 451
skin tumors, aggressive nonmelanomatous, photofrin-mediated photodynamic therapy for, in elderly, 395
Headache
after bexarotene, oral, for cutaneous T-cell lymphoma, 472
after Botox, 27
Healing
wound, in patients with calciphylaxis from secondary hyperparathyroidism, effect of parathyroidectomy on, 322
Health
care workers
artificial fingernails worn by, *Candida* osteomyelitis and diskitis after spinal surgery due to, 138
artificial fingernails worn by, microbial colonization of, effect of hand cleansing with antimicrobial soap or alcohol-based gel on, 139
with hand dermatitis, changing frequency of thiuram allergy in, 88
prick and patch testing results in, 89

expenditures, national, 1970 *vs.* 2000, 58
insurance
 coverage of U.S. population, 56
 nonelderly population with selected sources of, by family income, 56
 maintenance organization market penetration, in U.S., 57
Heart
 disease, serious coronary, risk with NSAIDs, 311
 failure, congestive, and itraconazole, 159
 variant of Fabry's disease, galactose infusion therapy for, 300
Helicobacter pylori
 eradication
  improvement of hereditary angioneurotic edema and, 65
  risk of peptic ulcers in patients starting long-term treatment with nonsteroidal anti-inflammatory drugs and, 308
 infection and NSAIDs, role in peptic ulcer disease, 307
Hemangioma
 capillary, high injection pressure during intralesional injection of corticosteroids into, 485
 congenital nonprogressive, clinicopathologically distinct from infantile hemangioma, 482
 cutaneous
  corticosteroids for, oral, 484
  cryogen spray cooling and pulsed dye laser treatment of, 486
 juvenile, microvascular phenotype shared by human placenta and, 481
Hematologic
 disease and cryoglobulinemia, 259
 malignancies after Merkel cell carcinoma, 406
Hematoma
 under flap, transposition, 3
 formation, postoperative, 2
Hemorrhagic
 rash and fever, diagnostic assessment, 127
 telangiectasia, hereditary, pulmonary hypertension in, clinical and molecular genetic features of, 301
Henoch-Schönlein purpura
 renal lesions in, acute and chronic, grading of, 263
 renal sequelae in adults with, predictive factors for, 262

Hepatitis
 C virus infection and cryoglobulinemia, 259
 G virus coinfection, effect on survival among HIV-infected patients, 178, 179
Herpes
 genital, recurrent, effect of resiquimod gel on recurrence rate of, 169
 simplex
  infection in children with organ transplants, 336
  infection in renal transplant recipients, 335
  labialis, docosanol for, 170
  reactivation after chemical peeling, 31
  reactivation after collagen implantation, 23
  virus 1716 injection, intralesional, in metastatic melanoma, 461
  virus type 2 transmission from men to women, effect of condoms on reducing, 168
 zoster
  as immune reconstitution disease after initiation of combination antiretroviral therapy for HIV infection, 185
  infection in children with organ transplants, 336
  infection in renal transplant recipients, 335
  pain in, acute, 172
Herpesvirus
 -6 infection and skin rash after allogeneic bone marrow transplantation, 174
 -8 infection and Kaposi's sarcoma in renal transplant recipients, 334
Hirsute
 women with normal menses, polycystic ovaries in, 219
Histidine
 decarboxylase specific antisense oligonucleotides, suppression of melanoma cell proliferation by, 463
Histiocytoma
 malignant fibrous, Mohs micrographic surgery for, 407
Histologic
 features of level 2 melanoma associated with metastasis, 421
 response to phototherapy with topical aminolevulinic acid for mycosis fungoides, 473
 study of electrosurgical *vs.* carbon dioxide laser peel, 347

Histology
predicts sentinel node status in
melanoma, 438
HIV
cases, worldwide, 45
infection, 177
antiretroviral therapy for,
combination, cost-effectiveness of,
184
antiretroviral therapy for,
combination, herpes zoster as
immune reconstitution disease after
initiation of, 185
expenditures for care in era of highly
active antiretroviral therapy, 183
risk of vulvovaginal and perianal
condylomata acuminata and
intraepithelial neoplasia and, 187
survival, effect of coinfection with GB
virus C on, 178, 179
warts in, oral, effect of highly active
antiretroviral therapy on frequency
of, 186
postexposure prophylaxis against, after
sexual or injection drug use
exposure, 177
HMO
market penetration, in U.S., 57
Hospital
admission for deep vein thrombosis and
pulmonary embolism, seasonal
variations in, 329
Hospitalization
risk due to upper gastrointestinal
bleeding among
corticosteroid-treated patients, 305
Hot-foot syndrome
pseudomonas, 135
House
dust mite control measures in adults
with atopic dermatitis, 74
Human immunodeficiency virus (see HIV)
Hyaluronan
gel, diclofenac in, for actinic keratoses,
368, 370
Hydroperoxides
lipid, vitamin C-induced decomposition
to endogenous genotoxins, 388
Hydroxychloroquine
vs. minocycline for early seropositive
rheumatoid arthritis, 254
Hydroxyurea
in sickle cell disease, cutaneous adverse
reactions to, 325
Hyperandrogenemia
acne and, 195

Hypercholesterolemia
after bexarotene, oral, for cutaneous
T-cell lymphoma, 472
Hyperesthesia
short-term, after Botox, 28
Hyperhidrosis
axillary, botulinum toxin A for, 343,
344
Hyperparathyroidism
secondary, calciphylaxis from,
parathyroidectomy for, 322
Hyperpigmentation
after laser resurfacing, 33
in pseudoporphyria, 288
Hypersensitivity
reactions to collagen implantation
localized, 19
systemic, 21
to yeast, IgE-mediated, systemic
ketoconazole for atopic dermatitis
with, 82
Hypertension
pulmonary, in patients with hereditary
hemorrhagic telangiectasia, clinical
and molecular genetic features of,
301
Hypertrichosis
in pseudoporphyria, 288
Hypertriglyceridemia
after bexarotene, oral, for cutaneous
T-cell lymphoma, 472
lipodystrophy and juvenile
dermatomyositis, 248
Hypertrophic
scars
myofibroblasts and apoptosis in,
effect of interferon-α2b on, 356
after tissue adhesive vs. suture for
closure of excisional wounds in
children and adolescents, 364
Hypertrophy
of masseter and temporal muscles,
botulinum toxin A for, 345
Hypopigmentation
after Jessner/trichloroacetic acid peel, 29
after laser resurfacing, 33
Hypothyroidism
after bexarotene, oral, for cutaneous
T-cell lymphoma, 472

I

Ibuprofen
antiplatelet effects of aspirin and, 310
risk of serious coronary heart disease
with, 311

Ichthyosis
  lamellar, autosomal recessive, TGM1
    gene mutations in, 297
Ig (*see* Immunoglobulin)
Iloprost
  suppresses connective tissue growth
    factor production in fibroblasts and
    skin of scleroderma patients, 236
Imaging
  central nervous system, and congenital
    melanocytic nevi, 410
  magnetic resonance (*see* Magnetic
    resonance imaging)
Imipenem
  for glanders, 137
Imiquimod cream
  for actinic keratoses, 371
  for basal cell carcinoma, superficial, 376
  for Bowen's disease, 374
Immune
  reconstitution disease, herpes zoster as,
    after initiation of combined
    antiretroviral therapy for HIV
    infection, 185
Immunobullous
  disease of childhood, mixed,
    antimicrobials for, 277
Immunodeficiency
  syndrome, acquired (*see* AIDS)
  virus, human (*see* HIV)
Immunoglobulin
  E-mediated hypersensitivity to yeasts,
    systemic ketoconazole for atopic
    dermatitis with, 82
  G1-Fc fusion complex therapy, tumor
    necrosis factor α (*see* Etanercept)
  IV
    high-dose, for toxic epidermal
      necrolysis, 275
    for pemphigus, 275
Immunologic
  features of cryoglobulinemia, 258
Immunosuppressed patients
  Trichophyton rubrum in, 151
Immunotherapy
  of alopecia areata with diphencyprone,
    predictive model for, 215
Impetigo
  contagiosum in children with organ
    transplants, 336
  in renal transplant recipients, 335
Inclusion
  cyst, inflamed epidermal, in posterior
    triangle of neck, 15
Inclusion-body
  myositis, malignancy incidence in, 245

Income
  family, nonelderly population with
    selected sources of health insurance
    by, 56
Indomethacin
  for parvovirus B19 infection with
    lupus-like presentation, 176
Induration
  after Zyderm I implant, 20
Infant
  acne in, clinical and therapeutic study,
    193
  eczema in, atopic, exposure to
    endotoxin decreases risk of, 71
  gangrene in, peripheral, 230
  hemangioma in
    congenital nonprogressive,
      clinicopathologically distinct from
      infantile hemangioma, 482
    cutaneous, oral corticosteroids for,
      484
Infarction
  myocardial, and oral contraceptives,
    197
Infection
  bacterial (*see* Bacterial, infection)
  fungal, 151
    of diabetic foot, 153
  mycobacterial, after liposuction, 37, 38
  skin, in renal transplant recipients, 335
  viral, 167
  wound, postoperative, 3
    with crust and exudates, 2
Infectious
  diseases
    cryoglobulinemia and, 259
    reportable, new cases in U.S., 44
Infestations, 189
Inflammation
  dense, residual primary basal cell
    carcinoma during Mohs
    micrographic surgery not masked
    by, 392
Inflammatory
  myopathy, biopsy-proven, malignancy
    incidence in, 245
  myositis syndromes, childhood, arthritis
    of, 248
  symptoms at test site of Zyderm
    collagen, 20
Infliximab
  in Behçet's disease, effect on
    sight-threatening panuveitis, 257
  in Behçet's syndrome, 256
  monotherapy for plaque psoriasis, 102
  for psoriatic arthritis, 101

for pyoderma gangrenosum and
psoriasis associated with Crohn
disease, 100
tuberculosis associated with, 104
Injection
drug use exposure, postexposure
prophylaxis against HIV infection
after, 177
Injuries
skin, recent, in normal children, 337
Insulin
-dependent diabetes and atopic
dermatitis, 76
resistance, lipodystrophy and juvenile
dermatomyositis, 248
Insurance
health
coverage of U.S. population, 56
nonelderly population with selected
sources of, by family income, 56
Integrins
mitogen-activated protein kinase
activation by, in pathogenesis of
psoriasis, 94
Interferon
α, high-dose, causing depression,
prevention with paroxetine, 457
α-2a and extracorporeal
photochemotherapy for stage II
cutaneous T-cell lymphoma, 475
α-2b
effect on myofibroblasts and
apoptosis in hypertrophic scars,
356
long-term adjuvant, for regional node
metastases from melanoma, 456
for melanoma, developing indications
for use of, 455
Interleukin
-1α activation of mitogen-activated
protein kinase in pathogenesis of
psoriasis, 94
-10 therapy, systemic, effects on
psoriatic skin lesions, 96
Interphalangeal
joint, distal, ganglion of, therapy by
identification and repair of leak of
joint fluid, 362
Intestinal
carriage after ingestion of
antibiotic-resistant *Enterococcus
faecium* from chicken and pork,
147
Intraepithelial
neoplasia, vulvovaginal and perianal,
risk with HIV infection, 187

Iodine-131
Mel-14 F(ab')$_2$, long-term response in
neoplastic meningitis secondary to
melanoma, 462
Irritability
after oral corticosteroids for cutaneous
hemangioma, 484
Ischemic
pain in scleroderma, surgery for, 239
Isotretinoin
depression and suicide in patients
treated with, 201
formulation, new micronized, for severe
recalcitrant nodular acne, 203
for infantile acne, 193
ocular side effects of, 200
teratogen warning symbol on,
interpretations of, 199
Itraconazole
heart failure and, congestive, 159
for onychomycosis of toenail
dermatophyte, in elderly, 157
long-term efficacy of, 158
Scopulariopsis brevicaulis, 156
vs. griseofulvin for *Trichophyton* tinea
capitis, 164
Ivermectin
for cutaneous larva migrans, 191
Ixodes scapularis
tick bite, single-dose doxycycline for
prevention of Lyme disease after,
123

J

Jessner/trichloroacetic acid peel
erythema after, persistent, 30
hypopigmentation after, 29
Joint
interphalangeal, distal, ganglion of,
therapy by identification and repair
of leak of joint fluid, 362
Journals
leading dermatology, 60
Juvenile
(*See also* Children)
dermatomyositis (*see* Dermatomyositis,
juvenile)
hemangiomas, microvascular phenotype
shared by human placenta and, 481

K

Kaposi's sarcoma
herpesvirus 8 infection and, in renal
transplant recipients, 334
Keloids
brachytherapy for, high-dose-rate, 360

earlobe
  recurrence rates after various
    postoperative therapeutic
    modalities, 359
  surgical excision and immediate
    postoperative adjuvant
    radiotherapy for, 357
Keratoconjunctivitis
  sicca, permanent, after isotretinoin use,
    201
Keratoses
  actinic
    counting, reliability of, 367
    diclofenac in hyaluronan gel for, 368,
      370
    imiquimod cream for, 371
    photodynamic therapy with topical
      aminolevulinic acid and fluorescent
      blue light for, 377
Ketoconazole
  for onychomycosis of toes,
    Scopulariopsis brevicaulis, 156
  systemic, for atopic dermatitis with
    IgE-mediated hypersensitivity to
    yeasts, 82
Kidney (*see* Renal)
Kif1C
  mediates macrophage resistance to
    anthrax lethal factor (in mice), 137
Klebsiella pneumoniae
  necrotizing fasciitis of head and neck
    due to, 130

L

Labial
  frenulum, inferior, absence in
    Ehlers-Danlos syndrome, 291
  herpes simplex, docosanol for, 170
Lactobacillus GG
  in primary prevention of atopic disease,
    72
Lamellar
  ichthyosis, autosomal recessive, TGM1
    gene mutations in, 297
Lamivudine
  prophylaxis against HIV after sexual or
    injection drug use exposure, 177
Larva
  migrans, cutaneous, in returning
    traveller, clinical features and
    management, 190
Laser
  carbon dioxide, peel with, *vs.*
    electrosurgical peel, clinical and
    histologic study, 347

dye
  flashlamp-pumped and long-pulsed
    tunable, for port-wine stains, 355
  pulsed, plus cryogen spray cooling for
    cutaneous hemangiomas, 486
microscopy, confocal scanning, in vivo,
    detection of clinically amelanotic
    melanoma and assessment of its
    margins by, 414
Nd:YAG, long-pulsed
  hair removal in pigmented skin with,
    352
  for reticular veins and venulectasias,
    clinical and pathophysiologic
    correlates of, 354
resurfacing
  acne after, 33
  complications of, 32
  complications of, reduction methods,
    35
  ectropion after, 34
  erythema after, 32
  hyperpigmentation after, 33
  hypopigmentation after, 33
  milia after, 33
  petechiae after, 34
  plus photothermolytic laser for
    difficult dermal pigmentation, 351
  scarring after, 33, 34
  swelling after, postoperative, 32
surgery, 343
  wiping away debris between passes
    during (in rat), 348
therapy, combined, for difficult dermal
    pigmentation, 351
Leg
  ulcers after hydroxyurea in sickle cell
    disease, 326
Leiomyosarcoma
  Mohs micrographic surgery for, 407
Leukocytoclastic
  vasculitis, cutaneous, in
    dermatomyositis, and malignancy,
    241
Leukopenia
  after bexarotene, oral, for cutaneous
    T-cell lymphoma, 472
Leukoplakia
  oral, DNA content as prognostic
    marker in, 397
Levamisole
  /cimetidine for recalcitrant warts in
    children, 167
Levonorgestrel
  /ethinyl estradiol in low-dose
    contraceptive for acne, 196

Lichen
  sclerosus
    incidence in men with squamous cell
      carcinoma of penis, 399
    vulgar, premenarchal, clobetasol
      propionate for, 318
Lichenoid
  reactions, oral, cutaneous, and genital,
    dental metal allergy in patients
    with, 91
Lidocaine
  toxicity in liposuction, 36
Lifestyle
  rheumatoid arthritis and, 253
Light
  blue, fluorescent, and topical
    aminolevulinic acid, photodynamic
    therapy of actinic keratoses with,
    377
  eruption, polymorphic, candidate gene
    analysis of, 227
  incoherent, photodynamic therapy of
    acne with δ-aminolevulinic acid
    and, 205
Limb
  infusion, isolated, for melanoma, 464
Lingual
  frenulum, inferior, absence in
    Ehlers-Danlos syndrome, 291
Lip
  hair, upper, prevalence in black and
    white girls during puberty, 218
Lipid
  hydroperoxides, vitamin C-induced
    decomposition to endogenous
    genotoxins, 388
Lipodystrophy
  dermatomyositis and, juvenile, 246
Liposomes
  topical T4 endonuclease V in, effect on
    skin cancer in xeroderma
    pigmentosum, 296
Liposuction
  complications of, 36
    rare, 37
    uncommon, 36
    very rare, 37
  mycobacterium after, atypical, 38
Lipotransfer
  bruising after, 39
  complications of, 38
Liver
  fibrosis, methotrexate-induced,
    amino-terminal propeptide of type
    III procollagen in routine screening
    for, 10-year follow-up, 112

Lung
  (*See also* Pulmonary)
  cancer in dermatomyositis and
    polymyositis, 242
Lupus
  erythematosus
    cutaneous *(see below)*
    discoid, causing depigmentation,
      epidermal grafting for, 229
    systemic, peripheral gangrene in
      infant with, 230
    timidus, phototesting in, 228
  erythematosus, cutaneous
    gene analysis of, candidate, 227
    subacute, association with terbinafine,
      160
    subacute, association with terbinafine,
      report of 5 cases, 161
    -like presentation of parvovirus B19
      infection, 175
Lyme disease
  case definition for national surveillance,
    119
  comparison in North America and
    Europe and Asia, 118
  epidemiology, clinical manifestations,
    diagnosis, 117
  patients with persistent symptoms and
    history, antibiotic treatment in, 124
  prevention, 119, 122
    after *Ixodes scapularis* tick bite,
      prevention with single-dose
      doxycycline, 123
    vaccine for, recombinant OspA, in
      children and adolescents, 125
  treatment, 119
Lymph node(s)
  metastases from melanoma, head and
    neck, clinically predictable pattern
    of, 451
  nonsentinel, reverse
    transcriptase-polymerase chain
    reaction analysis after completion
    lymphadenectomy for melanoma,
    447
  recurrence after lymphadenectomy for
    melanoma, risk factors for, 450
  regional, metastases from melanoma,
    effect of long-term adjuvant
    interferon α-2a in, 456
  sentinel (*see* Sentinel lymph node)
Lymphadenectomy
  completion, for melanoma, reverse
    transcriptase-polymerase chain
    reaction analysis of nonsentinel
    nodes after, 447
  for melanoma, risk factors for nodal
    recurrence after, 450

Lymphatic
  mapping and sentinel node biopsy in
    primary extremity melanoma, early
    recurrence after, 448
Lymphocyte
  T (*see* T cell)
Lymphoma
  non-Hodgkin's, in polymyositis, 242
  T-cell
    cutaneous (*see below*)
    transmission by allogeneic bone
      marrow transplantation, 478
  T-cell, cutaneous
    denileukin diftitox for, 476
    early-stage, refractory or persistent,
      oral bexarotene for, 471
    stage II, interferon-α2a and
      extracorporeal photochemotherapy
      for, 475
    staging classification for, modified,
      468
Lymphoproliferative
  disorders, 467
Lymphoscintigraphy
  in management of head and neck
    melanoma, 452
  preoperative, for identification of
    sentinel nodes in melanoma, 427
  reproducibility in melanoma, 429
Lysyl
  hydroxylase activity in type VI
    Ehlers-Danlos syndrome restored
    by adenoviral gene transfer (in rat),
    292

M

Macrophage
  granulocyte-macrophage
    colony-stimulating factor injection,
    perilesional, for cutaneous
    melanoma metastases, 459
  resistance to anthrax lethal factor
    mediated by Kif1C (in mice), 137
Maggot
  debridement therapy in outpatients, 191
Magnetic resonance imaging
  central nervous system, and congenital
    melanocytic nevi, 410
  for neurocutaneous melanosis in
    neurologically asymptomatic
    children with giant congenital
    melanocytic nevi, 409
  of perineural spread of squamous and
    basal cell carcinoma, 394
Malformations
  vascular, 481

Malignancy
  (*See also* Cancer)
  in dermatomyositis
    predicting factors of, 240
    risk and follow-up implications, 243
    vasculitis suggests, cutaneous
      leukocytoclastic, 241
  incidence in biopsy-proven
    inflammatory myopathy, 245
  in polymyositis
    predicting factors of, 240
    risk and follow-up implications, 243
  risk associated with psoriasis, 109
Mandibular
  nerve injury sequela, surgical, 15
Marrow (*see* Bone, marrow)
MART-1
  diagnostic accuracy for micrometastases
    in sentinel nodes of melanoma, 444
Masseter
  muscle hypertrophy, botulinum toxin A
    for, 345
Mast cells
  dermal, pimecrolimus inhibits mediator
    release from, 77
  role in neutrophil recruitment in bullous
    pemphigoid (in mice), 268
Mastocytosis
  cutaneous, bone marrow involvement
    in, 333
Meats
  ground, retail, isolation of
    antibiotic-resistant *Salmonella*
    from, 146
Meetings
  between general practitioners and
    pharmaceutical representatives,
    dramaturgical study of, 339
Mel-14
  F(ab')$_2$, iodine-131, long-term response
    in neoplastic meningitis secondary
    to melanoma, 462
Melan-A
  diagnostic accuracy for micrometastases
    in sentinel nodes of melanoma, 444
Melanocortin-1
  receptor gene variants determine risk of
    nonmelanoma skin cancer, 385
Melanocytic
  nevi (*see* Nevi, melanocytic)
  proliferations, benign, 409
Melanoma
  amelanotic, clinically, detection and
    assessment of margins by in vivo
    confocal scanning laser microscopy,
    414
  Apaf-1 inactivation in, 425

biopsy in, sentinel node, developing
indications for use of, 455
cell proliferation, suppression by
histidine decarboxylase specific
antisense oligonucleotides, 463
diagnosis, dermoscopy in, 413
differentiation of melanocytic nevi from,
automatic, 412
follow-up, ultrasound B-scan *vs.*
physical examination in, 453
head and neck
lymphoscintigraphy and PET in
management of, 452
metastases from, nodal, clinically
predictable pattern of, 451
incidence rates in U.S. whites, 50
recent trends in, 419
interferon α for, paroxetine for
prevention of depression induced
by, 457
interferon α-2b for, developing
indications for use of, 455
limb infusion for, isolated, 464
lymphadenectomy for
completion, reverse
transcriptase-polymerase chain
reaction analysis of nonsentinel
nodes after, 447
nodal recurrence after, risk factors
for, 450
lymphoscintigraphy reproducibility in,
429
meningitis secondary to, neoplastic,
long-term response to I-131 Mel-14
F(ab')₂, 462
metastases
cutaneous, perilesional GM-CSF
injection in, 459
gender and other survival predictors,
424
herpes simplex virus 1716 injection
in, intralesional, 461
lymph node, regional, effect of
long-term adjuvant interferon α-2a
in, 456
lymph node, sentinel,
micromorphometry-based concept
for routine classification, 430
micrometastasis in, sentinel node
diagnostic accuracy with Melan-A
and MART-1, 444
as predictor of outcome in patients
with thicker melanoma, 441
mortality
rates in U.S. whites, 50
related to early detection, 415
primary
biopsy in, sentinel node, 433

extremity, early recurrence after
lymphatic mapping and sentinel
node biopsy in, 448
in hidden sites, association with
thicker tumors, 420
level 2, associated with metastasis,
clinical and histologic features, 421
melanoma cells in sentinel nodes,
bone marrow and peripheral blood
detected by reverse
transcription–polymerase chain
reaction in, 445
prognosis, poor, increased soluble CD95
serum level correlates with, 426
risk after long-term exposure to PUVA,
107
sentinel node status in, melanoma
thickness and histology predict,
438
spindle cell, sentinel node status in, 443
stage I or II, sentinel node status as
predictor of clinical outcome, 439
surgical treatment, vertical dimension
in, 422
survival rates, 5-year, 51
thicker, sentinel node micrometastasis
and other histologic factors that
predict outcome, 441
ultraviolet radiation and, excessive
timing of, 418
vaccine, polyvalent shed-antigen, 458
Melanosis
neurocutaneous, significance in
neurologically asymptomatic
children with giant congenital
melanocytic nevi, 409
Melphalan
/actinomycin D in isolated limb infusion
for melanoma, 464
Meningioma
anaplastic, after Merkel cell carcinoma,
406
Meningitis
neoplastic, secondary to melanoma,
long-term response to I-131 Mel-14
F(ab')₂, 462
Meningococcal
disease, diagnosis in children with
hemorrhagic rash and fever, 127
Merkel cell carcinoma (*see* Carcinoma,
Merkel cell)
Metabolic
abnormalities in lipodystrophy and
juvenile dermatomyositis,
evaluation of, 246
Metabolism
phosphorus, role in development of
calcifications, 251

Metal
  allergy, dental, in patients with oral,
    cutaneous, and genital lichenoid
    reactions, 91
Metastases
  cutaneous, from melanoma, perilesional
    injection of GM-CSF for, 459
  lymph node
    from melanoma, head and neck,
      clinically predictable pattern of,
      451
    regional, from melanoma, effect of
      long-term adjuvant interferon α-2a
      in, 456
    sentinel, from melanoma,
      micromorphometry-based concept
      for routine classification, 430
  melanoma
    herpes simplex virus 1716 injection
      in, intralesional, 461
    level 2, clinical and histologic
      features, 421
  micrometastases, sentinel node
    of melanoma, diagnostic accuracy
      with Melan-A and MART-1, 444
    as predictor of outcome in patients
      with thicker melanomas, 441
Methotrexate
  for arthritis of inflammatory childhood
    myositis syndromes, 249
  for psoriasis
    liver fibrosis due to, amino-terminal
      propeptide of type III procollagen
      in routine screening for, 10-year
      follow-up, 112
    malignancy risk associated with, 109
  -responsive chronic idiopathic urticaria,
    63
Methylprednisolone
  high-dose pulse, for severe alopecia
    areata, 213
  IV
    with high-dose IV immunoglobulins
      for toxic epidermal necrolysis, 275
    pulse, for lipodystrophy and juvenile
      dermatomyositis, 248
Microbial
  colonization of artificial fingernails
    worn by health care workers, effect
    of hand cleansing with
    antimicrobial soap or alcohol-based
    gel on, 139
Microbiological
  study of Papillon-Lefèvre syndrome,
    302
Microbiologist
  military research, glanders in, 136

Microdermabrasion
  aluminum oxide crystal, for
    photodamage, 350
  complications of, 31
  epidermal and dermal changes after,
    349
Micrographic surgery
  Mohs (*see* Mohs micrographic surgery)
Micrometastasis
  sentinel node
    in melanoma, diagnostic accuracy
      with Melan-A and MART-1, 444
    as predictor of outcome in patients
      with thicker melanomas, 441
Micromorphometry
  -based concept for routine classification
    of sentinel lymph node metastases
    from melanoma, 430
Micronodular
  basal cell carcinoma, correlation of
    alpha-smooth muscle actin and
    invasion in, 390
Microscopy
  epiluminescence, in melanoma
    diagnosis, 413
  laser, confocal scanning, in vivo,
    detection of clinically amelanotic
    melanoma and assessment of its
    margins by, 414
Microvascular
  phenotype shared by juvenile
    hemangiomas and human placenta,
    481
Milia
  colored, after chemical peel, 31
  after laser resurfacing, 33
  in pseudoporphyria, 288
Military
  research microbiologist, glanders in,
    136
Mineral
  bone, density in patients receiving
    glucocorticoids, 2-year effects of
    alendronate on, 278
Minocycline
  for sarcoidosis, 321
  vs. hydroxychloroquine for early
    seropositive rheumatoid arthritis,
    254
Mite
  dust, house, control measures, in adults
    with atopic dermatitis, 74
Mitogen
  -activated protein kinase activation by
    integrins in pathogenesis of
    psoriasis, 94

Model
predictive, for immunotherapy of alopecia areata with diphencyprone, 215
Mohs micrographic surgery
dense inflammation does not mask residual primary basal cell carcinoma during, 392
risk of synchronous and metachronous second nonmelanoma skin cancer when referred for, 393
for spindle cell tumors of skin, 407
Molecular
genetic features of pulmonary hypertension in patients with hereditary hemorrhagic telangiectasia, 301
Molluscum
contagiosum in children with organ transplants, 336
Mometasone furoate
for radiation dermatitis, acute, 316
Monoclonal
antibody
anti-CD11a, for moderate to severe psoriasis, 99
anti-tumor necrosis factor α (*see* Infliximab)
Morphea
childhood, calcipotriol ointment plus low-dose UVA1 phototherapy in, 232
Mortality
from melanoma
metastatic, predictors of, 424
rates in U.S. whites, 50
related to early detection, 415
procedure-related, of autologous stem cell transplantation in systemic sclerosis, 237
Mouth
dry, after Botox, 28
MRI (*see* Magnetic resonance imaging)
Muscle
alpha-smooth muscle actin correlated with invasion in micronodular basal cell carcinoma, 390
hypertrophy, masseter and temporal, botulinum toxin A for, 345
Mycobacterial
infection after liposuction, 37, 38
Mycophenolate mofetil
for dermatitis, atopic, 81
for psoriasis, 110
Mycosis
fungoides
alcohol intake and smoking and, 467

extracutaneous, clinical characteristics and outcome, 470
photodynamic therapy with topical aminolevulinic acid for, 473
widespread plaque-type, nodular, and erythrodermic, high-dose UVA1 therapy of, 474
Myocardial
infarction and oral contraceptives, 197
Myofibroblasts
in hypertrophic scars, effect of interferon-α2b on, 356
Myopathy
inflammatory, biopsy-proven, malignancy incidence in, 245
Myositis
inclusion-body, malignancy incidence in, 245
syndromes, inflammatory childhood, arthritis of, 248
Myxoid
cyst, digital, therapy by identification and repair of leak of joint fluid, 362

N

Nail
fingernails, artificial, worn by health care workers
Candida osteomyelitis and diskitis after spinal surgery due to, 138
microbial colonization of, effect of hand cleansing with antimicrobial soap or alcohol-based gel on, 139
toenail onychomycosis (*see* Onychomycosis, toenail)
Naproxen
risk of serious coronary heart disease with, 311
Nasal
carriage as source of *Staphylococcus aureus* bacteremia, 129
Nasopharyngeal
carcinoma in dermatomyositis and polymyositis, 241
Nd:YAG
laser, long-pulsed
hair removal in pigmented skin with, 352
for reticular veins and venulectasias, clinical and pathophysiologic correlates of, 354
Neck
(*See also* Head and neck)
posterior triangle, inflamed epidermal inclusion cyst in, 15

Necrolysis
  toxic epidermal, high-dose IV
    immunoglobulins for, 275
Necrosis
  full- and partial-thickness, in distal flap,
    6
  graft, full-thickness skin, 11
  tissue
    grafted, after lipotransfer, 38
    local, after collagen implantation, 22
    local, after collagen implantation,
      management, 23
  wound edge, scar secondary to, 4
Necrotizing
  fasciitis of head and neck, 130
  infections due to group G streptococcus,
    and streptolysin S, 131
Neoplasia
  intraepithelial, vulvovaginal and
    perianal, risk with HIV infection,
    187
Neoplastic
  meningitis secondary to melanoma,
    long-term response to I-131 Mel-14
    F(ab')₂, 462
Nerve
  facial, in excisional and reconstructive
    surgery, 13
  mandibular, surgical injury sequela, 15
  temporal, surgical injury sequela, 14
Nervous
  system, central, imaging, and congenital
    melanocytic nevi, 410
Neurocutaneous
  melanosis, significance in neurologically
    asymptomatic children with giant
    congenital melanocytic nevi, 409
Neuropathy
  peripheral, and cryoglobulinemia, 259
Neutrophil
  recruitment in bullous pemphigoid, role
    of mast cells in (in mice), 268
Nevi
  congenital, combined laser therapy for,
    351
  melanocytic, 409
    congenital, central nervous system
      imaging and, 410
    congenital, giant, significance of
      neurocutaneous melanosis in
      neurologically asymptomatic
      children with, 409
    differentiation from melanoma,
      automatic, 412
  of Ota, combined laser therapy for, 351
Nickel
  allergy prevalence in adolescents, 67

sulfate patch testing with standardized
    ready-to-use test system, 86
Nodular
  acne, severe recalcitrant, new
    micronized isotretinoin formulation
    for, 203, 204
  granuloma formation after silicone
    implantation, 25
  mycosis fungoides, high-dose UVA1
    therapy of, 474
NSAIDs (*see* Anti-inflammatory, drugs,
    nonsteroidal)
Nuclear
  receptor corepressor, novel, *hairless*
    gene mutated in congenital hair
    loss disorders encodes, 212
  retinoid receptor decreases, progressive,
    during skin squamous
    carcinogenesis, 387

O

Occupation
  of patients evaluated in patch test
    clinics, 90
Octyl cyanoacrylate
  tissue adhesive *vs.* suture for closure of
    excisional wounds in children and
    adolescents, 364
Ocular
  side effects of isotretinoin, 200
Office
  -based physicians, non-federal, visits to,
    in U.S., 55
Oligonucleotides
  antisense, histidine decarboxylase
    specific, suppression of melanoma
    cell proliferation by, 463
Omalizumab
  effect on symptoms of seasonal allergic
    rhinitis, 64
Onychomycosis
  toenail
    antifungals for, long-term efficacy of,
      158
    dermatophyte, terbinafine and
      itraconazole for, in elderly, 157
    Scopulariopsis brevicaulis, efficacy of
      itraconazole, terbinafine,
      fluconazole, griseofulvin and
      ketoconazole for, 156
Oral
  leukoplakia, DNA content as prognostic
    marker in, 397
  lichenoid reactions, dental metal allergy
    in patients with, 91

pemphigus severity related to desmoglein 1 and 3 antibody levels, 272

warts, effect of highly active antiretroviral therapy on frequency of, 186

Organ
transplant recipients, pediatric, skin diseases in, 336

OspA vaccine
recombinant, for Lyme disease prevention, 119, 122
in children and adolescents, 125

Osteomyelitis
Candida, after spinal surgery, due to artificial nail use, 138

Ota's nevus
combined laser therapy for, 351

Outdoor
activities in childhood as protective factor for melanoma, 417

Outpatient
maggot debridement therapy, 191

Ovaries
adenocarcinoma after Merkel cell carcinoma, 406
cancer in dermatomyositis, 242
polycystic, in hirsute women with normal menses, 219

P

p53
involvement in control of hair follicle regression (in mice), 210
mutations in basal cell carcinomas from PUVA-treated patients with psoriasis, ultraviolet exposure as main indicator of, 388

Pain
acute, in herpes zoster, 172
after Botox, 27
ischemic, in scleroderma, surgery for, 239

Palmar
sympathectomy for ischemic pain and Raynaud's phenomenon in scleroderma, 239

Pamidronate
for calcinosis of juvenile dermatomyositis, 251

Pancreas
cancer in dermatomyositis, 242

Panuveitis
sight-threatening, in Behçet's disease, effect of infliximab on, 257

Papillomavirus
infection as risk factor for squamous cell carcinoma of head and neck, 396

Papillon-Lefèvre syndrome
microbiological study of, 302

Papulopustular
skin lesions in Behçet's syndrome with arthritis, 255

Parathyroidectomy
in patients with calciphylaxis from secondary hyperparathyroidism, 322

Paroxetine
for prevention of depression induced by high-dose interferon α, 457

Parvovirus
B19 infection, lupus-like presentation of, 175

Patch testing
clinics, occupation of patients evaluated in, 90
discordance alert, 87
of nickel sulfate and potassium dichromate with standardized ready-to-use test system, 86
prick testing with, results in health care workers, 89
results with standard series among whites *vs.* blacks, 85

Pathophysiologic
correlates of long-pulsed Nd:YAG laser treatment of reticular veins and venulectasias, 354

Peels
chemical
adverse reactions to, procedural, 31
complications of, 29
complications of, minimizing measures, 32
demarcation problems after, 31
erythema after, prolonged, 30
herpes simplex reactivation after, 31
infections after, superficial bacterial or yeast, 31
milia after, colored, 31
for photoaged skin, quantitative and qualitative effects of (in mice), 346
pigmentary changes after, 29
scarring after, 30
systemic effects of, 30
electrosurgical and carbon dioxide laser, clinical and histologic comparison, 347

Pemphigoid
bullous
corticosteroids for, oral *vs.* topical, 267

neutrophil recruitment in, role of
mast cells in (in mice), 268
treatment, think globally, act locally,
265
cicatricial, anti-epiligrin, and relative
risk for cancer, 270
Pemphigus
cutaneous, severity related to
desmoglein 1 and 3 antibody levels,
272
immunoglobulin therapy for, IV, 275
oral, severity related to desmoglein 1
and 3 antibody levels, 272
Penicillin
skin testing practice guideline improves
appropriateness of antibiotic
therapy, 143
Penis
carcinoma, squamous cell, high
incidence of lichen sclerosus in men
with, 399
Peptic
ulcer
disease, role of *Helicobacter pylori*
infection and NSAIDs in, 307
risk in patients starting long-term
treatment with nonsteroidal
anti-inflammatory drugs, effect of
eradication of *Helicobacter pylori*
on, 308
Peptide
antimicrobial
innate, skin protection from invasive
bacterial infection by (in mice), 141
secreted by sweat glands, dermcidin
as, 142
Perfume
allergy, prevalence in adolescents, 67
Perianal
condylomata acuminata and
intraepithelial neoplasia, risk with
HIV infection, 187
Perineural
spread of squamous and basal cell
carcinoma, CT and MR detection
of, 394
Periodontopathic
bacteria in Papillon-Lefèvre syndrome,
303
PET
in management of head and neck
melanoma, 452
Petechiae
after laser resurfacing, 34
Pharmaceutical
representatives, meetings between
general practitioners and,
dramaturgical study of, 339

Phenol
peel
for photoaged skin, quantitative and
qualitative effects of (in mice), 346
systemic effects of, 30
Phenotype
microvascular, shared by juvenile
hemangiomas and human placenta,
481
p-Phenylenediamine
sensitization rate for, in blacks *vs.*
whites, 85
Phosphorus
metabolism, role in development of
calcifications, 251
Photoaged skin
chemical peeling for, quantitative and
qualitative effects of (in mice), 346
Photobiology, 281
Photochemotherapy
extracorporeal, and interferon-α2a for
stage II cutaneous T-cell lymphoma,
475
Photodamage
microdermabrasion for, aluminum oxide
crystal, 350
Photodynamic therapy
for acne with topical δ-aminolevulinic
acid and incoherent light, 205
for keratoses, actinic, with topical
aminolevulinic acid and fluorescent
blue light, 377
for mycosis fungoides with topical
aminolevulinic acid, 473
photofrin-mediated, for aggressive head
and neck nonmelanomatous skin
tumors in elderly, 395
Photofrin
-mediated photodynamic therapy for
aggressive head and neck
nonmelanomatous skin tumors in
elderly, 395
Photosensitivity
disorders, 3, candidate gene analysis of,
227
in pseudoporphyria, 288
Phototesting
in lupus erythematosus tumidus, 228
Phototherapy
UVA, broad-band, in adult atopic
eczema, 80
UVA1
high-dose, for widespread
plaque-type, nodular, and
erythrodermic mycosis fungoides,
474
low-dose, plus calcipotriol ointment
in childhood morphea, 232

UVB
 narrow-band, for eczema, adult
  atopic, 80
 narrow-band, for vitiligo, 221
 skin carcinogenesis after, inhibitory
  effects of orally administered green
  tea, black tea, and caffeine on (in
  mice), 282
Photothermolytic
 plus resurfacing lasers for difficult
  dermal pigmentation, 351
Physical
 abuse and recent skin injuries in normal
  children, 337
 examination *vs.* ultrasound B-scan in
  follow-up of melanoma, 453
Physician(s)
 certified in dermatologic subspecialties,
  55
 office-based, non-federal, visits to, in
  U.S., 55
 specialty, effect on likelihood of
  tumor-free resection margins for
  basal cell carcinoma, 391
Pigmentary
 changes after chemical peel, 29, 31
Pigmentation
 dermal, difficult, combined laser therapy
  for, 351
 generalized, after minocycline for
  rheumatoid arthritis, 254
Pigmented
 skin, long-pulsed Nd:YAG laser-assisted
  hair removal in, 352
Pimecrolimus (*see* SDZ ASM 981)
Pincushion
 deformity, 7
 of transposition flap, 8
Pityrosporum ovale
 hypersensitivity to, IgE-mediated,
  systemic ketoconazole for atopic
  dermatitis with, 82
Placenta
 human, microvascular phenotype shared
  by juvenile hemangiomas and, 481
Plaque
 psoriasis (*see* Psoriasis, plaque)
 -type mycosis fungoides, high-dose
  UVA1 therapy of, 474
Platelet
 count, elevated, and risk of visual loss
  in giant cell arteritis, 261
Polycystic
 ovaries in hirsute women with normal
  menses, 219
Polymerase chain reaction
 reverse transcription-, in melanoma

of nonsentinel nodes after completion
 lymphadenectomy, 447
primary, detection of melanoma cells
 in sentinel nodes, bone marrow and
 peripheral blood by, 445
for TGM1 gene mutations in autosomal
 recessive lamellar ichthyosis, 297
Polymorphic
 light eruption, candidate gene analysis
  of, 227
Polymorphisms
 cytokine gene, in psoriasis, 95
Polymyositis
 malignancy in
  predicting factors of, 240
  risk and follow-up implications, 243
  risk of, 245
  specific types, frequency of, 242
  prognostic factors and short-term and
   long-term outcome, 244
Polyphenols
 green tea, cutaneous photoprotection
  from ultraviolet injury by, 281
Pork
 ingestion of antibiotic-resistant
  Enterococcus faecium from,
  intestinal carriage after, 147
Port-wine stains
 laser treatment of, flashlamp-pumped
  and long-pulsed tunable dye, 355
Positron emission tomography
 in management of head and neck
  melanoma, 452
Potassium
 dichromate patch testing with
  standardized ready-to-use test
  system, 86
Practice
 guideline for penicillin skin testing
  improves appropriateness of
  antibiotic therapy, 143
Practitioners
 general, meetings between
  pharmaceutical representatives and,
  dramaturgical study of, 339
Prednisone
 for hemangiomas, cutaneous, 484
 oral, *vs.* clobetasol propionate cream
  for bullous pemphigoid, 267
Premenarchal
 vulvar lichen sclerosus, clobetasol
  propionate for, 318
Prenatal
 probiotics in primary prevention of
  atopic disease, 72
Prescription
 products, spending on consumer
  advertising of, in U.S., 58

Prick testing
with patch testing, results in health care
workers, 89
Primary care
providers' skin cancer control practices,
impact of Basic Skin Cancer Triage
curriculum on, 378
setting, skin cancer screening and
prevention in, 379
Probiotics
in primary prevention of atopic disease,
72
Procollagen
type III, amino-terminal propeptide of,
in routine screening for
methotrexate-induced liver fibrosis,
10-year follow-up, 112
Propeptide
of type III procollagen, amino-terminal,
in routine screening for
methotrexate-induced liver fibrosis,
10-year follow-up, 112
Propionibacterium acnes
sciatica and, 206
Prostate
cancer and exposure to ultraviolet
radiation, 286
Protein
A, *Borrelia burgdorferi* outer surface
protein A vaccine in prevention of
Lyme disease in children and
adolescents, 125
kinase activation by integrins,
mitogen-activated, in pathogenesis
of psoriasis, 94
Proteoglycan
sulfate, antichondroitin, Mel-14 F(ab')₂,
I-131, long-term response in
neoplastic meningitis secondary to
melanoma, 462
Prurigo
actinic, candidate gene analysis of, 227
nodularis, topical capsaicin for, 317
Pseudomonas aeruginosa
hot-foot syndrome due to, 135
toe web infection due to, 134
Pseudoporphyria
clinical and biochemical study, 288
Psoralen
/UVA therapy (*see* PUVA therapy)
Psoriasis, 93
arthritis in, infliximab for, 101
childhood, 113
Crohn disease-associated, anti-tumor
necrosis factor α monoclonal
antibody for, 100
cytokine gene polymorphisms in, 95

guttate, streptococcal
superantigen-induced T-cell
proliferation patterns in, 93
lesions, effects of systemic
interleukin-10 therapy on, 96
malignancy risk associated with, 109
methotrexate for, liver fibrosis due to,
amino-terminal propeptide of type
III procollagen in routine screening
for, 10-year follow-up, 112
moderate to severe, anti-CD11a
antibody for, 99
mycophenolate mofetil for, 110
pathogenesis, mitogen-activated protein
kinase activation by integrins in, 94
plaque
chronic, streptococcal
superantigen-induced T-cell
proliferation patterns in, 93
chronic, treatment by selective
targeting of memory effector T
lymphocytes, 97
etanercept for, 104
infliximab monotherapy for, 102
pustular, generalized, low-dose
cyclosporine for, 114
PUVA therapy for, basal cell carcinomas
after, ultraviolet exposure as main
initiator of p53 mutations in, 388
refractory, thioguanine for, 111
Ptosis
after Botox, 26
methods of minimizing, 27
Puberty
lip hair prevalence in, upper, in black
and white girls, 218
Pulmonary
embolism
after isolated limb infusion for
melanoma, 465
seasonal variation in hospital
admission for, 329
severe, association with air travel,
331
hypertension in patients with hereditary
hemorrhagic telangiectasia, clinical
and molecular genetic features of,
301
Purpura
Henoch-Schönlein
renal lesions in, acute and chronic,
grading of, 263
renal sequelae in adults with,
predictive factors for, 262
PUVA therapy
with calcipotriol, topical, for vitiligo,
222, 224

cyclosporine and, squamous cell cancer
of skin after, 106
long-term, risk of melanoma after, 107
for psoriasis, basal cell carcinomas after,
ultraviolet exposure as main
initiator of p53 mutations in, 388
Pyoderma
gangrenosum associated with Crohn
disease, anti-tumor necrosis factor
α monoclonal antibody for, 100

Q

Quinupristin
-dalfopristin-resistant *Enterococcus
faecium* on chicken and in stool
specimens, 147

R

Race
patch test results with standard series
and, 85
Radial
arteriolysis with palmar sympathectomy
for ischemic pain and Raynaud's
phenomenon in scleroderma, 239
Radiation
dermatitis, acute, mometasone furoate
for, 316
therapeutic (*see* Radiotherapy)
ultraviolet (*see* Ultraviolet)
Radiotherapy
for Merkel cell carcinoma, 405
postoperative
adjuvant, immediate, for earlobe
keloids, 357
for keloids, earlobe, recurrence rates
after, 359
for Merkel cell carcinoma of head
and neck, effect on recurrence and
survival, 402
Rash
hemorrhagic, and fever, diagnostic
assessment, 127
skin, and HHV-6 infection after
allogeneic bone marrow
transplantation, 174
Raynaud's phenomenon
in systemic sclerosis
calcium channel blockers for, 236
surgery for, 239
Reconstructive
surgery
complications of, 1

complications of, acute, 1
facial nerve in, 13
5α-Reductase
testosterone and epitestosterone in male
pattern baldness, 216
Renal
failure
chronic, and acetaminophen and
aspirin, 309
diabetes and, perforating collagenosis
of, allopurinol for, 323
involvement in cryoglobulinemia, 259
lesions, acute and chronic, in
Henoch-Schönlein purpura, grading
of, 263
sequelae in adults with
Henoch-Schönlein purpura,
predictive factors for, 262
transplantation (*see* Transplantation,
kidney)
Reproductive
factors and rheumatoid arthritis, 253
Research
microbiologist, military, glanders in,
136
Resiquimod
gel, effect on recurrence rate of
recurrent genital herpes, 169
Resurfacing
laser (*see* Laser, resurfacing)
Reticular
veins, long-pulsed Nd:YAG laser
treatment of, clinical and
pathophysiologic correlates of, 354
Retinoid
receptors, nuclear, progressive decreases
during skin squamous
carcinogenesis, 387
Rheumatoid
arthritis (*see* Arthritis, rheumatoid)
Rhinitis
allergic
prevalence in adolescents, 66
seasonal, effect of omalizumab on
symptoms of, 64
RNA
component of telomerase mutated in
autosomal dominant dyskeratosis
congenita, 298
Rofecoxib
risk of cardiovascular events with, 312
Ropivacaine
as local anesthetic for skin infiltration in
skin surgery, 363
Rubber
additives, false-positive findings with
patch testing, 87

S

Salmonella
  antibiotic-resistant, isolation from retail
    ground meats, 146
Sarcoidosis
  tetracyclines for, 320
Sarcoma
  Kaposi's, and herpesvirus 8 infection in
    renal transplant recipients, 334
Scabies
  diagnosis in children, high-magnification
    videodermatoscopy in, 189
Scalp
  carcinoma, basal or squamous cell,
    perineural spread, CT and MR
    detection of, 394
Scanning
  microscopy, in vivo confocal laser,
    detection of clinically amelanotic
    melanoma and assessment of its
    margins by, 414
Scar
  formation, healed blisters with, in
    pseudoporphyria, 288
  hypertrophic
    myofibroblasts and apoptosis in,
      effect of interferon-α2b on, 356
    after tissue adhesive *vs.* suture for
      closure of excisional wounds in
      children and adolescents, 364
  secondary to wound edge necrosis, 4
Scarring
  after chemical peel, 30
  after laser resurfacing, 33, 34
Sciatica
  Propionibacterium acnes and, 206
Scleroderma (*see* Sclerosis, systemic)
Sclerosis
  systemic
    dermal fibroblasts in, decreased
      susceptibility to Fas-induced
      apoptosis of, 234
    functional ability related to skin score
      in, 234
    iloprost suppresses connective tissue
      growth factor production in
      fibroblasts and skin in, 236
    Raynaud's phenomenon in, calcium
      channel blockers for, 236
    stem cell transplantation in,
      autologous, 237
    surgery for ischemic pain and
      Raynaud's phenomenon in, 239

Scopulariopsis brevicaulis
  onychomycosis of toes, efficacy of
    itraconazole, terbinafine,
    griseofulvin and ketoconazole for,
    156
SDZ ASM 981
  for dermatitis, atopic, 78
    in children, 79
  inhibits mediator release from dermal
    mast cells and basophils, 77
Seasonal
  allergic rhinitis symptoms, effect of
    omalizumab on, 64
  variations in hospital admission for
    deep vein thrombosis and
    pulmonary embolism, 329
Seborrheic
  dermatitis
    antifungal agents for, topical, 316
    terbinafine for, oral, 315
Sentinel lymph node
  biopsy (*see* Biopsy, sentinel node)
  identification in melanoma, preoperative
    lymphoscintigraphy for, 427
  melanoma cells in, detection by reverse
    transcription–polymerase chain
    reaction, 445
  metastases, melanoma,
    micromorphometry-based concept
    for routine classification, 430
  micrometastasis
    in melanoma, diagnostic accuracy
      with Melan-A and MART-1, 444
    as predictor of outcome in patients
      with thicker melanomas, 441
  status in melanoma
    prediction by melanoma thickness
      and histology, 438
    spindle cell, 443
    stage I or II, as predictor of clinical
      outcome, 439
Sex (*see* Gender)
Sexual
  exposure, postexposure prophylaxis
    against HIV infection after, 177
Sickle cell
  disease, cutaneous adverse reactions to
    hydroxyurea in, 325
Sight
  -threatening panuveitis in Behçet's
    disease, effect of infliximab on, 257
Silicone
  implantation
    complications of, 24
    granuloma formation after, nodular,
      25

Skin
(*See also* Cutaneous)
adaptation, solar-stimulated, and its effect on subsequent UV-induced epidermal DNA damage, 284
carcinogenesis
squamous, progressive decreases in nuclear retinoid receptors during, 387
after UVB therapy, inhibitory effects of orally administered green tea, black tea, and caffeine on (in mice), 282
diseases
in organ transplant recipients, pediatric, 336
in systemic sclerosis, impact of autologous stem cell transplantation on, 237
fragility in pseudoporphyria, 288
graft (*see* Graft, skin)
infections in renal transplant recipients, 335
infiltration in skin surgery, ropivacaine as local anesthetic for, 363
injuries, recent, in normal children, 337
lesions, papulopustular, in Behçet's syndrome with arthritis, 255
photoaged, chemical peeling for, quantitative and qualitative effects of (in mice), 346
pigmented, long-pulsed Nd:YAG laser-assisted hair removal in, 352
protection from invasive bacterial infection by innate antimicrobial peptide (in mice), 141
rash and HHV-6 infection after allogeneic bone marrow transplantation, 174
of scleroderma patients, iloprost suppresses connective tissue growth factor production in, 236
score related to functional ability in systemic sclerosis, 234
surgery, ropivacaine as local anesthetic for skin infiltration in, 363
testing, penicillin, practice guideline improves appropriateness of antibiotic therapy, 143
tumors
head and neck, aggressive nonmelanomatous, photofrin-mediated photodynamic therapy for, in elderly, 395
spindle cell, Mohs micrographic surgery for, 407

xeroderma pigmentosum, DNA repair-deficient, reconstruction in vitro, clues to epidermal cancer proneness revealed by, 295
Smoking
acne and, 194
flap necrosis and, 5
grafts and, full-thickness skin, 11
mycosis fungoides and, 467
Smooth
muscle actin, alpha-, correlated with invasion in micronodular basal cell carcinoma, 390
Soap
antimicrobial, hand cleansing with, effect on microbial colonization of artificial fingernails worn by health care workers, 139
Solar
-simulated skin adaptation and its effect on subsequent UV-induced epidermal DNA damage, 284
Specialty
of treating physician affects likelihood of tumor-free resection margins for basal cell carcinoma, 391
Spending (*see* Expenditures)
Spinal
surgery, *Candida* osteomyelitis and diskitis due to artificial nail use after, 138
Spindle cell
melanoma, sentinel node status in, 443
tumors of skin, Mohs micrographic surgery for, 407
Spray cooling
cryogen, and pulsed dye laser treatment of cutaneous hemangiomas, 486
Squamous
carcinogenesis, skin, progressive decreases in nuclear retinoid receptors during, 387
cell carcinoma (*see* Carcinoma, squamous cell)
Stains
port-wine, laser treatment of, flashlamp-pumped and long-pulsed tunable dye, 355
Staphylococcus aureus
bacteremia, nasal carriage as source of, 129
necrotizing fasciitis of head and neck due to, 130
Statistics
of interest to dermatologist, 43
Stavudine
prophylaxis against HIV after sexual or injection drug use exposure, 177

Stem cell
transplantation, autologous, in systemic
sclerosis, 237
Sterile abscess
formation after collagen implantation,
21
management, 22
Steroids (*see* Corticosteroids)
Stomach
cancer in dermatomyositis, 242
Stool
specimens,
quinupristin-dalfopristin-resistant
Enterococcus faecium in, 147
Streptococcal
superantigen-induced T-cell proliferation
patterns in guttate *vs.* chronic
plaque psoriasis, 93
Streptococcus
group G causing necrotizing infections,
and streptolysin S, 131
Streptococcus
necrotizing fasciitis of head and neck
due to, 130
Streptolysin
S and necrotizing infections produced
by group G streptococcus, 131
Subspecialties
dermatologic, physicians certified in, 55
Suicide
in isotretinoin-treated patients, 201
Sulphonamides
for mixed immunobullous disease of
childhood, 277
Superantigen
-induced T-cell proliferation patterns,
streptococcal, in guttate *vs.* chronic
plaque psoriasis, 93
Surgery
cosmetic (*see* Cosmetic, surgery)
dermatologic, 343
excisional (*see* Excisional, surgery)
laser, 343
Mohs micrographic (*see* Mohs
micrographic surgery)
reconstructive (*see* Reconstructive,
surgery)
Suture
vs. Dermabond for closure of excisional
wounds in children and
adolescents, 364
Sweat
glands, antibiotic peptide dermcidin
secreted by, 142
Swelling
postoperative, after laser resurfacing, 32

Sympathectomy
palmar, for ischemic pain and
Raynaud's phenomenon in
scleroderma, 239

T

T4
endonuclease V, topical, in liposomes,
effect on skin cancer in xeroderma
pigmentosum, 296
T cell(s)
γδ, regulation of cutaneous malignancy
by (in mice), 386
lymphoma, cutaneous (*see* Lymphoma,
T-cell, cutaneous)
memory effector, treatment of chronic
plaque psoriasis by selective
targeting of, 97
proliferation patterns, streptococcal
superantigen-induced, in guttate *vs.*
chronic plaque psoriasis, 93
Tacrolimus
ointment for cutaneous graft-*vs.*-host
disease, 319
Targretin
capsules for early stage refractory or
persistent cutaneous T-cell
lymphoma, 471
Tea
black, orally administered, inhibitory
effects on skin carcinogenesis after
UVB therapy (in mice), 282
green
orally administered, inhibitory effects
on skin carcinogenesis after UVB
therapy (in mice), 282
polyphenols, cutaneous
photoprotection from ultraviolet
injury by, 281
Telangiectasia
hereditary hemorrhagic, pulmonary
hypertension in, clinical and
molecular genetic features of, 301
Telomerase
RNA component, mutation in
autosomal dominant dyskeratosis
congenita, 298
Temporal
arteritis, risk factors for visual loss in,
261
muscle hypertrophy, botulinum toxin A
for, 345
nerve injury sequela, surgical, 14
Tenascin-X
deficiency causing recessive form of
Ehlers-Danlos syndrome, 293

Teratogen
warning symbol, interpretations of, 199
Teratogenicity
of anticonvulsant drugs, 326
Terbinafine
-associated subacute cutaneous lupus
erythematosus, 160
report of 5 cases, 161
for onychomycosis of toenail
dermatophyte, in elderly, 157
long-term efficacy of, 158
Scopulariopsis brevicaulis, 156
oral, for seborrheic dermatitis, 315
vs. griseofulvin for tinea capitis, 163
Trichophyton, 164
Testosterone
biochemical role as indicator of male
pattern baldness, 216
Tetracyclines
for sarcoidosis, 320
TGM1 gene
mutations in autosomal recessive
lamellar ichthyosis, 297
Therapies
new and unusual, 315
Thiabendazole
cream for cutaneous larva migrans, 190
Thioguanine
for psoriasis, refractory, 111
Thiuram
allergy, changing frequency in
healthcare workers with hand
dermatitis, 88
Thrombosis
venous
deep, after isolated limb infusion for
melanoma, 465
deep, seasonal variation in hospital
admission for, 329
deep, symptomless, frequency and
prevention in long-haul flights, 330
risk with third-generation oral
contraceptives, 198
Tick
bite, *Ixodes scapularis,* doxycycline for
prevention of Lyme disease after,
123
Tinea
capitis
hair care practices and, 162
terbinafine *vs.* griseofulvin for, 163
Trichophyton, therapeutic options for,
164
versicolor in children with organ
transplants, 336

Tissue
adhesive, octyl cyanoacrylate, *vs.* suture,
for closure of excisional wounds in
children and adolescents, 364
connective tissue growth factor
production in fibroblasts and skin
of scleroderma patients, iloprost
suppresses, 236
fat, decreased after oral administration
of green tea, black tea, and caffeine
after UVB therapy, and skin
carcinogenesis (in mice), 282
grafted, necrosis after lipotransfer, 38
local, necrosis after collagen
implantation, 22
management, 23
Toe
ulceration associated with compression
bandaging, 332
web infection, gram-negative bacterial,
134
Toenail
onychomycosis (*see* Onychomycosis,
toenail)
Tomography
computed, of perineural spread of
squamous and basal cell carcinoma,
394
positron emission, in management of
head and neck melanoma, 452
Toxic
epidermal necrolysis, high-dose IV
immunoglobulins for, 275
Toxicity
lidocaine, in liposuction, 36
Toxin
botulinum (*see* Botulinum toxin)
Trainees
dermatology, in U.S., 54
Transglutaminase
1 mutations in autosomal recessive
lamellar ichthyosis, 297
Transplantation
bone marrow, allogeneic
HHV-6 infection and skin rash after,
174
transmission of T-cell lymphoma by,
478
hair, complications of, 34
kidney
Kaposi's sarcoma and herpesvirus 8
infection after, 334
skin cancer after, nonmelanoma,
annual incidence and predicted risk
of, 382
skin cancer surveillance after, 381
skin infections after, 335
organ, pediatric, skin diseases after, 336

stem cell, autologous, in systemic
sclerosis, 237
Traumatic
wound dehiscence, 5
Travel
air
long-haul, frequency and prevention
of symptomless deep vein
thrombosis in, 330
pulmonary embolism associated with,
severe, 331
Traveller
returning, clinical features and
management of cutaneous larva
migrans in, 190
Triamcinolone diacetate
injection, intralesional, high injection
pressure during, for capillary
hemangiomas, 485
Trichloroacetic acid
/Jessner peel
erythema after, persistent, 30
hypopigmentation after, 29
peel for photoaged skin, quantitative
and qualitative effects of (in mice),
346
Trichophyton
rubrum in immunosuppressed patients,
151
tinea capitis, therapeutic options for,
164
Trimethoprim
for acne, infantile, 193
TRUETest
patch testing of nickel sulfate and
potassium dichromate with, 86
Tuberculosis
infliximab-associated, 104
Tumor(s)
-free resection margins for basal cell
carcinoma, specialty of treating
physician affects likelihood of, 391
necrosis factor α
blocking therapy with infliximab (*see*
Infliximab)
monoclonal antibody against (*see*
Infliximab)
receptor IgG1-Fc fusion complex
therapy (*see* Etanercept)
post-tumor removal defect, 10
second, and Merkel cell carcinoma, 406
skin
head and neck, aggressive
nonmelanomatous,
photofrin-mediated photodynamic
therapy for, in elderly, 395
spindle cell, Mohs micrographic
surgery for, 407

U

Ulcer
leg, after hydroxyurea in sickle cell
disease, 326
peptic
risk in patients starting long-term
treatment with NSAIDs, effect of
eradication of *Helicobacter pylori*
on, 308
role of *Helicobacter pylori* infection
and NSAIDs in, 307
Ulceration
of glabellar area after Zyderm II
implantation, 22
toe, association with compression
bandaging, 332
Ulnar
arteriolysis with palmar sympathectomy
for ischemic pain and Raynaud's
phenomenon in scleroderma, 239
Ultrasound
B-scan, *vs.* physical examination in
follow-up of melanoma, 453
Ultraviolet
A
phototherapy, broad-band, in adult
atopic eczema, 80
plus psoralen (*see* PUVA therapy)
A1 phototherapy
high-dose, for widespread
plaque-type, nodular, and
erythrodermic mycosis fungoides,
474
low-dose, plus calcipotriol ointment
in childhood morphea, 232
B phototherapy (*see* Phototherapy,
UVB)
exposure as main initiator of p53
mutations in basal cell carcinomas
from PUVA-treated patients with
psoriasis, 388
-induced epidermal DNA damage, effect
of solar-stimulated skin adaptation
on, 284
photoinjury, cutaneous protection by
green tea polyphenols from, 281
radiation
excessive, timing of, and melanoma,
418
exposure and prostate cancer, 286
Urticaria
chronic idiopathic,
methotrexate-responsive, 63
Urticarial
disorders, 63

V

Vaccine
  melanoma, polyvalent shed-antigen, 458
  OspA, recombinant, for Lyme disease
    prevention, 119, 122
  in children and adolescents, 125
  varicella, effectiveness in clinical
    practice, 171
Valacyclovir
  for herpes simplex reactivation
    after chemical peel, 31
    after collagen implantation, 24
Varicella
  vaccine, effectiveness in clinical practice,
    171
Vascular
  cardiovascular events, risk with selective
    COX-2 inhibitors, 312
  disorders, collagen, 227
  endothelial growth factor-mediated
    angiogenesis, control of hair
    growth and follicle size by (in
    mice), 209
  malformations, 481
Vasculitis
  cutaneous leukocytoclastic, in
    dermatomyositis, and malignancy,
    241
VEGF
  -mediated angiogenesis, control of hair
    growth and follicle size by (in
    mice), 209
Vein
  reticular, long-pulsed Nd:YAG laser
    treatment of, clinical and
    pathophysiologic correlates of, 354
  thrombosis (see Thrombosis, venous)
Venulectasias
  laser treatment of, long-pulsed
    Nd:YAG, clinical and
    pathophysiologic correlates of, 354
Vertebral
  fracture in patients receiving
    glucocorticoids, 2-year effects of
    alendronate on, 278
Videodermatoscopy
  high-magnification, in diagnosis of
    scabies in children, 189
Virus
  antiretroviral therapy (see
    Antiretroviral, therapy)
  GB, C, coinfection, effect on survival
    among HIV-infected patients, 178,
    179
  hepatitis
    C, infection, and cryoglobulinemia,
      259

G, coinfection, effect on survival
    among HIV-infected patients, 178,
    179
herpes (see Herpes)
herpesvirus
  6 infection and skin rash after
    allogeneic bone marrow
    transplantation, 174
  8 infection and Kaposi's sarcoma in
    renal transplant recipients, 334
immunodeficiency, human (see HIV)
infections, 167
papillomavirus infection as risk factor
    for squamous cell carcinoma of
    head and neck, 396
parvovirus B19 infection, lupus-like
    presentation of, 175
Vision
  loss
    in giant cell arteritis, risk factors for,
      261
    unilateral, after collagen
      implantation, 24
  problems after isotretinoin use, 200
Visits
  to physicians, non-federal office-based,
    in U.S., 55
Vitamin
  C-induced decomposition of lipid
    hydroperoxides to endogenous
    genotoxins, 388
Vitiligo, 221
  calcipotriol for, topical, alone or with
    PUVA therapy, 222, 224
  UVB for, narrow-band, 221
Vulvar
  lichen sclerosus, premenarchal,
    clobetasol propionate for, 318
Vulvovaginal
  condylomata acuminata and
    intraepithelial neoplasia, risk with
    HIV infection, 187

W

Warts
  acuminate, vulvovaginal and perianal,
    risk with HIV infection, 187
  in children with organ transplants, 336
  oral, effect of highly active
    antiretroviral therapy on frequency
    of, 186
  recalcitrant, cimetidine/levamisole for, in
    children, 167
Wine
  consumption and mycosis fungoides,
    467

Women
  acne and hyperandrogenemia in, 195
  arthritis in, rheumatoid, and hair dye
    exposure, 253
  dermatitis in, acute radiation,
    mometasone furoate for, 316
  herpes simplex virus type 2 transmission
    from men to, effect of condoms on
    reducing, 168
  hirsute, with normal menses, polycystic
    ovaries in, 219
Workers
  health care (*see* Health, care workers)
Wound
  dehiscence, 4
    traumatic, 5
  edge necrosis, scar secondary to, 4
  excisional, closure, octyl cyanoacrylate
    tissue adhesive *vs.* suture for, in
    children and adolescents, 364
  healing in patients with calciphylaxis
    from secondary
    hyperparathyroidism, effect of
    parathyroidectomy on, 322
  infection, postoperative, 3
    with crust and exudates, 2

X

Xeroderma
  pigmentosum
    skin, DNA repair-deficient,
      reconstruction in vitro, clues to
      epidermal cancer proneness
      revealed by, 295

  skin cancer in, effect of topical T4
    endonuclease V in liposomes on,
    296

Y

Yeast
  IgE-mediated hypersensitivity to,
    systemic ketoconazole for atopic
    dermatitis with, 82
  infections, superficial, after chemical
    peel, 31

Z

Zidovudine
  prophylaxis against HIV after sexual or
    injection drug use exposure, 177
Zoster
  herpes (*see* Herpes, zoster)
Zyderm
  inflammatory symptoms at test site of,
    20
  I implant, induration and erythema
    after, 20
  II implant, ulceration of glabellar area
    after, 22
Zyplast
  instillation, sterile abscess formation
    after, 21

Author Index

A

Aberer W, 86
Acker S, 444
Acland KM, 347
Adachi JD, 278
Adam P, 164
Aegerter P, 413
Ahmad SR, 159
Ahmed AR, 275
Airò P, 474
Akabani G, 462
Algra A, 198
Allen J, 277
Allen MH, 93
Alpsoy E, 224
Alster TS, 352
Ameen M, 222
Amir A, 422
Andersen EA, 127
Andersen J, 127
Anderson R, 292
Andrés A, 360
Antoni C, 101
Appel T, 345
Archer DF, 196
Arlette J, 370
Arnold M, 110
Arvilommi H, 72
Asadullah K, 96
Asselineau D, 295
Aste N, 134
Atkins M, 455
Atzori L, 134
Avermaete A, 232
Aylett SE, 410

B

Bachelez H, 320
Bachter D, 401
Bäck B, 388
Bafounta M-L, 413
Bailey-King S, 330
Balda B-R, 430
Balicer RD, 422
Balslev E, 323
Barkovich AJ, 409
Barlow JO, 391
Baron SE, 193
Bast DJ, 131
Bastiaens MT, 385
Beauchet A, 413
Beaudoin GMJ III, 212
Beitz J, 201
Belli F, 456

Belsito DV, 87
Bennett Ml, 484
Benninghoff B, 371
Benson BG, 211
Berg KD, 478
Bernard L, 364
Bernerd F, 295
Berthier F, 329
Bhageshpur R, 359
Bilker W, 109
Billingsley EM, 392
Bindslev-Jensen C, 66
Bingham SF, 367
Binks M, 237
Birkebæk N, 76
Biro FM, 218
Bissonnette R, 99
Blackwell V, 190
Blaheta H-J, 445
Blair IA, 388
Blakely KW, 254
Blom M, 147
Bollero D, 275
Bolte G, 71
Bonsmann G, 160
Borron SW, 331
Borte M, 71
Boström A, 316
Botchkarev VA, 210
Boulay F, 329
Bourgeois P, 400
Bozzette SA, 183
Brady MS, 433, 448
Bramson HN, 211
Brand CU, 241
Brasch J, 86
Breedveld FC, 256
Brenner B, 406
Brewster D, 243
Brinster NK, 478
Brodland DG, 407
Brown LF, 209
Brown SM, 461
Bryan H, 352
Buchbinder R, 245
Busam KJ, 414
Bush TJ, 187
Butler PEM, 346
Bystryn J-C, 458

C

Cadranel J, 320
Callen JP, 161
Calonje E, 347
Caltabiano R, 189

Canchola AJ, 186
Caouette G, 337
Capodieci P, 425
Capuano M, 334
Caracciolo E, 214
Carmina E, 219
Cars O, 144
Casale TB, 64
Cascinelli N, 456
Cassano P, 275
Castro-Bohorquez FJ, 175
Catella-Lawson F, 309
Cattani P, 334
Çelebi S, 114
Cerio R, 163
Cetin L, 224
Chaine B, 325
Chamlin SL, 484
Chan CLH, 332
Chan FKL, 308
Chang C-J, 486
Charles C, 414
Chaudhari U, 102
Chen R, 268
Chen Y-J, 240
Cherpelis BS, 441
Chimenti C, 300
Choi CJ, 319
Choi EO, 351
Choi MH, 216
Choi PCL, 263
Chong S-U, 77
Christian MM, 390
Christiano AM, 297
Christos PJ, 379
Chu AC, 222
Chung BC, 216
Clary BM, 433, 448
Cochat P, 336
Cokgor I, 462
Cole DJ, 438
Cole GW, 367
Coleman D, 415
Coley SC, 410
Collin J, 343
Conley LJ, 187
Cornes PGS, 357
Cotellessa C, 214
Coull BA, 326
Coulson IH, 193
Cox A, 227
Cranston D, 399
Craven NM, 95
Cribier BJ, 158
Cserhalmi-Friedman PB, 297
Cullinan P, 68

Cunliffe WJ, 193
Cushing GL Jr, 383

D

Daniel KL, 199
Daniels SR, 218
Daoud MS, 288
Darling TN, 270
Datta V, 131
Davis ST, 211
Davison SC, 93
de Berker D, 362
de Berker DAR, 363
Dechant C, 101
de Coninck EC, 470
De Felice C, 291
de Lange-de Klerk ESM, 439
de Launey J, 374
Delmas PD, 278
DeRenzo CL, 212
DeShazer D, 136
Detmar M, 209
Devesa SS, 419
Dewar K, 137
de Winter S, 284
Dickel H, 85
Diekema DJ, 178
Di Maggio G, 291
DiNick V, 359
Diri E, 255
Dlova N, 164
Doherty VR, 243
Domingo P, 185
Domingo-Domènech E, 175
Doyle J, 364
Drucker DB, 302
Dubois W, 455
Düker I, 401
Dunne SM, 324
Dürr C, 241
Duvic M, 471, 476
Dworkin RH, 172

E

Edström DW, 473
Edwards MJ, 447
Edwards R, 200
Egan CA, 270
Egbert JE, 485
Ejerblad E, 309
Elbaum M, 412
Ellerbrock TV, 187
Ellis CN, 97

Elmets CA, 281
Eng CM, 299
Engel WK, 485
Ermis O, 224
Euvrard S, 336
Evans J, 124
Evey P, 85
Exarchou V, 222

F

Fahey T, 339
Fam AG, 324
Farkas H, 65
Fearfield LA, 333
Fekete B, 65
Feldman SR, 391
Finn J, 234
Fiorillo L, 135
Fischer G, 113
Fiveash J, 404
Flaherty LE, 424
Fleischer AB, 391
Fleischer AB Jr, 484
Foote JA, 384
Forbes A, 245
Fored CM, 309
Forrest DM, 143
Foster CL, 139
Foster RD, 409
Fowler JF Jr, 91
Francis N, 333
Frankel A, 476
Franklin V, 80
Fransway AF, 87
Fraunfelder FT, 200
Fraunfelder FW, 200
Freedberg KA, 184
Freedman BM, 349
French ME, 286
Friedlander SF, 364
Friedman HS, 462
Friedrich M, 96
Frustaci A, 300
Fryer AA, 286, 381, 382
Fuller LC, 163
Furst D, 237
Füst G, 65

G

Gach JE, 63
Galindo M, 234
Gambichler T, 232
García-Carrasco M, 258
García-Porrúa C, 262
García Rodriguez LA, 306

Gehring U, 71
Geilen CC, 110
Gershon AA, 171
Gershon S, 104
Gibbon K, 88
Gilead L, 191
Gillenwater AM, 402
Girardi M, 386
Girot R, 325
Girotto JA, 322
Giuliano AR, 384
Glattre E, 396
Glees JP, 357
Goettsch W, 335
Goitz RJ, 239
Goldberg L, 387
Goldman F, 298
Goldman GD, 393
Goldman KD, 199
Goldstein MG, 378
Gonzalez S, 346
González-Louzao C, 262
Goossens PH, 256
Gordon M, 100, 248
Graeber M, 78
Graffeo R, 334
Grant B, 138
Gratian MJ, 272
Gray JC, 80
Greaves MW, 63
Green A, 79
Greenberg ER, 383
Greenspan D, 186
Gregurek-Novak T, 156
Grobbee DE, 198
Grundmann-Kollmann M, 81
Grunow K, 77
Guix B, 360
Guler MM, 348
Gumnick JF, 457
Gupta AK, 156, 157, 164
Gupta S, 229
Gutgesell C, 74

H

Haase I, 94
Hachulla E, 244
Hacimustafaoğlu M, 114
Haddad F, 441
Hall K, 311
Hall S, 245
Hamuryudan V, 255
Hanneken S, 96
Harden PN, 381, 382
Harel G, 251
Harel L, 251

Harman KE, 272
Harmon JW, 322
Harper J, 79
Harris HM, 68
Harris RB, 384
Hartge P, 419
Harvey EA, 326
Hatron P-Y, 244
Hay RJ, 332
Heald AH, 153
Heckmann M, 344
Hedderwick SA, 139
Heenan PJ, 421
Heere-Ress E, 459
Hegyesi H, 463
Heickendorff L, 112
Heiken H, 179
Heise S, 74
Helm KF, 392
Henderson MA, 464
Henírquez I, 360
Hennessy S, 109
Henry K, 333
Henseler T, 86
Hernández-Díaz S, 306
Herrick A, 234
Herrmann F, 261
Hessel AC, 402
Hester K, 414
Hill CL, 242
Hipfel R, 142
Hobbs RM, 94
Hoeller C, 459
Hogewoning AA, 335
Holmes LB, 326
Holness DL, 89
Horev G, 250
Howard R, 162
Hu LT, 124
Huang J-Q, 307
Huemer C, 246
Huether MJ, 407
Hughes AP, 161
Huhn KM, 478
Humar D, 131
Hunger RE, 241
Hunt RH, 307

I

Iazzetta J, 324
Ihira M, 174
Itoh Y, 205

J

Jackson CW, 95

Jackson IT, 359
James CA, 482
James J, 302
Jansen B, 459
Jeffes EW, 377
Jemal A, 419
Jemec GBE, 323
Johnson RW, 172
Joly P, 267
Juneja A, 167
Juul S, 76

K

Kaerlev L, 467
Kahn JO, 177
Kalliomäki M, 72
Kanitakis J, 336
Kapoor SC, 309
Karacaoglu E, 348
Karagas MR, 383
Karon JM, 182
Kashani-Sabet M, 401, 468
Kaskel P, 417
Kässmann H, 429
Katsiari CG, 257
Katz KH, 392
Keene J, 104
Kelemen PR, 452
Kelly KM, 486
Kemmeren JM, 197, 198
Kennedy CTK, 363
Kielich C, 385
Kildal W, 397
Kiliç SS, 114
Kim JJ, 221
Kim YH, 470
Kinsler VA, 410
Kirby B, 95
Kirtschig G, 277
Kitson H, 246
Klempner MS, 124
Knapik-Botor A, 179
Kokoska MS, 452
Koller J, 429
Komarova EA, 210
Kondeatis E, 227
Konnikov N, 157
Koo SH, 351
Kopf AW, 412
Korenreich L, 251
Kortekangas-Savolainen O, 82
Kossard S, 374
Krämer K-U, 430
Kraus CN, 136
Kreimer-Erlacher H, 388

Kreuter A, 232
Krishnamurthy PN, 230
Kron M, 417, 453
Krueger GG, 97, 111
Krueger JG, 99
Kuhn A, 228
Kulp-Shorten C, 161
Kumpumäki S, 292

L

Labbé J, 337
Lacarrubba F, 189
Lachenmayr S, 199
Langenberg AGM, 168
Lapostolle F, 331
LaRussa PS, 171
Lauritsen JM, 66
Lauth X, 141
Lawrence C, 362
Lawson DH, 457
Lazarova Z, 270
Leali C, 474
Lebwohl O, 100
Lee LM, 182
Lee RJ, 450
Lee SH, 388
Lehoczky J, 137
Leissa BG, 159
Lemay A, 196
Leong SPL, 401
Lewis JJ, 433
Leyden JJ, 203
Lie AK, 396
Lim HW, 221
Lin C, 130
Lin J-T, 130
Lin Y, 282
Lindblad P, 309
Lindman H, 316
Link K, 168
Lintu P, 82
Liozon E, 261
Liu PY, 424
Llorca J, 262
Lobo RA, 219
Looks A, 475
Lorenz S, 355
Losina E, 184
Lou Y-R, 282
Lu Y-P, 282
Lubelsky S, 248
Lucky AW, 203, 218
Luger T, 78, 317
Luger TA, 160
Luscombe CJ, 286
Ly K, 261
Lynde CW, 157

M

MacDonald N, 215
Mace SR, 89
Machado RD, 301
Machin SJ, 330
Mackenzie-Wood A, 374
MacKie RM, 456, 461
Mackinson C, 147
MacPhail LA, 186
Mallek JA, 254
Malleson PN, 246
Mallon E, 93
Mancuso AA, 394
Mann B, 448
Marcil I, 106
Marghoob AA, 379
Margolis D, 109
Marie I, 244
Marks R, 376
Marrone A, 298
Martin JN, 177
Martini G, 236
Mason C, 111
Mat C, 255
Mathias CGT, 90
Mayer T, 453
McClay EF, 438
McCullough JL, 377
McDonald LC, 147
McFadden JP, 88
McMillan A, 468
McNeil SA, 139
Medina-Franco H, 404
Medsger TA, 239
Melander A, 144
Melia J, 415
Mellemkjoer L, 305
Mendenhall WM, 394
Messina J, 441
Metze D, 317
Meyer FJ, 332
Meyer J, 475
Meyer T, 371
Mikkilineni R, 378
Milan R, 464
Millard TP, 227
Milstone LM, 297
Mimouni M, 250
Mizeracki A, 481
Moffitt DL, 363
Mölstad S, 144
Monnet DL, 147
Morales Suárez-Varela
    MM, 467
Moran C, 195
Moreno-Picot S, 420
Morgan KW, 91
Mork J, 396

Morris A, 113
Morris T, 427
Morrison WH, 402
Mortz CG, 66
Moss S, 415
Moy RL, 390
Mukamel M, 250
Mukherjee D, 312
Mulcahy LD, 102
Muller MGS, 439
Munch M, 323
Musselman DL, 457
Musumeci ML, 189

N

Nadelman RB, 123
Nagasako EM, 172
Nagore E, 420
Narváez Garcia FJ, 175
Nedelec B, 356
Nelson JS, 486
Neonato M-G, 325
Ngheim P, 319
Nguyen CL, 438
Niederhagen B, 345
Nielsen GL, 305
Nielsen HE, 127
Nienhaus A, 194
Ning G, 268
Ninomiya Y, 205
Nissen SE, 312
Nizet V, 141
North PE, 481, 482

O

O'Brien CJ, 451
Ochsendorf F, 81
O'Dell JR, 254
Oe T, 388
Ogilvie ALJ, 101
O'Halloran DJ, 153
Ohashi M, 174
Ohtake T, 141
Olesen AB, 76
Oliver V, 420
Oliveria SA, 379
Olsen E, 476
Olsen J, 467
Olson G, 452
Olsson AR, 253
Oppenheim DE, 386
Oratz R, 458
Orfanos CE, 110

P

Pandhi R, 167
Papp K, 99
Park SH, 351
Parry MF, 138
Parsad D, 167
Passweg JR, 237
Pathak I, 451
Paul C, 158
Paul S, 485
Paul T, 445
Peris K, 214
Petersen-Schaeffer K, 451
Pfahlberg A, 418
Pidhorecky I, 450
Pires LM, 350
Pitts M, 201
Podda M, 81
Poland GA, 122
Polsky D, 425
Pommier RF, 427
Porwit A, 473
Potter GB, 212
Powell J, 277, 399
Prieto VG, 354
Proulx G, 450

Q

Qi DY, 444
Quadri G, 315
Quint EH, 318

R

Rabinovitz HS, 412
Rafiq M, 206
Ragoowansi R, 357
Rakowsky E, 406
Ramos-Casals M, 258
Randolph MA, 346
Rao S, 230
Rappl G, 426
Ratner LE, 322
Rauma T, 292
Ray WA, 311
Reece S, 382
Reece SM, 381
Reilly MP, 309
Reimer S, 271
Rettenbacher L, 429
Reynolds NJ, 80
Ricci R, 300
Richards K, 153
Richter-Hintz D, 228
Riedler J, 69

Rietschel RL, 90
Ris J, 185
Risberg B, 397
Rivero M, 234
Rivers JK, 370
Robertson KL, 302
Robson A, 399
Rodrigues LKE, 401
Rogers M, 113
Roland ME, 177
Romano P, 102
Romero MR, 94
Rooney B, 234
Ros A-M, 473
Rossiter S, 147
Roza L, 284
Rueda-Pedraza E, 349
Rycroft RJG, 88

S

Saag KG, 278
Sabroe RA, 63
Sacks SL, 170
Sadick NS, 354
Sagebiel RW, 443
Sales F, 400
Salminen S, 72
Sams WM Jr, 195
Sander S, 417
Santiago B, 234
Sauer B, 142
Savolainen J, 82
Sawyer D, 135
Scalf LA, 91
Scaparro E, 315
Schäfer T, 194
Schalkwijk J, 293
Schanbacher CF, 288
Schellenberg RR, 143
Scherer K, 355
Scherschun L, 221
Schiller M, 160
Schinstine M, 393
Schittek B, 142
Schmidt E, 271
Schoukroun G, 329
Schweitzer VG, 395
Scott G, 79
Scott PG, 356
Scurr JH, 330
Seed PT, 272, 347
Seidl H, 388
Seiter S, 213
Selik R, 182
Senet P, 320
Seubert S, 74
Sfikakis PP, 257

Shankowsky H, 356
Shapiro J, 215
Sharma V, 162
Shea B, 236
Shea CR, 354
Shear N, 370
Shen J-L, 240
Sherertz EF, 87
Sherman J, 191
Sherman RA, 191
Shetty VB, 230
Shidham VB, 444
Shiwen X, 236
Siebenhaar F, 210
Sigurgeirsson B, 242
Sikand VK, 125
Silverberg NB, 162
Singer SJ, 159
Singh D, 281
Skelton H, 151
Skelton HG, 105
Skogh T, 253
Slayden SM, 195
Smith CH, 163
Smith KJ, 105, 151
Smith MH, 169
Smith YR, 318
Soengas MS, 425
Søgaard H, 112
Somerset M, 339
Somlai B, 463
Sonntag M, 228
Sørensen HT, 305
Sørensen TL, 147
Sotlar K, 445
Speakman D, 464
Spencer JM, 350
Spruance SL, 169
Sridhar S, 307
Srinivasan A, 136
Ständer S, 317
Starz H, 401, 430
Steele CR, 386
Steere AC, 117
Steijlen PM, 293
Stein CM, 311
Stella M, 275
Stern RS, 106, 107, 265
Stevens JS, 427
Stewart B, 461
Stirling A, 206
Stockfleth E, 371
Stockton D, 243
Stratton R, 236
Strauss JS, 203
Sudbø J, 397
Sudler R, 146
Sulkes A, 406
Surget V, 331

Swartling C, 316
Swetter SM, 455
Szeto CC, 263

T

Tajima S, 205
Tan M-H, 100, 350
Tanis BC, 197
Taran JM, 421
Taylor JR, 368
Taylor JS, 85, 90
ter Huurne JAC, 385
Thelmo MC, 443
Theodossiadis PG, 257
Thiboutot D, 196
Thien VVS, 143
Thompson AE, 236
Thomson JR, 301
Tilgen W, 213, 426
Tillmann HL, 179
To KF, 263, 308
Tomaino MM, 239
Topol EJ, 312
Torres OH, 185
Toti P, 291
Trejo O, 258
Trembath RC, 301
Treseler PA, 443
Tschen E, 368
Tse S, 248
Tubesing K, 281
Tyring SK, 169

U

Ugurel S, 213, 426
Unger JM, 424
Urist MM, 404

V

van den Bosch MAAJ, 197
Vandeweyer E, 400
van Leent EJM, 78
van Leeuwen PAM, 439
van Loveren H, 335
Vanness ER, 288
Varga VL, 463
Varghese A, 470
Vázquez M, 171
Vega-Lopez F, 190
Verburg RJ, 256
Vieluf D, 194
Vink AA, 284
Vioux C, 295

Virno G, 315
Voit C, 453
von Eiff C, 129
von Lindern JJ, 345
Vulliamy T, 298

W

Waddell SP, 349
Wagner RF, 390
Wald A, 168
Waner M, 481, 482
Watters JW, 137
Weinstein GD, 377
Weinstein MC, 184
Weinstock MA, 367, 378
Weiss M, 339
Welch V, 236
Welsh M, 151
Whatling PJ, 343
White DG, 146
Williams CM, 352
Williams HC, 68
Williams LS, 394
Williams ML, 409

Wimmershoff M, 355
Wingren G, 253
Wise RP, 104
Wiseman MC, 215
Wolf JE Jr, 368
Wolf Y, 422
Wollina U, 475
Wong SL, 447
Wong WYL, 387
Worthington T, 206
Wrightson WR, 447
Wu C-Y, 240
Wu JCY, 308
Wünschmann S, 178
Wysowski DK, 201

X

Xiang J, 178
Xu X-C, 387

Y

Yano K, 209

Yarosh D, 296
Yeh F-L, 130
Yoo YS, 216
Yoshikawa T, 174
Yukna M, 138
Yuksel F, 348

Z

Zachariae H, 112
Zackheim HS, 468
Zane C, 474
Zeleniuch-Jacquotte A, 458
Zhang Y, 242
Zhao M-L, 268
Zhao S, 146
Zillikens D, 271
Zitelli JA, 407
Zuberbier T, 77
Zucca M, 134
Zucker M, 135
Zweers MC, 293

The year's best literature in one convenient volume!

YES! Please start my subscription to the *Year Book(s)* checked below with the current volume according to the terms described below.* I understand that I will have 30 days to examine each annual edition.

Please Print:

Name _____

Address _____

City _____ State _____ ZIP _____

Method of Payment

❑ Check (payable to **Mosby**; add the applicable sales tax for your area)

❑ VISA ❑ MasterCard ❑ AmEx ❑ Bill me

Card number _____ Exp. date _____

Signature _____

❑ **Year Book of Allergy, Asthma and Clinical Immunology (YALI)**
$91.00 (Avail. November)

❑ **Year Book of Anesthesiology and Pain Management (YANE)**
$96.00 (Avail. August)

❑ **Year Book of Cardiology® (YCAR)**
$96.00 (Avail. August)

❑ **Year Book of Critical Care Medicine® (YCCM)**
$94.00 (Avail. June)

❑ **Year Book of Dentistry® (YDEN)**
$89.00 (Avail. August)

❑ **Year Book of Dermatology and Dermatologic Surgery™ (YDER)**
$98.00 (Avail. October)

❑ **Year Book of Diagnostic Radiology® (YRAD)**
$98.00 (Avail. November)

❑ **Year Book of Emergency Medicine® (YEMD)**
$98.00 (Avail. May)

❑ **Year Book of Endocrinology® (YEND)**
$95.00 (Avail. July)

❑ **Year Book of Family Practice™ (YFAM)**
$83.00 (Avail. June)

❑ **Year Book of Gastroenterology™ (YGAS)**
$91.00 (Avail. December)

❑ **Year Book of Hand Surgery® (YHND)**
$99.00 (Avail. April)

❑ **Year Book of Medicine® (YMED)**
$91.00 (Avail. July)

❑ **Year Book of Neonatal and Perinatal Medicine® (YNPM)**
$99.00 (Avail. September)

❑ **Year Book of Neurology and Neurosurgery® (YNEU)**
$94.00 (Avail. January)

❑ **Year Book of Nuclear Medicine® (YNUM)**
$99.00 (Avail. June)

❑ **Year Book of Obstetrics, Gynecology, and Women's Health® (YOBG)**
$98.00 (Avail. February)

❑ **Year Book of Oncology® (YONC)**
$99.00 (Avail. November)

❑ **Year Book of Ophthalmology® (YOPH)**
$99.00 (Avail. September)

❑ **Year Book of Orthopedics® (YORT)**
$99.00 (Avail. October)

❑ **Year Book of Otolaryngology— Head and Neck Surgery® (YOTO)**
$91.00 (Avail. July)

❑ **Year Book of Pathology and Laboratory Medicine® (YPAT)**
$99.00 (Avail. March)

❑ **Year Book of Pediatrics® (YPED)**
$86.00 (Avail. January)

❑ **Year Book of Plastic and Aesthetic Surgery® (YPRS)**
$98.00 (Avail. March)

❑ **Year Book of Psychiatry and Applied Mental Health® (YPSY)**
$89.00 (Avail. March)

❑ **Year Book of Pulmonary Disease® (YPDI)**
$92.00 (Avail. April)

❑ **Year Book of Rheumatology, Arthritis, and Musculoskeletal Disease™ (YRHE)**
$99.00 (Avail. January)

❑ **Year Book of Sports Medicine® (YSPM)**
$93.00 (Avail. December)

❑ **Year Book of Surgery® (YSUR)**
$92.00 (Avail. September)

❑ **Year Book of Urology® (YURO)**
$99.00 (Avail. November)

❑ **Year Book of Vascular Surgery® (YVAS)**
$99.00 (Avail. April)

Order your *Year Book* today! Simply complete and detach this card and drop it in the mail to receive the latest information in your field.

*Your Year Book service guarantee:

When you subscribe to a *Year Book*, you will receive notice of future annual volumes about two months before publication. To receive the new edition, do nothing—we'll send you the new volume as soon as it is available. (Applicable sales tax is added to each shipment.) If you want to discontinue, the advance notice allows you time to notify us of your decision. If you are not completely satisfied, you have 30 days to return any *Year Book*.

VISIT OUR HOME PAGE!
www.mosby.com/periodicals

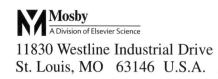

Mosby
A Division of Elsevier Science

11830 Westline Industrial Drive
St. Louis, MO   63146   U.S.A.